# CYCLOPÆDIA

or, an

Universal Dictionary of ARTS and SCIENCES

*(Chemistry, Medicine, Natural History, & Pharmacy)*

# CYCLOPÆDIA

or, an

*Universal Dictionary*

of the

ARTS and SCIENCES

Transcribed and abridged

by Anthony Charles Bravo

Bibliographical Note

This edition is an abridged republication of a work by Ephraim Chambers in two volumes, with some additional entries from the two volume addendum by Abraham Rees, published in 1749.

ISBN-10: 0-9814867-1-1
ISBN-13: 978-0-9814867-1-0



Published by Bravo Publishing.

## EDITORS PREFACE

This book is an abridged version of the Cyclopaedia published by Ephraim Chambers (1680 – 1740), in two volumes in 1728. A few additional entries have been added from the four volume set published by Abraham Rees (1743 – 1825), in 1774, to round out some of the sparser articles. The abridgement consists primarily of those entries referring to natural history, medicine and chemistry, thus providing an insight into the state of the medical arts in the seventeenth and early eighteenth centuries.

Many people, historical and current to the $17^{th}$ century, are referenced in the Cyclopaedia and this abridgment. However, in almost all cases only their last names are provided. In some cases, these are obvious to the modern-day audience, such as Newton and Des Cartes, but many are contemporary to the $17^{th}$ century and earlier. Most of these people have identified, although not all of them with complete certainty, and an index to the names has been provided. Note that the original spelling and punctuation in the Cyclopaedia has been retained.

Although we know little of Mr. Chambers life, he is credited with being the first to compile and publish an encyclopaedia. The Encyclopaedia Britannica, for example, was first published in 1771. Apparently, Mr. Chambers was inspired by John Harris' (1666 – 1719), Lexicon Technicum, published in 1704, which was considered more of a dictionary than an encyclopaedia, and decided he could improve upon the work. Abraham Rees added two more volumes, published as a supplement in one instance, and as a four-volume set re-arranged and re-written.

Mr. Chambers describes his Cyclopaedia in the preface to the work, "It may be even said, that if the System be an Improvement upon the Dictionary; the Dictionary is some Advantage to the System; and that this is perhaps the only Way wherein the whole Circle of Body of Knowledge can be deliver'd. In any other Form, many thousand Things must necessarily be hid and overlook'd : All the Pins, the Joints, the binding of the Fabrick must be invisible of course; all the lesser Parts whatsoever, must be in some measure swallowed up in the Whole. The Imagination, stretch'd and amplified to take in so large a Structure, can have but a very general, indistinguishing Perception of any of the Parts. Whereas the Parts are not less Matter of Knowledge when taken separately, than when put together. Nay, and in strictness, as our Ideas are all Singulars or Individuals, and as everything that exists is one; it seems more natural to consider Knowledge in its proper Parts, *i.e.* as divided into separate Articles denoted by different Terms; than to consider the whole Assemblage of it in its utmost Composition : which is a thing merely artificial and imaginary."

"And yet the latter Way must be allow'd to have many and real Advantages over the former; which in truth is only of use and significance as it partakes thereof : For this Reason, that all Writing in its own Nature is artificial; and that the Imagination is really the Faculty it immediately applies to. Hence it should follow, that the most advantageous way, is to make use of both Methods : To consider every Point both as a Part; to help the Imagination to the Whole : and as a Whole, to help it to every Part. Which is the View in the present Work – so far as the many and great Difficulties we have to labour under would allow us to pursue it."

"In this view we have endeavoured to give the Substance of what has been hitherto found in the several Branches of Knowledge both natural and artificial; that is, of Nature, *first*, as she appears to our Senses; either spontaneously, as in Natural History; or with the Assistance of Art, as in Anatomy, Chymistry, Medicine, Agriculture, &c. *Secondly*, to our Imagination; as in Grammar, Rhetorick, Poetry, &c. *Thirdly*, to our Reason; as in Physicks, Metaphysicks, Logicks, and Mathematicks. With the several subordinate Arts arising from each; as Architecture, Painting, Sculpture, Trade, Manu-factures, Policy, Law, &c. and numerous remote Particulars, not immediately reducible to any of these Heads; as Heraldry, Philology, Antiquities, Customs, &c."

TO THE

# K I N G

*S I R*,

The ARTS and SCIENCES humbly crave Audience of Your Majesty. The near Concern they have in the Happiness of a People, assures 'em of the favourable Attention of a Price who makes that Happiness his own. 'Tis by These, the Parsimony of Nature is supplied, and Life render'd easy and agreeable under its numerous Infirmities. By these the Mind is reclaim'd from its native Wildness; and enrich'd with Sentiments which lead to Virtue and Glory. 'Tis these, in fine, that make the Difference between your Majesty's Subjects, and the Savages of *Canada*, or the *Cape of Good Hope*.

THE Protection of the Arts has ever been esteemed the proper Province of the Great. 'Tis a Branch of the regal Office; which a Price, like Your Majesty, equal to the whole Charge of the Crown, will not suffer to be alienated into other Hands. From this, do the first and most distinguish'd Names in the List of Fame, derive a large Share of their Glory : and if there by any Age or Nation more conspicuous than the rest, and which is look'd on with Envy by our own; 'tis that wherein the Sovereigns have signaliz'd themselves most in this Quality. Indeed, the Time seems at hand, when we are no longer to envy Rome her AUGUSTUS and AUGUSTAN AGE, but Rome in her turn shall envy ours.

SOMETHING extraordinary is apparently intended by Providence in calling such a Prince, so such a People : A Prince who feels a generous Impulse to devote his Cares and all his Toils to the Welfare of Mankind; and a People conspiring with unexampled Ardor and Unanimity to all his glorious Views. Some of our best Princes have had their Hands ty'd down; check'd by reluctant Factions, who opposed every nobler Design : Your Majesty has found the happy Secret, to make even Contention do you Homage; and turn Opposition itself into Approbation, and Applause.

THERE is a Time reserv'd in Fate for every Nation to arrive at its Height; and the uppermost Place on the Terrestrial Ball is held successively by several States. May not the numerous Presages which usher in Your Majesty's Reign, give us room to expect that our Turn is next; and that what Greece was under *Alexander*, and *Rome* under *Augustus Caesar*, *Britain* shall be under GEORGE and CAROLINE?

BUT even this were to under-rate our Hopes, which are rais'd, by Your Majesty, to something still more truly glorious. Greatness, so fondly coveted, has already cost the World very dear; and, tho still pursued by unthinking Men under almost every Shape, is only desirable in a few. Of it self it is rather an Object of Terror and Alarm, than Delight; and at best only pleases, when joyn'd with something naturally amiable. From the Practice of your Majesty, Men may correct their Sentiments, and learn, that Greatness has no Charm except when founded in Goodness. To be Great, and a King, is but a small Matter with Your Majesty; 'tis a Quality many others enjoy in common with You, and to which some have even been doom'd, to their Infamy : 'tis what Herdo was, and Nebuchadnezzar was; and Nero and Domitian were. But, while other Princes chuse to be great in what is destructive, and others in things wholly indifferent; 'tis Your Majesty's Praise to be great in what is the Perfection of our Nature, and that whereby we approach nearest the Deity. Happy Choice! to use Power only as a Means of rendering your Beneficence more diffulsive : and thus make Power and Royalty minister to the Happiness of Mankind, which they have too often invaded.

THE Work I presume to lay at Your Majesty's Feet, is an Attempt towards a Survey of the Republick of Learning, as it stands at the Beginning of Your Majesty's auspicious Reign. We have here the Boundary that circumscribes our present Prospect; and separates the known, from the unknown Parts of the Intelligible World. Under Your Majesty's Princely Influence and Encouragement, we promise our selves this Boundary will be removed, and the Prospect extended far into the other Hemisphere. Methinks I see Trophies erecting to Your Majesty in the yet undiscover'd Regions of Science; an Your Majesty's Name inscribed to Inventions as present held impossible.

I am, with all Sincerity and Devotion,

*May it please Your MAJESTY,*

*Your Majesty's most Dutiful,*

*and Obedient Subject,*

*and Servant,*

Ephraim Chambers.

# CYCLOPÆDIA

A - Among physicians, ā or āā, is used in Prescription for *Ana*; to denote an equal Portion of divers Ingredients, whether in Respect of Measure or Weight. Lastly among Chymists, *AAA* signify an *Amalgama*, or the Operation of *Amalgamating*.

**ABACTUS**, among the ancient Physicians, *Abactus* was used for a Miscarriage procured by Art, or force of Medicines; in contra-distinction to *Abortus*, which is Natural. But the Moderns know no such distinction.

**ABLUENTS**, *Abluentia*, in Medicine, a Name some Authors give to those Remedies, better know under the Name of *Diluters*, and *Abstergents*.

**ABLUTION**, in Pharmacy, is a Preparation divers Remedies undergo, by washing them in Water, or some other Fluid, proper to cleanse and free them of their Impurities. The Word is sometimes also used, tho with less Propriety, for the washing, or infusing of certain Medicines in Water, to freshen them, and dissolve their Salts; called *Dulcifying*.

**ABORTION**, in Medicine, an immature Exclusion of the *Fœtus*; or the Delivery of a Woman with Child, before the legitimate Term; popularly called *Miscarriage*. This may happen at any time of Pregnancy; but if before the second Month after Conception, it is properly called a *false Conception*. We have Instances of *Abortions* by way of the Mouth, the *Anus*, the Navel, &c.

The usual Causes of *Abortion*, are immoderate Evacuations, violent Motions, sudden Passions, Frights, &c. Other Causes are the largeness and heaviness of the *Fœtus*, Irritations of the Womb, Relaxation of the Ligaments of the *Placenta*, Weakness, and want of Nourishment in the *Fœtus*; excess of eating, long fasting, or waking, the use of Busks for the Shape, offensive Smells, violent Purgatives; and, in the general, any thing that tends to promote the Menses. The Symptoms usually preceding are a Fever, either continual or intermitting; Pain in the Loin and Head, heaviness in the Eyes, a bearing down and Constriction of the Abdomen. When the Time of Miscarriage is just at hand, the Pains are much the same as those in Labour.

*Abortion* is dangerous where the Time of Pregnancy is far advanced so that the *Fœtus* must be large, where the Cause is very violent, the Patient strongly convulsed, a large Hemorrhage precedes or ensues, the *Fœtus* is putrify'd, &c. Under other circumstances it rarely proves mortal.

The Treatment is to be adapted to the particular Symptoms and Circumstances : If the Patient be Plethoric, as soon as the first Symptoms discover themselves, a Vein is to be opened : In case of Flooding, recourse is to be had to proper Astringents; of it those fail, to Fomentations, Injections, and Suffumigations : If a *Tenesmus* attend, Rhubarb is to be used; and if there be an habitual Laxity of the Uterine Vessels, Guaiacum.

*Abortion* is also used where the Child dies in the Womb; tho it remain there many Years, or even as long as the Mother lives.

**ABRASION**, is sometimes used among Medical Writers for the Act of wearing away the natural *Mucus* which covers the Membranes, and particularly those of the Stomach and Intestines, by sharp corrosive Medicines, or Humors. The Word is compounded of the Latin *ab*, and *rado*, I shave, or scrape off.

**ABSCESS**, in Medicine and Chirurgery, a Tumour arising on divers Parts of the Body, and tending to Suppuration. *Abscesses* arise from the Collections of peccant Humours in the internal Parts of the Body; and are also called *Imposthumes*. Their Name *Abcess* comes from the *Latin* Verb *abscedere*, to depart, or remove to another Place; in allusion to the morbid Humors being derived from elsewhere.

*Abscesses* arise ofteneth in Women after Delivery; and tho dangerous in themselves, yet appear to be the Crisis of the Disease that gave rife thereto. For the Cure, if they cannot be *discussed, i.e.* be carried off by proper artificial Evacuations, as Phlebotomy, Purging, &c. with the use of Calomel between while, and gentle perspirative Fotus's, Liniments, and Cataplasms; recourse is to be had to the contrary Method, and they must be brought to Suppuration. When the Matter is fully ripened, they are to be opened with a Lancet or Caustick, and their Cure attempted by Digestives and Incarnatives.

**ABSORBENTS**, in Medicine, Remedies which by the Softness of Porosity of their component Parts, become proper to sheath the Asperities of sharp pungent Humors; or to imbibe or dry away, as with a Sponge, superfluous Moistures. Such are the Testaceous Pouders, Hartshorn, Coral, Crabs Eyes and Claws, calcined Bones, burnt Ivory, &c. *Absorbents* are the same with what we otherwise call *Driers* and *Sweetners*. The Term *Absorbent* is frequently confounded with *Alcaly*; Alcalies having, really, the Effect of *Absorbents* with respect to Acids.

**ABSTERGENTS**, or *Abstersive Medicines*, a Class of Remedies, whose Effect is to abrade and wipe away such mucous Particles as they meet in their Passage; and thus cleanse the Parts of viscid or impure Adhesions, and carry off the morbid Matter of Wounds, Ulcers, &c. *Abstergents* are more usually called among Physicians *Detergents*.

*Abstergents* are of the Genus of Balsamicks; and only differ in their degree of Subtilty and Efficacy, from Vulneraries. The principal Simples in the Class of Detergents, are the Leaves of *Wormwood, Garlick, Leeks, Capers, Scurvygrass, Fumitory, Liverwort, Tansy,* and *Vervain; Bitter Almonds, Figs, Jujebs*[1]*, Raisins, Dates, Juniper-Berries; Gum Ammoniac, Balsam of Capivi*[2]*, Balm of Gilead, Tacamahaca*[3]*, Sapo; Turpentines; Barberries, Liquorice, Turmeric, Madder, Parmasitty*[4]*, Mummy, Sulphur, Salt, Mercury,* and *Native Cinnabar*.

The Word *Abstergent* is compounded of the Latin *abs*, from; and *tergo*, I wipe. Whence, also, *Abstersion* is sometimes used for the mechanical Act of

[1] Jujebs probably refer to the Jujube or Chinese date (*Ziziphus zizyphus*).

[2] Balsam of Copaiba, also known as Jesuit's Resin.

[3] The resin of the Balsam Poplar.

*Tersion*, or Wiping.

**ABSYNTHIUM**, *Wormwood*, a Medicinal Plant, of considerable Efficacy in quality of a Bitter and Stomachic. There are divers Kinds hereof enumerated by Botanists; at least 30. Those which obtain in Medicine, are,

1, the *Roman*, or small, called also *Pontic*; used as a Stomachic, Astringent, Discutient, and to prevent Putrefaction; *Etmuller*[1] says, there is not a chronic Distemper in which it is not serviceable. A Conserve of the *Roman Absynthium* is now also much used.

2, The *common* or large *Wormwood*, bitterer much than the former, and antiently used not only as a Stomachic and a Destroyer of Worms, but also a Detergent; and prescribed against the Jaundice and Dropsy : But it is now grown into disuse in those Intentions, as being prejudicial to the Eyes; and is now chiefly retained as an Ingredient in some of the Officinal Compositions; and particularly some cephalick distilled Waters.

Its Infusion in Wine, makes what they call *Vinum Absynthites*. The Pharmacopœias also mention an Extract of *Absynthium*, *Extractum Absynthii*; and a Syrup of *Absynthium*, *Syropus de Absynthio*. Some will have this to yield the *Semen Sanctum*, or *Santonicum*, i.e. *Wormseed*; but *Matthiolus*[2] affirms the contrary.

**ACACIA**, in Medicine, an inspissated Juice, of a Shrub of the Thorn kind; used as an Astringent. There are two Kinds, the *Vera* and the *Germanica*.

The *Acacia Vera*, is brought from the Levant; and supposed to be the Juice of the Pods of a large thorny Tree, growing in *Egypt* and *Arabia*. Some Naturalists will have it the same Plant that yields the Gum Arabick. It is very austere and binding; and on that account good against Fluxes. Chuse that of a tan-colour, smooth, and shining; and an astringent disagreeable in Taste. It is, or should be, an Ingredient in the *Theriaca Andromachi*.

The *German Acacia* is a Counterfeit of the former; being made of the Juice of unripe Sloes, boiled to the Consistence of a solid Extract; and put up in Bladders, like the former. It is distinguished from it chiefly by its Colour, which is as black as that of *Spanish* Liquorice. It is used as a Substitute to the true *Acacia*.

**ACANACEOUS**, among Botanists, a Term applied to a Class of Plants, popularly known under the Name of the *Thistle* Kind. The Word is formed of the Greek αχαζω, *Acuo*, I sharpen.

**ACATALEPSIA**, Acatalepsy, in Philosophy, Incomprehensibleness; or the Impossibility of comprehending or conceiving a thing. The *Pyrrhonians* and *Scepticks*, and even the Antient Academy, asserted an absolute *Acatalepsia* : All human Science or Knowledge, according to them, went no further than to Appearance and Verisimilitude.

[1] Michael Etmuller (1644-1683), a German physician.

[2] Pier Andrea Mattioli (1501 – 1577), an Italian physician who published commentaries on Dioscorides' Materia Medica.

**ACCENSION**, *Accensio*, in Physicks, the Act of *Kindling*, or setting a Body on Fire. *Accension*, on other Occasions, is called *Inflammation*, *Ignition*, *Conflagration*, &c. *Accension* stands opposite to *Extinction*. The Word is formed of the Latin *Accendo*, I kindle.

**ACCESS**, in Medicine, a Fit, or Return of some periodical Disease. Thus, we say, an *Access* of the Gout, an Ague, or an Intermitting Fever.

**ACERB**, *Acerbus*, a compound Taste, consisting of sour, with the Addition of a degree or Roughness. Such is the Taste of all Fruits before they are ripe. The Physicians usually make *Acerb* an intermediate Savour between Acid, Austere, and Bitter. All Matters which come under this Denomination are Astringent.

**ACETOUS** : The Chymists mention divers *Aceta*, or *Acetous* Liquors; as *Acetum Alcalizatum*; made of distilled Vinegar, with the Addition of some Alkaline, or Volatile Salt. *Acetum Philosophorum*, a sour kind of Liquor; made by dissolving a little Butter of Antimony in a great deal of Water. Acetum in Medicine, &c. the same with *Vinegar*; the Properties, Uses, and Preparations whereon, see under the article Vinegar. The word is pure *Latin*, formed of *Aceo*, I am sharp.

There are several Medicines in the Shops, whereon this Liquor is the Basis; as, *Acetum Distillatum*, distilled Vinegar, chiefly used in other Preparations for Dissolution, and Precipitation.

*Spiritus Acetia*, Spirit of Vinegar; made by drenching Copper Filings or Spittle Dust with distilled Vinegar, then evaporating it till the Fumes of the Vinegar cannot be smelt; the Saturation and Evaporation to be again repeated, till the Metal be satiated; which being then distilled, the Spirit comes over. Its Qualities and Uses are much the same with those of the former, only more powerful.

*Acetum Rosarum*, Vinegar of Roses; made of Rose-buds infused in Vinegar 40 or 50 Days; the Roses then pressed out, and the Vinegar preserved. It is chiefly used by way of Embrocation on the Head and Temples, in the Head-ach. After the same manner is made *Acetum Sambucinum*, Vinegar of Elders; *Acetum Anthosatum*, Vinegar of Rosemaries, &c.

The *German* Dispensatories abound with medicated Vinegars, chiefly used against pestilential Diseases : but they are not used among us.

**ACHILLES**. The ancient Botanists gave the Name *Achillæa* to several Plants; one of which is said to be the same with our Millefolium; and took its Name from *Achilles*, who, having been the Disciple of *Chiron*, first brought it into use for the Cure of Wounds and Ulcers.

**ACHOR**, *Achores*, in Medicine, the third Species or Degree of a *Tinea*, or Scald Head. *Achores* are a sort of spreading Ulcers, which break the Skin into a Number of little Holes, out of which oozes a viscid Humour. *Achores* only differ from *Favi* in this, that their Holes are smaller.

**ACID**, *Acidum*, any thing which affects the Tongue with a Sense of Sharpness, and Sourness. *Acids* are usually divided into *manifest* and *dubious*.

The *Manifest Acids*, are those above defined, which impress the Idea sensibly. Such are *Vinegar*, and its Spirit; the Juices *of Citrons, Oranges*; Spirit of *Nitre*, Spirit of *Alumn*, Spirit of *Vitriol*, Spirit of *Sulphur per Campanam*, Spirit of *Sea Salt*, &c.

*Dubious Acids*, are those which do not retain enough of the *Acid* Nature to give sensible Marks thereof on the Taste, but agree with the *Manifest Acids* in some other Properties, sufficient to refer them to the same Class. Hence it appears that there are some Characters of *Acidity* more general than that of the sharp Taste; tho 'tis that Taste is chiefly regarded in the Denomination.

The great and general Criterion, then, of *Acids*, is that they make a violent Effervescence, when mixed with another sort of Bodies, called *Alkalies*. Yet is not this Property alone universally to be depended on to determine a Body an *Acid*, without the joint Consideration of the Taste, and the Changes of Colour produced on other Bodies thereby. To distinguish *dubious Acids* from Alcalies, mix them with a blue Tincture of Violets : If the turn it red, they are of the *Acid* Tribe; if green, Alkaline.

*Acids* are all of the Tribe of Salts; and compose a particular Species thereof, called *Acid Salts*. Add, that the *Acid* Salts are all found to be volatile; by which they are distinguished from the rest, which are either fixed, or at least have a urinous, instead of an *acid* Taste.

Some late Chymical Philosophers have even made it very probable, that 'tis the *Acid* is the saline Part or Principle in all Salts. They consider it as a subtile, penetrating Substance, diffused thro' the several Parts of the Globe; which, according to the different Matters it happens to be united withal, produces different Kinds of Bodies : If it meets a fossil Oil, it converts it into Sulphur; if it be received into the *Lapis Calcarius*, it coagulates with it and becomes Alumn; with Iron it grows into green Vitriol; with Copper, into blue Vitriol, &c.

Of this Sentiment is Sir. *I. Newton*. "In decompounding Sulphur," says that Author, "we get an *Acid* Salt of the same Nature with Oil of Sulphur *per Campanum*; which same *Acid* abounding in the Bowels of the Earth, unites sometimes with the Earth, and thus makes Alumn; sometimes with Earth and Metal, and makes Vitriol; and sometimes with Earth and Bitumen, and thus compounds Sulphur." *Opticks*.

In effect, all our native Salts, tho without any Mixture from Art, are yet found to be real Mixtures; and their Composition and Decomposition is easily made. "As many as they are, they may be all reduced," according to M. *Homberg*[1], "to three Kinds, *viz*. Salt-petre, Sea-Salt, and Vitriol; each whereof has its several Species. Of the Combination of these with different oily Matters, are all the other Salts produced. By the Analyses we have made of 'em, they all appear to be composed of an aqueous, an earthy, a sulphurous, and an acid Part; but the *Acid* was hold the pure Salt : This makes our Chymical Principle Salt, the common Basis of all Salts; and which, antecedent

[1] Wilhelm Homberg (1652 – 1715), a Dutch natural philosopher

to its Determination to any particular Species, appears to be one familiar, uniform Matter, tho never found alone, but always accompany'd with some sulphureous Mixture or other; which determine sit to some one of the three sorts of Fossil Salts abovemention'd." *Mem. de l'Acad. R. des Sciences.* An. 1708.

The *Acid*, accompanied with its determining Sulphur, never becomes sensible to us, except when lodged either naturally in some earthy Matter, or artificially in an aqueous one. In the first Case, it appears under the Form of a crystallized Salt; as Salt-petre, Sea Salt, &c. In the second, it appears in form of an *Acid* Spirit; which, according to the Determination of the Sulphur accompanying it, is either Spirit of Nitre, or Spirit of Salt, or Spirit of Vitriol.

What is here spoke of the three simple fossil Salts, may be equally applied to all the compound Salts of Vegetables and Animals, with this difference, that the latter have always a larger Proportion of the earthy Matter than the simple ones, when in the form of a concrete Salt; and a larger Proportion of the aqueous Matter, when in the form of an *acid* Spirit. And hence we account for two important Phænomena; 1, That the *acid* Spirits of Animal and Fossil Salts, are always weaker, and less penetrating, as well as lighter in Weight, than those of the Fossil Salts : 2, That after a vehement Distillation, they leave a larger quantity of earthy Matter behind them than the Fossil do.

The Salt naturally contained in Plants, may be considered as a Mixture of Earth, Oil, a little Water, and an *acid* Salt : This last Ingredient being separated from the Plant with a vehement Fire, shoots into a new Salt, which sometimes retains an *acid* Taste, as in the Tartar of Wine; sometimes it assumes a Sweetness, as in Sugar; sometimes is bitter, as in Quinquina; and sometimes almost insipid, as in Sage. This, M. *Homberg* calls the essential Salt of the Plant; which, by a gentle Distillation, resolves into an insipid Water, an *acid* Liquor, and a ruddy fetid one; containing part of the *acid* Salt, and part of the fetid Oil of the Plant : of the Combination of which, is composed a particular Kind of fetid Salt, smelling like Urine, called the Volatile Salt or Volatile Alcaly Salt of the Plant : And the *Caput Mortuum* remaining, being reduced into Ashes, is separate by Lixiviation into one Part of fixed Alcaly Salt, and another of the insipid Alcaline Earth. Add, that the essential Salt always dissolves entirely in Water, even the earthy Part joined with it. But if the same Salt have been robbed, by means of Fire, of a great part of its *Acid*; the earthy Part will not wholly dissolve, but a Sediment of insipid Earth, indissoluble in Water, will be found at the bottom; to which, if an *acid* Spirit be added, it then becomes entirely dissoluble in Water : Whence it may be fairly concluded, that the other Part of the Ashes, before dissolved in the Water, and which after Evaporation appears in form of a fixed lixivial Salt, was only dissolved by Virtue of the *Acid* it contained; or as having retained enough of the *Acid* to effect a Dissolution.

Again, when the Earth of the Plant, satiated with its *Acid*, becomes a crystallized Salt; no more of the same *Acid* can be introduced into it : whereas the lixivious Salt drawn from the Ashes, does not crystallize, but still greedily imbibes the *Acid* Spirits.

Hence it may be probably concluded, that the Lixivious, or fixed Alcaly Salt, is not other than the Earth of the plant, which notwithstanding the Violence of the Fire, has retained a little Portion of its *acid* Salt, sufficient to dissolve it in Water; still reserving a sufficient Number of *Loculi* or Pores, to lodge the first *Acid* that shall offer it self, in lieu of that driven out of it by the Fire. And as the Name *Alcaly* is only given to a Salt, in respect of its imbibing and retaining an Acid presented to it, in order to the producing a crystallized Salt; the Lixivious Salts of the Plants may be said to be more or less Alcaline, as they absorb more or less *Acid*; or, which amounts to the same, as they contain more of fewer Vacuities to be filled with *Acids*.

An Alcaly, after it has been fully satiated with one sort of *Acid*, will yet sometimes admit and retain part of another *Acid* : This is chiefly observed where a Vegetable *Acid* has been received first, and a Fossil one is offered after. And it seems owing to this, That the Vegetable *Acid* having undergone a greater degree of Fermentation in the Body of the Plant, is become rare and pervious, in respect of the more solid and weight Particles of the Mineral *Acid*; which therefore force a way in.

The same is always the Case, where an *Acid* appears an Alcaly with respect to another *Acid*; that is, where, of two *Acid* Spirits, one whereof has a Mixture of some Alcaly; the rarer of the two having possessed the Pores of the Alkaly, is compressed by the other denser *Acid*. Thus, a Pin-cushion, tho ever so full of Cotton, will admit a good Number of Pins.

Now, urinous Salts are Alkalies as well as the Lixivious Kind, *i.e.* they greedily imbibe Acids, retain them, and together with them compose Salts which crystallize. But their Volatility seems to make it plain, that they are not, like the former, a Composition of a mere earthy Matter, with a little Acid; in regard a mere Earth can never become Volatile by such Admixture. Yet is there a great deal of Reason to imagine, that this Composition is no other than a Part of the same Matter, which would have produced the Lixivious Salt, intimately mixed with a deal of the fetid Oil of the Plant; and that the Oil is the sole Cause of the Volatility of these Salts.

M. *Homberg*, in his *Essai du Sel principe*, makes three Classes of *Acid* Salts, corresponding to the three Species of Sulphurs wherewith the primitive Acids may be combined. The first Class consists of such as contain an Animal, or a Vegetable Sulphur, which amount nearly to the same. To this Class belong all the distilled Acids of Plants, Fruits, Woods, &c. which must necessarily retain part of the Oil of the Plant, which is their Sulphur. To this Class also belongs Spirit of Nitre; as being a Substance procured from the Excrements of Animals, &c.

The second class is of those which contain a bituminous Sulphur. Such are Vitriol, common Sulphur, and Alumn; which are all usually procured from a Mineral Stone, wherein Bitumen is the prevailing Ingredient. The third is of such as contain a more fixed Mineral Sulphur, approaching the Nature of a metalline one. Such are the *Acids* drawn from Sea Salts and Sal Gemma's; the latter of which is chiefly found in Places near Mines of Metals, and the former probably arises from Rocks, or Veins of Sal Gemmae running into the Sea, and there dissolved.

From the peculiar Nature and Properties of the Sulphur thus accompanying the several Kinds of *Acid* Salts, their different Phænomena and Effects are to be accounted for.

The *Acids* of Animals are doubtless chiefly derived from Plants, in the ordinary way of Food and Nutrition; and those of Plants, again, from those of Minerals. So that there should seem to be but one Spring of *Acidity* : The Diversities arise from what happens to them in passing thro' the organized Bodies of Plants and Animals. Hence it is, that Plants and Animals especially, yield a very volatile Alkaly Salt; whereas, the Salts of Minerals are found altogether *acid*, and much more fixed and concrete; tho 'tis the same Matter in both Cases, under different assumed Forms.

Thus, the younger *Lemery*[1] argues, that as Animals feed on Plants, and reciprocally, in the Instance of Salt-petre, &c. Plants feed on Animals; inasmuch as their Vegetation is excited by Manure; it happens, that what was real Salt-petre in Plants, becomes only a nitrous Sal Ammoniac in Animals, and vice versa. The same Author accounts for this double Metamorphosis, by supposing that the nitrous Principle remains the same in both Cases, and in both Cases is attached to the same Matrix, with this only difference, that the Matrix becomes more earthy in Plants, and by that means, fixed; and in Animals, loses its earthy Parts, and assumes other oily ones, which render it volatile. *Mem. De l'Acad.* An. 1717.

As to the Manner wherein *Acids* act on Alcalies, the great Number of little Bubbles produced during their Action, and the Heat arising thereupon – M. *Homberg* explains it thus – The Matter of Light, which he supposes to be the chymical Principle, Sulphur, and to possess the whole Extent of the Universe; is kept in a perpetual Motion by the continual Impulses which the Sun and Fixed Stars give it : But this Motion, happening on some Occasions to be slackened, may be retrieved again, and augmented by the near Approach of Flame, which that Author supposes the only Matter capable of giving Motion to Light. This Motion of Light cannot proceed, without continually striking against the solid Bodies, and even passing thro' all the porous ones, it meets in its way.

Suppose, now, *Acids* to be little, solid, pointed Bodies, swimming at liberty in an aqueous Fluid, and kept in continual Motion, by the repeated Impulses of the Matter of Light; and Alcalies, to be spongious Bodies, whose Pores have formerly been filled with the Points of *Acids*, and which still retain the Dents of Impressions thereof, and are ready to receive the like Points when driven within them. 'Tis easy to conceive, that if some of those porous Alcalies float in the same Liquor wherein the solid *Acids* float; these latter, being impelled by the Matter of Light, will enter the Cavities of the former, which are framed as it were on purpose for their Reception; and that they will do it the more readily, if the Motion of the Matter of Light, wherewith they are impelled, have been accelerated by external Heat.

This Introduction of *Acids* into the Body of Alcalies, is, in all appearance, effected with a great Velocity and a deal of Friction; inasmuch as it produces so considerable a degree of Heat : And as the Pores of the Alcalies were before filled with an aerial Matter, which is now expelled by the Points of the *Acids*; that Air is put into Motion, and produces the Bubbles, which are so much the more sensible, as the Heat accompanying the Action is the greater.

Sir *I. Newton* accounts for the Effects of Acids in a different manner, *viz.*

[1] Louis Lemery (1677 – 1743), physician and son of Nicolas Lemery

from the great Principle of Attraction. "The Particles of *Acids*," he observes, "are of a size grosser than those of Water, and therefore less volatile; but much smaller than those of Earth, and therefore much less fix'd than they. They are endu'd with a very great attractive Force, wherein their Activity consists; it being by this that they affect and stimulate the Organ of Taste; and by this also, that they get about the Particles of Bodies, either of a metalline or a stony Nature, and adhere closely to 'em on all sides; so as scarce to be separable from them by Distillation or Sublimation : and when thus gather'd about the Particles of Bodies, by the same Power they raise, disjoin, and shake them one from another; that is, dissolve 'em."

"By their attractive Force, also, wherewith they rush towards the Particles of Bodies, they move fluid ones, and excite Heat; shaking asunder some Particle, so as to turn them into Air, and generate Bubbles : and hence all violent Fermentation; there being in all Fermentation a latent *Acid*, which coagulates in Precipitation. Acids, also, by attracting Water as much as they do the Particles of other Bodies, occasion the dissolv'd Particles readily to mingle with Water, or swim or float in it; after the manner of Salts : And as this Globe of Earth, by the Force of Gravity, attracting Water more strongly than it does lighter Bodies, cause those Bodies to ascend in Water, and go upwards from the Earth; so, the Particles of Salts, by attracting the Water, mutually avoid and recede from one another as far as they can; and are thus diffus'd throughout the whole Water."

"The Particles of Alcalies consist of earthy and *acid* Parts united together; but these *Acids* have so great an attractive Force, that they can't be separated therefrom by Fire; and that they even precipitate the Particles of dissolv'd Metals, by attracting from them the acid Particles, which before had dissolv'd, and kept them in Solution."

"If these *acid* Particles be join'd with earthy ones, in a small Quantity; they are so closely retain'd by the latter, as to be quite suppress'd and lost, as it were, in them; so that they neither stimulate the Organ of Sense, nor attract Water; but compose Bodies which are not *acid*, *i.e.* fatty and sweet Bodies; as *Mercurius Dulcis*, Brimstone, *Luna Cornea*, &c. From the same attractive Force in these *acid* Particles thus suppress'd, arises that Property of Bodies, that they stick or adhere to almost all Bodies, and are easily inflammable. Thus, the *Acid* that lies suppress'd in sulphureous Bodies, by more strongly attracting the Particles of other Bodies (earthy ones for instance) than its own; promotes a gentle Fermentation, produces and cherishes natural Heat, and carries it on so far sometimes, as to the Putrefaction of the Compound; Putrefaction arising hence, that the *acid* Particles which have long kept up the Fermentation, at length insinuate into the little Interstices that lie between the Particles of the first Composition; and so intimately uniting with those Particles, produce a new Mixture or Compound, which cannot be return'd into its original form."

"Water has no great dissolving Force, because there is but a small Quantity of *Acid* in it; for whatever strongly attracts, and is strongly attracted, may be reputed an *Acid*: But in such things as are dissolved in Water, the Dissolution is slowly perform'd, and without any Effervescence. When these *Acids* are applied to the Tongue, or any excoriated Part of the Body; leaving the subtile Earth wherewith they were before united, they rush into the Sensory, act there as Menstruums, and disjoin its Parts; thus causing a painful Sensation."

The illustrious Author, it must be own'd, here carries the Notion of *Acidity* a great length : Dissolution, according to him, is only effected by Attraction, and is proportional to the degree of attractive Power in the Dissolvent; but all Bodies which attract much are *Acids*, on his Principle; and consequently all powerful Menstruums must belong to that Class. And yet Spirit of Urine, which readily dissolves Iron or Copper, even in the Cold, is allow'd an Alcaly; and accordingly makes a vehement Conflict with *Aqua fortis*.

Some chymical Philosophers, the last Century, endeavour'd to derive the Qualities of Bodies, and the other Phænomena of Nature, from the Consideration of Alcaly and *Acid*.

If has been a Point much controverted among the Physicians, whether or no there be any sincere *Acid* in human Blood? The generality stand for the Negative; and all Mr. *Boyle's*[1] Experiments, in his History of Blood, seem to give the thing on that side. But the accurate M. *Homberg* has at last turn'd the Scales the other way; and shewn, by repeated Experiments, that an *Acid*, or what is commonly call'd so, and judg'd such by the Change of Colour it causes in Tincture of Violets, may be drawn from the Blood of all Animals in general, and human Blood in particular. *Mem. de l'Acad. Roy. des. Sciences*. An. 1712.

Hence, and from the careful Analyses that Author *Boyle* has made of the Flesh and Excrement of divers Animals, particularly Man; he infers, that the *Acid*, or Sea Salt of the Aliment taken into the Bodies of Animals; is not destroyed therein, but passes into the Substance of them : the superfluous Portion being returned unaltered along with the Excrements.

*Acids* are prescribed in Medicine, as Coolers, Antifebrisicks, Antiscorbuticks, Diaphoreticks, Alexipharmicks, &c.

"*Acids*," Mr. *Boyle* observes, "not only disturb the Body while they continue sensibly *acid*; but in many Cases create Distempers, whereof they should seem the Remedies. Tho they be reputed to have an incisive and resolutive Virtue, and accordingly are prescribed to cut tough Phlegm, and dissolve coagulated Blood : yet there are some *Acids* which must evidently coagulate the animal Fluids, and produce Obstructions, with all their Train of Consequences. Thus, it is known, that Milk readily curdles with Spirit of Sea Salt, &c."

**ACIDITY**, *Aciditas*, *Acor*, the Quality which constitutes, or denominates, a Body, *Acid*; or that Sensation of Sharpness and Acrimony which *Acids* excite upon the Taste. A little Vitriol leaves an agreeable *Acidity* in Water. Vinegar and Verjuice have different sorts of *Acidity*. The Predominance of *Acidities* in the Body, and their ill Effects, in coagulating Blood, &c. is prevented by either repelling and mortifying them with Lixivious or Urinous Salts; or sheathing and absorbing them, with Alcalious Bodies. Thus, Minium destroys the *Acidity* of Spirit of Vinegar; Lapis Calaminaris that of Sea Salt, &c.

**ACIDULÆ**, in Natural History, a Species of Mineral Waters, which discover a degree of Acidity to the Taste. *Acidulæ* are native Waters, impregnated

[1] Robert Boyle (1627 – 1691), Irish scientist, natural philosopher and inventor.

with Particles of some acid Mineral; as Vitriol, Alumn, Nitre, or Salt. Sometimes there is also a vinous Flavour joined with the Acid; by which they become peculiarly denominated *Vinous Waters.*

The Class of *Acidulæ* are usually very cold; whence some Authors define *Acidulæ* to be all such Mineral or Medicinal Waters as are not hot. The Physicians also frequently include Chalybeat or Ferruginous Waters, under the Class of *Acidulæ.*

The Word is a Diminutive of *Acidum*; which is formed from the *Greek* αχις, *Point, Edge*; in regard the Points of acid Substances prick and vellicate the Tongue. We sometimes also meet with *Acidulated, q.d.* something wherein acid Juices have been put, in order to give it a Coolness, and Briskness.

**ACINI**, in Botany, small Grains, growing in Bunches; after the manner of Grape-stones. The word is *Latin*, and literally signifies *Grape-stone.* Hence, Anatomists have called some Glands of a similar Formation, *Acini Glandulosi.*

**ACONITE**, *Aconitum*, a Plant, famous among the Antients, both in quality of a Poison, and a Remedy. The antient Botanists give the Name *Aconite* to several Plants of different Kinds. One Species they called *Lycoctonum*, Λυχεχγνεν, *Wolfs-bane* or Κυνοχτενεν, *Dogs-bane*; from its Effects : Of this they had likewise their Divinations; as the *Napellus*, thus called *à Napo*, because its Root resembled the Turnip-Kind : another called *Anthora, Anti-Thora, q.d.* good against Disorders of the *Thora.*

The whole Class of *Aconites* is held extremely caustic and acrimonious, in Virtue whereof they produce mortal Convulsions, or Inflammations which end in Mortification; with which the Antients were so surprised, that they were afraid to touch them : And hence a thousand superstitious Precautions about the manner of gathering them. The Roots are held of service in Malignant Fevers; and accordingly make an Ingredient in some Orvietans, and other Alexipharmic Compositions.

*Aconite* is aid to take its Name from *Acona*, a City in *Bithynia*[1], where it grows in great abundance : tho it is also found in other Places, particularly the Mountains about *Trent.* Some derive its Name from αχονεν, *a Rock naked or bare of Earth*, whereon the Plant readily thrives. It was also called μυοχτοιΘ; as killing Mice with its bare smell, according to *Pliny*[2]. The Poets feign it to have arose from the Foam of the Dog *Cerberus*, when *Hercules* dragged him out of Hell.

The Antients used this Plant against the Sting of the Scorpion, which is said to be deadened by the Touch of the *Aconite*, and restored to its Vigour by that of Hellebore. *Theophrastus*[3] relates, that they had a way of preparing it in those Days, so as it should only destroy at the End of one or two Years. Arrows dipt in its Juice prove mortal wherever they wound. The *Indians* use *Aconite*, corrected in Cows Urine, with good success against Fevers.

[1] A Roman province in Turkey bordered by the Black Sea and the Bosphorus.

[2] Gaius Plinius Secundus (23 – 79), or Pliny the Elder, the Roman natural philosopher.

[3] Theophrastus (ca. 381 – 287 BC), a Greek philosopher and botanist.

**ACORUS**, a Medicinal Plant, of the Rush or Flag Kind; frequently confounded by the Antients, and also by the modern Apothecaries, with the Calamus Odoratus. There are two Species of *Acorus*; the *Verus*, or true, and the *false*. They are distinguished by this, that from the middle of some of the Leaves of the former, there arises a longish Cluster of an Infinity of little Flowers, the Thickness of the little Finger, and resembling Macropiper, or Long Pepper. The *false Acorus* is the common Swordgrass.

'Tis only the Root of the *Acorus* that is used in Phsyick; and 'tis this we usually call *Acorus*. The *true* is brought from *Lithuania* and *Tartary* : It is knotty, reddish, without, and white within; as thick as the little Finger, and half a foot long. It is spicey and bitterish; and used in Cephalic and Stomachic Compositions. It is also an Ingredient in the *Theriaca Andromachi*. Some rank Galangals as a Species of *Acorus*.

**ACRASIA**, αχρασια, is used by some Writers in Physick, for the Excess or Predominancy of one Quality above another; either in a Mixture, or in the Constitution of a human Body.

**ACRIMONY**, Asperity or Sharpness, expresses a Quality in Bodies, by which they corrode, destroy, or dissolve others. Salts are only caustic in Virtue of the *Acrimony*. The *Acrimony* of the Bile is supposed the Cause of divers Disorders. A Catarrh is a Defluxion of *Acrimonious* Humour.

**ACTIVE** *Principles*, in Chymistry, are those which are supposed to act of themselves, and do not need to be put in action by others. Salt, Sulphur, and Mercury, are usually considered by the Chymists as *Active* Principles; and Phlegm and Earth, as Passive ones.

M. *Homberg*, and some late Chymists after him, only make one *Active* Principle, *viz*. Sulphur, or Fire; which they take to be the Source or Principle of all the Motion and *Action* of the Universe. The Term *Active Principles*, says Dr. *Quincy*[1], has been used to express some Divisions of Matter, that are, by some particular Modifications, comparatively *active*, in respect of others; as, *Spirit*, *Oil*, and *Salt*, whose Parts are better fitted for Motion, than those of Earth and Water; but with how much Impropriety, will easily appear.

For, in a strict Sense, all Motion in Matter is rather Passion; and there is no Active Principle, unless we call so that known Property of Gravitation, on which the *Newtonian* Philosophy is founded; which is a mutual Inclination of Bodies towards one another, in proportion to the Quantity of Matter, in all Bodies : so that let them exist under what Modifications soever, there can be no Alteration made of this universal Property. Hence, the Division of Matter into what, for Distinction sake, may be called Spirit, does not give it any Properties inconsistent with this general Law.

**ACUTE** *Disease*, is that which terminates, or comes to its Period, in a few Days; or, as the Physicians express it, *cito & cum periculo terminator*. In this Sense, the Word stands opposed to *Chronical*. All Diseases which hold above forty Days, are reputed Chronical. Dr. *Quincy* thinks an *Acute Disease* may

[1] John Quincy, M.D., (d. 1722) apothecary and iatrophysical writer.

be defined, that which is attended with an increased Velocity of Blood. *Acute Diseases* are the more dangerous, in that, beside the Violence of the Symptoms, if there be not time to empty the *Primæ Viæ*, 'tis very difficult to stop their Progress, and save the Patient. *Acute Diseases* are usually divided into those properly called *Acute*; and those, which by reason of the Vehemence of the Symptoms, are called *Most Acute.*

**ADAMANT**, *Adamus*, in Natural History, &c. an ancient Name for a Precious Stone, by us called a *Diamond.*

**ADEPS**, in Anatomy, a Species of *Fat*, found in the Cavities of the Abdomen. The *Adeps* differs from the common *Fat*, called *Pinguedo*; in that it is thicker, harder and of a more earthy Substance. The *Adeps* is much the same with what we call *Sevium, Suet*, or *Leaf. Adeps* is used by the Physicians, as a general Name for Fat or either Kind.

The *Adeps Anseris*, Goose's Fat; *Adeps Canis*, Fat of a Dog; *Adeps Hominis*, Fat of Man; *Adeps Vipere*, Vipers Fat; and *Adeps Ursi*, Bears Fat, are all used in Medicine, in quality of Ripeners, or Drawers; as being of a penetrating Nature, and thereby suited to dissolve and rarify the Tumors, and bring them as it were to Maturity. The specific Virtues ascribed to certain of them, do not seem well warranted.

**ADIAPHOROUS**, Adiaphorus, *q.d. Indifferent or Neutral*; a Name given by Mr. *Boyle* to a Kind of Spirit distilled from Tartar and some other Vegetable Bodies; and which is neither Acid, Vinous, nor Urinous; but in many respects different from any other sort of Spirit.

**ADRAGANT**, or Tragacanth. A sort of Gum. See Tragacanth.

**ADUST**, *Adustus*, is applied, among Physicians, &c. to such Humours, as by long Heat become of a hot and fiery Nature. Such is Choler supposed to be. Melancholy is usually considered as black and *adust* Bile. *Adust* Blood, says *Blanchard*, is when by reason of extraordinary Heat, its more subtile Parts are all evaporated, leaving the grosser, with all the Impurities therein, half rorrify'd, as it were. The Word is formed of the *Latin aduro*, I burn.

**ÆGILOPS**, a Tumor, or rather Ulcer, in the great Canthus or Angle of the Eye, by Root of the Nose; either with or without an Inflammation. The Word, in its original Greek, αιγιλωψ, signifies a Goat's Eye; in regard, Goats are supposed extremely liable to this Distemper.

If the *Ægilops* be neglected, it bursts, and degenerates into a Fistula, which eats into the Bone. Authors frequently use *Ægilops*, *Anchylops*, and *Fistula Lachrymalis* promiscuously : But the more accurate, after *Ægineta*, make a difference. The Tumor, ere it becomes ulcerous, is properly called *Anchylops*; and after it has rendered the *Os Lachrymal* carious, *Fistula Lachrymalis.*

If the *Ægilops* be accompanied with an Inflammation; it takes its Rise from the Abundance of Blood, which the too great Plenitude discharges upon the Corner of the Eye. If it be without an Inflammation, it is supposed to proceed from a viscous pituitous Humour, thrown upon this Part.

**ÆGYPTIACUM**, in Pharmacy, a kind of detersive Unguent; so called from its dusky Hue or Colour, which resembles the swarthy Complexion of the Ægyptians. It is composed of Verdigrease, Vinegar, and Honey, boiled to a Consistence. The Prescription is *Mesue's*[1]. It is chiefly used for eating off rotten Flesh, and cleansing foul Ulcers; particularly Venereal ones in the Throat, &c. It also destroys those cancerous Erosions apt to grow in Childrens Mouths.

**ÆSCHYNOMENOUS** Plants, among Botanists, are those popularly called Sensitive Plants.

**ÆSTUARY**, is sometimes also used in Pharmacy, for a Vapour-Bath, *Balneum Vaporosum.*

**ÆS** *Ustum*, called also *Crocus Veneris*, a Chymical Preparation, made of Copper cut into thin Plates, put into a Crucible with Sulphur and Salt, *stratum super stratum*, and thus set in a hot Charcoal Fire, till the sulphur be consumed. It is very detersive; and is used for eating off dead Flesh. They who make this use of it, are to heat it red hot in the Fire nine times; and quench it as often in Linseed Oil.

**ÆTHER**, is usually understood of a thin, subtile Matter, or Medium, much finer and rare than Air; which commencing from the Limits of our Atmosphere, possesses the whole heavenly Space. The Word is *Greek*, αιθυρ, supposed to be formed from the Verb αιθεον, *to burn, to flame*; some of the Antients, particularly *Anaxagoras*[2], supposing it of the Nature of Fire.

The Philosophers cannot conceive that the largest Part of the Creation should be perfectly void; and therefore fill it with a Species of Matter under the Denomination of *Æther*. But they vary extremely as to the Nature and Character of this *Æther*.

Some conceive it as a Body *sui generis*, appointed only to fill up the Vacuities between the heavenly Bodies; and therefore confined to the Regions above our Atmosphere. Others suppose it of so subtile and penetrating a Nature, as to pervade the Air, and other Bodies; and posses the Pores and Intervals thereof. Others deny the Existence of any such specific Matter; and think the Air it self, by that immense Tenuity and Expansion it is found capable of, may diffuse it self thro the interstellar Spaces, and be the only Matter found therein.

In effect, *Æther*, being no Object of our Sense, but the mere Work of Imagination, brought only upon the Stage for the sake of Hypothesis, or to solve some Phænomenon, real or imaginary; Authors take the Liberty to modify it how they please. Some suppose it of an elementary Nature, like other Bodies, and only distinguished by its Tenuity, and the other Affections consequent thereon : which is the *Philosophical Æther*. Others will have it of another Species, and not Elementary; but rather a sort of fifth Element, of a purer, more refined, and spirituous Nature than the Substances about our

[1] Yuhanna ibn Masawaih (777 – 857), an Assyrian physician, aka Johannes Mesue.

[2] Anaxagoras (500-428 BC), Greek natural philosopher.

Earth; and void of the common Affections thereof as Gravity, &c. The heavenly Spaces, being supposed Regions or Residence of a more exalted Class of Beings; the Medium must be mire exalted in proportion. Such is the antient and popular Idea of *Æther*, or *Æthereal Matter*.

The Term *Æther* being thus embarrassed with a Variety of Ideas, and arbitrarily applied to so many different things; the later and severer Philosophers chuse to set it aside : and in lieu thereof, substitute other more determinate ones. Thus, the *Cartesians* use the Term *Materia Subtilis*; which is their *Æther*: And Sir. *I. Newton*, sometimes, a *Subtile Spirit*, as in the Close of his *Principia*; and sometimes a *Subtile* or *Æthereal Medium*; as in the *Opticks*.

The Truth is, there are abundance of Considerations, which seem to evince the Existence of some Matter in the Air, much finer than the Air it self. There is an unknown something, which remains behind when the Air is taken away; as appears from certain Effects which we see produced *in Vacuo*. Heat, Sir *I. Newton* observes, is communicated thro a Vacuum, almost as readily as thro Air: But such Communication cannot be without some interjacent Body, to act as a Medium. And such Body must be subtile enough to penetrate the Pores of Glass; and may be very well concluded to permeate those of all other Bodies; and consequently be diffused thro all the Parts of Space : Which answers to the full Character of an *Æther*.

The Existence of such *Æthereal* Medium being settled; that Author proceeds to its Properties; inferring it to be not only rarer and more fluid than Air, but exceedingly more elastic, and active : In Virtue of which Properties, he shews, that a great part of the Phænomena of Nature may be produced by it. To the Weight, *e.g.* of this Medium, he attributes Gravitation, or the Weight of all other Bodies; and to its Elasticity, the elastic Force of the Air, and of the nervous Fibres, and the Emission, Refraction, Reflection, and other Phænomena of Light; as also, Sensation, Muscular Motion, &c. In fine, this same Matter seems the *Primum Mobile*, the first Source or Spring of physical Action in the modern System.

The *Cartesian Æther* is supposed not only to pervade, but adequately to fill all the Vacuities of the Bodies; and thus to make an absolute Plenum in the Universe. But Sir *I. Newton* overturns this Opinion, from divers Considerations; by shewing, that the Celestial Spaces are void of all sensible Resistance : For, hence it follows, that the Matter contained therein, must be immensely rare, in regard the Resistance of Bodies is chiefly as their Density; so that if the Heavens were thus adequately filled with a Medium or Matter how subtile soever, they would resist the Motion of the Planets and Comets much more than Quicksilver or Gold.

**ÆTHEREAL**, *Æthereus*, something that belongs to *Æther*, or is of the Nature of *Æther*. Thus, we say, the *Æthereal* Space; *Æthereal* Regions, &c. Some of the Antients divided the Universe, with respect to the Matter contained therein, into *Elementary* and *Æthereal*. Under *Æther*, or the *Æthereal* World, was included all that Space above the upper Element, *viz.* Fire. This they supposed to be perfectly, homogeneous, incorruptible, unchangeable, &c.

'Twas a Point controverted among them, Whether or no the *Æthereal*

Matter had the Property of Gravity? Many late Philosophers, not only at home but abroad, contend for its Gravity; and even for its being the Cause of Gravity in all other Bodies. In effect, says *Chauvin*[1], Bodies do not descend by any inherent Principle; but by the Impulse or Trusion of something eternal : which can be nothing but *Æther*; in regard they fall *in Vacuo* as readily, nay more so, than in open Air : From the same Principle arises the Cohesion of Bodies.

*Æthereal Oil*, is a fine, subtile Oil, approaching nearly to the Nature of a Spirit. Thus, the pure Liquor rising next after the Spirit, in the Distillation of Turpentine, is called the *Æthereal Oil* of Turpentine. Some Chymists distinguish two Principles in Urine; the one a volatile urinous Salt, resembling Spirit of Nitre; the other an *Æthereal Oil*, or *Sulphur*; partaking of the Nature of Spirit or Wine.

**ÆTHIOPS** *Mineral*, a Preparation of Mercury, made by grinding equal Quantities of crude Quicksilver and Flower of Sulphur, in a Stone or Iron Mortar; till they become incorporated into a black Pouder. It is prescribed for the Worms, and all Crudities and Acrimony of the Humours; and is reputed infallible against the Itch, and other cutaneous Diseases.

**ÆTIOLOGY**, *Ætiologia*, a Rationale, or Discourse of the Cause of a Disease. In this Sense, we say, the of the Small Pox, of the Hydrophobia, of the Gout, the Dropsy, &c. The Word is com-pounded of the *Greek* αιτια, *Cause*, and λογος, *Sermo, Discourse.*

**ÆTITES**, in Natural History, the *Eagle-Stone.* The *Ætites*, or *Lapis Ætites*, is a kind of Stone, vulgarlarly said to be found in the Eagle's Nest; but this, as well as many of the Virtues ascribed to it, seem to be fabulous. It is found under ground in several Parts : Near *Treves* in *France*, one can scarce dig a few feet, without finding considerable Strata or Beds thereof. The Word is formed of the *Greek* αετος, *Aquila*, Eagle.

'Tis usually hollow, and has a kind of Core or Kernel in it, which, upon shaking, rattles : Some have two, and others three such Cores. It is found of various Forms, and Sizes; but its Texture or Consistence is pretty uniform; consisting of two or three Lays or Coats of a Matter resembling baked Earth : Especially the innermost. They are originally soft, and of the Colour of yellow Oker. *Dioscorides*[2] says, it is of use in discovering a Thief; for by mixing it with his Meat, he'll be unable to swallow it. *Matthiolus* informs us, that Birds of Prey never hatch their young without this Stone; and that they seek it as far as the *Indies.*

The Use now made of the Stone, is to assist Women in Labour; to which end, they fasten it about the Knee : it being a Tradition, that according as it is applied above or below the Matrix, it has the Faculty of retaining or excluding the Child. Hence, it is sometimes directed to be bore about the Arm to prevent *Abortion.*

[1] Etienne Chauvin (1640 - 1725), a Cartesian philosopher.

[2] Pedanius Dioscorides (ca. 40-90 BC), a Greek physician who wrote *De Materia Medica.*

**AGARIC**, or *Fungus Agarici*, in Pharmacy, a kind of fungous Excrescence growing on the Trunks, and large Branches of several Trees; but chiefly on the Larch-Tree, and certain Oaks. *Dioscorides* derives its Name from a Province of *Sarmatia*[1], called *Agaria*; whence it was first brought. Several Authors, and among the rest, *Galen*[2], take it for a Root; but the common Opinion is for its being of the Mushroom kind. It is brought from the *Levant*. It is white, light, tender, brittle, of a bitter Taste, pungent, and a little Styptic. This is what the Antients called the *Female Agaric* : As for the Male, it is usually yellowish and woody; and is generally excluded out of Physick, being only used in Dying.

*Agaric* was a Medicine in mighty use among the Antients; not only for the purging of Phlegm, but in all Distempers proceeding from the gross Humours and Obstructions; as the Epilepsy, Madness, Asthma, &c. Yet they complained, that it weakened the Bowels, and purged too violently. They had divers Corrections for it; chiefly of the Aromatic kind : But Dr. *Quincy* says, the best way is to banish it for good, as the present Practice has almost done: for that it rather makes People sick, than purges them; being very nauseous, and but a little cathartic.

By a chymical Solution, it passes almost wholly into Oil : It yields no volatile Salt; but abounds with a sort of scaly Earth, and an acid Phlegm. We read of *Pillulæ de Agarico*, and *Troches of Agaric* : but they are disused. Some Authors also mention a *Mineral Agaric*; which is a whitish Stone, found in the Clefts of Rocks in *Germany*; called also *Lac Lunæ*, and by some Naturalists, *Lithomagra*, and *Stenomagra*.

**AGENT**, *Agens*, in Physicks, that whereby a thing is done or effected; or that which has a Power whereby it acts on another; or by its Action induces some Change in another. The Word *Agent* is used promiscuously with *Efficient*; and in contraindication to *Patient*.

The Schools divide *Agents* into *Natural* and *Free*. *Natural* or *Physical Agents*, are those immediately determined by the Author of Nature, to produce one sort of Effect; with an Incapacity to produce the contrary thereto. Such is Fire, which only heats, and does not also cool.

*Free* or *Voluntary Agent*, is that which may equally do any thing, or the opposite thereof; as acting not from any Pre-determination, but from Choice. Such is the Mind supposed to be; which may either will or nill the same thing.

*Natural Agents*, again, are subdivided into *Universal*; which are such as produce Effects of the same Kind and Denomination with the *Agents* themselves : and *Equivocal*, whose Effects are of a different Kind, &c. from the *Agents*.

The Schoolmen reckon the following Circumstances necessary to the Being of an *Agent*, *viz.* That it be contiguous to the Object, distinct from it, have a Power over it, a Sphere of Activity, and a Proportion or Rate of acting.

**AGGLUTINANTS**, *Agglutinantia*, in Medicine, a Species of strengthening Remedies, whose Office and Effect is to adhere to the solid parts of the Body,

[1] Sarmatia was a Roman territory encompassing parts of Russia and the Ukraine.

[2] Claudius Aelius Galenus (129 – 200), a Greek philosopher and physician.

and thus recruit and supply the Place of what is wore off and wasted in the animal Actions. These are most of them of the glutinous Kind, or such as easily form themselves into Gellies and gummy Consistencies; whence the Name *Agglutinant*, which is formed of *ad*, to, and *gluten*, glue. The principle Simples which come under this Class, are Ising-glass[1], Olibanum[2], Gum Arabic, Dragons Blood[3], Cassia, Sago, Vermicelli, Pulse, Comfrey, Plaintain, &c.

**AGGLUTINATION**, literally, denotes the Act of joining, or cementing two Bodies together, by means of a proper Gluten, or Glue. In Medicine, the Term is peculiarly used for the Addition of a new Substance; or the giving a greater Consistence to the Animal Fluids, to fit them the more for Nourishment.

**AGNUS** *Castus*, a Shrub, famous among the Antients as a Specific for the Preservation of Chastity, and the preventing of all Venereal Diseases, Pollutions, &c. The *Greeks* called it Αγνος, *Chast*; to which has since been added the Reduplicative *Castus*, q.d. *Chast, chast*. The *Athenian* Ladies, who made Profession of Chastity, lay upon leaves of *Agnus Castus*, during the Feasts of *Ceres*. It is reputed a Cooler, and particularly of the Genital Parts; and was antiently used in Physick, to allay those inordinate Motions arising from seminal Turgescences : But it is out of the present Practice.

**AGUE**, a periodical Disease, consisting in a cold shivering Fit, succeeded by a hot one; and going off in a Diaphoresis, or Sweating. According to the Periods or Returns of the Fits, the Disease is either a *Quotidian, Tertian*, or *Quartan Ague*, or *Fever*.

The next Cause of *Agues*, seems to be an obstructed Perspiration, or whatever by overloading the Juice, retards their Motion, or occasions a Lentor in the Blood. The Symptoms are Heaviness and Reaching; a weak, slow Pulse; Coldness, and Shivering, felt first in the Joints, thence creeping over the whole Body; Pain in the Loins, and an involuntary Motion of the Jaw.

A *Vernal Ague* is easily cured; but an *Autumnal* one is more obstinate, especially in aged and cachectical Persons. If complicated with a Dropsy, Peripneumony, &c. dangerous. When an *Ague* proves fatal, it is usually in the cold Fit. The Cure is usually begun with an Emetic of Ipecacuanha, an Hour before the Access; and compleated with the Cortex Peruvianus, administered in the Interval between two Fits; and continued at times, to prevent a Relapse.

Dr. *Quincy* endeavors to account for the Effect of the Bark, from the Irregularity, Asperity, and Solidity of its Particles, which fit it to break those Viscidities in the Juices whereby the Capillaries where obstructed, and to draw up the Solids into a Tension, sufficient by the vigorous Vibrations thereof. The first Intention, he observes, is answered by its corrugating the Nerves, and rendering the Contractions of the Vessels more brisk and forc-

[1] Ichthycolla, a glue made from a fish, possibly the Sturgeon.

[2] Frankincense.

[3] A red resin probably from the plant *Dracaena cinnabari*.

ible. Hence also its Effects upon such as are apt to sweat immodestly.

**ALABASTRA**, in a Plant, are those little green Leaves which compass in the bottom of the Flower.

**ALBUM** *Græcum*, or *Stercus Canis Officinale*, Dogs white Dung, is a Medicinal Drug, in the present Practice, used with Honey, to cleanse and deterge, chiefly in Inflammations of the Throat; and that principally outwardly, as a Plaster.

**ALBUMEN** *Ovi*, the White of an Egg. It is used in Medicine, as being of a glutinous or binding Nature, on which Account it is often mixed with Bole Armoniac, &c. to prevent any strained Part from rising into a Tumor, and restore it to its Tone or Elasticity. It is also an Ingredient in some Mixtures for consolidating fresh Wounds, and preventing too great a Loss of Blood.

**ALCHYMY**, or Alchemy, a higher or more refined kind of Chymistry, employed in the more mysterious Researches of the Art. The Word is compounded of the Arabic Particle of Augmentation, *Al*, and the Latin *Chymia*, Egyptian *Kemia*, or *Greek* χιμια, *Chymistry*.

The Name *Alchymy* is of long standing : The first time it occurs, is in *Julius Firmicus Maternus*, an Author who live under *Constantine* the Great, and who in his *Mathesis*, C. XV. speaking of the Influences of the Heavenly Bodies, affirms, "that if the Moon be in the House of *Saturn*, at the Time a Child is born, he shall be skilled in *Alchymy*."

The great Objects or Ends pursued by *Alchymy*, are,

1, The making of Gold; which is attempted three different ways : by Separation; by Maturation; and by Transmutation; which last is to be effected by means of what they call the *Philosopher's Stone*.

2, An Universal Medicine, adequate to all Diseases.

3, An Universal Dissolvent, or *Alkehest*.

4, An Universal Ferment; or a Matter which being applied to any Seed, shall increase its Fecundity to Infinity : If, *e.g.* it be applied to Gold, it changes the Gold into the Philosopher's Stone of Gold; if to Silver into the Philosopher's Stone of Silver; if to a Tree, the Result is the Philosopher's Stone of the Tree, which transmutes everything it is applied to into Trees, &c.

The Origin and Antiquity of *Alchymy* are much controverted. If regard may be had to Legend and Tradition, it must be as old as the Flood; nay, *Adam* himself is represented by the *Alchymists* as an Adept. A great part, not only of the Heathen Mythology, but of the *Jewish* and Christian Revelations, are supposed to refer hereto: Thus, *Suidas* will have the Secret of the Philosopher's Stone couched in the Fable of the *Argonauts*; others find it in the Books of Moses, &c.

But, if the Æra of the Art be examined by the Monuments of History; it will lose a deal of this fancied Antiquity. The learned *Dane, Ol. Borrichius*[1], has

[1] Olau Borrichius (1626 – 1690), a Danish physician.

taken immense Pains to prove it known to the antient *Greeks* and *Egyptians*. *Her. Conringius*[1], on the contrary, with equal Address, undertakes to shew its Novelty.

In effect, not one of the antient Poets, Philosophers, or Physicians, from *Homer* till 400 Years after Christ, mention any such thing. The first Author who speaks of making Gold, is *Zosimus* the *Panopolitan*, who lived towards the Beginning of the Vth Century, and who has an express Treatise, περι της ιερας τεχνης του χρυσου και του αργυρου ϖοιητιος, *Of the divine Art of making Gold and Silver*, still extant in manuscript in the *French* King's Library. The next is *Æneas Garæus*, another *Greek* Writer, towards the Close of the same Century, in whom we have the following Passage : "Such as are the skilled in the Ways of Naturem can take Silver and Tin, and changing their Nature, turn them into Gold." The same Writer tells us, he was "wont to style himself χρυςιχος, *Gold-finder*, and χημευς, *Chymist*." Hence we may gather, there was some such Art in being in that Age; but, as neither of these Authors relate how long it had been known before, their Testimony will not carry us back beyond the Age wherein they lived.

Nor do we find any earlier, plainer Traces of the Universal Medicine : not a Syllable of any such thing in all the Physicians and Naturalists, from *Moses* to *Geber*[2] the *Arab*, who is supposed to have lived in the VIIIth Century. In that Author's Work, entitle, *The Philosopher's Stone*, mention is made of "a Medicine which cures all Lepras:" This passage some Authors suppose to have given the first Hint of the Matter; tho *Geber* himself, perhaps, meant no such thing : For, by attending to the *Arabick* Stile and Diction of this Author, which abounds in Allegory, it appears highly probable, that by *Man* he means Gold, and by Lepras or Diseases, the other Metals, which are all impure in comparison of Gold.

*Suidas* accounts for this total Silence of Authors in respect of *Alchymy*, by observing, that *Diocletian*[3] procured all the Books of the antient *Egyptians* to be burnt; and that it was in these the great Mysteries of Chymistry were contained. *Conringius* calls this History in question, and asks how *Suidas*, who lived but 500 Years before us, should know what happended 800 Years before him? To which *Borrichius* answers, that he learnt it of *Eudemus*, *Helladius*, *Zozimus*, *Pamphilus*, and &c. as *Suidas* himself relates.

*Kircher*[4] asserts, that the Theory of the Philosopher's Stone is delivered at large in the Fable of *Hermes*; and that the antient *Egyptians* were not ignorant of the Art, but declined to prosecute it. They did not need to transmute Gold, they had ways of separating it from all kinds of Bodies, from the Mud of the *Nile*, and Stones of all Kinds. But, he adds, these Secrets were never wrote down or made publick, but confined to the Royal Family, and handed down traditionally from Father to Son.

The chief Point advanced by *Borrichius*, and on which he seems to lay the

[1] Hermann Conring (1606 – 1681), a German physician and professor of medicine.

[2] This is probably Abu Musa Jabir ibn Hayyan (ca. 721 – 815), a Persian philosopher and alchemist.

[3] Gaius Aurelius Valerius Diocletianus (244 – 311), a Roman emperor who reigned from 286 through 305.

[4] Anathasius Kircher (1601 – 1680), a German scholar who wrote extensively on Egyptology.

greatest Stress, is the Attempt of *Caligula*, mentioned by *Pliny*, for procuring Gold by Distillation from Orpiment. *Hist. Nat.* L. XXXIII. c. 14. But this, it may be observed, makes very little for that Author's Pretensions; there being no Transmutation, no Hint of any Philosopher's Stone, but only a little Gold extracted or separated from the Mineral.

The principal Authors in *Alchymy* are *Geber, Friar Bacon, Ripley, Lully, John* and *Isaac Hollandus, Basil Valentine, Paracelsus, Van Zuchten,* and *Centiveglio.*

**ALCOHOL**, or rather *Alkool*, in Chymistry, an *Arabic* Term, chiefly understood of the purest Spirit of Wine, raised or rectified by repeated Distillations to its utmost Subtility, and Perfection; so that if Fire be set thereto, it burns wholly away, without leaving the least Phlegm or Fæces behind. The Word is formed from the *Arabic* or *Hebrew* קאל, Kaal, to lessen, attenuate, subtilize.

**ALE**, *Cerevisia*, is also a Denomination given to divers medicated Liquors, or Diet-Drinks, whereof *Ale* is the Basis, or Vehicle. The medicated Wines, Waters, and *Ales*, make a large Article in our Dispensatories. Such are the *Cerevisia Oxydorica*, for the Eyes; *Cerevisia Anti-Arthritica*, against the Gout; *Cerevisia Cephalica*, for the Head; *Cerevisia Epileptica*, &c.

*Gill Ale* is prepared by infusing the dry Leaves of *Hedera Terrestris*, *i.e.* Ground-Ivy, in Malt-Liquor; which hereby becomes impregnated with the Virtues of the Simple; and is therefore reputed Abstersive, and Vulnerary; good in Disorders of the Breast, and against Obstructions of the Viscera.

*Dr. Butler's*[1] *Purging Ale*, is prepared of Polypody, Sena, Sarsaparilla, Aniseeds, Scurvygrass, Agrimony, and Maindenhair, put up in a Bag, and hung in a Vessel of *Ale*.

We also meet in some Dispensatories with *Syrop of Ale*, made by boiling that Liquor to a Consistence; used against Obstructions in the Kidneys, &c.

**ALE**-*Berry*, is *Ale* boiled with Bread and Mace; sweetened, strained, and drank hot.

**ALECTORIA**, in Natural History, a Stone sometimes found in the Stomach, Liver, or rather Gall-Bladder of old Cocks. It is ordinarily of the Figure of a Lupine, and seldom exceeds the Bigness of a Bean. It has abundance of Virtues attributed to it, but most of them are fabulous. The Word Is derived from αλιχτορ, a *Cock*.

**ALEMBICK**, or *Limbeck*, a Chymical Vessel, consisting of a Matrass, fitted with a roundish Head, perforated in a sloping Tube, for the condensed Vapours to pass thro in Distillation. *Alembick* is popularly understood of the whole Instrument of Distillation with all its Apparatus; but in the proper sense of the Word, it is only Part hereof, *viz.* a Vessel usually of Copper, whereto a concave, globular, metalline Head is closed luted; so as to stop the rising Vapours, and direct them into its Rostrum or Beak.

[1] William Butler (1535 – 1618), an English physician.

The Heat of the Fire raising the volatile Parts of the Subject, exposed in the bottom of the Vessel; they are received into its Head, where they are condensed, either by the Coldness of the ambient Air, or by Water externally applied; and become a Liquor, which runs out at the Beak into another Vessel, called the *Recipient*. The Head or Capital of the *Alembick*, is sometimes incompassed with a Vessel full of cold Water, by way of Refrigeratory; tho this Intention is now more commonly answered by a *Serpentine*.

There are divers Kinds of *Alembicks* : An *Open Alembick*, where the Capital and Cucurbit are two separate Parts; a *Blind Alembick*, or Blind Head, where the Capital is sealed Hermetically upon the Cucurbit, &c. The Word is formed of the *Arabick* Particle *Al*, and the Greek αμβιξ, a sort of earthen Vessel, mentioned by *Atheneus*, and *Hesychius*[1]. Tho, *Matthew Silvaticus*[2], in his *Pandect Medicine*, asserts the Word *Alembick* to be *Arabick*, and that it literally denotes the upper part of a distilling Vessel.

**ALEXIPHARMIC**, in Medicine, expresses that Property which a Remedy, either simple or compound, hath to resist or destroy every thing of a poisonous Nature : For the Antients had a Notion, that there was Poison in all malignant Diseases, and in the generality of those whose Cause is unknown.

*Alexiterial, Cardiac, Antidote, Alexipharmic*, and *Counterposion*, are all Terms of the same Signification. *Alexipharmics* are ordinarily divided into such as are general; and those more particular, supposed only to combat some particular Disease. But this Division is founded more on Speculation than Experience.

*Alexipharmic* Medicines, contain a great Number of volatile Parts, and such as render fluid the Mass of Blood. The greatest part of them are aromatick, and pungent to the Taste. Among the rest, it is true, there are some acid Plants and Juices; but these are only reckoned in the Number, on account of their Use in malignant, colliquative Fevers. *Alexipharmics* chiefly act by exciting or increasing a Diaphoresis, or Perspiration; by which the noxious Matter is thrown off.

*Alexipharmics*, whether simple or compound, are also esteemed Preservatives against malignant, and pestilential Fevers : But they are to be used with Caution; some being only proper in Condensations, and others in Colliquations of the Blood. The Word is derived from the Greek αλεξω, *arceo*, to drive out, or expel; and οαρμαχον, *Venenum*, Poison.

**ALEXITERIAL,** in Medicine, a Term of the same import with Alexipharmic.

**ALGAROT**, or Algarel, in the *Arabian* Chymystry; a Pouder prepared of Butter of Antimony; being in reality no more than the Regulus of that Mineral, dissolved in Acids, and separated again by means of several Lotions with lukewarm Water, which imbibes those Acids. This is also called *Mercurius Vitæ*, or simply Emetic Pouder. It purges violently both upwards

[1] Hesychius of Alexandria (ca. 5th cent.) who compiled a Greek lexicon.

[2] Matteo Silvatico (1285 - 1342), an Italian physician in Salerno.

and downwards. By collecting all the Lotions, and evaporating two third Parts, what remains is a very acid Liquor, called *Spirit of Philosophical Vitriol.*

**ALHANDAL**, a Term in the *Arabian* Pharmacy. The Troches of *Alhandel, Trochisci Alhandelæ*, are a kind of Troches, composed of Colocynthis[1], Bdellium[2], and Gum Tragacanth[3]. They are esteemed good Purgatives, and are used on divers Operations. The Word is formed of the *Arabic Handel*, or *Handhal*, a Name for Colocynthis.

**ALIMENTARY**, Alimental, something that relates to *Aliment*, or Food. The antient Physicians hold that every Humour consists of two Parts; an *Alimentary*, and an Excrementitious one.

**ALKAHEST**, or *Alcahest*, in Chymistry, an universal Menstruum or Dissolvent, wherewith some Chymists have pretended adequately to resolve all Bodies into their first Matter.

Those two eminent Adepts, *Paracelsus*[4] and *Helmont*[5], expressly declare, that there is a certain Fluid in Nature, capable of reducing all sublunary Bodies, as well homogeneous as mixed, into their *Ens primum*, or Original Matter whereof they are composed; or into an uniform equable and potable Liquor, that will unite with Water and the Juices of or Bodies, yet retain its seminal Virtues; and if mixed with it self again, thereby be converted into pure elementary Water. Whence they also imagined, it would at length reduce all Things to Water.

This Declaration, seconded by the Asseveration of *Helmont*, who religiously swears himself possessed of the Secret, has excited the succeeding Chymists and Alchymists to the Pursuit of so noble a Menstruum. Mr. *Boyle* was so fond of it, that he frankly acknowledges he had rather have been Master thereof than of the Philosopher's Stone.

Indeed, 'tis not difficult to conceive, that all Bodies might originally arise from some first Matter, which was once in a fluid Form. Thus, the primitive Matter of Gold is, perhaps, nothing more than a ponderous Fluid, which from its own Nature or a strong Attraction between its Parts, afterwards acquires a solid Form. And hence, there does not appear any Absurdity in the Notion of an universal Ens, that resolves all Bodies into their *Ens genitale.*

The *Alkahest* is a Subject that has been canvassed by an infinite Number of Authors; as, *Pantaleon, Philalethes, Tachenius, Ludovicus*, &c. *Boerhaave* says, a Library might be collected out of them. *Weidenfelt*[6], in his Treatise *de Secretis Adeptorum*, has given us all the Opinions that have been entertained about it.

[1] Bitter Apple or Wild Gourd (*Citrullus colocynthis*) is a purgative.

[2] A gum or resin, similar to myrrh, from trees of the genus *Commiphora*.

[3] The dried sap of several plants of the genus *Astragalus*.

[4] Phillip von Hohenheim(1493 – 1541), a Swiss physician and alchemist.

[5] Jan Baptist van Helmont (1580 – 1644), a Flemish physician and chemist.

[6] Johann Seger von Weidenfeld (Johannes Segerus Weidenfeld), alchemical writer in the mid-sixteenth century.

The Term *Alkahest* is not peculiarly found in any Language : *Helmont* declares he first observed it in *Paracelsus,* as a Word that was unknown before the Time of that Author, who in his second Book, *De viribus Membrorum,* treating of the Liver, has these Words : *Est etiant* Alkahest *liquor, magnam hepatis conservandi & confortandi,* &c. "There is also the Liquor *Alkahest,* of great efficacy in preserving the Liver; as also in curing hydropical and all other Diseases arising from Disorders of that Part. If it have once conquered its like, it becomes superior to all other hepatick Medicines; and tho the Liver it self were broken and dissolved, this Medicine should supply its Place." 'Tis this single Passage of *Paracelsus,* that excited the succeeding Chymists to an Inquiry after the *Alkahest*; there being but one other indirect Expression about it in all his Works.

Now it is being a frequent Practice with this Author to transpose the Letters of his Words, and to make use of Abbreviations, and other ways of Concealment; as in Tartar, which he would write *Sutratar*; for *Nitrum, Mutrin,* &c. 'tis supposed *Alkahest* may be a Word thus disguised. Hence some imagine it formed of *Alkali est*; and accordingly, that it was the Alkaline Salt of Tartar volatized. This seems to have been *Glauber's*[2] Opinion; who indeed performed surprizing things with such a Menstruum upon Subjects of all the three Kingdoms.

Others will have it the *German* Word *Algeist, q.d.* wholly spirituous, or volatile : Others are of Opinion, that *Alkahest* is taken from *Salls-geist,* which signifies Spirit of Salt; for the Universal Menstruum, 'tis said, is to be wrought from Water; and *Paracelsus* himself calls Salt the Centre of Water, wherein Metals ought to die, &c. In effect, Spirit of Salt was the great Menstruum he used on most Occasions. The Commentator on *Paracelsus,* who gave a Latin Edition of his Works at *Delft,* assures that the *Alkahest* was Mercury, converted into a Spirit. *Zwelfer*[3] judg'd it to be a Spirit of Vinegar rectified from Verdi-grease. And *Starkey*[4] thought he discovered it in his Soap.

There have been some synonymous and more significant Words used for the *Alkahest.* The elder *Helmont* mentions the *Alkahest* by the compound Name of *Ignis-aqua,* Fire-Water : But he here seems to mean the circulated Liquor of *Paracelsus*; which he terms Fire, from its Property of consuming all things; and Water, on account of its liquid form.

The same Author called it *Ignis-gehennæ,* infernal Fire; a Word also used by *Paracelsus* : He also intitles it "*Summum & felicissimum omnium salium,* the principal and most successful among Salts, which having obtained the highest degree of Simplicity, Purity, and Subtility, alone enjoys the Faculty of remaining unchanged and unimpaired by the Subjects it works on, and of dissolving the most stubborn and untractable Bodies, as Stones, Gems, Glass, Earth, Sulphur, Metals, &c. into real Salt, equal in weight to the Matter dissolved; and this with as much ease as hot Water melts down Snow. This Salt," continues he, "by being several times cohobated with *Paracelsus's Sal*

[2] Johann Rudolph Glauber (1604 – 1668), a German chemist and alchemist.

[3] Johann Zwelfer (1618 – 1668), a German chemist and doctor.

[4] George Starkey (1628 – 16665), also known as Eirenaeus Philalethes, an American doctor and alchemist.

*circulatum*, loses all its Fixedness; and at length becomes an insipid Water, equal in quantity to the Sal it was made from."

*Helmont* is express that this Menstruum is intirely the Product of Art, and not of Nature. "Tho," says he, "a homogeneal Part of elementary Earth may be artificially converted into Water, yet I deny that the same can be done by Nature alone; for no natural Agent is able to transmute one Element into another." And this he offers as a Reason why the Elements always remain the same. It may let some light into this Affair, to observe that *Helmont*, as well as *Paracelsus*, took Water for the universal Instrument of Chymistry, and Natural Philosophy; and Earth for the unchangeable Basis of all Things : That Fire was designed as the efficient Cause of all Things; that seminal Impressions were lodged in the Mechanism of the Earth; and that Water, by dissolving and fermenting with this Earth, as it does by means of Fire, brings every thing to light; whence originally proceeded the Animal, Vegetable, and Mineral Kingdoms; even Man himself being thus at first created agreeably to the account of *Moses*.

The great Character or Property of the *Alkahest*, we have observed, is to dissolve, and change all sublunary Bodies; Water alone excepted. The Changes it induces proceed thus :

1, The Subject exposed to its Operation, is converted into its three Principles, Salt, Sulphur and Mercury; afterwards, into Salt alone; which then becomes volatile; and at length is wholly turned into insipid Water. The manner of Application is by touching the Body proposed to be dissolved, *e.g.* Gold, Mercury, Sand, or the like, once or twice with the pretended *Alkahest*; and if the Liquor be genuine, the Body will be converted into its own Quantity of Salt.

2, It does not destroy the seminal Virtues of the Bodies dissolved thereby. Thus, Gold is, by its Action, reduced to a Salt of Gold; Antimony to a Salt of Antimony; Saffron to a Salt of Saffron, &c. of the same seminal Virtues, *Helmont* understands those Virtues which depend upon the Construction or Mechanism of a Body, and which make it what it is. Hence, as actual and genuine *Aurum potabile* might readily be gained by the *Alkahest*, as converting the whole Body of Gold into a Salt, retaining its seminal Virtues, and being withal soluble in Water.

3, Whatever it dissolves, may be rendered volatile by a Sand-heat; and if after volatizing the Solvend, it be distilled therefrom, the Body is left pure insipid Water, equal in quantity to its original self, but deprived of its seminal Virtues. Thus, if Gold be dissolved by the *Alkahest*, the Metal first becomes Salt, which is potable Gold; but when the Menstruum is distilled there from, 'tis left mere Elementary Water. Whence it appears, that pure Water is the last Production or Effect of the *Alkahest*.

4, It suffers no Change or Diminution of Force by dissolving the Bodies it works on, and therefore sustains no Reaction from them; being only immutable Menstruum in Nature.

5, 'Tis incapable of Mixture, and therefore remains free from Fermentation and Putrefaction; coming off as pure from the Body it has dissolved, as when first put thereon; without leaving the least Foulness behind.

**ALKALY**, *Alkali*, Alcaly, in Chymistry, a Name originally given, by the *Arabians*, to a Salt extracted from the Ashes of a Plant called *Kali*; and by us Glass-wort, because used in the making of Glass. Afterwards, the Term *Alkaly* became a common Name for the lixivious Salts of all Plants; that is, for such Salts as are drawn by Lotion from their Ashes. And hence, again, in regard the original *Alkaly* was found to ferment with *Acids*; the Name has since become common to all volatile Salts, and all terrestrial Substances which have that effect.

*Alkaly*, then, in its modern extensive Sense, is any Substance, which being mixed with an *Acid*, an Ebullition and Effervescence ensues thereon. And hence arises the grand Division of Natural Bodies into the two opposite Classes of *Acids* and *Alkalies*.

*Boerhaave*[1] scarce takes this Circumstance to be enough to constitute any determinate Class of Bodies. In effect, *Alkalies* are not of one familiar homogeneous Nature : but there are two several sorts. The first obtained from Vegetable and Animal Substances, by Calcination, Distillation, Putrifaction, &c. The second are of the terrestrial Kind; as Shells, Bole, &c.

The two species, *Boerhaave* observes, differ widely from each other; having scarce any thing in common, but their being effervescible with Acids. The one is a Class of native, fixed, scentless, insipid, mild, astringent, fossil Bodies : The other a Set of such as are volatile, odorous, sapid, caustic, aperitive, and procured by Art.

Hence, adds the same Author, mere Effervescence with Acids, must be allowed to be of it self insufficient to determine the Nature of an *Alkaly* : and that such a Name, which properly denotes a caustic fiery Substance, should not be affixed to any mild and gently Body, as Chalk, &c. but other Properties and Considerations are to be taken in, and particularly their Taste, manner of procuring, and the Change of Colour they produce in Bodies.

With regard to this last Circumstance, those Liquors which being poured on Syrup of Violets, change it of a green Colour, are *Alkalies*; as those which turn it red, Acids. This Oil of Tartar turns it of a kindly green; and Oil of Vitriol of a Carmine red : And if to the Syrup thus made red by Oil of Vitriol, Oil of Tartar be poured, it turns that part wherewith it comes in contact, green; leaving the rest red : and the like holds of Oil of Vitriol, poured on Syrup made green by Oil of Tartar.

To the like effect M. *Homburg* observes that "a mere heat and bubbling arising upon the Admixture of a Body with an Acid, does not seem an adequate Criterion of the *Alkaline* Nature; since distilled Oils of all kinds are found to do thus much; and many of them with more vehemence than *Alkalies* themselves, so as sometimes even to take fire, which *Alkalies* never do."

All lixivious Salts have these Characters of *Alkaly*. And not only lixivious, but also all urinous Salts; which are constantly found to imbibe Acids with great eagerness, and after Ebullition, to unite and crystallize with them. Hence we have two Kinds of Alkaly Salt, *viz*. Fixed or Lixivious Alkalies; and Volatile, or Urinous ones. But beside *Alkaly* Salts, there are an Infinity of

[1] Herman Boerhaave (16668 – 1738), a Dutch physician and botanist.

other bodies, not saline; which answer to the Characters of *Alkaly*, *i.e.* produce much the same Effects with Acids, as the *Alkaly* Salts above mentioned. And these alkaline Matters are in other respects of different Natures.

Some, *e.g.* are merely *Earthy*; as Quick-lime, Marble, Sealed Earths, &c. Others are *Metalline*; among which, some have their peculiar and appropriate Acids to act on them, as Gold, Tin, and Antimony, which only dissolve with Aqua Regia; Silver, Lead, and Mercury, with Aqua fortis; and the others with other sorts of Acids, as Iron, Copper, Zink, Bismuth; &c. There are others of the Animal Class; consisting, 1, Of stony matters found in the Viscera of certain Species; as the Calculus humanus, Bezoards, Crabs Eyes, &c. 2, Testaceous Matters and Shells; as Pearls, Oyster-shells, Cuttle-fish, Bones, the Shells or Coats of Lobsters, Crabs, &c. 3, The Parts of Animals which by length of time, or some other Cause, are become stony, or even earthy; as the fossil Unicorn's Horn, &c. Lastly, almost all Stone Marine Plants, as Coral, &c.

After all, the *Alkaline* Property does not appear to be native, but rather producible by Art. This Opinion seems to have been first started by *Helmont*: before him, it was the standing Opinion, that Fixed *Alkalies* pre-existed in mixed Bodies; and were only separated or extricated from the Parts of the Compound. *Helmont* advanced, that they did not this pre-exist in their alkaline Form, but were Productions of the Fire, by whose violent Action, part of the Salt which in the Concrete is all volatile, lays hold of some part of the Sulphur of the same Body; and both melting together, are fixed into an *Alkaly* : which Fixation he exemplifies, by what happens when Salt-petre and Arsenick, tho both volatile, being exposed to Fire, are fluxed by the Operation thereof, and made to fix each other.

Some late Chymists, and particularly M. *Geoffroy*[1], carry the Point something further, and assert, that all *Alkaly* Salts whatever, both Fixed and Volatile, are wholly the Effect of Fire; in that before any Action of the Fire, they did not pre-exist in the Mixt wherein they afterwards appeared.

Notwithstanding all the seeming Opposition and Hostility between Acids and *Alkalies*, they may be converted into one another; at least, Acids are convertible into *Alkalies*; as is shewn at large by M. *Geoffroy* in a Discourse express, in the *Mem. de l'Acad. An.* 1717, where the Nature and Origin of *Alkalies* is excellently explained.

*Alkaly* Salts, according to this Author, are only Acids concentrated in little Molecules of Earth, and united with certain Particles of Oil, by means of Fire. When an Acid, which we conceive in the general as a small, solid, pointed Spiculum, happens to be absorbed or concentrated in a proper Portion of Earth; the whole becomes denominated a *Saline , Compound, Neutral,* or *Intermediate Salt*; by reason the Acid, thus inclosed in a Sheath, cannot excite the same Savour as when disengaged therefore; and yet excites a saline Taste : and for this reason is compound, &c.

Now, Fire is the only Agent capable of disengaging the Acid, from the Earth

[1] Etienne Francois Geoffroy (1672 – 1731), French apothecary and chemist, or possibly his brother Claude Joseph.

it is thus invested withal. Upon this, the Acid being lighter than the Earth, rises, and evaporates; leaving the Earth at the bottom of the Vessel; which for this Reason is called *Fixed*, in contradistinction to the Acid, which is *Volatile*. This Earth, thus bereaved of its Acid, is left with its Pores open and empty, which before were filled; and withal, in sustaining the Action of Fire, it necessarily retains some of the Particles thereof, which give it an acrimonious Taste, that mere Earth could never have. Form this Taste it is called Salt; and from its Pores being open, and thus disposed to admit and imbibe new Acids, it is called *Alkaly Salt*.

Now, it is not to be imagined, that an Earth which has once been impregnated with Acids, can ever be perfectly divested thereof; there will still remain some, tho much less than before. So that an *Alkaly* may be conceived as only a too small Quantity of Acid, inclosed in too large a Quantity of Earth.

The visible and sensible Fire is not the only Agent capable of separating Acids from their Earth; Fermentation has the same Effect, in virtue of that pure active Fire produced or concerned therein. *Alkalies*, therefore, are the Production, either of one, or the other Fire, and the same may be said of the Acids disen-gaged therefrom; it being Dis-union of the Parts of the same Salt occasioned by Fire, that yielded both the Acids as well as the *Alkalies*.

On this principle every Acid is volatile, and every *Alkaly* should be fixed, if the *Alkaly* were only Earth : But, in regard the little *Acid* remaining in the *Alkaly*, may be united with a Portion of Oil, as well as a Portion of Earth; and Oil is known to be volatile; the Compound, that is, the *Alkaly*, must be volatile, in case the Oil prevail therein. In this Case, the *Alkaly* is found to have a strong, penetrating, urinous Taste and Smell; and is what we call a *Volatile Urinous Alkaly Salt*. These things well considered; it will be easy to assign what must ensue upon the Separations, or new Unions of the Parts of a Mixt.

An *Acid*, 'tis evident, may become an *Alkaly*, in that after having been separated from its Matrix, it may be restored in a small Quantity to another Matrix, either wholly earthy or earthy and oleaginous. In the first Case, it will become a *Fixed Alkaly*; in the second, it must be, a *Volatile Alkaly*, if in the supposed Matrix the operation of Oil prevail over that of Earth; and in this Case it will be urinous. Again, what before was a fixed *Alkaly*, may become Volatile and Urinous, by depositing or letting go part of its Earth, and taking Oil in its stead.

These Transmutations are not found equally easy and practicable in the three different Kinds of Mixts, or the three Kingdoms; by reason of the Diversity of Circumstances that must concur thereto. They are much the most rare and difficult in the Mineral Realm; by reason, no doubt, that the Parts of Minerals are more closely tyed together, and have, as it were, less play. The only instance Chymistry hath hitherto produced, of a Mineral Acid's being converted into a Fixed *Alkaly*, is in the Operation of fixing Salt-petre.

The Vegetable Kingdom, it is observed, furnishes a large Quantity of fixed *Alkaly* Salt; and a little volatile *Alkaly* : The Animal Kingdom, on the contrary, affords a deal of volatile *Alkaly* Salt, and but little fixed. The Fossil Kingdom affords a very little native fixed *Alkaly* Salt, as the *Egyptian* Natrum, and the Salts procured by Lotion from saline Earth about *Smyrna* and some other Places of the East; and the Chymists have also found a

Method of converting Nitre into a fixed *Alkaly* : But no body hath hitherto produced a volatile *Alkaly* from the Acids of the Mineral Kingdom. And yet, if Acid Salts of the Vegetable Kind be convertible either into fixed or volatile *Alkalies*, why may not Mineral Acids be susceptible of the same Change? since Vegetable Acids are originally no other than Mineral ones : For, from whence but the Earth should Plants derive their acid Juice?

In effect, M. *Geoffroy* has at length shewn the Operation feasible, by an actual Transformation of the same Acid, Nitre, into a volatile urinous *Alkaly*. By the way, it is to be noted, that the Instance of *Egyptian Natrum* or Nitre, furnishes an Objection against the general Assertion of all *Alkalies* being artificial, or produced by Fire : Mr. *Boyle*, who had some of this Salt sent him by the *English* Ambassador at the Porte; found that Vinegar would work briskly on it, even in the Cold; "Whence," says he, "it appears, that the *Egyptian* Nitre, acknowledged to be a native Salt, and made only by the Evaporation of superfluous Water of the *Nile*, is yet of a lixivious Nature, or at least abounds with Particles that are so, tho produced without any precedent Incineration, and the Matter of it exposed to no Violence of the Fire, to make it afford an *Alkaly*." He adds, "However, he does not know any other Body in Nature, except this, wherein the *Alkaline* Properties are not produced." *Ibid.* – And proceeds to give Instances of *Alkalies* being made from Sea Salt, and other Acids; and shews, "how the same Body, without the Addition of any other Salt, may be varying the manner of the Fire's Application, be made either to afford little else than Acids, or a greater or less Quantity of *Alkaly*." *Id. ibid.*

### *Hypothesis of* Alkaly *and Acid.*

*Tachenius*[1] and *Sylvius de la Boe*[2], followed by the Tribe of vulgar Chymists, strenuously assert Sal *Alkaly* and Acid to be the only universal Principles of all Bodies; and by means hereof, account for the Qualities of Bodies, and the rest of the Phænomena of Nature; particularly those in the Animal Œconomy. In a word, *Alkaly* and Acid are substituted in the stead of Matter, and Motion. Mr. *Boyle* attacks this Hypothesis with great force of Argument. In effect, 'tis at best but precarious to affirm, that Acid and *Alkaline* Parts are found in all Bodies.

When the Chymists see Aqua fortis dissolves Filings of Copper, they conclude, that the acid Spirits of the Menstruum meet in the Metal with an *Alkaly*, upon which they work; but how unsafe a way of arguing this is, appears hence, that Spirit of Urine, which is allowed a volatile *Alkaly*, and accordingly makes a great Conflict with Aqua fortis, readily dissolves filings of Copper, and more genuinely than the acid Liquor. So, when they see the Magistery of Pearl or Coral, prepared by dropping Oil of Tartar into the Solution of those Bodies made with Spirit of Vinegar; they ascribe the Precipitation to the fixed *Alkaly* of the Tartar, which mortifies the Acidity of the Spirit of Vinegar : whereas, the Precipitation would no less ensue, if, instead of the *alkalizate* of Oil of Tartar, that strong Acid, Oil of Sulphur *per*

[1] Otto Tachenius (ca. 1620 – 1690), a German physician and chemist.

[2] Franciscus Sylvius, born Franz de le Boe, (1614 - 1672), a German physician and chemist.

*Campanam*, were used.

It may also be doubted, whether it be just to suppose, that when an Acid is discovered in a Body, the Operation of that Body on another, abounding with an *Alkaly*, must be the Effect of a Conflict between those two Principles. For, an acid Body may do many things, not simply as an Acid, but on account of a Texture or Modification, which endows it with other Qualities as well as Acidity. Thus, when the Chymists see an acid Menstruum, as Aqua fortis, Spirit of Salt, Oil of Vitriol, &c. dissolve Iron, they presently ascribe the Effect to an Acidity in the Liquors; tho well dephlegmed urinous Spirits, which they hold to have a great Antipathy to Acids, will readily dissolve crude Iron even in the Cold.

Further, the Patrons of this Hypothesis, seem arbitrarily to have assigned Offices to each of their two Principles, as the Chymists do to each of their *tria prima*; and the Peripateticks to each of their four Elements. But 'tis not enough to say, that an Acid, for instance, performs these things, and an *Alkaly* those; and that they divide the Operations and Phænomena of natural Bodies between them : Assertions of such moment ought not to be received, without further Proof. Indeed, the very Distribution of Salts into Acids and *Alkalies*, has somewhat arbitrary in it; there being not only several things wherein each differs from its self. To say nothing of the Diversity of fixed and volatile *Alkalies* abovementioned; some, as Salt of Tartar, will precipitate the Solution of Sublimate into an Orange-tawny; others, as Spirit of Blood and Hartshorn, precipitate such a Solution into a milky Substance; and Oil of Tartar very slowly operates upon Filings of Copper, which Spirits of Urine and Hartshorn will readily dissolve in the Fire.

And among Acids themselves the difference is not less; for some of them will dissolve Bodies that others will not : and this even where the Menstruum that will not dissolve the Body, is reputed much stronger than that which does; as dephlegmated Spirit of Vinegar will dissolve Lead reduced to minute Parts in the cold, which is an Effect that Chymists expect not from Spirit of Salt. Nay, one Acid will precipitate what another has dissolved, and *e contra*; as, Spirit of Salt will precipitate Silver out of Spirit of Nitre. Add, the Properties peculiar to some particular Acids, as that Spirit of Nitre or Aqua fortis, dissolves Camphire into an Oil, and coagulates common Oil into a constituent Substance like Tallow; and tho it will both corrode Silver, Copper, Lead, and Mercury, and keep them dissolved, it quickly lets fall almost the whole Body of Tin.

'Tis no wonder that the Definitions given of Acid and *Alkaly* should be inaccurate and superficial; since the Chymists themselves do not seem to have any determinate Notion of sure Marks, whereby to know them distinctly. For, to infer, that, because a Body dissolves another, which is dissoluble by this or that known Acid, the Solvent must also be Acid; or to conclude, that, if a Body precipitates a dissolved Metal out of a confessedly acid Menstruum, the Precipitate must be an *Alkaly*, is precarious : since Filings of Spelter will be dissolved by some *Alkalies*, *viz.* Spirit of Sal Ammoniac, &c. as well as by Acids; and Bodies may be precipitated out of acid Menstrua, by other Acids, and by Liquors wherein there appears not the least *Alkaly*. Add, that a Solution of Tin-glass, made in Aqua fortis, would be precipitated both by Spirit of Salt, and by common Water. Nor does that other Criterion of Acids and *Alkalies, viz.* The Heat, Commotion, and Bubbles excited upon their being put together, appear more determinate; since almost any thing fitted variously and vehemently to agitate the minute Parts of a Body, will produce heat in it. Thus, tho Water be neither an Acid nor an *Alkaly*, it will quickly grow very hot, not only with the highly acid Oil of Vitriol, but with the *alkalizate* Salt of Tartar.

Neither is the Production of Bubbles, tho accompanied with a hissing Noise, a certain Sign; such Production not being a necessary Effect of Heat, excited by Conflict, but depending on the peculiar Disposition of the Bodies put together, to extricate, produce, or intercept Particles of Air. Hence, as Oil of Vitriol, mixed in a due Proportion with fair Water, may be brought to make the Water very hot, without exciting Bubbles : so Mr. *Boyle* has found, that *alkalizate* Spirit of Urine, drawn with some kinds of Quick-lime, being mixed with Oil of Vitriol moderately strong, would afford an intense heat, whilst it produced either no manifest Bubbles at all, or scarce any; tho the urinous Spirit was strong, and in other Trials operated like an *Alkaly* : and tho with the Spirit of Urine made *per se*, in the common way, Oil of Vitriol will produce a great hissing, and a multitude of conspicuous Bubbles. On the other side, some acid Spirits, as of Verdegrease, made pure, poured on Salt of Tartar, will frequently make a Conflict, and produce a large froth; tho not accompanied with any manifest heat.

Many make the Taste the Touchstone whereby to try Acids and *Alkalies* : But there is a multitude of Bodies, wherein we can so little discern by the Taste which of the Principles is predominant, that one would not suspect there was a Grain of either of them therein : Such are Diamonds, most Gems, and many ignobler Stones; Gold, Silver, Mercury, &c. There are also Bodies abounding with acid or *alkalizate* Salts; which either have no Taste, or a quite different one from that of the chymical Principles. Thus, tho Venice-glass be in great part composed of a fixed *Alkaly*, it is insipid on the Palate : And Crystals of Silver and Lead, made with Aqua fortis, and containing numerous acid Particles of the Menstruum, manifest nothing of Acidity in the Mouth; the latter having a saccharine Sweetness, and the former an extreme Bitterness. And even in Vegetable Substances of a manifest Taste, 'tis not easy to know by that, whether it be the Acid or the Alkaline Principle which predominates in 'em : As, in the essential Oils of Spices, and the gross empyreumatical Oils of Wood; and even in Alcohol of Wine, which some contend to be an Acid, and others, an *Alkaly*.

**ALKALIZATE**, or Alkaline Bodies, among Chymists, are such as have their Pores naturally so formed, that they are fit to be pierced, and put into Motion by the Points of an Acid poured upon them.

**ALKEKENGI**, a Medicinal Fruit, produced by a Plant of the same Denomination, and popularly called *Winter-Cherry*. The Plant bears a near resemblance to Solanum or Nightshade; whence it is frequently called in Latin by that Name, with the addition or Epithet of Vesicarium. It is sometimes also called *Halicacabum*. The Fruit is celebrated for its lithontriptic Quality; and prescribed to cleanse the Urinary Passages of Gravel, and other Obstructions. Its detersive Quality also recommends it against the Jaundice, and other Disorders of the Viscera. The *Trochischi*

*Alkekengi*, prepared from it, are but little prescribed in the modern Practice.

**ALKERMES**, in Medicine, &c. a Term borrowed from the Arabs. The *Confection of Alkermes*, is a celebrated Remedy, of the Form and Consistence of a Confection; whereof the Kermes Berries are the Basis. The other ingredients, as prescribed by the College, are Pippin-Cyder, Rose-Water, Sugar, Amber-grease, Musk, Cinnamon, Aloes Wood, Pearls, and Leaf Gold. But tho Sweets are usually omitted. It is much used as a Cordial; especially, says Dr. *Quincy*, among Female Prescribers, and in compliance to them : But that Author decries its Value in that Intention, and thinks it ought only to be regarded as a Sweetner.

**ALLUM**, or Alum, *Alumen*, a kind of Mineral Salt, of an acid Taste, leaving in the Mouth a Sense of Sweetness accompanied with a considerable Degree of Astringency. The antient Naturalists allow of two sorts of *Allum*; the one *Native*, the other *Factitious*. The Natural is founding the Island of *Milo*, being a kind of whitish Stone, very light, friable and porous; and streaked with Filaments resembling Silver.

The Factitious *Allum*, is prepared in different manners, according to the different materials whereof it is made. *Allum* is of divers Kinds, *Red, Roman, Citron, Plumose, Saccharine*, and *Burnt*. The three last of which, are not properly *Allums*.

*England, Italy*, and *Flanders*, are the Countries where the *Allum* is principally produced. The English *Allum*, called also *Roche-Allum, Allumen Rupeum*, is made from a blueish mineral Stone, frequent in the Hills in *Yorkshire* and *Lancashire*. This Stone they calcine on a Hearth or Kiln; then steep it successively in several Pits of Water : then boil it for about 24 Hours : Lastly, letting it stand for about two Hours; the Impurities subside, and leave a pure Liquor; which, removed into a Cooler, and some Urine added to it, begins, in three of four Days, to gather into a Mass; which being taken out, washed, and melted over again, is fit for use.

The Mineral Stone, before it is calcined, being exposed to the Air, will moulder in pieces, and yield a Liquor whereof Copperas may be made; but being calcined it is fit for *Allum*. As long as it continues in the Earth, or in Water, it remains a hard Stone. Sometimes a Liquor will issue out of the Side of the Mine, which by the Heat of the Sun is turned into a Natural *Allum*.

In the *Allum*-Works at *Civita Vecchia*, the Process, as described by M. *Geoffroy*, is somewhat different. The Stone, which is of a ruddy hue, being calcined, they boil and dissolve the Calx in Water; which imbibing the Salt, *i.e.* the *Allum*, separates it from the useless Earth. Lastly, leaving the Water thus impregnated with Salt to stand for some Days, it crystallizes of it self, like Tartar about a But, and makes what they call *Roche* or *Roman-Allum*.

At *Solsatara*, near *Puzzuoli*, is a considerable oval Plain, the Soil whereof is wholly saline; and so hot, that the Hand cannot long bear it. From the Surface hereof, in Summertime, there arises a sort of Flour, or saltish Dust; which being swept up, and cast into Pits of Water at the bottom of the Plain; the Heat of the Ground, without any other Fire, evaporates the Water, and leaves an *Allum* behind.

*Allum* dissolves in Water, and what remains undissolved at bottom, is a sort of Calx, which dissolves readily enough in Oil, or Spirit of Vitriol. And hence there arises some doubt, whether *Allum*, as it does not leave an Earth behind, does properly belong to the Class of Salts. Mr. *Boyle* assures us, that *Allum* ore robb'd of its Salt, does in tract of Time recover it again in the Air.

The Swedish *Allum* is made of a Mineral which contains a great deal of Sulphur and Vitriol, not to be taken away but by Calcination or Distillation. The Matter remaining in the Iron Vessels used in separating the Sulphur from the Mineral, being exposed to the Air for some time, becomes a kind of blueish Ashes, which they lixiviate, crystallize, and convert into *Allum*.

The Word *Allum* comes from the *Greek* αλς, *Salt*; or perhaps from the Latin *Lumen*, Light; because it adds a Lustre to Colours.

*Allum* is of some use in Medicine, in quality of an Absorbent; but being apt to excite Vomiting, is not much used inwardly, and rarely without some smooth Aromatick, as a Corrector. 'Tis used outwardly in astringent Lotions, and is an Ingredient in several Dentifrices.

It is a principal Ingredient in Dying and Colouring; neither of which can be well performed without it. It serves to bind the Colour upon the Stuffs, and it has the same Uses there, that Gum-water and glutinous Oils have in Painting. It likewise disposes Stuffs to take the Colour, and adds a degree of Briskness and Delicacy to it; as we see visibly in Cochineal, and the Grains of Scarlet.

The Effects of *Allum* seem owing to its styptick, or astringent Quality, by which it binds the finer Parts of Colours together, and prevents their exhaling. Hence also it preserves Paper that has been dipp'd in its Water, from sinking when wrote upon.

*Saccharine* Allum bears a near resemblance to Sugar. It is a Composition of common *Allum* with Rose-water, and Whites of Eggs, boil'd together to the Consistency of a Paste, and thus moulded at pleasure. As it cools, it grows hard as Stone.

*Burnt* Allum, *Alumen Ustum*, is *Allum* calcined over the Fire, and thus render'd whiter, more light, and easily pulveriz'd.

*Plumose* Allum, *Alumen Plumosum*, is a sort of saline, mineral Stone, of various Colours, most commonly white bordering on green; resembling *Venetian* Talc, except that instead of Scales, it rises in Threads or Fibres, resembling those of a Feather; whence its name, from *Pluma*, Feather.

Some will have this to be the *Lapis Amianthus* of the Antients.

**ALMOND**, *Amygdala*, a kind of Fruit, inclosed with a thick Stone, and under a thin Skin. The *Almond* is the Produce of a pretty tall Tree, resembling a Peach Tree; frequent in *Germany*, *France*, and the neighbouring Countries; as also in *Barbary*, &c. Its Flowers are pentapetalous, and ranged in the Rose manner : The Pistil becomes a fleshy Fruit, containing a Seed, which is the Almond; and which drops out when the Fruit is arrived at Maturity. *Almonds* are chiefly of two Kinds, Sweet and Bitter.

The *Sweet Almonds*, *Amygdalæ Dulces*, are of a soft, grateful Taste; and are reputed cooling, heating, emollient, and nutritive : are much prescribed in Emulsions, and found of good effect in all Disorders from cholerick and acrimonious Humours. The *Oil of Sweet Almonds*, drawn without Fire, is a safe and useful Remedy in nephritick Pains. It is also of good repute for Costiveness and Gripes in Children.

*Bitter Almonds, Amygdalæ Amaræ,* are held aperient, detersive, and diuretick; and those Accounts commended in Obstructions of the Liver, Spleen, Uterus, &c. Some esteem 'em good to take off the Effects of Drunkenness. Accordingly, *Plutarch* relates that *Drusus's* Physician, a stout Drinker, took down at every Cup five *Bitter Almonds,* to allay the Heat and Fumes of the Wine.

The express'd *Oil of Bitter Almonds,* is much used to soften and deterge the Wax out of the Ear. Some affirm, that *Bitter Almonds* bruis'd, kill or stupefy Fowl; so that they may be taken with the Hands : which, they say, is a Secret practis'd among the *Bohemians* : And that the Husks remaining after the Oil is express'd, have the same Effect.

The Word *Almond* comes from the French *Amande*; which *Menage*[1] derives from the Latin *Amandala,* a Term occurring in the Capitulars of *Charlemagne* : Others rather derive it from the *Greek* αμυγδαλον, which signifies the same thing.

**ALMONDS** *of the Throat,* called also *Tonsillæ,* and improperly *Almonds of the Ears.* They are two round Glands, placed on the Sides of the Basis of the Tongue, under the common Membrane of the *Fauces*; wherein are contain'd a great Number of lesser ones, which discharge thro' the great Sinus a mucous and slippery Matter into the Fauces, Larynx, and Oesophagus, for the moistening and lubricating of those Parts. When the Oesophagus Muscle acts, it compresses the *Almonds*; and as they are subject to Inflammation, they frequently are the Occasion of what the common People call a *sore Throat.*

**ALMOND**, or *Almond-Furnace,* is a peculiar kind of Furnace, used in Refining; to separate all kinds of Metals from Cinders, parts of Melting-Pots, Tests, Bricks, &c. The *Almond-Furnace,* called also the Sweep, is usually six Foot high, four wide, and two thick; built of Brick, and having a Hole in the middle of the Top, eight Inches over; which grows narrower towards the bottom, where, on the Fore-part it ends in a Point, encompass'd with a Semicircle of Iron, to keep the melted Metal. About the middle of the Back, there is another Hole, to receive the Nose of a pair of Bellows, which require the continual Strength of two Men to work.

The Matter, then, on which the Operation is to be perform'd, being beat small, they kindle Charcoal in the Furnace, to anneal it; and when hot, they throw in two or three Shovelfuls of Coals to one of the forementioned'd Stuff; and so proceed during the whole Work, putting Lay upon Lay of one and the other. After eight or ten Hours the Metal beings to run; and when the Receiver below is pretty full, they lade it out with an Iron Ladle, and cast it in Sows, in Cavities, or Forms made with Ashes.

**ALOES**, *Aloe,* in Medicine and Pharmacy, the inspissated Juice of a ferulaceous Plant of the same Name; much used as a purgative Remedy. The

[1] Gilles Ménage (1613 – 1692), a French scholar and philologist.

*Aloe*-Plant grows in divers Parts of the *East* and *West-Indies*; and is also found in some Countries of *Europe*, as *Spain*, and particularly the Mountains of *Siera Morena*. Its Leaves are green, very thick, hard, and prickly; yielding a kind of Cotton, whereof Laces may be made. Out of the middle of the Leaves arises a Stem, which bears the Flower, and the Fruit, the Seed whereof is very light and hemispherical.

*Dioscorides, Pliny,* and the antient Naturalists, seem only to have been acquainted with one Species of *Aloes*; which is the *Aloe Vulgaris* above described : But the late Travels into *Asia, Africa,* and *America,* have occasion'd the Discovery of forty more sorts, unknown to Antiquity. M. *Bradley*[1] assures us, he has seen above sixty several Kinds in the Physick-Garden at *Amsterdam*. So that *Aloe* is now become the Denomination of a Genus. Among the Number, however, there are not above twelve that yield the purgative Juice above mentioned.

The Juice or Extract of *Aloes*, is usually distinguish'd into three Kinds. The first, which is called *Succotrine* as being brought from *Succotra*, is the purest and most transparent; being friable, inodorous, black in the Lump, but of a beautiful yellow Colour when bruis'd. It is brought in Skins from the *Levant* and *East Indies*. The second is called *Hepatic*, because of its Liver-colour : It is resinous, smells like Myrrh, has a yellow Colour when pounded, and is bright from *China*. Some confused this with the following sort; as, in effect, there are but two sorts commonly known in our Shops.

The third is the most impure, the blackest, and the strongest. It was formerly used by the *Indians* to pitch their Vessels withal : and is of little Use among us, excepting for Horses and Cattle; for which reason it is call'd *Caballine*, *i.e.* Horse-*Aloes*.

Besides these, some mention another kind of Aloes prepared in Barbadoes, and brought over in large Gourds : but most Writers make this the Caballine kind. Some have imagin'd, that these differences of *Aloes* were owing only to the greater, or less Purification of the Juice: But this is a Mistake; it having been found that no Dissolutions, how often soever repeated, will change Hepatic into Succotrine, nor Caballine into Hepatick *Aloes*.

The manner of preparing *Aloes* is very easy, there being nothing to do but to cut the Leaves of the Plant, and to expose the Juice that spontaneously oozes out of them to the Sun, till it becomes of a proper Consistence.

*Aloes* is extremely bitter, and purgative; externally applied, either in Substance or Tincture, it prevents Putrefaction and Gangrene. Its Bitterness makes it so nauseous, that it is rarely used in liquid Forms, but is generally made into Pills, whereof half a Dram is an ordinary Dose. Scarce any of the Officinal Pills are without this in their Composition.

Its cathartic Virtue, is best employ'd in watery, cold, and corpulent Constitutions, as it heats and attenuates; being bad for thin and hectick Constitutions. It is accounted efficacious in promoting the Menses; and is also good to destroy Worms.

[1] Richard Bradley (1688 – 1732), an English botanist and horticultural writer.

M. *Boulduc*[1], by his Analysis of *Aloes*, has found that the Succotrine scarce contains half the Resin or sulphurous Part, but one third more of the saline Part, found in the Hepatic. Hence the Succotrine comes to be preferable for internal Uses, and the Hepatic for external.

*Aloe Rosata*, is a Preparation of the *Aloes* Juice, made by dissolving it in Juice of Damask Roses, and evaporating it to the Consistence of Paste. Then, more Juice is added, and the Evaporation repeated, again and again. This is held a gentler and safer Cathartick than the *Aloes* alone.

*Aloes* is also a kind of fragrant Indian Wood; thus called from its exceeding Bitterness, which resembles that of the *Aloes* Juice. This *Aloes*, called also *Agallochum*, is infinitely valued; and divers strange Fables have been invented as to the Origin of the Tree that yields it: Some feign that it grew in Paradise, and was only convey'd to us by means of the Rivers overflowing their Banks, and sweeping off the Trees in their way.

Others suppose it to grow on inaccessible Mountains; where it is guarded by certain wild Beasts, &c. The *Siamese* Embassadors to the Court of *France*, in 1686, who brought a Present of this Wood from their Emperor, first gave the *Europeans* any consistent Account of it.

The Tree grows in *China, Lao*, and *Cochinchina*[2]; and is much about the Size and Figure of our Olive Trees. The Trunk consists of three sorts of Wood, very different in Colour, and Properties : Immediately under the Bark it is black, compact, and heavy, call'd by the *Portugueze, Pao d'Aquila, q.d.* Eagle-Wood. That next under this, is of a Tan colour, light and veiny, resembling rotten Wood; and called *Calambou.*

The Heart, or innermost part is called *Tambac*; and more valued by the Indians than Gold it self. It affords a very strong, but agreeable smell; and is used as a Perfume; and is withal held a sovereign Remedy against the Palsy, Deliquiums, Weaknesses, &c.

'Tis the *Calambon* alone that is known among us. It is brought in small bits of a very fragrant scent; especially when cast on the Fire, where it melts like Wax. The best is of a blackish purple Colour, and so light as to swim on Water: It is hot and drying; and esteem'd a great Strengthener of the Nerves.

Some pharmaceutical Writers make a Distinction between *Aloes, Lignum Aloes*, and *Xylo Aloes*; which may amount to the three Orders of Wood above mention'd. Tho' among us they are the same thing.

**ALOPECIA**, or Alopechy, in Medicine, &c. a Falling of the Hair, from what Cause soever that arise. The Word is form'd from αλοπυξ, Vulpes, a Fox; whose Urine, it is said, will occasion Baldness; or because such a Disease is common to that Creature.

**ALPHOS**, in Medicine, a Distemper described by Celsus, under the Name of Vitiligo; wherein, the Skin is rough and looks as if it had Drops of white upon it, not much differing from Morphew.

[1] Gilles-Francois Boulduc (1675 – 1742), a French apothecary and scientist.

[2] The southern part of Vietnam including the city of Saigon.

**ALTERANT**, or Alterative, in Medicine, a Property, or Power in certain Remedies, whereby they induce an Alteration in the Body, and dispose it for Health or Recovery, by correcting some Indisposition; without occasioning any sensible Evacuation.

Under *Alterants*, therefore, come all Medicines which are not Evacuants. 'Tis a Point much question'd by some, whether there really be any such thing as an *Alterant* in this Sense; *i.e.* any thing which tends to cure a Disease otherwise than by eliminating or expelling some peccant Matter.

Dr. *Quincy* has made it probable, that Remedies usually reputed *Alterants*, act in the same manner on the remoter and more intimate Parts of the Habit, as Emeticks, Purgatives, &c. do on the Stomach and Intestines.

*Alteratives*, therefore, are better defined, such Medicines as have not immediate sensible Operation, but gradually gain upon the Constitution, by changing the Humours from a State of Distemperature to Health.

**ALUDELS**, in Chymistry, Subliming Pots. *Aludels*, are a Range of earthen Tubes, or Pots without bottoms; fitted, one over another, and diminishing as they advance the Top. The lowest is adapted to a Pot, placed in the Furnace, wherein the Matter to be sublimed is lodg'd. And at the Top is a Head, to retain the Flowers which ascend.

**AMALGAM**, or *Amalgama*, in Chymistry, a Mass of Mercury, united and incorporated with a Metal. The *Amalgam* of Mercury with Lead, is a soft, friable Substance, of a Silver Colour. The Word *Amalgama* is form'd of the *Greek* αηα, *simul*, together, and γαηειν, *jungere*, to join.

By washing and grinding this *Amalgam* with fair warm Water in a glass Mortar, the Impurities of the Metal will mix with the Water : and by changing the Water, and repeating the Lotion again and again, the Metal will be further and further purified. *Boerhaave* mentions it as one of the greatest secrets in Chymistry, to contrive to bring off the Liquor at last as clear and unsully'd as when first pour'd on the *Amalgam*; which might afford a Method of making the nobler Metals, or procuring them from the Baser.

This philosophical way of purifying Metals, may be applied to all the Metals, except Iron and Copper.

**AMALGAMATION**, in Chymistry, the Operation of making an *Amalgama*; *i.e.* of calcining, or rather dissolving some Metal, especially Gold, by means of Mercury. *Amalgamation* is performed by fusing, or at least igniting the Metal; and in this State adding a proportion of Mercury thereto; upon which they mutually attract, and incorporate with each other. All Metals, except Iron and Copper, unite and *amalgamate* with Mercury; but Gold with greatest facility; Silver the next, then Lead, and Tin.

The *Amalgamation* of Gold is usually perform'd by heating the Laminae or Plates of Metal red hot; after which, Quicksilver is to be pour'd upon 'em, and the Mixture stirr'd with a little Iron Rod, till it begins to rise into Smoke. It is then thrown into a Vessel full of Water, where it coagulates and becomes manageable.

This Calcination is in great use among Goldsmiths, and Gilders, who by this means render Gold fluid and ductile for their Purposes. Such Mixture or *Amalgama* being laid on any other Metal, for instance, Copper; and this afterwards placed on the Fire to evaporate; the Gold will be left alone on the Surface of the Copper : which makes what we call *Gilding*. Gold retains about thrice its own weight of Mercury.

The Blackness adhering to the *Amalgama* may be washed away with Water; and a deal of the Mercury press'd out thro' a linen Cloth: The rest being evaporated in a Crucible, the Gold remains behind in an impalpable Pouder.

This Operation is denoted among Chymists by the letters AAA.

**AMAUROSIS**, in Medicine, a Deprivation of Sight; the Eyes remaining fair, and seemingly unaffected. *Amaurosis* is the same with what the *Latins* more usually call Gutta Serena. The Word is *Greek*, αμαυρωσις, *q.d. Darkness*; form'd of αμαροω, *obscuro*.

**AMBER**, *Succinum*, *Carabe* or *Karabe*, *Glessum*, *Electrum*, *Chrysolectrum*, in Natural History, &c. a yellow transparent Substance, of a gummous or bituminous Form and Consistence, but a resinous Taste, and a smell like Oil of Turpentine; chiefly found in the *Baltick Sea*, along the Coasts of *Prussia*, &c.

Naturalists are infinitely divided as to the Origin of *Amber*, and what Class of Bodies it belongs to : some referring it to the Vegetable, others to the Mineral, and some even to the Animal Kingdom. Its Natural History, and its Chymical Analysis, afford something in favour of each Opinion.

*Pliny* describes it as "a resinous Juice, oozing from aged Pines, and Firs; (others say, from Poplars, whereof there are whole Forests on the Coasts of *Sweden*); and discharged thence into the Sea; where undergoing some Alteration, it is thrown in this form upon the Shores of *Prussia*; which lies very low : They add, that it was hence the Antients gave it the Denomination *Succinum*; from *Succus*, Juice." *Nat. Hist.* Lib. XXXVII.

This Opinion of the antient Naturalist, is confirmed by the Observation of many of the modern ones; particularly the learned Father *Camelli*[1] *Philosoph. Transact.* No. 290.

Some have imagin'd it a Concretion of the Tears of Birds; others, the Urine of a Beast; others, the Scum of the Lake *Cephiside*, near the *Atlantick*; others, a Congelation form'd in the *Baltick* Sea, and in some Fountains where it is found swimming like Pitch. Others suppose it a Bitumen, trickling into the Sea from subterraneous Sources; there concreted into this form, and thrown ashore by the Waves.

This last Opinion was a long time the most popular; and seem'd to have the best Ground : but this, too, is now discarded; as good *Amber* having been found in digging at a considerable distance from the Sea, as that gathered on the Coast.

Others suppose *Amber* a compound Substance. *Prussia* say they, and the

[1] Georg Joseph Kamel, Camellus, (1661 – 1706), a Jesuit missionary and botanist.

other Countries which produce *Amber*, are moistened with a bituminous Juice, which mixing with the vitriolick Salts abounding in those Places, the Points of those Salts fix its Fluidity, whence it congeals : and the Result of that Congelation makes what we call *Amber*; which is more or less pure, transparent, and firm, as those Parts of Salt and Bitumen are more or less pure, and mix'd in this, or that Proportion.

The Chymists are as much divided as the Naturalists. *Amber* being found by Distillation to yield an acid Spirit, which precipitates into a Salt; is inferr'd, by some, to be of a mineral Nature; this being a Circumstance peculiar to that Kingdom, and never found in the Distillation of Vegetables : To which may be added, that *Amber* dissolves in Alcohol, not in Water; melts at the Fire, and is inflammable; which are Characters, that seem to refer it to the Class of Sulphurs, or Bitumens. Others, on the contrary, argue it of the Vegetable Kind, from its resolving into the same Principles with Vegetables; *viz.* Water, Spirit, Salt, and Oil. *Boerhaave* resembles it to Camphire, which is a concreted Oil of the aromatic Plants of that Country, elaborated by Heat into a crystalline Form.

There are several Indications which discover where *Amber* is to be found. The Surface of the Earth is there cover'd with a soft scaly Stone; and Vitriol in particular abounds there, which is sometimes found white, sometimes reduced into a Matter like melted Glass, and sometimes figur'd like petrify'd Wood.

*Amber* assumes all Figures in the Ground; that of a Pear, an Almond, a Pea, &c. Among others, there have been found Letters very well formed; and even *Hebrew* and *Arabick* Characters. Within some pieces of *Amber*, have likewise been found Leaves, Insects, &c. included; which seems to indicate either that the *Amber* was originally in a fluid State; or that having been exposed to the Sun, it was soften'd, and render'd susceptible of the Leaves, Insects, &c. which came in its way. The latter of these seems the more agreeable to the Phænomenon, in regard those Insects, &c. are never found in the Centre of the piece of *Amber*, but always near the Surface.

'Tis observed by the Inhabitants of the Places where *Amber* is produc'd, that all Animals, whether terrestrial, aerial, or aquatick, are extremely fond of it; and that they frequently find Pieces of it in the Excrements, and in their Bodies when open'd.

The most remarkable Property of *Amber*, is, that, when rubbed, it draws or attracts other Bodies to it; and this, 'tis observ'd, it does, even in those Bodies which the Antients thought it had an Antipathy to; as oily Bodies, Drops of Water, the Basilisk, Sweat of human Body, &c. Add, that by Friction it is brought to yield Light pretty copiously in the dark; whence 'tis reckon'd among the native *Phosphori*.

*Amber* is reputed of some medicinal Efficacy; being used in Suffumigations, to remove Defluxions; and in Pouder as an Alterant, Absorbent, Sweetner, and Astringent. In times of Plague, those who work in *Amber* at *Koningsberg* are said to be never infected; whence it is held a Preservative. It is esteem'd a Lithonthriptick, Diuretick, and Promoter of the Menses.

Some distinguish *Amber* with regard to its Colours, into *yellow, white, brown*, and *black*. But the two latter are supposed of a different Nature and Denomination; the one call'd *Jet*, the other *Ambergrease*. The *white* is most valued for Medicinal Uses, as being best digested, of the most odoriferous Smell, and containing the greatest Quantity of Volatile Salt. The yellow is most prized by those who work it into Beads, and other Toys, by reason of its transparency.

*Kerkrig*[1] pretends to be Master of the Secret of making Coffins of *Amber*, without destroying its Transparency. 'Tis probable he took the Hint from the *Ethiopians*, who bury their Dead in Glasses. An *Ethiopian*, tho black, makes a fine Figure in a Venice Crystal; much more would he do in a Cover of yellow *Amber*.

The *Amber* gather'd on the *Prussian* Coasts, yields that Prince a handsome Revenue. Authors make mention of other Places where it is found, as on the Banks of the *Po*; the Coasts of *Marseilles*; and divers Parts of *Asia, Africa*, and even *America* : But *Hartman*[2], who has wrote the History of the *Prussian Amber, Succini Prussici Historia*, &c. treats all these Accounts as Fables, and denies *Amber* to be found any where but in the Northern Countries of *Europe, viz.* in *Poland, Silesia*[3], and *Bohemia*[4], rarely; *Jutland*[5], *Holstein, Denmark*, oftener; more frequently still on the Coasts of *Samogitia*[6], *Courland*[7], *Livonia*[8], and *Pomerania*[9]; but most of all, in *Prussia*, in the Country called *Sambia*[10], from *Neve Tiff* to *Urantz Urug*.

The Word is originally *Arabick, Ambar*, or *Anbar*, which signifies the same thing.

*Spirit of Amber*, is an acid Liquor, procur'd from *Amber*, by pulverizing and distilling it by a Sand-heat, with or without the Addition of Tobacco pipes, Bricks, Sand, &c. It is chiefly used externally in Rheumatick Pains and Aches; and internally, in inveterate Gleets, &c.

*Oil of Amber*, is a fine, transparent, ponderous, yellow Oil; procured after the Spirit, by increasing the degree of Fire. This, by Rectification, becomes a good Anti-hysteric, and Emmenagogue; being very subtile and penetrative.

*Volatile Salt of Amber*. The principal Chymical Production of this Substance, is a peculiar white, transparent, acid Salt; which rises after the Oil, and fixes in the Neck of the Retort, &c. It is a good Cephalic, and Detergent : Dr. *Quincy* says, it extremely attenuates, cuts and penetrates the most remote and minute Recesses; and thus scours, as it were, the whole nervous System. Its chief tendency, he adds, is to Secretion; and what it

[1] This might be Theodor Kerkring (1640 – 1693), a Dutch physician and alchemist.

[2] Philipp Jakob Hartmann (1648 – 1707), a German physician.

[3] Silesia was an area in Europe encompassing mainly present day Poland.

[4] Bohemia is now primarily the Czech republic.

[5] Jutland is now Denmark and parts of northern Germany.

[6] Samogitia is now Lithuania.

[7] Courland is now primarily Latvia.

[8] Livonia is now mainly Estonia and parts of Latvia.

[9] Pomerania now consists of parts of Germany and Poland near the south coast of the Baltic Sea.

[10] Sambia was a region in present-day Russia on the south-east of the Baltic Sea.

carries along with it, is by Urine. It also contributes, with Alexipharmicks, to promote a Diaphoresis; and is scare ever omitted in Prescription for chronic Cases, as Epilepsies, Palsies, &c.

The great Consumption of this Medicine, and the small Proportion that *Amber* yields of it, occasion it to be frequently adulterated with Sal Ammoniac, Nitre, Cream of Tartar, Salt of Coral, &c.

*Tincture of Amber*, is procured by Digestion in Spirit of Wine with a Sand-heat. It is prescribed with the same Intentions as the *Salt of Amber*.

*Liquid Amber*, is a kind of native Balsam, or Resin, like Turpentine; clear, reddish or yellowish; of a pleasant Smell, almost like Ambergrease. It flows liquid, from an Incision made in the Bark of a fine large Tree in *New Spain*; but hardens as it grows older into a solid form, and is brought to us in Barrels. It is reputed an excellent Balsam; mollifies, consolidates, and is a good against the Sciatica, Weakness of the Nerves, &c.

**AMBERGREASE**, Ambergris, *Ambra Grisia*, *Ambarum*, a fragrant Drug, that melts almost like Wax; commonly of a grayish or ash-colour, used both as a Perfume and a Cordial. It is found on the Sea-Coasts, in several Countries; as, along the Southern and Eastern Parts of *Africa*, *Madagascar*, the *Maldives*, some Parts of the *Mediterranean*; and in the *West Indies*, about the Islands of *Bermudas*, &c. It is of divers Colours, whitish, brownish, streak'd with yellow, blackish, &c. There is a great variety of Opinions among Naturalists with regard to its Origin and Production : To rehearse 'em all, would make a Volume. The principal may be reduced to these which follow.

1, Some take it for the Excrement of a Bird, which being melted by the Heat of the Sun, and wash'd off the Shore by the Waves; is swallow'd by Whales; who return it back in the Condition we find it. Or, as *Barbosa*[1] relates, from the *Moorish* Inhabitants of the *Maldives*; the Excrements abovemention'd are alter'd and refin'd by lying on the Rocks, exposed to the Sun, Moon, and Air; from whence they are afterwards wash'd off by the rising Sea. They add, that the Whales frequently swallow pieces hereof : that those Pieces we meet withal of a black Colour, took that Hue in the Stomach of those Animals; that the brown are such as have floated long on the Water; and the white, such as have only been a short time there, which they value the most. *Ramusio*, Tom. I. fol. 313.

2, Others speak of it as the Excrement of a Cetaceous Fish; because sometimes found in the Intestines, and sometimes in the Faeces themselves of such Animals. *Justus Klobius*[2], in his History of *Amber*, describes the Animal; which he says is a Whale, and called the *Trunk* : Adding, that the Sperma Ceti is taken out of the Head of the same Creature. Others, with the *Persians*, suppose the Fish that yields the *Ambergrease*, a Sea-Calf; others, with the *Africans*, a peculiar Species of Fish, named *Ambracan*; others a Crocodile, by reason its Flesh is perfumed, &c.

But, to both these Hypotheses it is objected, That we have no Instance of any Excrement capable of melting like Wax. Add, that if it were the

[1] Duarte Barbosa (ca. 1480 – 1521), a Portuguese writer and trader who travelled with Ferdinand Magellan.

[2] Justus Fidus Klobius (d. 1670), a German professor of medicine.

Excrement of a Whale, it should rather be found in such Places where those Animals abound, as about *Greenland*, &c. than about the *Maldivy* Islands, *Soffala*, *Melinda*, *Cape Comorin*, &c. where not Whales are found.

3, Others take it for a kind of Wax, or Gum, which distils from Trees and drops into the Sea, where it congeals and becomes *Amber-grease*.

4, Others, and particularly many of the Orientals, imagine it springs out of the bottom of the Sea, as Naptha does out of some Fountains. They add, that the only Springs hereof are in the Sea of Ormus, between the *Arabian* and *Persian* Gulphs. *Edrissi*[1], who is of this Opinion, in the first Climate of his Geography, mentions pieces of *Ambergrease*, on those Coasts, weighing a full Quintal. *Paludanus*[2] and *Linschoot*[3] speak of it as a sort of Pitch, gradually working up from the bottom of the Sea, and hardening in the Sun.

5, Others take it for a Sea-Mushroom, tore up from the bottom by the Violence of Tempests; it being observ'd, that *Ambergrease* is never found but after Storms.

6, Others assert it a Vegetable Production, issuing out of the Root of a Tree, whose Roots always shoot toward the Sea, and discharge themselves into the same. This Account we have in the *Philosophical Transactions*, from one of the *Dutch* Factors at *Batavia* : And the same is confirmed by Mr. *Boyle. Of Tastes and Odors.*

7, Others suppose it a spongious kind of Earth, which the working of the Sea washes from off the Rocks, where, being lighter than Water, it floats. Others are of the Opinion that it is a bituminous Matter; that it is at first liquid, and runs into the Sea, and that it is there condensed and reduced into a Mass.

8, Lastly, others maintain, that *Ambergrease* is made from the Honey-Combs which fall into the Sea from the Rocks, where the Bees had formed their Nests. This Opinion has something of Experience on its side, and begins now to be generally allow'd; several Persons having seen Pieces that were half *Ambergrease*, and half plain Honey-Comb : and others, again, having found large Pieces of *Ambergrease*, which when broke, Honey-Comb, and Honey too, were found in the middle.

The Pieces frequently seem composed of divers Strata, laid one over another; with Stones and other Bodies inclosed therein; and the Strata are sometimes full of little Shells, which seem a Species of Concha Anatifera : Whence it may be conjectur'd, that the *Ambergrease* has originally been in a fluid State; or at least, that it has been melted; and in that State has form'd it self afresh, and invelop'd such Bodies as happen'd to be in its way.

It is of considerable use among Perfumers, who melt it over a gentle Fire, and make Extracts, Essences, and Tinctures of it. It would be of more use in Physick too, were not its Smell so rank and offensive, and on that account apt to occasion Vapours.

[1] Al Sharif El Edrissi (ca. 12th cent.), an Arab geographer and cartographer.

[2] Barnhard Paludanus (1550 - 1633), a Dutch physician and collector.

[3] Joan Hughes van Linschooten, a Dutch traveller who lived around the beginning of the seventeenth century.

We have various Instances in Authors, of huge Pieces of this Matter : The largest that has been known in Europe, was brought by the *Dutch East-India* Company, toward the Close of the last Century; and kept in their House for some Years. It was almost round; measured two Foot in Diameter, and weigh'd an hundred eighty two Pounds. The great Duke of *Tuscany* offer'd fifty thousand Crowns for it.

**AMBER**-*seed*, or *Musk-seed*, is a Seed somewhat like the Millet, of a bitterish Taste, and brought dry to us from *Martinico* and *Egypt*. The *Egyptians* use it internally, as a Cordial, to fortify the Heart, Stomach, and Head, and to provoke Lust. It gives a grateful Scent to the Breath, after eating; but is not proper for those who are inclined to Vapours.

**AMBLYOPY**, *Amblyopia*, in Medicine, a Disease of the Eyes; otherwise called *Gutta Serena* and *Amaurosis*. The Word comes from αμβλυς, *obtusus*, dull, and οπτομαι, *video*, I see.

**AMIANTHUS** *Lapis*, in Natural History, the same with Asbestos

**AMMI**, or *Semen Ammeos*, a kind or aromatick Seed, of considerable use in Medicine; the Produce of a Plant of the same Name. The Seed is brought from the *Levant* : it is found to contain a great deal of essential Oil, and volatile Salt; and to be attenuating, aperitive, hysterick, carminative, cephalick, and alexi-pharmick being one of the four lesser hot Seeds. It expels Wind, provokes the Menses, &c. According to *Lemery*, the Plant takes its Name *Ammeos* from αμμος, *arena*; its Seed being very like Grains of Sand. It is also called *Ammi Creticum*, or *Ethiopicum*, to distinguish it from the vulgar *Ammi*, or Bishops-weed. It is sometimes also called *Cuminum Ethiopicum*.

**AMMONIAC**. *Gum Ammoniac*; or, as it is sometimes, tho improperly called, Armoniac, is a kind of Gum, brought from the East Indies; supposed to ooze from an umbelliferous Plant. It ought to be in dry Drops, white within, yellowish without, easily fusible, resinous, somewhat bitter, and of a very sharp Taste and Smell, somewhat like Garlick.

*Dioscorides* says, it is the Juice of a kind of Ferula growing in *Barbary*; and that the Plant that produces it, is called *Agasyllis*. *Pliny* calls the Tree whence it grows, *Metopion*; and says, the Gum takes its Name from the Temple of *Jupiter Ammon*, nigh which the Tree grows. Some say, this Gum served the Antients for Incense in their Sacrifices.

The good *Ammoniac* is of a high Colour, and not mixed with any Scrapings of Wood, Stone, or Sand; it is called θραυαμα, *Fracture*. The other, which is full of Stones or Sand, is called φυραμα, that is, *Mixture*.

It enters several medicinal Compositions, as an Attenuant, and Detergent, against Disorders arising from Viscidities, and Grumes. Outwardly applied, it is resolutive and suppurative; and, as some say, will of it self draw out Splinters, &c. Some dissolve the Gum in Vinegar, and others Liquors, and call it *Lac Ammoniacum*; much used in Asthmas, and Obstructions of the Lungs. But the more usual form of prescribing it is in Pills.

**AMMONIAC**. *Sal Ammoniac*, is also a kind of Salt; more usually wrote *Armoniac.*

**AMOMUM**, a Medicinal Fruit, called also *Amomum Racemosum*, *Amomum Verum*, and *Elaterii Pomum*. It resembles the Muscat Grape; and grows, like it, in Clusters; is about the bigness of a Chich-Pea, round, membranous, and divided into three Cells, which contain several brown, angular Grains; of a very strong aromatick Taste, and Smell.

This Fruit is brought from the *East Indies*; and makes part of the Composition of Treacle; and is thought to be the *Sison*, or *Sinon*, of the Antients. Besides this, there is likewise another paler Seed, which bears the Name, *Amomium*; but neither of them are in much repute in Physick.

The Commentators on *Pliny*, and *Dioscorides*, have never been able to agree upon the antient *Amomum*; the generality of 'em pitch on Fruits different from this. Some will have the Rose of *Jericho* pass for it. F. *Camelli* is positive he has discover'd the real *Amomum* of *Dioscorides*, and that it is the *Tugus*, or *Birao*, or *Caropi*, growing in the *Philippine* Islands; the Grains or Berries whereof, are worn by the Natives about their Necks; both on account of their Agreeable Odour, and of their supposed Virtue in preserving from Infection, curing the Sting of the Scolopendria, &c. *Phil. Trans*. No. 248.

*Scaliger*[1] is confident, that the *Amomum* of the Antients was not a Fruit; but the Wood it self, which bore some resemblance to a Bunch of Grapes, and was particularly used in embalming of Bodies : and hence, says he, the Term *Mummy* was given to the Bodies of *Egyptians* embalm'd with it.

**AMULET**, *Amuletum*, a kind of Medicament, hung about the Neck, or other part of the Body; to prevent, or remove Diseases. The Word *Amulet* is form'd of the Latin *Amoletum, Amolimentum*; of *amoliri*, to remove, drive away.

Such as Quills of Quick-silver or Arsenic, which some hang on the Neck, or wear under the Shirt against the Plague, and other contagious Diseases; the Blood stones worn by others against Hemorrhages; and that wore by the Women of the *East Indies* to bring down the Menses.

*Amulets* are frequently no other than a sort of Spells or Charms; consisting of quaint Words and Characters, supposed to have the Virtue of warding off ill. *Pliny* makes frequent mention of 'em.

The *Greeks* called these kind of Remedies φυλαχτηρια, *Phylacteries*; πριπτα, *Periapta*; αποτελεσματα, πιτρημματα, πιαμματα, βρεβια. The *Latins* call 'em *Amuleta, Appensa*, &c. The Council of *Laodicea* forbids Ecclesiasticks to wear such *Amulets* and Phylacteries, on Pain of Degradation. St. *Chrysostom* and St. *Jerom* are likewise zealous against the same Practice. *Hoc apud nos*, says this last Father, *superstitiosae mulierculae, in parvulis Evangeliis & in crucis lingo & istiusmodi rebus quae habent quidem zelum Dei sed non juxta scientiam, usque hodic facticant.*

*Amulets* are now fallen from the great Repute they were Antiently in; yet

[1] Joseph Justus Scaliger (1540 – 1609), a French humanist and scholar.

the great Mr. *Boyle* alledges 'em as an Instance of the Ingress of external Effluvia into the Habit; in order to shew the great Porosity of the Human Body. He add, that he is perswaded some of these external Medicines do answer; for that he himself having once been subject to bleed at the Nose, and reduced to use several Remedies to check it; found that Moss of a dead Man's Skull, tho only applied so as to touch the Skin till the Moss was warm thereby, the most effectual of any. A memorable thing of this kind was communicated to *Zwelfer* by the chief Physician to the States of *Moravia*, who having prepared some Troches of Toads after *Helmont's* manner, not only found that being worn as *Amulets* they preserv'd him and his Domesticks and Friends from the Plague; but being put on the Plague-Sores of others, they were greatly reliev'd, and even saved thereby.

The same Mr. *Boyle* shews how the Effluvia even of cold *Amulets*, may in tract of Time pervade the Pores of a living Animal; by supposing an Agreement between the Pores of the Skin, and the Figure of the Corpuscles. *Bellini*[1] has demonstrated the Possibility of the Thing in his last Propositions, *De Febribus* : And the like is done by Dr. *Wainwright*, Dr. *Keil*[2], &c.

**AMURCA**, in Pharmacy, a Medicine made of the Lees of Sediment of Olives. It is an Astringent.

**ANA**, or āā, in Medicine, denotes an equal Quantity of any Thing, whether in liquid or dry Measure. Hence *Anatica Proportio* is used by some Writers to signify the Ratio, or Proportion of Equality.

**ANABROSIS**, in Medicine, the issuing of Blood at a Hole wore in a Vein by Corrosion. The Word is *Greek*, αναβρωσις, *crosio*.

**ANACATHARTIC**, is understood of a purging Medicine, that works upwards. The Word comes from ανα, *supra*, upwards; and χαθαιρω, *purgo*, I purge.

**ANALEPTICKS**, in Medicine, *Restoratives*; or Remedies proper to restore the Body, when wasted or emaciated, either by the Continuance of a Disease, or the Want of Food. The Word is *Greek*, Αναλογια, derived of Αναλαμβανο, *I re-establish, restore.*

**ANANAS**, in Natural History, by some called *Nanas*, by others *Jayama*, and by us popularly the *Pine-Apple* on account of the resemblance it bears to the Cones of Pines or Firs; is a fine *Indian* Fruit, which grows on a Plant like the Fig-tree, and of the Size of an Artichoke.

The Fruit is adorned on the Top with a little Crown, and a bunch of red Leaves resembling Fire; having the delicious Taste of the Peach, the Quince, and the Muscadine Grape, all together. M. *du Tertre*[3] describes three Kinds of *Ananas*.

[1] Lorenzo Bellini (1643 – 1704), an Italian physician and anatomist.

[2] James Keil (1673 – 1719), a Scottish physician and anatomist.

[3] Jean-Baptiste du Tertre (1610 – 1687), a French missionary and botanist.

They make a Wine from the Juice, which is almost equal to Malmsy Sack, and will intoxicate as soon.

It is good to strengthen the Heart and Nerves, against nauseating, to refresh the Spirits, and excites Urine powerfully; but it is apt to occasion Abortion in Women. They make a Confection of the *Ananas* on the Spot, which they bring hither whole; and is found of good service to restore a decay'd, or aged Constitution.

The *Ananas*, or *West-Indies* Pine-Apple, is generally allow'd, both for its rich and delicious Flavour, and its beautiful Colour, for the King of Fruits. Great Endeavours have of late been used to cultivate the Plant in *Europe*; in which they have succeeded, and there are now produced delicious Fruits of this kind, in some of the fine Gardens in *England*. They are usually about the Size of a Tennis-Ball.

**ANAPLEROTICKS**, in Medicine, such Remedies as incarnate, and fill up Ulcers and Wounds with new Flesh. *Anapleroticks* are the same with what we otherwise call Incarnatives. The Word comes from the *Greek* αναπλρουν, *to fill up*.

**ANASARCA**, in Medicine, a sort of universal Dropsy, wherein the whole Substance of the Body is stuffed, or bloated with pituitous Humours. The *Anasarca* is otherwise called *Leucophlegmatia*. The Word is form'd of the *Greek* ανασαρχα. The *Anasarca* is a further degree of a *Cachexia*. In an *Anasarca*, the Legs swell at the beginning, especially towards Night, and then pit remarkably : The Urine is pale, the Appetite decays; at length the Swelling rises higher, and appears in the Thighs, Belly, Breast, Arms. The Face becomes pale and cadaverous; the Flesh soft and lax; a difficulty in Respiration comes on, attended with a slow Fever, &c.

**ANASTOMATICS**, or Anastomatic Medicines, are such as have the Faculty of opening, and dilating the Orifices of the Vessels; and by that means of making the Blood circulate the more freely. The Word comes from the *Greek* αναστομοω, *I open, unstop*.

**ANATRON**, or Natron, a kind of native Salt-petre, or Nitre, found in *Egypt*. Anatron, is also a volatile Salt, skimm'd from the Composition of Glass, when in fusion. When pounded, it yields a kind of Pouder; which being dissolv'd in Air, or in a proper Liquor, becomes common Salt, after Coagulation. *Anatron* is likewise the Name of a nitrous Juice which condenses in Vaults, Arches, and other subterraneous Places. *Anatron* is also used by some Writers for a compound Salt, made of Quick-lime, Alum, Vitriol, common Salt, and Nitre.

**ANCHYLOPS**, in Medicine, a Species, or rather Degree of Fistula Lacrymalis; frequently confounded with Ægilops, &c.

**ANEURISM**, *Aneurisma*, in Medicine, a soft yielding Tumor, form'd of Blood extravasated and spread under the Flesh, by the Rupture or Dilatation of an Artery. *Aneurisms* usually proceed from an Artery being accidentally cut, or prick'd in bleeding; or from some preternatural Distention, or a Corrosion of its Coats, &c. The Word comes from the *Greek* ανευρευω, *dilato*, I dilate.

If an Artery happens to be cut, the Blood gushes out impetuously, by starts; and is not easily stopp'd : an Inflammation and Discolouration of the Part succeeds, with a Tumor, and Inability to move the Part. The Symptoms are nearly the same in case of a Corrosion of the Coats of the Artery, only less violent.

If the Blood cease to flow from the wounded Artery, and pour it self between the Interstices of the Muscles; recourse is had to manual Operation; which being neglected, the Extirpation of the Limb frequently becomes unavoidable. An *Aneurism* from a Distention of the Canal, is seldom fatal; tho reckon'd, when large, incurable : The chief Inconveniencies are the Magnitude of the Tumor, and the Pulsation.

M. *Littre*[1] give us the History of an *Aneurisma* of this kind, in the Aorta; the Cause whereof he attributes to an extraordinary Diminution of the Cavity of the Axillary and Subclavian Arteries. *Hist. de l'Acad.* R. An. 1712. Another History of an *Aneurisma* of the same Part, we have in the *Philosophical Transactions.* It was occasioned by some violent Shocks the Patient receiv'd on the Breast, which threw him into spitting of Blood, and soon after form'd the Tumor, whereof he dy'd. Upon Dissection, the *Aneurisma* was found so big, that it filled the whole Cavity of the Thorax on the right Side. No. 265.

**ANGELICA**, called also Archangelica, and *Radix Siriaca*, a medicinal Plant, thus named, on account of its great Virtue as an Alexipharmic or Counterpoison. It is of a sweet Smell, and aromatick Taste; and is loaded with highly exalted Oil, and volatile Salt. It is reputed cordial, stomachick, cephalick, aperitive, sudorifick, vulnerary, resists Poison, &c. tho the chief Intention wherein it is now prescribed among us, is as a Carminative. Its Root is in the most esteem; tho the Leaves are also used. Angelica-*Water*, is one of the compound Waters of the Shops; thus called from the *Angelica* Roots, which are the Basis thereof.

**ANGINA**, in Medicine, a Disease, popularly call'd the *Quincy, Squinancy*, or *Esquinancy*. Angina is a Difficulty of Respiration and Deglutition, from a Disease in the Muscles and Glands about the Throat and Larynx. The Word is formed from the *Greek* αγχειν, *strangulare*, to strangle, suffocate.

If any symptoms appear on the outside of the Throat, the *Angina* is said to be *external*; if none appear, *internal.* It is sometimes supposed to be *epidemical.* In the *external Angina*, before any Suppuration appears, recourse is had to repeated Venæsection in the Jugulars. Vesicatories and Cuppings are also used; with Purgatives, emollient Gargles, &c.

**ANHELITUS**, signifies a shortness and thickness of Breath; as in an Asthma. The Word is *Latin*, form'd of the Verb *anbelo*, I puff and blow.

[1] Alexis Littre (1658 – 1726), a French anatomist and Surgeon.

**ANIMA**, a Soul; whether Rational, Sensitive, or Vegetative. The Word is pure *Latin*, form'd of the Greek ανεμος, *Ventus*, Wind, Breath.

**ANIMA MUNDI**, q.d. *Soul of the World*, or *of the Universe*, is a certain pure, ethereal Substance or Spirit, diffused, according to many of the antient Philosophers, thro the Mass of the World, informing, actuating, and uniting the divers parts thereof into one great, perfect, organical, vital Body of Animal.

*Plato* treats at large of the ψυχη του χοστμου, in his *Timæus*; and is even supposed to be the Author of the Dogma : Yet are Interpreters much at a loss about his Meaning. *Aristotle*, however, taking it in the common and obvious sense, strenuously opposes it.

*Serranus*[1], on *Plato's Timæus*, explains this Doctrine thus : "Our Philosopher will have the Universe ζωον εμψυχον εννουν, consisting of Body and Spirit; the Spirit he makes to be that Analogy, or Symmetry, whereby things of different Nature, are amicably associated in the grand Compages of all things. In which sense the *Anima Mundi* signifies as much as the Form of the Universe."

Others will have the *Anima Mundi* to signify I know not what ignific Vertue, or vivific Heat, infused into the Chaos, and disseminated thro its whole Frame; for the Conservation, Nutrition, and Vivification thereof.

Others suppose *Plato*, by his *Anima Mundi*, to have meant God, or the Spirit of God; and to have taken the Hint from Moses, who in his Account of the first Day's Creation, says, *The Spirit of God moved on the Face of the Deep*.

The modern *Platonists* explain their Master's *Anima Mundi* by a certain universal, ethereal Spirit, which in the Heavens exists perfectly pure, as retaining its proper Nature; but on Earth, pervading elementary Bodies, and intimately mixing with all the minute Atoms thereof, assumes somewhat of their Nature; and becomes of a peculiar Kind.

They add, that this *Anima Mundi*, which more immediately resides in the Celestial Regions as its proper Seat, moves and governs the Heavens in such manner, as that the Heavens themselves first received their Existence from the Fœcundity of the Spirit : For that this Anima, being the primary Source of Life, every where breathed a Spirit like itself, by virtue whereof various kinds of things were framed conformable to the Divine Ideas.

The Notion of an *Anima Mundi* is rejected by most of the modern Philosophers; tho M. *du Hamel*[2] thinks, without any great reason; for the generality of them admit something very much like it. The *Peripatetics* have recourse to celestial Influxes, in order to account for the Original of Forms, and the secret Powers of Bodies.

The *Cartesians* have their subtile Matter, which answers to most of the Uses, and Intentions of *Plato's Anima Mundi*; being supposed to flow from the Sun and the other heavenly Bodies, and to be diffused thro all the Parts of the World, to be the Source or Principle of all Motions, &c. Some later

[1] Johannes Serranus, born Jean de Serres (1540 - 1598), a French historiographer.

[2] Jean Baptiste du Hamel (1624 - 1706), a French natural philosopher.

Philosophers substitute Fire; and others a subtile elastic Spirit or Medium diffused thro all the Parts of Space.

The principle thing objected, on the Christian Scheme, against *Plato's* Doctrine of the *Anima Mundi*, is, that it mingles the Deity too much with the Creatures; confounds, in some measure, the Workman with his Work, making this, as it were, a part of that, the several Portions of the Universe so many parts of the Godhead.

**ANIMA** *Hepatis, q.d.* the Soul of the Liver; a Term applied by Chymists, to the *Sal Martis*, Salt of Iron or Steel; on account of its Use in Distempers of that Part. It is sometimes also prescribed under the Name of *Vitriolum Martis*.

**ANIMA** *Pulmonum*, is used for Crocus or Saffron; by reason of its great Use in Diseases of the Lungs.

**ANIMA**, or Gum *Animæ*, in Pharmacy, a kind of Gum or Resin; whereof there are two kinds, *Western* and *Eastern*. The first flows from an Incision of a Tree in *New Spain*, called *Courbati*; it is transparent, and of a Colour like that of Frankincense : its Smell is very agreeable, and it easily consumes in the Fire.

The Eastern Gum *Anima* is distinguished into three Kinds; the first white; the second blackish, in some respects like Myrrh; the third pale, resinous, and dry.

All the several Kinds of *Anima* are used in Perfumes, by reason of their charming Smell; they are also applied externally in cold Disorders of the Head and Nerves, in Palsies and Catarrhs; but are little known among us; insomuch that our Apothecaries usually sell Bdellium for Gum *Animæ*.

**ANKYLOSIS**, a Disease of the Juncture of an human Body; where the nervous Liquor that shou'd lubricate the Bones, and make their Motions more easy, growing too thick, clog up, and as it were, cement the Bones within one another. The Word is derived from the *Greek* αγκυλωσις, which comes from αγκυλη, a Hardness, or Callus in a Juncture.

**ANNIS SEED**, or Aniseed, a medicinal Seed or Grain; produced by an Umbiliferous Plant of the same Name, common in our Gardens. It has a sweetish Taste, intermix'd with something pungent and bitter : It is reputed an Aromatic, and prescribed not barely as a Carminative against Wind; but also as a Pectoral, Stomachic and Digestive.

It also yields by Distillation, a white cordial Oil call'd *Essence of Anis seed*; of a very strong penetrating Smell, and efficacious in its medicinal Operation: It being also used by the Confectioners to scent their Pomatums, &c. In distilling the *Annis-seed* for the Oil; there is procured a limpid Water call'd *Annis-seed* Water; which has much the same Virtues with the Oil.

**ANODYNE**, in Physick, is understood such Remedies, as by their gentle Heat and temperate Moisture, calm and assuage Pain. These are also called *Paregoricks*. There are others, which bear the same Name, but improperly, *viz.* such as occasion a Stupor, Drousiness, and Sleep, properly called *Narcoticks, Hypnoticks*, or *Opiates*.

The true *Anodynes* are applied externally, to the part affected. Such among the Class of Simples are the Onion, Lilly, Root of Mallows, Leaves of Violet, &c. The Word is derived from the privative Particle α and ωδυνω, *doleo*, to be in pain.

We have also certain compound Medicines in the Shops prepared with this Intention; and all called by this Name. Such is the *Anodyne Balsam*, made of *Castille* Soap, Camphir, Saffron, and Spirit of Wine; digested in a Sand-heat. It is recommended not only for procuring Ease in the most racking extremities of pain, but for assisting in discharging the peccant matter that occasion'd it.

**ANOREXY**, *Anorexia*, in Medicine, an Inappetency, or Loss of Appetite. *Anorexia* is properly a longer continuance than is natural, without a desire to eat. If the Thought, or Sight of proper Food, create a Sickness in the Stomach, or a Tendency to vomit; it is called a Nausea. *Anorexia*, is chiefly considered as a Symptom of some other Disorder, from which the curative Indications are to be taken, and afterwards Stomachics used. The Word is compounded of the privative Participle α and ορεχθεω, *Cupio*, I desire.

**ANTHELMINTICKS**, Medicines good to destroy Worms. The Word is compounded of αντι, *contra*, against, and ελμινδ, *Vermis*, Worm.

**ANTHERA**, in Pharmacy, a Term used by some Writers for the Yellow part in the Middle of a Rose. It is reputed more astringent than the rest.

**ANTHERÆ**, among Botanists, those little Tufts, or Knobs which grow on the Tops of the Stamina of Flowers; more usually called *Apices*.

**ANTHORA**, or *Healing Wolfs-bane*, a Species of *Aconite*, whose Root is useful in Physick; being reputed a good Antidote, and a certain Counter-poison to the *Thora*, whence its Denomination *Anthora*. The Root contains a great deal of volatile Salt and essential Oil. It is alexipharmick, cardiack, stomachick, and good against the Wind-Cholick.

**ANTHOS**, Ανθοδ, in its original *Greek*, signifies *Flower*; but by way of Excellency is appropriated to *Rosemary*, so as to express only Flowers of Rosemary.

**ANTHRACOSIS**, a Disease of the Eyes, occasion'd by a corrosive Ulcer, cover'd with Skin, and attended with a general Swelling; especially of the Parts about the Eye. The Word is Greek ανθρακωσις, and *denotes* an Inflammation resembling a Coal; ανθραξ signifying a Coal.

**ANTHRAX**, ανθραξ, strictly signifies a *live Coal*; and figuratively, a Scab or Blotch, made by a corrosive Humour, which, as it were, burns the Skin, and occasions sharp pricking Pains. The Anthrax is also called *Carbo* and *Carbunculus*. The Cure is attempted with Cataplasms of *Thoriac. Lond.*

*Allium, Cepae coct. Sapo Nig.* &c.

**ANTIHECTICKS**, *Antihectica*, Remedies against *Hectical* Disorders.

**ANTIHECTICUM** *Poterii*, in Pharmacy, a celebrated Chymical Preparation, made of equal quantities of Tin, and chalybeated Regulus of Antimony, by melting 'em in a large Crucible, and putting to them, by little and little, three times the quantity of Nitre : the Detonation being over, the whole is wash'd with warm Water till no saltness remains.

It is very penetrating Medicine, making way into the minute Passages, and searching even the nervous Cells; whence its use in *Hectic* Disorders, from which it derives the Name.

It is applied to good purpose in Heaviness of the Head, Giddiness, and Dimness of Sight, whence proceed Apoplexies and Epilepsies; And in all Affections and Foulnesses of the Viscera of the lower Belly is reckoned inferior to nothing. Thus it obtains in the Jaundice, Dropsies and all kinds of Cachexies. Dr. *Quincy* adds, that there is scarce a Preparation in the Chymical Pharmacy of greater efficacy in most obstinate chronick Distempers.

**ANTIMONIALS**, in Medicine, Preparations of Antimony; or Remedies whereof Antimony is the Basis, or principal ingredient. *Antimonials* are chiefly of an emetic tendency : tho' they may be so qualified as to become either Cathartic, or Diaphoretic, or even only Alterative.

Dr. *Quincy* assures, that there are no Medicines in Pharmacy to be compared with these in Maniacal Affections : for that there are of Emetics or Cathartics of any other Tribe that are strong enough for such Patients, unless in an Overdose which might be dangerous.

An *Antimonial Cup*, made either of Glass of *Antimony*, or of *Antimony* prepared with Salt-petre, tho' a Substance indissoluble by the Stomach, will give a strong Cathartic, or Emetic Quality to any Liquor poured into it ; without any diminution of its own weight.

**ANTIMONY**, *Antimonium*, in Natural History, a Mineral Substance, of a Metalline Nature, having all the seeming Characters of a real Metal, excepting Malleability. *Antimony* is what we properly call a Semi-Metal : being a Fossil Glebe, composed of some undetermined Metal, combined with a sulphurous and stony Substance.

It is found in Mines of all Metals; but chiefly those of Silver and Lead: that in Gold Mines is usually held the best. It has also his own Mines; particularly in *Hungary*, *Transylvania*, and *Germany*, and several Provinces of France. *Antimony* is found in Clods or Stones of several sizes, bearing a near resemblance to black Lead; only that it is lighter and harder : whence also it is called Marcasite of Lead; and its metalline part supposed to be of that Species.

Its Texture is somewhat particular, being full of little shining Veins of Threads, like Needles; brittle as Glass - sometimes there are Veins of a red of golden Colour, intermixed, which is called Male Antimony; that without 'em being denominated Female. It fuses in Fire, tho' with some difficulty; and dissolves more easily in Water.

When dug out of the Earth, it is put into Cones, or *Antimonial* Horns; which makes the common or crude *Antimony* of the Shops, the Apex whereof is always the best and purest part, as the Basis or broadest Part is the foulest.

*Antimony* is supposed by many of the Chymists to contain the seminal Principles of all kind of Bodies; and accordingly the Character whereby it is denoted in their Writings, is the same with the Character of the Earth; to denote that *Antimony* is a kind of Microcosm.

The Uses of *Antimony* are very Numerous, and Important. It is a common ingredient in Specula, or burning Concaves, serving to give them a finer Polish. It makes a Part in Bell-Metal; and renders the Sound more clear. It is mingled with Tin to make it more hard, white, and sounding; and with Lead, in the casting of Printer's Letters, to render them more smooth and firm. It is a general Help in the melting of Metals, and especially in casting of Cannon Balls.

*Antimony* is the *Stibium* of the Antients; by the *Greeks* called στιμμ. The reason of its modern Denomination is usually referr'd to *Basil Valentine*[1], a *German* Monk, who having thrown some of it to the Hogs, observ'd that after purging them violently, they immediately grew fat upon it. This made him think that by giving his Fellow-Monks a like Dose, they would be the better for it. The Experiment however succeeded so ill, that they all died of it; and the Medicine thenceforward was called *Antimony, q.d. Anti-Monk.*

Its singular Properties and Effects have occasion'd it various other Denominations, as Proteus, by reason of its various forms and appearances, *Lupus, Devorator, Saturn of the Philosophers, Balneum Solis, Lavacrum Leprorum*, &c. all chiefly respecting its Faculty of destroying, and dissipating whatever Metals are fused along with it, all except Gold; whence its great Use in refining and purifying.

*Antimony* is particularly used in Pharmacy, under various Forms, and with various Intentions. Its medicinal Virtue is supposed to arise from the sulphurous part in its Composition, which being dissolved by any proper Menstruum, sets at liberty an active volatile Salt, or other unknown Principle, to which the Operation is chiefly owing.

Before the XIVth Century, *Antimony* had no place in Medicine; otherwise than as an Ingredient in some Cosmeticks : but about that time, *Basil Valentine* having found a method of preparing, and correcting he dangerous Qualities of its Sulphur, published a Book, entitled *Currus Triumphalis Antimonii*, wherein he maintained it a sure Remedy for all Diseases. But, in spight of all he could say in its behalf, tho' confirmed by Experience, *Antimony* remained in a general Neglect, upwards of 100 years; till about the beginning of the XVIth Century, when it was brought into Vogue by *Paracelsus*. The Parliament of *Paris*, immediately upon this Restoration, condemned the use of it in form; and a Physician named *Besnier*, having been found delinquent herein, was excluded the Faculty. It seems, a deal of Mischief had been done by it, for want of knowing the proper ways of

[1] Basil Valentine (ca. 15th cent.), also known as Basilius Valentinus, a German Benedictine monk and alchemist.

Application; so that the Arret of Parliament represents it as a mere Poison.

Several learned Men complained of so severe and unjust a Prohibition; and by a Course of happy Experiments brought it into Esteem again : whence in spight of all the Invectives made against *Antimony*, by divers Authors, it was at length replaced in the Year 1637, by Public Authority, among the Number of Purgative Drugs; and was inserted accordingly in the Pharmacopœia, published by the Faculty the same year.

*Patin*[1] did all he could to decry *Antimony* : in his Letters we find an unusual Vehemence express'd against it. He had even compiled a large Register of Persons whom the Physicians had kill'd by it; which he called the *Martyrology of Antimony.*

*Crude* Antimony, or *Antimony in Substance,* is the Native Mineral *Antimony,* melted down and cast in Cones, as abovementioned. It is much used in Diet-drinks and Decoctions of the Woods, and Compositions against the Scurvy, as a Diaphoretic, and Deobstruent.

*Prepared* Antimony is that which has undergone some Chymical Process, whereby its Nature and Powers are altered or abated; and this differently, according to the Circumstances of the Preparation.

*Antimony,* says Mr. *Boyle,* alone, or associated with one or two other Ingredients, by a variety of Operations and Compositions, might be brought to furnish a whole Apothecary's Shop : It will answer the Physicians Intention whether he wants to employ a Cathartic, or an Emetic, a Diuretic, Diaphoretic, Deobstruent, Bezoardic, Cordial, &c.

*Glass of* **ANTIMONY**, *Vitrum Antimonii,* is crude *Antimony* ground and calcined by a vehement Fire, in an earthen Crucible; till it cease to fume, which is a Proof that its Sulphur is evaporated. This Calx is then vitrified in a Wind Furnace; upon which it becomes transparent, ruddy, and shining. This is the strongest Emetic of any Preparation of *Antimony.* Yet, if dissolved in Spirit of Urine, it ceases to be either Emetic, or Cathartic; even tho' the Menstruum be drawn from it.

*Flowers of* **ANTIMONY**, is *Antimony* pulverized, and sublimed in an Aludel; the volatile Parts whereof stick to the subliming Pot. This is also a powerful Vomitive; of singular Efficacy in maniac Cases; being the *Herculean* Remedy by which some have gain'd so much Reputation. Another sort of Flowers are made of Regulus of *Antimony* with Sal-Ammoniac sublimed as before; which make a Remedy somewhat gentler than the former. *Helmont* also gives us a Preparation of *purging Flowers of Antimony.*

*Butter of* **ANTIMONY**, is a white, gummous Liquor; otherwise call'd *Icy Oil of Antimony.* It is usually prepared of crude (tho' sometimes of Regulus of) *Antimony,* and corrosive Sublimate, by pulverizing, mixing and distilling 'em by a gentle Heat : upon which the Butter rises into the Neck of the Retort; from which, when full, it is to be melted down into the Receiver by the Application of live Coals. It is of a very fiery, corrosive Nature, so as to be a Poison when used internally. Externally it is applied as a Caustic, to stop

[1] Guy Patin (1601 - 1672), a French phlebotomist and professor in the University of Paris.

Gangrenes, cure Carie's Cancers, &c.

This Butter may be converted into an Oil, called also *rectified Butter of Antimony*; by gently distilling it a second time; which renders it more fluid, subtile, volatile, and efficacious. This digested with thrice its Weight of Alcohol, makes the purple *Tincture of Antimony*, a Secret highly valued by Mr. *Boyle*, as an excellent Vomit. The same Butter precipitates by warm Water, into a white, ponderous Powder, or Calx, call'd *Mercurius Vitae*, and Powder of *Algarot*; reputed a violent Emetic.

Of Butter of *Antimony* is also prepared the Bezoar Mineral; by dissolving the rectified Butter with Spirit of Nitre; then drying the Solution, and applying more Spirit of Nitre; and repeating this a third time. The white Powder remaining at last, kept nearly red hot for half an Hour, is the Bezoardicum Mineral.

*Cinnabar of* **ANTIMONY**, is prepared of Mercury, Sulphur, and *Antimony* mixed and sublimed in a luted Bolt-head, and a naked Fire. It is a good Diaphoretic and Alterative. There is also a Cinnabar of *Antimony* procured after the Butter of *Antimony* has done rising, by increasing the Degree of Fire. This sublimed a second time, makes a yet better Cinnabar.

*Crocus*, or *Liver of* **ANTIMONY**, is the same with what we otherwise call *Crocus Metallorum*; excepting that this latter is more mild and less emetic; being made by repeated Lotions of the former, in warm Water, and then drying it again to a Powder. It is also call'd *Terra Sancta Rulundi, Terra Aurea, Terra Rubra*, &c.

*Diaphoretic* **ANTIMONY**, is prepared of *Antimony* powder'd and mixed with three time the Quantity of Nitre; and the Mixture thrown at several times into an ignited Crucible : upon which, a Detonation ensures. What remains being kept in Fusion a quarter of an Hour, turns into a white Mass call'd *Antimony Diaphoreticum Nitratum*, or *Diaphoretic Antimony* with Nitre; being hereby bereaved of its emetic and purgative Virtue, and rendred only Diaphoretic. If the Air can have Access to it, it will again become emetic.

There is also a kind of sweet *Diaphoretic Antimony*; made of the former, by pulverizing, boiling it in Water, and filtrating the Decoction : Upon which, a white Powder will be left in the Filtre; which being washed by repeated Effusions of warm Water, and dried, is the *dulcified* or *common Diaphoretic Antimony*. This is given as an Alexipharmic in malignant Fevers, Small Pox, &c. particularly in case of Deliriums. It is also applied in scorbutic and venereal Disorders : Though the learned *Boerhaave* absolutely decries it, as a mere metallic Calx, destitute of all medicinal Virtue, and only fit to load and choak up the Body, by its Inactivity and Weight.

*Diaphoretic Nitre of* **ANTIMONY**, is made by exhaling the Solution of the preceding Preparation over a gentle Fire to a dryness; upon which, there remains a Salt composed of Nitre the Sulphur of the *Antimony*, call'd *Nitrum Antimoniatum*. It is no other than a sort of *Sal Prunellæ*, or *Sal Polychrestum*; and accordingly is found aperitive, cooling, diuretic; good in inflammatory Fevers, &c.

*Golden Sulphur of* **ANTIMONY**, is made of the Scoria which arises in preparing the Regulus; by boiling it, filtrating the hot Decoction, and adding distilled Vinegar : Upon which the whole coagulation changes into a brown Powder. The whole Mass being wash'd by repeated Affusions of Water, till the Liquor come away scentless and insipid, and then dried, it becomes a red Powder, called the *Golden Sulphur*, or *Precipitate of Antimony*; either on account of its own Colour, or the yellow one it gives to Glass, Metals, &c. It either proves emetic, cathartic, diuretic, or sudorific, as its Force happens to be determined.

*Crocus*, or *Calx of* **ANTIMONY**, is the Regulus distilled with Spirit of Nitre, in a Sand-Furnace; what remains after the Fumes are all spent, is a white Powder; which being wash'd sweet, is the Crocus required. It is diaphoretic; and by many set on a footing with the Mineral *Bezoard*.

*Magistery of* **ANTIMONY**, is crude *Antimony* digested with *Aqua Regia* eight or ten Days; to which, Water is then put, but pour'd off again e'er it settle : This to be repeated till there remains nothing behind but a yellowish Powder; which, being suffer'd to settle, and the Water decanted off, becomes by repeated Ablutions, an insipid Magistery. Its Operation is rather cathartic than emetic, tho' sometimes sudorific.

**ANTIMONY** *revivified, Antimonium resuscitam*, is prepared of Flowers of *Antimony* and Sal-Ammoniac, digested in distill'd Vinegar; then exhaled, and the remainder sweetened by Ablution. It is emetic, and sometimes also sudorific; good in Maniacal Cases, &c.

All these Preparations of Antimony, how severe soever alone, may yet be so managed, as to operate little or nothing at all in the *Primæ Viæ*, nor be perceived till they are qualified into the smallest Vessels. And then it is they are qualified to combat the Gout, Pox, Evil, &c.

**ANTIPERISTALTIC**, in Anatomy, a Motion of the Intestines contrary to the Peristaltic Motion. The Peristaltic Motion is a Contraction of the Fibres of the Intestines from above, downwards; and the *Antiperistaltic* Motion is their Contraction from below, upwards. The Word is derived from the Greek ανη, against, πιρι, about, ςαλθιχος, that which hath the Power compressing.

**ANTISCORBUTICKS**, Remedies against the Scorbutus or Scurvy.

**APEPSY**, *Apepsia*, in Medicine, a want of Digestion. *Apepsia*, is a Defect in the Stomach, which prevents the Aliment taken in from affording a proper Chyle for supplying the Blood and nourishing the Body. The Word is form'd from the privative Particle α, and πεπτω, *coquo*, I boil, or concoct.

**APERIENS**, or Aperient, or Aperitive, in Medicine. The Word is *Latin*; being the Participle of the Verb *Aperire*, to open; *q.d. opening*. *Crocus Martis* Aperiens, *opening Saffron of Iron*, is a Preparation of Iron-Plates or Filings, made by exposing them to the Rain or Dew, till they contract a Rust; which is the Medicine required. It is a good *Aperient*.

**APERIENTS**, or Aperitive *Medicines*, are such as open the obstructed Passages of the small Vessels, Glands, and Pores; and by that means promote a due Circulation of the contained Juices. *Aperients*, then, coincide with Deobstructants. The five lesser *Aperient*, or opening Seeds, are Grass, Madder, Eryngo, Capers, and Cammock. The greater opening Seeds are Smallage, Fennel, Asparagus, Parsly, and Butcher's Broom.

**APETALOUS**, in Botany, something without Petala or Leaves. The Word comes from the privative Participle α, and πεταλον, *Folium*, a Leaf.

**APHRONITRE**, *Aphronitrum*, a kind of Nitre, mention'd by the Antients; supposed to be the Spume, or the lightest and subtilest Part thereof, emerging to the top. Some modern Naturalists rather take the antient *Aphronitre* to have been a Native Salt-Petre; now call'd *Salt-Petre of the Rock*. The Word is compounded of the *Greek* αφρος, Froth, and νιτρον, Nitre.

**APHTHÆ**, in Medicine, little Ulcers or Pimples rising in the Mouth, the Palate, Gums, at the Root of the Tongue, &c. The Word seems derived from the *Greek* φθιω, to corrupt; or from απτω, *accendo*, I kindle.

Sucking Children are particularly subject to these *Aphthæ*, when either the Nurse's Milk is corrupted or the Child's Stomach becomes unfit for Digestion: for in these cases, the sharp acrimonious parts of the Milk rising up, easily exulcerate those tender and delicate parts.

There are some of these *Aphtha* white, others red, others livid and blackish: The white and red are the least dangerous, and the most easily cured; the livid and black often prove mortal.

When they happen in grown Persons, they are owing to thin, serous, and sharp Humours returned from the several parts of the Body to the Mouth.

A Liniment of *Mel Rosatum* and Oil of Vitriol, is esteem'd a good Remedy for the *Aphthæ*.

**APICES**, in Botany, little Knobs growing on the Tops of the Stamina, in the middle of Flowers. They are commonly of a dark, purplish Colour. By the Microscope they have been discover'd to be, as it were, a sort of *Capsulæ seminales*, or Seed-Vessels, containing in them small globular, and often oval Particles of various Colours, and exquisitely formed; called the *Farina Fœcundans*. What the Uses of these are, is not entirely agreed : Some have guessed them to be a kind of male Sperm which falling down into the Flower, fœcundates and ripens the Seed. The Word is *Latin*; being the Nominative plural of *Apex*, the Top or Summit of any thing.

**APOCHYLISMA**, among Physicians, *Inspissation*; the boiling and thickening of any Juice with Sugar and Honey, into a kind of hard Consistence.

**APOCROUSTICS**, Medicines intended to stop the Flux of malignant Humours, to a part diseased. They are usually cold, astringent, and consisting of large Particles; wherein they differ from drawing Medicines, which are hot, and consist of more subtile parts. The Word is derived from αποκρουω, *pulso, pello*, I drive.

**APOPHLEGMATISMS**, are Medicaments, chew'd in order to draw away Phlegm, and Humours from the Head and Brain. Of this kind is Tobacco; which is as excellent as any, abating that it spoils the Teeth; and Sage has almost the same Virtues without the same Defects. The Word comes from the *Greek* απο and φλεγμα.

**APOPLEXY**, in Medicine, a sudden Privation of all Senses, and all the sensible Motions of the Body, excepting that of the Heart and Lungs; attended with a great Depravation of the principle Faculties of the Soul.

It differs from a *Carus*, a *Lethargy*, and a *Coma*, in regard that in these three Distempers, the Stupor is not so profound, nor all Sensation quite destroy'd. It differs from a *Syncope*, in that there is no sensible Pulse in this last; whereas in an *Apoplexy*, the Pulse is perceptible almost till Death. It differs from an Epilepsy, in regard all Motion is not abolish'd in that as in this: and it differs from the Palsy, inasmuch as the Palsy is not attended with any Stupor, nor does it deprive the Patient of Sense and Perception.

The *Apoplexy* may be occasion'd by an Interruption of the Passage of the Blood towards the Brain; or by any thing that hinders the Influx of the animal Spirits into the Organs of Sense, and the Parts of voluntary Motion : Sometimes it is owing to an abundance of Phlegm, and sometimes to a viscid *Pituita*, wherewith the Brain is oppress'd; as is observable in Winter *Apoplexies*, and in those of old People.

It sometimes also comes from too gross a Lympha, which stops up the Nerves; or a Plethora, which oppresses them; or Excrescencies withinside the Cranium, pressing the Vessels; or a Polypus, blocking up the Carotids, &c. In dissecting Persons dead hereof, clotted extravasated Blood is usually found in one or both Ventricles of the Brain. See *Philos. Transact.* No 173, 313, &c.

*Hippocrates* distinguishes two kinds of *Apoplexies*, the one *strong*, the other *weak*; only differing in the greater, or less Difficulty of Respiration. The more modern Authors distinguish *Apoplexies*, from their Cause, into *Sanguineous* and *Pituitous*; to which may be added *Lymphatic, Polypous*, &c. The Fit is usually preceded by a violent Pain in the Head, Dimness and Loss of Sight or Memory : Sometimes by an universal Indolence; and sometimes by a Flux of pituitous Matter by the Nose and Mouth. It is attended with a roaring and difficulty of breathing; sometimes with a Fever, rarely with a foaming at the Mouth, frequently with a Sweat, Hemorrhoids, or Diarrhæa; and so goes off.

To prevent *Apoplexy*, Wine and hard Liquor are to be avoided; no eating to excess; nor no sleeping after Dinner : Exercise to be kept up, and Care and Chagrin to be kept under.

To cure an *Apoplexy*, Medicines must be used that occasion large Evacuations; and nothing of opiate or astringent meddled withal. During the Fit, copious bleeding in the Jugulars to be used, and the Patient laid on his back; applying strong Volatiles to the Nose; blow up strong Sternutatories, and rub the Temples with Cephalic Mixtures. A hot Iron may also be apply'd near the Vertex or Occiput; an Epispastic to the Neck; to which are to be added powerful Purgatives, Clysters, &c. Cupping and Scarrification on the Head, are commended by some in lieu of Venæfication.

The Disease sometimes degenerates into a Paralysis. Sometimes only half the Head is affected; in which Case the Disease is called *Hemiplagia.* The Word *Apoplexy*, comes from the *Greek*, αποπληττειν, to strike or astonish; this Distemper striking suddenly, and, as it were, like a Thunder-bolt.

**APOSTEME**, *Apostema*, Apostume, in Medicine, a preternatural Tumor; call'd also *Abscess* and *Imposthume.* The Word is form'd of the *Greek* αποστημαι, which comes from the Verb αφισταθαι, *abscedere*, to depart from one place and fix in another; alluding to the manner wherein the Tumor is usually form'd of a translated Humour.

**APOSTOLORUM** *Unguentum*, the *Apostles Ointments*, in Pharmacy, is a kind of detergent, or cleansing Unguent, composed of twelve Drugs; the Number of the *Apostles*, whence its Name. It was invented by *Avicenna*, and is otherwise called *Unguentum Veneris.* The principal ingredients are Turpentine, Resin, Wax, Gum Ammoniac, Birth-wort Roots, Olibanum, Bdellium, Myrrh, and Galbanum, Opopanax, Verdegrease, Litharge, Oil of Cloves and Vinegar.

**APOTHECARY**, a Person who practises Pharmacy, or that part of Physick which consists in the Preparation and Composition of Medicines. The Word is derived from the *Greek* ατοθηκη, *Shop*, by way of Eminence. *Nich. Langius*[1] has wrote a large Volume expressly against the *Apothecaries*, their *quid pro quo's*, ignorance in the *Materia Medica*, and suffering themselves to be so easily imposed on by foreign Merchants, Druggists, &c. who supply 'em with adulterated Drugs, one sort for another, old Effœte exhausted ones, for new ones just imported from the Levant, &c.

The *Apothecaries* in *England* are obliged to make up their Medicines, according to the Formula's prescribed in the College Dispensatory. Their Shops are subject to the Visitation of the Censors of the College; who are empowered to destroy such Medicines as they think good.

*Bartholin*[2] complains of the too great number of Apothecaries in *Denmark*; tho' there were but three in *Copenhagen*, and four in all the Kingdom beside : What would he have said of *London*, where there are upwards of 1300?

**APOZEM**, in Medicine, a Form of Remedy, otherwise call'd a *Decoction. Apozems* are a Class of liquid Medicines, compos'd of Decoctions of divers Plants, Roots, Flowers, Leaves, Fruits, and Seeds, sweetened and clarified.

It differs from *Syrup*, in Thickness and Consistence; the Syrup being more dense and viscous than the *Apozem.* It differs from a *Julep*, in that it is thicker and more viscous; and is not made with distill'd Waters, as Juleps are, but only with Decoctions.

[1] This may be Charles Nicholas Langius (1670 – 1741), a Swiss naturalist.

[2] Caspar Bartholin (1558 – 1629), a Danish physician and anatomist.

There are purging *Apozems*, Cephalic *Apozems*, Hepatic *Apozems*, &c. The Word is derived from the *Greek* αποζεω, *deservesco*, I grow hot, I boil.

**APYREXY**, in Medicine, the Intermission of a Fever or Ague. The Word is formed of the privative Particle α, and πυρ, *Ignis*, Fire or Heat, or πυραιοτο, *febrecito*, to be feverish.

**AQUA FORTIS**, is a corrosive Liquor, serving as a Menstruum wherewith to dissolve Silver, and all other Metals except Gold. *Aqua fortis* is made of Salt-Petre, which is the only Salt that will act on Silver.

To prepare *Aqua fortis*, they mix either Sand or Alum, or Vitriol, or the two last together, with the Salt-Petre; then distill it by a violent Fire; and catch the Fumes; which condensing in the Receiver, are the *Aqua fortis*. If some of those Matters be not added to the Nitre, it runs too readily, and thus prevents the Evaporation; but when the Fusion is prevented, the parts of the Salt receiving more violent Impressions from the Fire, are converted into a volatile Spirit.

If to the Spirit of Nitre thus distilled, Sea-Salt or Sal Ammoniac be added; it commences *Aqua Regia*, and will no longer dissolve Silver, but Gold. Hence, to try whether or no *Aqua fortis* be pure; put a Grain of a Solution of Silver in *Aqua fortis*, into a like Quantity of the Water in question : and if the Solution remains without either the Water's turning milky, or the Silver precipitating, the *Aqua fortis* is pure.

*Aqua fortis* is commonly held to have been invented about the Year 1300; tho others will have it to been known in the Time of Moses.

*Aqua fortis* is a Liquor of various and extensive Use. It is very useful to Refiners for parting or separating Silver from Gold and Copper. To the Workers in Mosaic, for staining and colouring their Woods. To Dyers in their Colours, and particularly Scarlet.

To other Artists, for the colouring of Bone and Ivory; which is done by steeping the Matters therein, after first tinging it with Copper or Verdigrease, &c. Some also turn it into *Aqua Regia*, by dissolving in it a fourth of its weight of Sal-Ammoniac, and then stain therewith Ivory Hafts and Bones, of a fine purple Colour. There are, also, Book-Binders, who throw it on Leather, and thereby make fine Marble Covers for Books. And there are Diamond-Cutters, who use it to separate Diamonds from metalline Powders. 'Tis, farther, of service in etching Copper, or Brass Plates.

Lastly, Mr. *Boyle* assures us he has caused Canes to be stained like Tortoise-Shell, by a mixture hereof Oil of Vitriol, laid on them at several times, over live Coals, to cause it to penetrate the deeper; and, afterwards, giving them a Gloss with a little soft Wax and a dry Cloth.

**AQUA** *omnium storum*, in Pharmacy, signifies the distilled Water of Cows-Dung, when they are at Grass.

**AQUA** *Regalis*, or Regia. It is thus called, because it dissolves Gold, which is vulgarly esteemed the King of Metals. It is sometimes also called *Aqua Chrysulea* and *Stygia*.

**AQUA** *Vitæ*, is commonly understood of what we otherwise call Brandy. Some, however, distinguish between them; appropriating the Term Brandy to what is procured from Wine, or the Grape; and *Aqua Vitæ* to that drawn after the same manner from Malt, &c.

**AQUEOUS**, *Aquosus*, something that partakes of the Nature of Water, or abounds therein. Thus Milk is said to consist of an *Aqueous* or serous, and a butyrous Part. The Chymists separate the *Aqueous* Part or Phlegm from all Bodies by Distillation.

*Aqueous Humour*, is the first or outermost of the three Humours of the Eye. It lies immediately under the Cornea, which it causes to protuberate a little; and is supposed to be furnished by certain Ducts provided for the purpose.

Anatomists are divided about the Origin and Conveyance of this Humour. 'Tis certain, the Source must be pretty plentiful, inasmuch as, if by any Accident the Coats it is contain'd in be wounded, so that the Humour runs out, and the Cornea falls or collapses; the Wound readily heals, by only closing the Eye, and the Humour recruits : of which we have numerous Instances among Physicians.

Dr. *Nuck*[1] thinks he has discover'd the Ducts whereby the Humour is furnish'd. Others denying the reality of those Ducts, suppose it immediately derived from the Arteries. Dr. *Drake*[2] admits the Ducts, and takes 'em to be only Branches of the excretory Ducts of the *Glandular Innominata*, and *Lachrymalis*; which piercing the Tunicks of the Eye, deliver their Liquor by ways hitherto unknown.

*Gum* **ARABICK**, is the Name of a Gum which distils from a Species of Acacia, growing in *Egypt* and *Arabia*. It is very common among us, but little is to be met with which is genuine; it is suspected to be adulterated with our common Plumb-tree Gums. That is accounted best, which is in smallest Pieces, and almost of a white Colour. It dissolves easily in any aqueous Liquor, and is good in all kinds of Fluxes.

**ARÆOTICKS**, or Areoticks, in Medicine, such Remedies as tend to open the Pores of the Skin, and render them large enough for the morbifick Matter's being carried off by Sweat or insensible Perspiration. To the Class of *Aræoticks* belong Diaphoreticks, Sudorificks, &c.

**ARBOR** in Chymistry. *Arbor Philosophica*, is a Name common to several Metalline Crystallizations; thus call'd from their Ramifications resembling a Tree. *Arbor Diane*, Diana's Tree. *Arbor Martis*, Tree of Mars.

**ARBOREUS**, Arboreous, is applied by some Naturalists to such Excrescencies, Fungus's, Mosses, and other Parasites as grow on Trees.

[1] Anton Nuck (1650 – 1692), a Dutch anatomist, also known as Antonius Nuck van Leiden.

[2] James Drake (1667 – 1707), an English physician and anatomist.

**ARCANUM** literally signifies a Secret; and is therefore very pertinently applied by Quacks and Impostors in Medicine, who conceal their Ignorance and Fraud under a pretence of Secrecy. Hence Legions of *Arcana*. There are also standing officinal Compositions, under the Denomination of *Arcana* : such are

The *Arcanum Corallinum*, a Preparation of red Precipitate; made by distilling it with Spirit of Nitre, and repeating Distillation again and again, till a red Powder be procured. This Powder boiled in Water, and the Water poured off, and tartariz'd Spirit of Wine put to the Powder; two or three Cohobations are made : which leave a Powder, much like the Prince's Powder; of good use in the Gout, Dropsy, Scurvy, &c. It operates chiefly by Stool.

*Arcanum Joviale*, is made of an Amalgam of Mercury and Tin, digested in Spirit of Nitre : the Nitre being drawn off, the remaining matter is wetted with Spirit of Wine, and Spirit burnt away; and this for several times till the pungent taste has gone: what remains is used much with the same Intentions as the *Antihecticum Poterii*, and is recommended by some as a Sudorific.

*Arcanum duplicatum* is prepar'd of Caput Mortuum of Aqua fortis, by dissolving it in hot Water, filtrating, and evaporating it to a Cuticle; then leaving it to shoot. The *Arcanum duplicatum*, or *Panacea duplicata* is extolled as a Diuretic, and Sudorific. The Recipe was purchased at the expense of 500 Dollars, by that great Virtuoso the Duke of *Holstein*. *Schroder*[1], that Prince's Physician, writes wonders of its great uses in Hypochondriacal Cases, continued and intermitting Fevers, Stone, Scurvy, &c.

**ARCHÆUS**, an obscure Term, used chiefly among the Antient Chymists, to express I know not what principle of Life and Motion; the Cause of all the Effects which we observe in Nature. Hence, as they differ in their Ideas of a vitalCause; the Term *Archæus* becomes applied to very different Things : Tho most of 'em conceive it of the Nature of Fire.

Some use *Archæus* to denote the Fire lodg'd in the Centre of the Earth; to which they ascribe the Generation of Metals and Minerals, and which they mean a certain universal Sprit, diffused throughout the whole Creation, the active Cause of all the Phænomena in Nature. Others, instead of *Archæus*, chuse to call it the Anima Mundi; and others the Vulcan or Heat of the Earth.

They add, that all Bodies have their Share of this *Archæus*; and when this is corrupted, it produces Disease, which they call *Archæal*-Diseases. They likewise attribute Ideas to it; which for this Reason they call *Archæal* Ideas.

The Word is derived from αρχη, Principle; this Fire being the Principle and Source of all the Effects in Nature.

*Helmont* is a great Asserter of the Dogma of an *Archæus*. "No Poison," says he, "can act on a Carcass : if, therefore it have any Effect, 'tis by means of the *Archæus*." He adds, "that if an heterogeneous Body happen to be present to the *Archæus*; it rises into a fervour, endeavours to expel the hostile matter; and, in order to that, exerts all the force of the Body. To cure any Disease,

[1] This is probably Johann Christian Schröder (1600 -1664), a German physician.

therefore, is to pacify, and compose this *Archæus*."

This *Archæus*," he holds, "is irritated at the least appearance of any thing heterogeneous; and as its Office is to watch over Health, and Safety of the whole Body; it is excited at the very Shadow of the Enemy, calls its Forces to the Charge, raises Fevers, &c. All, therefore, required to an universal Medicine, is something that may readily pacify and lay this Unnatural Fever upon all occasions."

This Doctrine of *Helmont*, *Boerhaave* observes, would not be so absurd, did he not ascribe Understanding to this *Archæus* : setting this aside, the principle which renders Poisons deadly, and Remedies beneficial, is the Circulation of the Blood.

**ARCHE**, among Physicians, the beginning of a Disease.

**ARDENT**, Ardens, something hot, and, as it were, burning. The Word is form'd of the Latin *Ardere*, to burn. *Ardent* Fever, is a violent burning Fever.

**ARDENT** *Spirits*, are those distill'd from fermented Vegetables; thus call'd because they will take Fire and burn. Such are Brandy, Spirits of Wine, &c.

**ARDOR** *Ventriculi*, a Heat in the Stomach, usually expressed by the Word Heart-burn, or Cardialgy.

**ARGILLA**, or Argil, a white Earth, like Chalk, but more brittle; of some Use in Physick. The Word is sometimes also used for Potters Earth, or Clay.

**ARGYROPÆA**, in Alchemy, the Art of making Silver. The Scope or Design of Argyropæa and Chrysopæia, is to make Gold and Silver. The Word is formed of αργυρος, Silver, and ποιεω, I make.

**ARISTA**, in Botany, a long needle-like Beard, that grows out from the Husk of Corn, or Grass; called also the Awn.

**ARISTOLOCHIA**, popularly call'd *Birthwort*; a medicinal Plant, used as an Ingredient in Treacle, &c. *Cicero* derives its Name from its Inventor *Aristolochus*; others, from its Virtues. These last suppose it form'd from αριϛος, *optimus*, and λοκεια, bringing forth young; in regard it is found of excellent Use in bringing down the Lochia, or Menses of Women newly deliver'd.

There are four Kinds of *Aristolochia, viz.* the *round*, *long*, *rampant* or creeping, and the *slender*; but only the two former are used among us. The *round* is of a sub-acrid aromatic Taste, found very common in *Languedoc, Spain*, and *Italy* : Its Root is of particular Use in facilitating Delivery, provoking the Menses, and bringing down the After-Birth; and is externally applied in vulnerary Tinctures, and in Waters for Gangrenes.

The *long Aristolochia* likewise grows in *Languedoc*; its Root is used in Opiates, and in Tinctures for the Asthmas, and to excite Menses; its Decoction, in Lotions, to facilitate the Delivery of the After-Birth, &c.

Besides these, there are several other Kinds of *Aristolochia* in *America*;

one particularly found in *Virginia*, whose Roots are used against the Bites of venemous Beasts, in malignant Fevers, and the Small-Pox. Its alexipharmachick Virtue has occasion'd it to be called *Viperinum Virginiæ*.

**ARMARIUM** *Unguentum*, in antient Writers, a sympathetick Ointment, or Weapon Salve, whereby Wounds are said to have been cured at a Distance, by only dressing the Weapon.

**ARMONIACK**, or rather Ammoniac, in natural History, a sort of volatile Salt; whereof there are two Kinds, ancient and modern.

The antient *Sal Ammoniac*, called also *Sal Cyrenaic*, described by *Pliny* and *Dioscorides*, was a native Salt, generated in the Earth, or rather the Sands, in those large Inns or Caravanseras, where the Crouds of Pilgrims coming from all Parts to the Temple of *Jupiter Ammon*, used to lodge. The Method of Conveyance in those Parts being on Camels; and those Creatures when in *Cyrene* a Province of Egypt wherein that celebrated Temple stood, urining in the Stables, or say some in the parched Sand: Of this Urine, which is remarkably strong, sublimed by the Heat of the Sun, arose a kind of Salt, denominated sometimes from the Temple *Ammoniac*, and sometimes from the Region *Cyrenaic*.

This Salt being no longer found in those Places, some Authors suspect there was never any such thing; and that the antient as well as the modern *Sal-Armoniac* was factitious. What pleads for the contrary, is, that the Salt frequently belched out large Quantities from Mount *Aetna*, appears much of the same Nature, and answers to most of the Characters of the antient *Sal-Armoniac*. The Reason no more is produced in *Egypt*, is the Cessation of Pilgrimages to that ancient Idol. Its Characters are, that it cools Water, turns *Aqua Fortis* into *Aqua Regia*, and consequently dissolves Gold; that it sublimes by a large Fire, and affords a pungent urinous Savor.

The modern *Sal-Armoniac*, called also *Aqua Cælestis*, is held by some to be native, and to trickle out of the Ground about Mount *Vesuvius, Aetna*, &c. in Form of a Liquor; which, when filtered and inspissated, becomes *Sal-Armoniac*. But 'tis certain, all the modern *Sal-Armoniac* is compound and factitious; consisting of a Mineral, a Vegetable, and an animal Salt combined together.

Indeed, though there scarce be any Drug more common than *Sal-Armoniac*, the Public has been entirely at a Loss, both as to the Place whence it comes, and how it was made; all we know for certain, was that it came from the *Levant*, and was a volatile urinous Salt, penetrated by an Acid. Father *Sicard*[1], the Jesuit, has at length removed the Veil, in the Memoirs of the *Journal de Trevoux*, for September 1717. This Salt, says that Father, in a Letter to the Count de *Tholouse*, is made in *Egypt*, in a sort of Ovens contrived for the Purpose, the Tops whereof are perforated with several longitudinal Clefts; and on these Clefts are laid several long-necked Glass-Bottles, filled with Soot, a little Sea-Salt, and the Urine of Cattle; well stopped.

[1] Claude Sicard (1677 – 1726), a French Jesuit priest and missionary.

This done, they cover them up with a Body of Clay and Brick, all but the Necks, which lie open to the Air; and put the Fire in the Oven, which they keep up for 3 Days and Nights. The Phlegm of the Materials contained in the Bottles, being thus exhaled by the Heat of the Fire; and the acid and alkaline Salts abounding therein, being thus brought together near the Necks of the Bottles, they coalesce, harden, and form a whitish Mass, which is the *Sal-Armoniac*. It must be added, that all Soot is not fit for the Purpose, but only that exhaling from a sort of Fuel made of Dung.

Our Chymists have divers Ways of preparing a *Sal-Armoniac*, in Imitation of this. The common Way is by putting one part of common Salt, to five of Urine; to which some add half that Quantity of Soot : The whole being put in a Vessel, they raise from it by Sublimation a white friable farinaceous Substance, which they call *Sal-Armoniac*. M. *Lemery* suspected, that what is imported to us from Abroad, must be made after a different Manner; he even concluded that it was made as our common Salt is, by Lotion, and Evaporation : In which Suspicion, it appears from the foregoing Account, he is far from the Truth. They purify it by Dissolution in hot Water; which being filtered, and evaporated to a Cuticle, shoots into a fine white Salt, used in Medicine both as a Sudorific and a Diuretic; and proving a good Aperient in all Obstructions.

There are various Preparations of this Salt, in the modern Pharmacy; as, Sublimate of *Sal-Armoniac*, of like Virtue as the purified. *Volatile Sal Armoniac*, made by subliming the *Sal-Armoniac* with Salt of Tartar; used against malignant Fevers as a Sudorific; as also in Pocket Smelling-Bottles.

*Flowers of Sal-Armoniac*; made of *Sal-Armoniac*, with Sea-Salt decrepitated. Its Vertues are much the same as of the sublimated *Sal-Armoniac*. Sometimes, instead of the Sea-Salt, Iron or Steel are used; which makes what they call *Martial Flowers of Sal-Armoniac*, of a very penetrating and deobstructant Nature, and recommended in all Kinds of Obstructions, Cachexies, Jaundice, Dropsie, &c.

*Spirit of Sal-Armoniac* – Of this we have various Kinds, which derive different Denominations and Properties from the different additional Ingredients the Salt is distilled withal: As, *Spirit of Sal-Ammoniac with Tartar*, with *Quicklime*; with *Amber*; with *Steel* or *Iron* : *Sweet* Spirit of *Sal-Ammoniac*; *Acid* Spirit of *Sal-Armoniac*; *Diuretic* Spirit of *Sal-Armoniac*, &c.

**AROMATIC**, *Aromaticus*, is understood of a Drug, Plant, or the like, which yields a brisk, agreeable Smell, and a warm, spicy Taste. Such are Frankincense, Storax, Benjoin, Cinnamon, Mace, Cloves, Nutmeg, Pepper, &c. Such also are Lavender, Marjoram, Sage, Thyme, Rosemary, &c. The Word is form'd of the Greek αρωμα, of αρω, to make fit, accommodate; in regard Spices, which are all *Aromatic*, are used for the seasoning and preparing of Meats.

**AROMATICKS**, or *Aromatic* Medicines, are either simple or compound. To this Class belong most Cardiac, Cephalic, and Carminative Remedies, with many stomachic ones.

The *Aromaticum Rosatum*, is a compound officinal Powder, made of Red

Roses, Liquorice, Aloes Wood, Yellow Sanders, Cinnamon, Cloves, Mace, Gum Tragacanth, Nutmegs, Cardamums, Galangals, Spikenard, Ambergrease and Musk mix'd together. It is chiefly prescribed in Cordial and Cephalic Boles and Electuaries, to strengthen the Stomach and Head, which all *Aromaticks* have a Tendency to.

*Aromaticks* are particular Service in cold cachectic Habits, where the Load of Humours has been forced away by strong Detergents and Catharticks; as they tend to strengthen the Fibres, and prevent a Relapse. Hence they become of absolute Use after Purging, and carrying off the Waters of a Dropsy; or in the Intervals thereof, to fortify the Springs, and prevent a filling again.

**ARSENIC**, *Arsenicum*, in natural History, a ponderous mineral Substance, extremely caustic or corrosive, to the Degree of a violent Poison. The Word is compounded of the Greek ανερ, Man, and νιχαω, I overcome, kill; alluding to its poisonous Quality. *Arsenic* is rank'd among the Class of Sulphurs. There are divers Kinds of *Arsenic*; *viz.* Yellow, or Native; Red, and Crystalline.

Native *Arsenic* is of a Yellow, or Orange-colour; whence it is also denominated *Auripigmentum*, or *Orpiment*. It is chiefly found in Copper-Mines, in a sort of Glebes or Stones, of different Figures and Size.

In Colour, tho' always Yellow, yet admits of divers Shades and Mixtures, as a golden Yellow, reddish Yellow, green Yellow, &c. It is found to contain a Portion of Gold, but so little, as not to quit the Cost of separating it. Of this are prepared two other Kinds of *Arsenic*, viz. *White* and *Red*. This, sublimed with some other Matters, is the *Sandaracha Græcorum*.

Tho' some Naturalists will have Red *Arsenic*, and *Realgal*, two distinct Drugs, taking the latter for a native Mineral, and the former for a Preparation of a native *Arsenic*. *Red Arsenic*, called also *Realgal*, is only the native Yellow rubified by Fire.

The White, or Crystalline, is drawn from the Yellow, by subliming it with a Proportion of Sea-Salt. 'Tis this Species is chiefly in Use among us for real *Arsenic*. Some Authors give it a different Origin, and maintain it a native Matter, found in white scaly Glebes in the Mines.

White and Yellow *Arsenic* are also procurable from Cobalt : The Method of which, as practised in Hungary, is given us by Dr. *Krieg*[1], in the *Philosophical Transactions*, No 293. The Cobalt being beat to Powder, and the light sandy Part washed off, by a Current of Water, they put what remains in a Furnace; the Flame of which passing over the Powder, takes along with it the Arsenical Part, in Form of a Smoak; which being receiv'd by a Chimney, and carried thence into a close Brick Channel, sticks by the Way to the Sides; and is scraped off, in form of a whitish or yellowish Powder. From what remains of the Cobalt, they proceed to make *Smalt*.

The smallest Quantity of any of these *Arsenics*, being mixed with any Metal, renders it friable, and absolutely destroys its Malleability. Hence, the Refiners dread nothing so much as *Arsenic* in their Metals; nor could any thing be so advantageous to them, were such a thing to be had, as a

[1] David Krieg (1669 – 1710), a German surgeon and naturalist

Menstruum that would absorb, or act on *Arsenic* alone; for them their Metals would be readily purified, without flying off, or evaporating.

A single Grain of *Arsenic* will turn a Pound of Copper into a beautiful seeming Silver. This Hint many Persons have endeavoured to improve on, for the making of Silver, but in vain, as it could never be brought to sustain the Hammer : Some have been hang'd for coining Species of this spurious Silver.

The Chymists furnish several Preparations of *Arsenic*, which all turn on repeated Ablutions and Sublimations, to blunt the corrosive Salts thereof, and change them into a safe Medicine, after the Manner of Sublimate. Such are Ruby of *Arsenic*, &c.

But it scarce appears worth the Pains : And whatever some may urge, *Arsenic* should never be used inwardly in any Form, as gnawing and tearing the Parts, and occasioning mortal Convulsions. Its Fume taken into the Lungs kills instantly : And the oftner it is sublimed, says *Boerhaave*, the ranker it grows. Butter and Cow's Milk taken in large Quantities, prove good Antidotes against *Arsenic*.

*Regulus of* Arsenic, is the most fix'd and compact Part thereof, prepared by mixing it with Pot-ashes and Soap, dissolving the whole, and casting it into a Mortar; upon which the heaviest Part falls to the Bottom.

*Caustic Oil of* Arsenic, is a Butyrous Liquor, like Butter of Antimony, prepared of *Arsenic* and corrosive Sublimate. It serves to eat off fungous Flesh, cleanse carious Bones, &c.

*Arsenical* Magnet, *Magnes Arsenicus*, is a Preparation of Antimony with Sulphur and White *Arsenic*.

**ARTHRITIS**, in Medicine, a Disease better known under the name of the Gout. The Word is form'd from the Greek αρθρον, Articulus, a Joint; in regard the chief Seat of that Distemper is in the Joints.

**ARTIFICIAL**, *Artificialis*, something made by Art; not produced naturally, or in the common Course of Things.

"Art is usually consider'd as Thing very different from Nature; and *artificial* Things from natural ones : Whence arises another more grievous Error, *viz.* that Art is a different Principle built upon Nature, and of such Power, as to be able, either to prefect what Nature had begun, to rectify and amend her when disordered, or to free her when confined; tho' not utterly to divert or transmute her. But the Truth is, *artificial* Things do no differ from natural one in Nature or Form, but only in the Efficient : Man has no Power over Nature, beside what he has by Motion; in virtue whereof, he can apply natural Bodies to, or remove them from, one another. Where such Application, or joining of active Things to passive ones, is practicable, there may Man do any thing; where it is not, nothing. Gold we sometimes see purified by the Chymist's Fire; and sometimes find it perfectly pure in the Sands, Nature herself having done the Business : So the Rainbow is sometimes form'd on high in the Water of a Cloud; and some times here below by a sprinkling of Water. Nature, therefore, governs all Things; under this Subordination, of the Course of Nature, the Latitude or Evagation of Nature, and *Art*, or Man super-added to her other Works."

*Bacon*[1], *de Augmen.*

**ARYTHMUS**, in Medicine, a Sinking or Failure of the Pulse, so as it can no longer be felt. The Word is form'd from the privative Particle α, and ρυθμος, *Modulus*, or *Pulsus*.

**ASBESTINE** *Paper* or *Cloth*, is such as will burn in the Fire, be purified by it, and yet not consume. It is made of the *Asbestos*, or *Lapis Amianthus*; and is by some called *Linum Vivum*. The Antients are said to have made Napkins and towels of it, which, when foul, instead of Washing, they threw into the Fire to cleanse.

**ASBESTOS**, or *Amianthus Lapis*, in natural History, called also *Carystius Lapis*, in incombustible Matter; supposed by some to be a sort of Flax, growing on the *Pyreneans*; whence it is also called *Linum vivum*, *Linum incombustibile*, &c.

The *Asbestos*, or *Lapis Asbestos*, is really a sort of native fissile stone, which one may split into Threads of Filaments, very fine, brittle, yet somewhat tractable, silky, and of a greyish silver Colour, not unlike Talc of Venice.

It is almost insipid to the Taste, indissoluble in Water; and expos'd to the Fire, neither consumes nor calcines. A large Burning-glass, indeed, reduces it into little Glass Globules, in proportion as the Filaments separate; but common Fire only whitens it.

These Filaments are of different Lengths, from one inch to ten. The Stone is found inclosed within other very hard Stones, and is brought from the Isles of the *Archipelago*, the *Pyreneans*, and from *Montauban* in *France*. We have seen Instances of it in *Scotland, Wales*, &c.

Several Persons have pretended to the Secret of spinning the *Asbestos* : *B. Porta*[2] assures, that in his Time, 'twas a thing known to every Body in Venice: And yet this should seem hardly practicable. Without the Mixture of some other very pliant Matter, as Wool, Line, or Hemp along with it; the Filaments of the *Amianthus* it self being too brittle to make any tolerable fine Works.

The Works made of *Asbestos*, were heretofore held in so great Esteem, that they were of equal Price with Gold; and none but Emperors and Kings had Napkins made of it. Some Antiquaries are of Opinion, that the Antients made Shrouds of the *Asbestos*, wherein they burnt the Bodies of their Kings, in order to preserve their *Ashes* entire, and prevent their being mix'd with those of Wood, and other combustible Matters, whereof the common Funeral Piles were form'd. Others assert, that the Antients used the *Asbestos*; to make perpetual Wicks for sepulchral Lamps.

However this be, there are some at this Day who use the *Asbestos* for the Wicks of such Lamps as they would not have any trouble withal; because the *Amianthus* never wasting, there is no occasion for shifting the Wick.

[1] Sir Francis Bacon (1561 – 1626), an English philosopher, lawyer, and scientist.

[2] Jean Baptista Porta, or Giambattista della Porta (1535 – 1615), Italian physician and scientist.

The Word ασβεστος, *Asbestos*, properly signifies an *incombustible Body*; being formed of the privative Particle α, and σβεννυμαι, *extinguo*. Notwithstanding the common opinion that Fire has no Effect on the *Asbestos*; yet, in two Trials before the Royal Society, a Piece of incombustible Cloth made of this Stone, a Foot long, and a half a Foot broad, weighing about an Ounce and a half, was found to lose above a Dram of Weight, each time.

The *Asbestos* applied to any Part of the Body, excites an Itching; and yet we read of it as antiently prescribed for Diseases of the Skin, and particularly for the Itch : Unless it were rather the *Alumen Plumosum* that was meant hereby; for even at this Day, they are frequently confounded.

**ASCARIDES**, in Medicine, a kind of little Worms, sometimes found in the Rectum, and adhering to the Fundament. They are thus called from the Greek ασκαριζω, I leap, on account of their continual troublesome Motion, causing a most intolerable Itching.

**ASCITES**, in Medicine, a Species of Dropsy, affecting chiefly the Abdomen, or Lower Belly. The *Ascites* is the ordinary Water-Dropsy. The Word is borrowed from the Greek ασκος, *Uter*, Belly.

**ASHES**, *Cineres*, the terrene or earthy Part of Wood, and other combustible Bodies, remaining after they are burnt or consumed with Fire. *Ashes* are properly the Earth, and fix'd Salts of the Fuel, which the Fire cannot raise, all the other Principles being gone off in the Smoak. The Chymists frequently call the *Ashes* of a Body its *Calx*.

*Ashes*, if well burnt, are usually pure White, by reason the Oil to which they owe their Blackness when in a Coal, is supposed quite evaporated. The *Ashes* of Kali, Fern, or the like, are a principal Matter in the Composition of Glass.

The *Ashes* of all Vegetables are found to contain Iron, insomuch that M. *Geoffroy* makes it a chymical Problem, which he proposes to the Public, *To find Ashes without any Particles of Iron therein*. Whether the Metal existed in the Plants themselves, or is produced in 'em by the Operation of Calcination, is a Point very ingeniously controverted between Mess. *Geoffroy* and *Lemery* the younger, in the Memoirs of the Royal Academy.

*Ashes*, are of considerable Use in making Lixiviums, or Lyes, for the Purposes of Medicine, Bleaching, Sugar-Works, &c. The Antients preserved the *Ashes* of their dead Ancestors, with great Care and Piety, in Urns, for the Purpose. *Ashes*, of all Kinds, in Virtue of their Salt, make an excellent Manure for cold and wet Grounds.

In the *Philosophical Transactions*, N°. 21. we have an Account of a Shower of Ashes in the Archipelago, which held several Hours, and extended to Places distant above 100 Leagues.

**ASPALATH**, *Aspalathum*, in Pharmacy, the Wood of a prickly Tree, heavy, oleaginous, somewhat sharp and bitter to the Taste, of a strong Smell and Purple Colour.

The *Aspalath* is otherwise called Rhodium, or Rosewood, and was antiently in much Repute, as an Astringent or Dryer, but now disused. In Virtue, Taste, Smell, and Weight, it resembles the Lignum Aloes; and in Physick they are frequently substituted the one foe the other.

There are four Kinds of *Aspalath* – the first, of the Colour of Box; hard, solid, heavy, and of a Smell like Roses, whence its Appellation *Rosewood*. The second, red, like Yew, and of a very agreeable Smell. The third, hard, twisted, knotty : It has a rank Smell, like that of a Goat, and a disagreeable Taste. The fourth, has an ash-colour'd Bark, and it's a Wood of a Purple Dye.

The Rose wood is what the inhabitants of *Martinico* call *Cypress-wood*. It affords an Oil of admirable Scent; reputed one of the best Perfumes, chiefly used in scenting Pomatums and Liniments.

**ASPERIFOLIÆ**, in Botany, one of the Divisions or Kinds of Plants. The Characters of the *Asperifolious* Kind, are, that the Leaves stand alternately, or without any certain Order on the Stalks : The Flowers are monopetalous, but have the Margin cut into five Divisions, sometimes deep, sometimes shallow; and the upper Spike or Top of the Plant, is often curved back, something like a Scorpion's tail. They are called *Asperifoliæ*, because they are usually *rough-leav'd*, but not always so.

After each Flower there are usually succeed four Seeds; Mr. *Ray*[1] reckoning the *Cerinthe* the only Plant of this Genus, that hath less than four Seeds at the Root of each Flower; this, indeed, hath but two. The Herbæ Asperifoliæ, are the *Pulmonaria Maculosa, Cynglossa, Borago, Buglossa, Anchusa, Echinum, Linum Umbilicatum, Heliotropium majus, Aparine major, Consolida major, Lithospermum, Echium Scorpoides*, and *Cerinthe*.

**ASPIC**, *Oil of Aspic*, vulgarly called Oil of Spike, is an inflammable Oil drawn from the Leaves and Flowers of a Plant frequent on the Southern Parts of France, resembling Lavender, and by the Botanists called *Lavandula Mas*. It is much used by Painters and Farriers; and sometimes also in Medicine. The true Oil of *Aspic*, is of a white Colour, and an aromatic Taste; and is held the only Thing capable of dissolving Sandarach : By which it is easily distinguish'd from the Counterfeit, which is only Oil of Turpentine mixed with a little Petrol.

**ASSA-FOETIDA**, or Asa-Foetida, a Gum or Resin, brought from the *East Indies*, of a brownish Colour, a sharp Taste, and a very strong, offensive Smell; whence it is also called *Stercus Diabolis*, or Devil's Dirt.

'Tis not known from what Plant this Gum is procured : all that has been advanced on that Point by the Botanists and the Writers of Pharmacy, amounts to no more than Conjectures, founded on the different Relations of Travellers. They who after the Antients, suppose it drawn from the *Laser*, or *Laserpitium*, would be hard put to it to get clear of those many Disputes which have so often divided the Botanists on the Subject of the true *Laser*, and the *Succus Cyrenaicus*, so infinitely prized among them. Indeed there seems but little Resemblance between the Gum described by M. *Furetierre*[2],

[1] John Ray (1627 – 1705), the English botanist who wrote the *Historia generalis plantarum*.

[2] This may be Antione Furetiere (1619 – 1688), a French scholar.

out of *Pliny*, lib. Xix. C. 3 and our *Assa-Fœtida* : If they be the same, 'tis certain we are not acquainted with half its Virtues.

The modern *Assa-Fœtida*, which is little used but by the Farriers, is a Gum said to distil during the Summer's Heats, from a little Shrub, frequent in *Persia, Media, Assyria*, and *Arabia*. It is at first white, bordering on yellow, then on red, and lastly on Violet; and melts under the Fingers like Wax.

It is of known Efficacy in some uterine Disorders; but the Rankness of its Smell occasions it to be seldom used; yet in the *East-Indies* it makes an Ingredient in their Ragouts.

**ASSA-DULCIS**, a Name sometimes given to Gum Benjoyn.

**ASSARABACKA**, or Assara-Bacara, a Plant mentioned by *Pliny* and *Dioscorides*, under the Name of the *Wild Nardus*; by us called Asarum. *Avicenna* relates, that it is brought from *China*; that its Roots resemble those of Gramen, or Dog's-Tooth; but that it has a pretty brisk Smell, and bites the Tongue when tasted. Its Leaves were antiently much in Use, as an Emetic, and Cathartic; and in some Authors we find a superstitious Observance in the gathering 'em : They alledge, that if the Plant be pull'd forward it becomes vomitive, but if backwards purgative. *Rulandus*[1] and *Fernelius*[2] frequently describe it as a Diuretic. But it is chiefly used among us as a Sternutatory, in order to which, it is dried and reduced to Powder, to be taken as Snuff; in which Quality it drains the Head of mucous Humours.

**ASSATION**, the preparing or dressing of Medicaments, or Foods, in their own Juices, without Addition of any foreign Moisture. *Assation*, in respect of culinary Matters, is more frequently call'd *Roasting*; and in Pharmacy, *Ustion* or *Torrefaction*. The Word is form'd of the Latin *assare*, to roast.

**ASTHMA**, in Medicine, a Disease of the Lungs, accompanied with a Shortness, and Difficulty of Respiration. Or, *Asthma* is a Difficulty of Breathing, arising from a Disorder of the Lungs; and usually attended with violent Motions of the Diaphragm, Abdominal and Intercostal Muscles, as also a rattling in the Throat. The Word is Greek, αστθμα, form'd of the Verb αιο, *Spiro*; I breath.

If Respiration be only thick and quick, without the other Symptoms, it is call'd a *Dyspnæa*. If it be so intense as to occasion a violent Motion of the Muscles of the Thorax; so that the Patient cannot be tolerably easy, except in an erect Posture, it is call'd an *Orthopnæa*.

The *Asthma* is usually divided into *Moist* and *Dry*, or *Manifest* and *Occult*, or *Pneumonic* and *Convulsive* : The first attended with a Expectoration of Purulent Matter; the latter without. The true *Asthma* is occasioned by an abundance of Serosities, or of gross viscous or purulent Humours, collected in the Cavities of the Lungs, which stop up or straighten the Passages of the Air, and compress the Bronchia. It is also owing to Empysema's, Phthisis's,

[1] Martin Ruland the Elder (1532 – 1602), a German alchemist and physician.

[2] Jean Francois Fernel (1497 – 1558), a French physician.

Crudities in the Stomach, Cachexies, &c.

The Compulsive *Asthma* is supposed to be occasioned by an irregular Motion of the Animal Spirits; and happens when the Spirits do not show fast enough, or in sufficient Quantity, into the Muscles of the Breast, either by reason of an Obstruction, or of some other Obstacle; The necessary Consequence whereof is a violent and painful Respiration. The *Asthma*, again, either continual, or periodical, and intermitting; which last returns chiefly where a sober Regimen is no observed.

The *Asthma* is found to be the most violent when the Patient is in Bed, and in a prone Posture; the Contents of the lower Belly, in that case, bearing against the Diaphragm, so as to lessen the Capacity of the Breast, and to leave the Lungs less room to move.

The Cure of the true or pneumonic *Asthma*, is by bleeding; after which Emeticks may be used; and if the Paroxysm returns, Epispasticks, with Glysters instead of Purges. Infusions of Fim. Equin. or the Juice thereof, being detersive and attenuating, are reputed excellent. Linctus's also contribute to the Cure, Millepedes, Spirit of *Gum Armoniac*, with *Sal Armoniac*, Coffee, Tincture of Sulphur, &c. are commended in *Asthmatick* Cases. For the convulsive Kind, the Cure is attempted by *Antiepilepticks*, *Antihystericks*, *Antispasmodicks*, &c.

**ASTRINGENTS**, *Astringentia*, in Medicine, *binding Remedies*; or such as have the Power of contracting the Parts and diminishing the Pores thereof. *Astringents* act either by the Asperity of their Particles, whereby they corrugate the Membranes, and make them draw up closer; or by thickening Fluids, whereby they cannot run off so fast as before. *Astringents* therefore stand opposed to Laxatives. The Word is compounded of the Latin *ad* and *stringo*, I bind.

Hence, *Astringents* are of the Class of Strengtheners, or Corroborants; the Nature and Operation whereof, see under the Article Strengthener. *Astringents* only differ from *Stypticks*, in Degree of Efficacy. Among Simples, Mint, red Roses, Nettles, Sanicle, Barbaries, Quinces, Pomegranates, Sloes, Cinnamon, Blood-stone, Alum, Chalk, Boles, Coral, Tutty, &c. are principal *Astringents*.

**ATAXY**, *Ataxia*, a want of Order or Regularity. The Term is chiefly used in Medicine, where the Order of the Critical Days, or other Phænomenon of a Disease, is inverted. The Physicians have frequent recourse to an *Ataxy* or Irregularity of the Spirits, when at a loss to account for any Disorder in the Body. The Spirits, Dr. *Drake* observes, being always at Hand, are forced to bear the blame of a thousand things they are innocent of. The Word is compounded of the privative Particle α and ταξις, Order.

**ATHANOR**, in Chymistry, a large immoveable Furnace, built of Brick or Earth, and cover'd with a Tower a-top; proper to maintain a temperature and equable Degree of Heat for a considerable time. The Heat of the *Athanor* is intended or remitted by opening or shutting a Register.

It is made to communicate its Heat by Tubes or Apertures at the Side of the Hearth or Fire-Place, to several adjacent Vessels; by which means different

Operations are carry'd on at the same time. We meet with divers Forms and Constructions of this Furnace, in the Writers of Chymistry.

The *Athanor* is also call'd *Piger Henricus*, flow Harry; because chiefly used in the flower Operation; and because when once filled with Coals, it keeps burning a long time; whence the Greek call it ακηνετν, *q.d.* giving no trouble, as it does not need to be continually attended. It is also call'd the *Philosophical Furnace*, or *Furnace of Arcana*; and popularly, the *Tower Furnace*.

The Word *Athanor* is borrowed from the *Arabs*, who call an Oven, *Tanneron* from the Hebrew חניד, *Tannour*, an Oven, or Furnace; whence, with the additional Particle *al*, אלחניר, *Altannour*, &c. Others chuse to derive the Name from the *Greek* αθανατος, Immortal; because of its durable Fire.

**ATHEROMA**, in Medicine, a Kind of a Tumour or Swelling, of a pappy Consistence, without pain, or discolouring the Skin. The *Atheroma* is contain'd in a Cystis or membranous Bag; and does not give way when touched with the Finger, nor retains any dent after pressure. The *Atheroma* is thus call'd from the *Greek* αθηρα, a Kind of Pap or Pulp which the Matter of this Tumour resembles. It is near a-kin to the *Meliceris* and *Steatoma*; and cured like them.

**ATOM**, *Atomus*, in Philosophy, a *Corpuscle*; or a Part or Particle of Matter so minute as to be invisible. The Word is *Greek*, ατομος; form'd of the privative α and τεμνω, I cut, I divide. *Atoms* are properly the *minima Naturæ*, the last or ultimate Particles into which Bodies are divisible; and are conceived as the first Rudiments, or component Parts of all physical Magnitude or the pre-existent and incorruptible Matter whereof Bodies were form'd.

The Notion of *Atoms* arises hence, that Matter is not divisible, *in infinitum*. And hence many Authors are led to deny the reality of *Atoms*, together with that of Mathematical Points : An *Atom*, say they, either has Parts, or it has none : If it has none, it is a mere Mathematical Point : It if have, then do these Parts also consist of others and so to Infinity. But this is to recede from the genuine Character of Atoms, which are not esteemed indivisible particles, because of their want of Bigness, or Parts; (for all physical Magnitude must have three Dimensions, Length, Breadth, and Thickness; and all Extension is divisable) but they are indivisible on account of their Solidity, Hardness, and Impenetrability, which precluded all Division, and leave not Vacancy for the Admission of any foreign Force to separate or disunite them.

As *Atoms* are the first Matter, 'tis necessary they shou'd be indissolvible, in order to their being incorruptible. Sir *Isaac Newton* adds, that 'tis also required they be immutable, in order to the World's continuing in the same State, and Bodies being of the same Nature now as formerly. Hence the Antients were also led to maintain *Atoms*, eternal; for that what is Immutable must be Eternal.

They also added Gravity, and in Consequence thereof, Motion, to their *Atoms:* And further, observing that Atoms thus falling perpendicularly, cou'd not join or unite together; they super-added a fortuitous or side

Motion, and furnish'd them with certain hooked Parts, in order to enable them to catch and hang the better together. And from a casual or fortuitous Jumble of these hamous *Atoms*, they supposed the whole Universe to be formed.

**ATOMICAL** *Philosophy*, the Doctrine of *Atoms*; or a Method of accounting for the Origin and Formation of all things, from the Supposition of *Atoms*, endued with Gravity and Motion. The *Atomical* Philosophy was first broach'd and taught by *Moschus, Leucippus*[1], and *Democritus*[2]: It was cultivated by *Epicurus*[3]; whence it became also denominated the *Epicurean Philosophy*. It has been since retrieved by *Gassendus*[4], and others; and is now espoused and adhered to by a great Part of the philosophical World, under the Denomination of the *Corpuscular Philosophy*.

**ATONY**, *Atonia*, in Medicine, &c. a want of Tone or Tension; or a Relaxation of the Solids of a human Body; occasioning a loss of Strength, Fainting, &c. The Word is compounded of the privative α, and τεινω, *tendo*, I stretch.

**ATRABILIS**, in the antient Medicine, black or adult Bile. *Atrabilis* was one of the great Humours of the antient Physicians; whence arose the *Atrabilary*, one of their Temperaments; answering to what we call *Melancholy*.

**ATROPHY**, *Atrophia*, an Indisposition or Disease, wherein the Body or some of its Parts, do not receive the necessary Nutriment, but dwindles or wastes insensibly. Such are what we commonly call *Consumptions, Phthises*, &c. An *Atrophy* is natural in old Age, call'd *Atrophia Senilis*. The Word is compounded of the privative Particle α, and τρεφω, I feed, nourish.

**ATTENUANTS**, Attenuatives, or Attenuating Medicines, such as subtilize or break the Humours into finer Parts; and thus dispose them for Motion, Circulation, Excretion, &c. *Attenuants* stand opposed to *Thickeners*, or Medicines which condense, inspissate, &c.

**ATTENUATION**, *Attenuatio*, the Act of attenuating; that is, of making any Fluid thinner, and less consistent than it was before. The Word is compounded of the *Latin ad*; and *tenuis*, thin, slender, weak. *Attentuation* is defined more generally by *Chauvin*, the dividing or separating of the minute Parts of any Body, which before, by their mutual Nexus or Implication, form'd a more continuous Mass. Accordingly, among the Alchymists, we sometimes find the Word used for Pulverization, or the act of reducing a Body into an impalpable Powder.

**ATTIRE**, in Botany, is used to denote the third Part or Division of the Flower of a Plant; the other two being the Empalement and the Foliation. This *Attire* is of two Kinds; Semini-form, and Florid. The *Semini-form Attire* consist of

[1] Leucippus (ca. 5th cent. BC), a Greek philosopher.

[2] Democritus (ca. 460 370 BC), a Greek philosopher.

[3] Epicurus (341 – 270 BC), a Greek philosopher.

[4] Petrus Gassendus, born Pierre Gassendi (1592 – 1655), a French philosopher.

two Parts; Chives, or the Stamina; and Semets, or Apices; one upon each *Attire*.

The *Florid Attire* is usually call'd *Thrums*, as in the Flowers of Marigold, Tansy, &c. These Thrums are called *Suits*, which consist of two, but most times of three Pieces. The outer Part of the Suit is the Floret, whose Body is divided at the top, like a Cowslip Flower, into five Parts or distinct Leaves.

**ATTRAHENTS**, *Attrahentia*, or Attractive *Remedies*, such Medicines, externally applied, as by their Activity and Warmth penetrate the Pores; and mix with and rarefy any obstructed Matter; so as to render it fit for Discharge, upon lying open the Part by Caustick or Incision. *Attrahents* are the same with what we otherwise call *Drawers, Ripeners, Maturantia, Digestives*, &c.

The principal Simples belonging to this Class, are the several Kinds of Fats, or *Adipes*; the Dungs of Pidgeons and Cows; Bran, Yest, Herring, the Sucking of a Leech, Melilot, Tobacco, Oil, Pitch, Rosin, Frankincense, &c.

In many Instances, as the Matter rarefies and grows more fluid by means of such Medicines; the refluent Blood is apt to wash it back into the common Mass; which sometimes does a deal of Mischief; or by making it take up more room upon its Rarefaction, occasions it to distend more the Parts in which it is contained : Upon which a Sense of Pain is excited, and thereby a greater Concourse of fluid, and consequently a needless Increase of the Tumor. So that Medicines under this Denomination require the most careful Management.

**AVIGNON**-*Berry*, call'd also, *French Berry*, is the Fruit of a Shrub, by some Authors call'd *Licum*; growing plentifully near Avignon, &c. in *France*. The Berry is somewhat less than a Pea; its Colour Green, approaching towards a Yellow; of an astringent and bitter Taste. It is much used by the Dyers who stain a yellow Colour with it; and by the Painters, who make a fine golden Yellow of it.

**AUREA** *Alexandrina*, in Pharmacy, a kind of Opiate or Antidote, in great Fame among the antient Writers. It is called *Aurea*, from the Gold which enters its Composition; and *Alexandrina*, as having been first invented by a Physician name *Alexander*. It is reputed a good Preservative against the Colick and Apoplexy.

**AURICULA** *Judæ*, or *Jew's Ear*, a kind of Fungus or Mushroom, resembling in Figure, a human Ear. It grows on old Elder Trees, which is the Tree whereon, 'tis pretended, *Judas* hang'd himself; which has given occasion to the Name. The Fungus steep'd in Water, and applied to the Eyes, frees them of Inflammations : 'Tis also used Gargle-wise in Decoctions, against Inflammations of the throat, or swelling of the Tonsils.

**AURUM**, in Natural History, Gold. The Word is chiefly applied to certain Chymical Preparations, whereof Gold is the Basis or principal Ingredient. Such are the *Aurum potabile, Aurum fulminans*, &c.

**AURUM** *fulminans*, fulminating or thundering Gold. It is inflammable, not only by Fire, but also by a gentle Warmth; and gives a Report much louder than that of Gunpowder. Its Effect is commonly said to be principally downwards; in opposition to Gun-powder, which is chiefly upwards; but this rather seems a vulgar Error. A Scruple of this Powder acts more forcibly than half a Pound of Gun-powder : a single Grain laid on the Point of a Knife, an lighted at the Candle, goes off with a greater Noise than a Musket. It is said to consume even to the very last Atom.

**AURUM** *potabile, Potable Gold*, is a Composition made of Gold, by reducing it, without any Corrosive, into a Gum, or Substance like Honey, of the Colour of Blood; which Gum steep'd in Spirit of Wine, acquires a Ruby-colour, and is call'd Tincture of Gold.

An Ounce of this Tincture, mix'd with sixteen Ounces of another Liquor, is call'd *Aurum potabile*, because of its Gold-colour; and is said to be a sovereign Remedy against several Diseases.

A modern Physician has asserted that Gold is a Resin drawn from the Earth; and that the grand Secret of rendering Gold *potable*, does not consist in dissolving this Resin by means of Corrosives, but by a Water, wherein it melts like Ice or Snow in hot Water; and this Water must be nothing but a Water extracted from Gold, agreeable to an Axiom that he lays down, which is, that Matters of different Natures have no Ingress into one another; but that every Menstruum or Dissolvent ought to be taken from Bodies of the same kind with those it is to act upon.

The same Author observes, that Blood and Urine furnish a *Sal Armoniac*, which mingled with *Aqua-fortis*, acts upon Gold : whence he conjectures, that there may be a conformity of Nature between Gold and Blood; and that by consequence, Gold well open'd and subtiliz'd, might produce a Resin, and a Fire that wou'd augment the Blood.

**AWN**, in Botany, *Arista*; the Beard growing out of the Husk of Corn or Grass.

**AXUNGIA**, a kind of Fat, the softest and moistest of any in the Bodies of Animals. It is different from *Lard*, which is a firm Fat; and from *Suet* Leaf, or Adeps, which is a kind of dry Fat. The Word is supposed to be form'd, *ab Axe Rotarum quae unguntur*. The *Latins* distinguish Fat into *Pinguedo*, call'd also *Axungia*; and *Adeps*, or *Sevum*; but many of our modern Writers confound them.

The Physicians make use of the *Axungia* of the Goose, the Dog, the Viper, and some others, especially that of Man, which is of extraordinary Service in the drawing and ripening of Tumors.

**AXUNGIA** *of Glass*, call'd also the *Gall*, and *Salt of Glass*, is a Scum taken from the Top of the Matter of Glass before it be vitrified.

**AZOTH**, among the antient Chymists, signified, sometimes, the first Matter of Metals; sometimes an universal Medicine; and sometimes the Mercury of a Metal. But the Term is now disused.

**BACCIFEROUS** Plants, whether Trees, Shrubs, or Herbs, are such as bear Berries, *i.e.* Fruit cover'd with a thin Membrane, wherein is contained a Pulp, which grows soft and moist when ripe, and encloses the Seed within its Substance. The *Bacciferous* Trees Mr. *Ray* divides into four Kinds:

1. Such as bear a caliculate or naked Berry; the Flower and Calix both falling off together, and leaving the Berry bare, as the Sassafras Tree, &c.

2. Such as have a naked monopyreneous Fruit, that is, containing in it only one Seed, as the *Arbutus, Terebinthus, Lentiscus*, &c.

3. Such as have a naked but polypyreneous Fruit, that is, containing two or more Kernels or Seeds within it, as the *Jasaminum, Ligustrum*, &c.

4. Such as have their Fruit composed of many Acini, or round soft Balls set close together like a Bunch of Grapes, as the *Uva marina*[1], *Rubus vulgaris*[2], *Rubus Idaeus*[3], and the *Rubus minor fructu caruleo*[4].

**BACILLI**, in Medicine, such Compositions as are of a cylindrical Figure, like a Stick; call'd also Lozenges : from the Latin Word *Baculus*, a Staff.

**BALAUSTINES**, in Pharmacy, are the Flowers of the Pomegranate, which are very rough to the Tongue and Palate, and very astringing; they are therefore used in Diarrhæas, and other Fluxes, Hernias, &c.

**BALLON**, in Chymistry, a French Word for a large round short-neck'd Matrass, or Vessel used in Chymistry, to receive what is distilled or drawn off by the means of Fire. *Ballon* is also used in Architecture for a round Globe placed a-top of a Pillar, or the like, by way of a Pillar.

**BALM**, or *Balsam*, a kind of Gum, in very great Reputation in Medicine and Chirurgery; used to be liquefied by means of Spirit of Wine or Oil, and found a sovereign Remedy in the Cure of Wounds and several Diseases. The Ladies set a particular Value on it, in regard when mix'd with the Yolk of an Egg and Spirit of Wine, it makes an admirable Paint.

There are various Kinds of *Balms* or *Balsams*, if into the Number hereof we take all those which Empires, or even Physicians and Chirurgeons call by this Name; such are *Apoplectic Balsams, Stomachic Balsams, Bezoardic, Hysteric, Vulnerary, Magisterial*, &c. But the Genuine, that us, the Natural *Balsams*, come in a little Compass, being in great measure reducible to these two, the *Balm* of *Gilead*, and *Balm* or *Balsam* of *Peru*.

*Balm of Gilead*, or of the *Levant*, is held in the greatest Esteem, tho there are some who hold that of *Peru* equal to it in Virtue. 'Tis drawn by Incision from a Tree called *Balsamum*, growing in *Egypt* and *Judea*, and which is held so precious, that it makes Part of the special Revenue of the *Grand*

[1] Shrubby horsetail, or Joint-Fir, a species of *Ephedra*.

[2] The blackberry.

[3] The raspberry.

[4] The dewberry or lesser bramble.

*Signior*, with out whose Permission none are allowed to be planted or cultivated. The Incision through which this admirable Juice flows, is made in the Dog-Days : *Theophrastus* says it must be made with Iron Nails; *Pliny* with Glass, because, says he, Iron makes the Plant die : *Tacitus*[1] tells us, that when the Branches are full of Sap, their Veins seem to apprehend the Iron, and stop when the Incision is made with that Metal, but flow freely when opened with a Stone, or a Piece of broken Pitcher : Lastly, *Marmol*[3] says, the Veins must be opened with Ivory or Glass. The Juice is white at first, afterwards becomes green, by degrees a Gold Colour, and when old the Colour of Honey. It is at first muddy, but by degrees grows clear, and of the Consistence of Turpentine. Its Smell is agreeable, and very brisk; its Taste bitter, sharp and astringent; it easily dissolved in the Mouth, and leaves no Stain on Woollen Cloth.

The *Balsam* commonly in Use is brought hither from *Cairo*, and is not properly the Gum, or Tears of the Tree, flowing by Incision, for it yields but little that way; but is prepared from the Wood and the green Branches of the Tree distilled; and yet even this is frequently adulterated with *Cyprus Turpentine* : Besides which, there is likewise a Liquor extracted from the Seed of the Plant, which is frequently passed off for the true *Balsam*, tho its Smell is much weaker, and its Taste much bitterer. The Tree is about the Height of a *Granada* Tree; its Leaves like those of the Rue, always green; its Flowers white, and in form of Stars, whence spring out little pointed Pods, inclosing a Fruit like an Almond, called *Carpobalsamum*, as the Wood is called *Xylobalsamum*, and the Juice *Opobalsamum*.

The Carpobalsamum enters the Composition of Treacle, having little other Use in Medicine : It must be chosen of an aromatick Taste and agreeable Smell. The Xylo-balsamum, which like the other Products of the Balsam-Tree, is brought from Cairo, is used in Troches of Hedycrum. 'Tis in little Faggots, the Bark red, the Wood white, and resinous, and aromatick. There is likewise a Balm of Mecca, which is a dry white Gum resembling Copperas, especially when old. 'Tis brought from Mecca by the Return of the Caravans of Pilgrims and Mahometan Merchants, who travel there out of Devotion to the Birth-Place of their Prophet. It has all the Virtues of the Balm of Gilead, or Judea; and is probably the same, only harden'd, and its Colour alter'd.

*Balsam of Peru* is of three Kinds; or rather, one and the same Balsam has three several Names, *viz. Balsam of Incision*, which is a white glutinous Resin ouzing at an Incision in the Tree, and afterwards thicken'd and harden'd. This is excellent for green Wounds, and much resembles the *Opobalsamum*, excepting in Smell, which distinguishes it.

*Dry Balsam*, which is distill'd from the Tips of Branches cut off, to which are fasten'd little Vessels to receive the Liquor, which at first is like Milk, but reddens by being exposed to the Sun. Its chief Use is in the Composition of the *Lac Virginale*, which is made much better with this, than with Styrax or Benjoin.

Lastly, *Balsam of Lotion*, which is blackish, and is drawn from the Bark, Roots, and Leaves of the Tree minced and boiled together. This is used

[1] Gaius Cornelius Tacitus (ca. 56 – 120), a Roman historian.

[2] Luis del Marmol (ca. 1520 – 1600), a Spanish historian and geographer.

in Wounds like the *white Balsam*; and on account of its excellent Smell, by the Perfumers.

Besides these two *Balsams*, which alone are to be esteemed genuine ones, Naturalists reckon *Balsam of Copais* or *Copayba*, of *Tolu* or *liquid Amber*, and a *New Balsam*. *Balsam of Copa, Copais, Campais*, or *Copayba*, comes from *Brasil* in earthern Bottles, pointed a-top. 'Tis a kind of Oil, either clear or thick; the first white, of a resinous Smell: the other a little more on the yellow; both are admirable for Wounds : The *Jews* use it after Circumcision to stop the Blood.

*Balsam of Tolu* is a liquid Resin, which as it grows old becomes of the Colour and Consistence of *Flanders* Size. It comes by Incision from some Trees growing in *New Spain*; where the Inhabitants receive it in little Vessels of black Wax : In Taste and Smell it resembles *Balm of Gilead*; as it grows old it takes the Consistence of *dry Balm*.

*Balsam of liquid Amber* is a clear reddish Resin, produced by a Tree in *New Spain*, called by the Natives *Ososol*, much resembling Ambergrease, especially in Smell, whence it Name. The New Balsam is liquid; when new it is called *Oil of liquid Amber*, and when old *Balsam of liquid Amber*; it comes from both the *Spains*, in Barrels; and is very rare among us : 'Tis found sovereign for Wounds, especially in *Fistulas in Ano* : It resembles *Balsam of Tolu* in Smell and Colour, and is express'd in the manner of *Oil of Laurel*, from a red Fruit in the Island of *St. Domingo*.

*Artificial* **BALSAMS**, in Pharmacy, are Medicines usually employ'd externally : In Consistence they somewhat exceed a common Unguent, and are prepared principally to recreate the nobler Parts, by their excellent Odor. There are some also of a more liquid Consistence, between an Oil and Liniment; the principle Use whereof is in Wounds : They are made various Ways, and of various Aromaticks and distill'd Oils; Oil of Nutmegs, or white Wax, are usually the Basis of *Balsams*; with these are mixed Deer's Grease, Manna, &c.

According to the different Intentions they are to answer, they acquire different Names, as *Apoplectick, Stomachick*, &c. *Balm* or *Balsam of Sulphur* is of two kinds, viz. that of *common Sulphur*, and that of *Sulphur with Anise* : the first is drawn by Fire from a Composition of Nut Oil drawn without Fire, Flowers of Sulphur, Oil of Tartar, and White Wine mix'd. This is used to digest and resolve crude Matters gathered in any Part of the Body : 'tis applied externally, and serves for the Basis of the Plaister of *Sulphur*.

*Balsam of Sulphur anisated*, is drawn from the Oil of green Anise and Flower of Sulphur dissolved together. *Balm of Saturn*, is a *Salt of Saturn*; Dr. *Harris* says, a *Sugar of Saturn*, dissolved in Oil or Spirit of Turpentine digested, till the Matter have acquired a red Tincture. This is found to resist the Putrefaction of Humours, and is good to cleanse and cicatrize Ulcers

**BALM** or **BALSAM**, among the Chymists, is the Spirit of common Salt extracted by Art. The Preparation is this : They dissolve the Salt, and place its Dissolution, well clarified, in Horse-Dung to purify, for the Space of two or three Months, and then distil it strongly with a Sand-Heat; upon which there arises a pretious Unctuosity, wherein Things the most corruptible being steep'd, are said to remain entire, eternally. 'Tis said, that 'twas by this means some of the Antients preserved dead Bodies entire without reducing 'em to Mummy, and particularly that of the Women mentioned by *Volaterran*[1] to be found in a Mausoleum near Albania, in the Time of Pope *Alexander* VI. which was by his Order thrown secretly into the *Tiber*, to prevent Idolatry; she being found as fresh as when alive, tho she had been dead 1300 Years.

**BALNEUM**, a Word much used by Chymists, generally signifying a Vessel of Water, in which another is placed that requires a more gentle Heat than the naked Fire.

*Balneum Mariæ*, is by some so called, as being supposed to have been first invented by the Blessed Virgin; but by others with more Propriety, *Balneum Maris*, or *Sea-Bath*, in regard the Vessel here floats on a kind of Sea. Here the Cucurbit is placed in hot Water, which warms the Matter contain'd. A Sand Heat is sometimes also called *Balneum siccum*, or *cineritium*, or *arenosum*.

**BALSAMICK**, a Term in Physick, signifying that Property in Medicine, whereby 'tis render'd soft, gently attenuating, and somewhat agglutinant.

**BARBOTINE**, a Grain, otherwise call'd *Semen Santonicum*, and *Semen contra Vermes*, or *Worm-Seed.*

**BASILICON**, in Pharmacy, is an Unguent so call'd, compos'd of Rosin, Wax, Pitch, and Oil; which the Surgeons use for a *Supperative.*

**BATRACHITES**, a Stone supposed to be found in Frogs, to which the antient Physicians and Naturalists attribute the Virtue of resisting Poison. The Word is form'd from the *Greek*, βατραχος, *rana*, a frog.

**BDELLIUM**, or *Bedellium*, a kind of Gum. The Name is well known among the Learned; but they can't agree what it is. 'Tis mention'd in *Genesis*[2], c. 2. c. 12. and *Josephus*[3] explains the Passage, by saying 'tis the Gum of a Tree resembling the Olive-Tree; and that the Manna wherewith the *Jews* were fed in the Desert, resembled this Drug : But *Scaliger* and others set aside this Explanation, and own, they don't know what the *Bdellium* mention'd in Scripture is.

The *Bdellium* in use among us, seems again to have been unknown to the Antients : Some say it distils from a kind of Thorn; others from a Tree resembling that which produces Myrrh. Some say it is produced on the Banks of the River *Senegal* in *Africa*; others, near the City *Saraca* in *Arabia Felix*[4]. When good, 'tis in clear transparent Pieces, of a reddish Grey without; when touch'd with the Tongue, yellow, bitter, soft, and odoriferous. It enters the Composition of *Mithridate*, and the *Emplastrum divinum*.

[1] Aulus Caecena de Volaterrae (ca. 69 BC), an Etruscan historian.

[2] "And the gold of that land is good : there is bdellium and the onyx stone." KJV

[3] Yosef ben Matityahu (ca. 37 – 100), a Jewish historian.

[4] The present-day country of Yemen.

**BEATING**, in Medicine, a Term applied to the Agitation or Palpitation of the Pulse or Heart. Some Physicians distinguish 81 different Kinds of Simple Beatings, and 15 Compound ones. They compute about 60 Beats in the Space of a Minute in a temperate Man.

**BECHICA**, Medicines proper for Diseases of the Lungs and Breast; frequently also call'd *Pectorals*. *Bechick* is also used for any thing relating to a Cough, &c. The Word comes from the Greek, βηξ, βηχος, *Cough*.

**BEN**, or *Behen*[1], a Name given to a Medicinal Root, rank'd among the Cardiacs and Counter-Poisons; and to an Oil express'd from this Root, used by Perfumers, &c. The Root of Ben is divided into white and red : The first is insipid, leaving only a little Bitterness behind it on the Tongue; the red is fibrous, brown without, and reddish within. They are both brought from Syria, and have the same Virtues, being substituted for each other; they must be chosen dry, and are of an aromatick, astringent Taste.

**BENJOYN**, or, as 'tis commonly called, *Benjamen*, an excellent kind of Resin, imported from the Kingdom of *Lao*, and other Parts of the *East-Indies*. 'Tis procured by a Wound or Incision in a Tree, whose Leaves resemble those the Lemmon-Tree. 'Tis of a yellowish Colour, of an agreeable Scent, and easy to melt. There are three Sorts of it : The first is call'd *Amygdaloides*, because of its being interspers'd with several white Spots which resemble broken Almonds : This comes from *Siam*. The second is black and very odoriferous; it drops from young Trees, and comes from *Sumatra*; 'tis call'd *Benzoinum de Boninas*. The third Sort is also black, but less odoriferous; this is found in the Islands of *Java* and *Sumatra*. 'Tis used in Physick, as a Pectoral and Anti-Asthmatick; and thrown on live Coals, it serves to perfume Houses, &c.

**BERGAMOT**, is a kind of Essence, drawn from a Fruit, produc'd by ingrafting the Lemmon-Tree on the *Bergamot-Pear* Stock. 'Tis no more than the oily Fluid of these Lemons express'd by the Fingers. There is likewise a kind of Snuff of the same Name, which is only clean Tobacco, with a little of the Essence rubb'd into it.

**BEZOAR**, or Bezoard, a Medicinal Stone, esteem'd a Sovereign Counter-Poison, and an excellent Cardiac. 'Tis also given in Vertigo's, Epilepsies, Palpitation of the Heart, Jaundice, Cholick, and so many other Diseases, that were its real Virtues answerable to its reputed once, it were doubtless a *Panacea*. Indeed, its Rarity, and the peculiar Manner of its Formation, have, perhaps, contributed as much to its Reputation, as any intrinsick Worth. At present it begins to be prized less, and a great many able Physicians discard it, as of no use or Efficacy at all.

There are several Kinds of *Bezoar*; the Chief are the *Oriental*, the *Occidental*, and that of *Germany*. The *Oriental* is in the most Esteem, and is brought from several Parts of the *East-Indies*, chiefly *Golconda*[2] and

[1] The kelor, or horseradish, tree (*Moringa oleifera*).

[2] Golconda, or Golkonda was an ancient Indian city in Andhra Pradesh, west of Hyderabad.

*Cananor*[1] : 'Tis there found mingled with the Dung of an Animal of the Goat Kind call'd *Pazan*; in the Belly whereof this Stone is found : The Buds of a certain Shrub which the Animal uses to brouze, are usually found in the middle of it, and supposed to be the Seed whence it arises. The *Bezoar* ordinarily grows of the Bigness of an Acorn, sometimes of that of a Pigeon's Egg. It is composed of several shining Skins, or Coats, like an Onion, sometimes of a Blood-Colour, sometimes a pale yellow, a brownish red, and Honey-Colour. The Number of *Bezoards* produced by each Animal is various, some yielding one, two, &c. to fix, and others none at all. The larger the Stone the more valuable its Price increasing like that of the Diamond. A Stone of one Ounce is sold in the *Indies* for 100 Franks, and one of four Ounces for 2000 Livres. *Oriental Bezoar* must be chose shining, of a Smell like that of Ambergrease, smooth to the Touch, and in large Pieces; its Figure is indifferent, its Colour usually Olive.

*Bezoar* is easily sophisticated, and the Deceat is easily discover'd. The Methods of proving it are, *1st*, to steep it three or four Hours in lukewarm Water; if the Water ben't ting'd, nor the *Bezoar* lose of its Weight, 'tis pure. *2dly*, To try it with a sharp, red hot Iron; if it enters the Stone, and the Heat makes it fry and shrivel, 'tis factitious. *3dly*, To rub it over a Paper smear'd with Cerusse; if it leave a yellow Teint, 'tis good.

*Occidental Bezoar*, or *Bezoar of Peru*, is very different from the first. 'Tis found in the Belly of several Animals, peculiar to the Country : In some 'tis the Bigness of a Nut, in others of a Pullet's Egg; in some 'tis oval, in others flat, in others round; 'tis usually of an Ash-Colour, sometimes dusky; and form'd of Scales, like the *Oriental*, but much thicker; 'tis smooth and even without-side, but when broke, looks as if it had been sublimated, by reason of the little shining Needles whereof it appears to be composed. The Animals that produce it are the Guanaco's, Jacho's, Vicunna's, and Taragua's; the *Bezoar* of which last is the most esteemed, this Animal being much like the Goat that produces the Oriental.

The *German Bezoar*, which some call *Cow's Eggs*, is found in the stomach of some Cows, but more frequently in that of the Chamois or Isard. These are supposed to be nothing else but the Hair of those Animals, which being occasionally lick'd off by the Tongue, is swallow'd down, and being impregnated with the Saliva, &c. is condens'd into Balls. Some of these *Bezoars* weight 18 Ounces, but they are not much esteem'd, tho they are useful in some Medicines, and by the Painters in Miniature, to make their yellow Colours.

Besides these three Kinds of *Bezoar* which the Shops afford, there are three other Kinds much rarer, *viz.* the *Stone of the Hog*, that of *Malacca* or *Porcupine*, and that of the Ape. The first call'd by the *Dutch*, *Pedro de Porco*, and by the *Portuguese*, who first brought it into *Europe*, *Pedro de Vaporis*, found in the Gall-Bladder of a Boar in the East-Indies. In Figure and Size it resembles a Filbert, tho more irregular; its Colour not fix'd, but most commonly white with a Teint of blue; it is smooth and shining. The *Indians* attribute infinite Virtues to this *Bezoar* : They call it *Mastica de Soho*, and prefer it to the *Oriental Bezoar*; not so much on account of its being

[1] Cananor, or Kannur, a town in south-east India in the state of Kerala.

supposed the best Preservative in the World against Poisons, as on account of its being Sovereign in the Cure of the *Mardoxi*, a Disease they are very liable to, and which is not less dangerous than the Plague in *Europe*. The other Properties they ascribe to it are, that 'tis admirable against malignant Fevers, Small Pox, and most Diseases of Women not with Child; Experience shewing that it promotes Abortion in those who use it indifferently. To use it, they infuse it in Water, or Wine, till it has communicated a little Bitterness to it. To facilitate the Infusion, and at the same time preserve so precious a Stone, they usually set it in a gold Case pierced with Holes.

*Bezoars of Porcupines* and *Monkies* only differ from those of the *Hog*, in that they are found in the Gall-Bladder of those Animals; unless we say with *Tavernier*[1], that these two, which he calls *Malacca-Stones*, are not taken from the Gall-Bladders, but the Head of the Monkey and Porcupine; and that they are held in such esteem by the Natives of *Malacca*, that they never part with 'em, unless as Presents to Ambassadors, or the greatest Princes of the East. Some add, that they are likewise found in Siam. Indeed, the Form, Colour and Properties of these three Bezoars are so near a-kin, that 'tis more than probable, that 'tis the same Stone under three different Names.

*Bezoar* is applied by the Chymists, to several of their Preparations, on account of the *Bezoardick* Qualities they are suppos'd to have.

*Animal* Bezoar is the Heart and Lungs of the Viper pulverized together.

*Mineral* Bezoar is an Emetick Powder of Antimony corrected with Spirit of Nitre, and softened by repeated Lotions, which carry off the purgative Virtue of the Antimony, and substitute a Diaphoretick one. It promotes Sweat like the Stone of that Name.

**BEZOARDICUM** *Joviale*, or *Bezoar of Jupiter*, a Regulus made by melting three Ounces of Regulus of Antimony and two of Block-Tin, which, powder'd and mix'd with six Ounces of Corrosive Sublimate, and distill'd off in a kind of Butter, and that dissolv'd in Spirit of Nitre, the Solution is distill'd three times; the *Bezoar* remaining at bottom, to be powder'd, wash'd, and mingled with Spirit of Wine, till it grow insipid.

**BEZOARDICUM** *Lunale*, or *of the Moon*, is made by mixing eight Ounces of rectified Butter of Antimony with one of fine Silver. This is dissolved in Spirit of Nitre, by gently pouring it on, fresh and fresh, till the Ebullition cease; when, the Spirit is drawn off by a gentle Heat, and the Bezoar manag'd as the former.

**BEZOARDICUM** *Martiale*, a Dissolution of *Crocus Martis* by Reverberation in Butter of Antimony, with Spirit of Nitre pour'd on it; the rest as in the first.

**BILE**, a yellow, bitter Juice separate from the Blood in the Liver, collected in the *Porus Bilarius*, and Gall-Bladder, and thence discharged by the Common Duct into the *Duodenum*.

The Bile is of two Kinds, *Hepatick* and *Cystick* : The first, properly call'd

[1] Jean-Baptiste Tavernier (1605 – 1689), a French traveller.

*Bile*, separated immediately from the Glands of the Liver into the *Porus Bilarius* : The second, call'd *Gall*, separated likewise from the Glands of the Liver into the Gall Bladder, by Roots or Ducts proper to itself. The *Cystick Bile* is thicker, a deeper yellow, and bitterer; is not evacuated continually, but only when its Receptacle is replete; in which Case the Contraction of the irritated Fibres propels it into the *Duodenum*. The *Hepatick* is thinner, more mild and pellucid, and is continually oozing out; being expell'd by the sole Actions of the neighbouring Humours.

The *Cystick Bile*, or Gall, resists Acids, and, mix'd with other Fluids, gives 'em the like Property : It absterges like Sope, and renders Oils capable of mixing of Water; it resolves and attenuates Resins, Gums, and other tenacious Bodies, rendering 'em homogeneal to itself. 'Tis neither alcalious nor acid, but seems a Concretion of Oil, Salt, and Spirits diluted with Water.

By a Chymical Analysis Dr. *Drake* observes, it affords some Sulphur, or Oil, some volatile Salt, a good deal of fix'd Salt, (in which particularly it differs from all other animal Liquors) and a pretty Quantity of *Caput Mortuum*, or Earth : the Basis is Phlegm. The Effect of the *Bile* is, by mixing with the Chyle and the Fæces, to attenuate, resolves, absterge, and stimulate the *Fibræ motrices*, to mix together things very different, to bruise and blunt those that are sharp and saline, to divide those that are coagulated, to open the Passages for the Chyle, to excite Appetite, to act the Part of a Ferment, and to assimilate crude things to things concocted. These Effects the *Cystick Bile* has in a greater, the *Hepatick* in a less Degree.

Dr. *Quincy* thinks their principal Use is to sheath and blunt the Acids of the Chyle, entangling them with its Sulphurs, so as to prevent their being sufficiently diluted in the Pancreatick Juice to enter the Lacteals : Which he thinks confirmed by this, that notwithstanding the great Quantity of acid Salts in the Aliment in the Stomach, there are never any found in the Chyle after it has pass'd the Duodenum, and been impregnated with the Chyle continually oozing out from the *Porus Bilarius*.

*Borelli*[1] asserts, that Part of the *Bile* discharged into the Intestines, re-enters the *Mesaraick* Veins, and mixing with the Blood of the *Vena Porta*, is again percolated thro the Liver; and *Boerhaave* seems of the same Opinion; Some will have the *Cystick Bile* brought to its Receptacle three different Ways, and that 'tis even composed of three different Kinds of *Bile*, whence its new Properties. *Boerhaave* takes those Properties to result from its stagnating in the Gall-Bladder; and, with *Malpighi*[2], thinks the bitter Part may probably take that Property in the Glandules between the Coats of the Gall-Bladder, which are furnish'd from the *Cystick* Arteries; whence it proceeds bitter, and mixes with the rest in the Bladder.

The *Bile* is the Juice of very great Importance, with regard to the good or ill Habitude of the Animal. Dr. *Woodward*[3] has traced its Effects throughout the Body very minutely, and makes no Scruple to ascribe most of the Diseases thereof to some Disorder of the *Bile*. This he takes to be the chief Spring in

[1] Giovanni Alfonso Borelli (1608 – 1679), an Italian physicist and anatomist.

[2] Marcello Malpighi (1628 – 1694), an Italian physician.

[3] John Woodward (1665 – 1728), an English physician and natural philosopher.

the Animal Machine, and from this accounts for most of the Phænomena of a Body, whether healthy or diseas'd : And yet the Antients took it to be no more than an Excrement, for which they could not find any Use. Many of the Moderns, from the small Quantity of *Bile* secern'd, have been led into a Mistake, that this Secretion is not the sole End of so considerable a Viscus as the Liver. Dr. *Keil* observes, that in a Dog whose common Duct was near as big as that of a Man, he gather'd at the Rate of about two Drams an Hour; tho in a human Body, there is Reason to think the Quantity secreted to be greater.

Sometimes the *Bile* from yellow becomes greenish, like Verdigreese, and frequently pale, like the Yolks of Eggs, and that without any other apparent Cause than a little Motion, a Convulsion, or a violent Passion of the Mind. This occasions many and terrible Diseases, as Nausea's, an Abhorrence of Food, Anxiety, Sighing, Cardialgia's, Wind, Diarrhea's, Dysenteries, acute Diseases, Fevers, and Convulsions. Sometimes it becomes black, and takes the Name of *Choler* : In this Case it sometimes tastes like a very sharp Vinegar; sometimes like putrified Blood, gnawing, burning, dissolving, consuming, occasioning Inflammations, Gangrenes, Mortifications, violent Pains, and terrible Fermentations.

Of *black Bile*, *Boerhaave* distinguishes three Kinds : First, the mildest, arising from the Matter of the Blood put in too great Motion, which hence takes the Name of *Adust* : The second is an Aggravation of the first arising from the same Causes, only heighten'd : The Third is a corrupt, parch'd *Bile*, which, if it arose from a greenish, or palish *Bile*, is still worse. Too great an Evacuation of the *Bile*, either upwards or downwards, robs the Chilefaction of its main Ingredient; hence it prevents Digestion, Secretion, Excretion of the Fæces, produces an acid Temperament, Cold Weakness, Paleness, Swoonings, &c. If when prepare it be prevented its Discharge into the Intestines, it produces a Jaundice.

For the Manner in which the Secretion of the *Bile* in the Liver is effected, there are various Opinions. Some maintain, that the Pores of the Secretory Glandules of the Liver, have a certain Configuration and Magnitude, to which the Particles of the *Bile* flowing in the Blood being just answerable, both in Bulk and Figure, are admitted in, and all the rest excluded. Others, with *Silvius* and *Lister*[1], not allowing any Difference in the Configuration, as knowing that the Pores of all Vessels are Circular, and that Particles of all Kinds will be admitted, if small enough, have recourse to a Ferment which they suppose to reside in the Liver, by means whereof the Particles of the Blood, in their Passage thro the Secretory Ducts, assume the Form of *Bile*. But as this is little else than begging the Question, others have recourse to another Hypothesis; maintaining, that the Fluids contain'd in the Blood of the *Vena Porta*, while that enters the Substance of the Liver in its way to the Extremities of the *Vena Cava*, indifferently apply to the Apertures of the Secretory Tubules contiguous to the extreme Branches of the *Porta*, which are wide enough, and to the Roots of the *Cava*, which are not wide enough, to receive 'em; by which means being separated from the Society and the intestine Motion of the other and the essential Parts of the Blood, and being

[1] Martin Lister (1638 – 1711), an English physician and naturalist

no longer agitated by the Vital Action of the Blood-Vessels, and exposed to the Action of the *Bilary* Vessels, they constitute a new Humour distinct from the Blood, call'd *Bile*, &c.

Lastly, Dr. *Keill* accounts for this Secretion of the *Bile* from the strong Attraction between the Particles whereof the *Bile* is composed. He observes, that the Heart and Liver being so near each other; were the *Cœliack* Artery to have carried all the Blood to the Liver, considering the Velocity of the Blood, so viscid a Secretion as the Bile cou'd never have been effected. Nature therefore forms a Vein for that purpose, *viz.* the *Porta*, and by its sends the Blood from the Branches of the *Mesenterick* and *Cœliack* Arteries to the Liver; by which the Blood is brought a great way about, passing through the Intestines, Stomach, Spleen, and Pancreas, e'er it arrives at the Liver : Thus its Velocity is exceedingly diminish'd, and the Particles that are to form the Gall have a sufficient time to attract one another, and unite before they come to their secerning Vessels. But, as if this Diminution of Velocity were not sufficient for the purpose, Nature has gone further; having made the Cavities of all the Arteries increase as they divide: thus the Sum of the Branches arising from the *Aorta*, is to the *Aorta* itself as 102740 to 100000.

And yet, as if that Proportion were to little for the present Purpose, Nature has here taken a further Step, and increas'd the Branches springing from the *Mesenterick* Artery in the greater Ratio. Thus, in a Body which he examined, he found the Sum of the Branches more than double that of the Trunk; and therefore the Velocity of the Blood in the former, must be less than half that of the latter. He further shews, from a just Calculation, that the Time the Blood now takes in its Passage from the *Aorta* to the Liver is at least 26 Minutes: whereas, had an Artery gone directly from the *Aorta* to the Liver, it would have passed in little more than half a Second, *viz.* in 2437 times the Space it now takes up in its Passage. Whence it appears, that the Blood was not in a Sate fit to yield *Bile*, had it gone directly from the *Aorta* to the Liver; and that a longer Time, and more languid Motion, was necessary to have the *Bilious* Particles in a readiness to the separated. He adds, that were the Humours separated by the Glands at all Times and Places the same in the Blood, and not form'd after this manner, Nature wou'd not have been at so much expence to retard the Blood's Velocity : Besides that, the *Bile* has another Advantage from the Use of the *Porta*; for, by running thro so many Parts e'er it reach the Liver, it leaves behind it most of its Lympha; by which means the Particles being brought nearer each other, are, by their mutual Attraction, sooner united.

The Word Bile comes from the *Latin Bilis*, which some fetch further from the *Greek* Βια, Violence, because *Bilious* People are inclined to Anger. Others fetch it from the *Latin bullire*, to boil. The *Bile* is a Part founding all Animals: even Pigeons, &c. which have no Gall-Bladder, yet have *Bile*; their Liver being found very bitter. M. *Tauvry*[1] observes, that the *Bile* becomes one of the principal Causes of Thirst, by mixing with the Salival Juice.

**BISMUTH**, a Mineral Body, half Metallick; compos'd of the first Matter of Tin, while yet imperfect; and found in Tin Mines. Its substance is hard,

[1] Daniel Tauvry (1669 – 1701), a French physician and anatomist.

heavy, sharp, and brittle, of a large Grain, polish'd white, and shining. 'Tis also call'd *Tin of Glass*; because, when broke, it shews a vast Number of little polish'd Substances like Glass: 'Tis also call'd *Marchasite*, by way of Excellence, because surpassing all others in Whiteness and Beauty. It contains an Arsenical Salt, very dangerous to take inwardly. Its Precipitate is a very white Magistery, which is mix'd with Waters and Pomatums to make a Fucus to beautify the Complexion, and preserver the Skin. There are also Flowers prepar'd from it, which take away Spots in the Face; whence 'tis otherwise call'd *Blanc de Perle*.

*Alonso Barba*[1] says, there has been lately found a Mine of *Bismuth* in *Bohemia*; and ranks it among the Metals : But *Bismuth* is properly the Regulus of the Stone call'd *Cobalt*; whence is prepar'd *Arsenick*, *Lapis Lazuli*, and *Bismuth*. M. *Stahl*[2], a *German* Physician, gives us its Preparation.

There is also an *Artificial Bismuth*, which is that ordinarily used, made by reducing Tin into thin *Laminæ*, or Plates, and cementing them by a Mixture of *white Tartar*, *Salt-Petre*, and *Arsenick*, stratified in a Crucible over a naked Fire. The same is also made of a Stone call'd *Zin*, using Lead instead of Tin, and a little Calamine Stone.

**BLEEDING**, an Operation in Chirurgery, consisting in the opening of a Vein with a Lancet, for the evacuation of corrupted or redundant *Blood*. *Bleeding* is the surest and most efficacious Species of Evacuants. It was very rare among the Antients, but is frequent among the Moderns. *Ostiensis* observes, that at Rome Persons of Quality are not allow'd *to be let blood*, even in their most dangerous Diseases, without Leave from the Pope. The *Hippopotamus* is said to have first taught Men the Use of *Bleeding* : For that Animal being overcharg'd with *Blood*, rubs herself against a pointed Bulrush, and opens a Vein; till finding her Plenitude discharged, she welters in the Mire to staunch the *Blood* again.

**BLOOD**, a warm, red Liquor or Humour, circulating, by means of Arteries and Veins, through every Part of the Body. While in its Vessels, it appears to the naked Eye, uniform and homogeneous; but, when let out and cold, separates spontaneously into two different Parts; the one red and fibrous, which coheres into a Mass, and is call'd the *Cruor*; the other thin and transparent, which retains its Fluidity when cold, and, being suppos'd specifically heavier than the other, sustains and bears it up, and is call'd the *Serum*. The Proportion of the *Serum* to the *Cruor*, Dr. *Drake* makes at a Medium, as one and half to one : But Mr. *Boyle*, more accurately, makes the Serum 11/15 of the whole *Blood*; and Dr. *Jurin*[3] 15/17 of the whole Weight, or 1/4 of the Bulk.

By the Microscope, the *Blood* appears to consists of little red Globules, swimming in an aqueous Liquor, suppos'd to be the Curor and Serum, that appear so distinct when let out. M. *Leewenhoeck*[4] computes these Globules to

[1] Alvaro Alonso Barba (1569 – 1662), a Spanish priest and metallurgist.

[2] Georg Ernst Stahl (1659 – 1734), a German physician and chemist.

[3] James Jurin (1684 – 1750), an English physician and scientist.

[4] Antony van Leeuwenhoeck (1632 – 1723), a Dutch scientist.

be twenty five thousand times smaller than the smallest Grains of Sand; and Dr. *Jurin* makes 'em still less. Upon an accurate Mensuration, he found the Diameter of one, equal to 1/1240 of an Inch, or 1/124 of an ordinary Hair of the Head. Dr. *Drake* thinks, that tho the rapid Motion of the *Blood* may make the *Cruor* appear round, and perhaps, by a kind of Whirling, or Rotation, really convolute 'em; yet that their Figure is not naturally Globular, when let out, as appears from their Cohesion, or hanging together in a Lump; which spherical Bodies, touching in a very few Points, are not apt to do : But, on the contrary, this Property, he thinks, argues an Implication of their Fibres within one another : Which is confirm'd by what Dr. *Adams*[1] observ'd by his Microscope, *viz.* that immediately after Emission of *Blood*, 'tis so far from exhibiting any red Globules, that it appears to consist of infinite Branches, running in no certain Order, and variously colour'd.

By a Chymical Analysis, the *Blood* is found to consist of *Phlegm*, as the Basis or Vehicle of Volatile Salts; of Oil, which, by some nice Examiners, has been found of two Kinds; and of *Caput mortuum*, or Earth; which, tho it may consist of divers Substances, essentially different from each other, yet all we get out of it is a little fix'd Salt. From the best Experiments in this kind it appears, that in seven Ounces of human Blood, there are five Ounces two Drachms of Phlegm, three Drachms of a subtile, spirituous Oil, two Grains of a thicker Oil, two Drachms of Salt, and about two of Earth. Dr. *Jurin* adds, that the *Serum*, upon a Chymical Analysis, exhibits a great deal of Phlegm, and of the other Principles a small Quantity; and, on the contrary, the *Cruor* yields less Phlegm, but the other Principles much more copiously than the Serum. From which Data he concludes, that the Globules consist of some Phlegm united with the Oil and Salts, and a small Quantity of Earth; but in what Proportion, and how, and in what Parts they are form'd, &c. is not determin'd.

Indeed, it must be consider'd, that the Principles which the Chymists thus produce separate, may possibly be much alter'd by the Fire. Thus, 'tis past doubt, the Oils drawn from the *Blood* by Fire, are vastly different from the natural Oil which circulates with the *Blood*. To which may be added, that the *Caput mortuum* remaining after Distillation, may, possibly, be a new Production, which had no Existence under any Form resembling that in the *Blood*.

**BOLE**, in Medicine, is us'd, in the general, for several Kinds of Earths that enter Galenical Preparations, and are used by Painters and other Artists.

*Bole-Armoniac*, or *Ammoniac*, is a kind of Earth, of considerable Medicinal Virtue, brought from *Armenia*. The Physicians sometimes call it *Rubrica Synopica*, from the City of *Synope*, where it is suppos'd to be found. 'Tis of a pale red Colour, and partakes much of the Nature of Stone; but soft, fat, friable, easily pulveriz'd, and sticks to the Tongue. 'Tis esteem'd Desiccative and Stiptic; in which Quality 'tis us'd in several Diseases, both internal and external. This *Bole* is easily falsify'd, and the Merchants frequently sell *Lemnian-Earth* in lieu thereof. *Matthiolus* says, 'tis found in Gold, Silver, and Copper Mines.

[1] George Adams Sr. (ca. 1730 – 1773), an English optician and instrument maker.

*Bole of the Levant*, is a Medicinal Earth brought from the Levant; nearly of the same Nature, and having the same Uses with the *Bole-Armoniac*. *Pomet*[1] says, there is no such thing among us, as either true *Bole-Armoniac*, or *Bole of the Levant*; and that all the *Boles* now in use, are brought either from the Provinces of *France*, or the neighbouring Countries. But this does not seem sufficiently warranted; and the New *Tarifs*, or Duties on Goods imported into *France*, which mention 'em both, make it credible that there are of either kind imported into that Kingdom. Indeed, it appears, that 'tis the *Levant Bole* which passes among us for the *Armoniac* : It enters several Compositions, particularly *Diascodium*, to give it the Colour, &c.

**BOLT-HEAD**, the same as Matras; a Vessel used by the Chymists.

**BORAX**, a Mineral Salt, used in soldering, brazing, and casting Gold and other Metals; known to the Antients under the name of *Chrysocolla*. *Pliny* divides *Borax* into Natural and Artificial : The *Natural*, according to him, is only a flimsy Humor running in Mines of Gold, Silver, Copper, and even Lead; which being congeal'd and harden'd by the Winter's Cold, becomes of the Consistence of Pumice-Stone. For *Artificial Borax*, he says, 'tis made by letting Water run in the Veins of the Mine, all the Winter long, till *June*; and letting the Mine dry, the rest of the Year. So that Artificial *Borax*, according to him, is no more than the Mineral putrify'd and corrupted. The same Author distinguishes *Borax* into Black, Green, Yellow, and White; assuming their several Colours, as well as Values, from the several Mines whereof they are form'd. The Natural, according to him, is heavier than the Factitious.

The Moderns, in like manner, distinguish two Kinds of *Borax*; *Natural*, call'd Crude; and *Artificial*, which is purify'd and refin'd. The Natural is a Mineral Salt, of the common Form, dug out of the Earth in several Parts of *Persia*; and found also at the Bottom of a Torrent, running in the Mountains of *Purbeth*, near the *Frontiers* of *White Tartary* : When taken up, 'tis expos'd to the Air; where it acquires a kind of reddish Fat, which serves to feed it, and prevent its calcining. When in its Perfection, 'tis sent to *Amadabat*, in the Territories of the Great *Mogol*, where the *European* Merchants buy it. There is another kind of *Artificial Borax*; drier, and of a greyish Colour, like *English* Copperas; only differing from the former, by its being longer expos'd to the Air.

For Artificial *Borax*, it was the *Venetians* who first found out the Art of preparing it; or, rather, of purifying the Natural : 'Tis done by dissolving it in Water; then filtrating and crystallizing it : using, for that purpose, Cotton Matches; about which the *Borax* crystallizes, like Sugar candy and Verdigrease on Wood. The *Dutch*, after refining it, reduce it into little Pieces, like tagged Points; and 'tis thus commonly us'd.

*Borax*, refin'd either in the *Dutch* or *Venetian* manner, should be clear and transparent, almost insipid to the Taste; and above all, Care must be taken it have no Mixture of *English* Allom. *Borax* is of some use in Medicine, as it enters the Composition of the Unguent *Citrin*. 'Tis also used in the

[1] Pierre Pomet (1658 – 1699), a French apothecary, chemist and botanist.

Prepararation of a Fucus for the Ladies.

*Agricola*[1] says, there is a fossile Nitre, as hard as that whereof the *Venetians* make *Borax* : In which he has Reason; this Nitre being nothing but the *Persian Borax* abovemention'd. What he adds, that the *Venetian Borax* is made of the Urine of young People who drink Wine, beat in a Mortar to the Consistence of an Unguent; then mix'd with Iron Rust and Nitre : is not only false, but it is a Misrepresentation of a Passage in *Pliny, Hist. Nat.* L. 33. c. 5.

**BRASIL** or Brazil, a Wood so call'd, because first brought from *Brasil*, a Province of *S. America* : It is denominated variously, according to the Places whence it is brought. Thus we have *Brasil* of *Fernambouc*[2], *Brasil* of *Japon*, of *Lamon*, of St. *Martha*; and lastly *Brasillet*, brought from the *Antilles*.

The *Brasil* Tree ordinarily grows in dry barren Places, and in the middle of Rocks; it is very thick and large, usually crooked and knotty : Its Flowers, which are of a beautiful red, exhale a very agreeable Smell, which strengthens the Brain. Tho the Tree be very thick; it is cover'd with so thick a Bark, that when the Savages have taken it off the Wood, a Trunk, which before was the Thickness of a man, is scarce left equal to that of his Leg.

*Brasil* Wood is very heavy, dry, crackles much in the Fire, and scarce raises any Smoak, by reason of its extreme Dryness. None of the several Kinds have any Pith, except that of the *Japon* : that of *Fernambouc* is esteem'd the best. It must be chosen in thick Pieces, close, sound, without any Bark; and such as, upon splitting, of pale becomes reddish; and when chew'd has a sugar Taste. It is much us'd in Turned Works, and takes a good Polish; but its chief use is in Dying, where it serves for a read Colour : 'Tis a spurious Colour, however, it gives; and easily evaporates and fades : Nor is the *Wood* to be us'd without Allum and Tartar. From the *Brasil* of *Fernambouc*, is drawn a kind of *Carmine*, by means of Acids. There is also a liquid *Lacca* made of it, for Miniature.

**BRASS**, *Orichalcum*; or as the *French* call it, *Yellow Copper*; a factitious Metal, compos'd of Copper, and *Lapis Calaminaris*. The Method of Preparation is as follows. The *Lapis* being calcin'd, and ground fine as Flour, is mix'd with ground Charcoal; and incorporated, by means of Water, into a Mass : Thus prepar'd, about seven Pounds of the *Calamine* is put into a Melting-Pot of about a Gallon; and over it, about five Pounds of *Copper*; which is let down into a Wind-Furnace eight Foot deep, remaining there about 11 Hours; in which Time 'tis converted into *Brass*. After melting, it is cast into Plates, or Lumps : 45 Pounds of crude *Calamine*, produces 30 Pounds burnt, or calcin'd. The sometimes use *Brass-shruff* instead Copper; but that is not always to be procur'd in Quantities sufficient, being no more than a Collection of Pieces of old *Brass*.

Pure *Brass* is not malleable unless hot; when cold it breaks : After melting twice, 'tis no longer in a Condition to bear the Hammer at all : to work it, they put 7 Pounds of Lead to 100 of *Brass*; which renders it more soft and pliable. *Brass* is us'd in the casting of Guns : The best Proportion for Gun-Metal, 'tis

[1] Georgius Agricola, born Georg Bauer (1494 – 1555), a German physician and scientist.

[2] Pernambuco is a state in the north-east of Brazil.

said, is for 11 or 12 thousand Weight of Metal, to use ten thousand Pound of *Brass*.

The best *Brass* Guns are made of malleable Metal, not of pure Copper and *Calamine* alone; but it is necessary to add coarser Metals, to make it run close and sounder, such as Lead and Pot-Metal. Bell-Metal is a Composition of *Brass* and Tin : and Pot-Metal of *Brass* and Lead; 20 Pound of Lead, is usually put into 100 Pound of Pot-Metal. The Manufacture of *Brass*, was kept a Secret in *Germany* for many Ages.

*Brass of Corinth*, has been famous in all Antiquity : *L. Mummius*[1] having sack'd and burnt that City, 146 Years before our Saviour's Time, 'tis said this precious Metal was form'd from the immense Quantities of Gold, Silver, and Copper wherewith *Corinth* abounded, thus melted and run together by the Violence of the Conflagration. The Statues, Vessels, &c. form'd of this Metal were inestimable. Those who speak of it accurately, distinguish it into three Kinds; in the first, Gold is the prevailing Metal, in the second Silver; in the third, Gold, Silver, and Copper, are equally blended.

*Oil of* **BRICKS**, is an Oil of Olives, imbib'd by the Substance of *Bricks*, and afterwards distill'd from it. The Pieces of *Brick* being heated red hot in live Coals, are extinguish'd in an Earth half saturated with Oil of Olives : Being then separated and pounded grossly, the *Brick* imbibes the Oil. 'Tis then put in a Retort, and plac'd in a Reverberatory Furnace; and by Fire is drawn an Oil, which the Apothecaries call *Oleum de Lateribus*; and the Chymists, *Oil of Philosophers*, us'd to resolve Tumors, in the Spleen, in Palsies, and Epilepsies.

**BRONCHOCELE**, a Tumor, with a large round Neck, rising on the *Bronchial* Part of the *Trachea*, very frequent in the *Alps* : The *Latins* call it *Hernia Gutturis*. The Word is form'd from the *Greek* βρογχος, *Bronchia*, Windpipe; and κηλη, swelling.

**BRYONY**, the Root of a Plant of the same kind with the *Mechoaca* : It was formerly in great Reputation as a Purgative; but has now lost the greatest part thereof; yet it evacuates pretty strongly, sometimes by Vomiting, but more frequently by Urine : Whence some Authors recommend it, as excellent for purging Serosities; and even as a Specifick in the Dropsy.

M. *Boulduc* found, by a Chymical Analysis, that it consisted only of saline Principles, without any Resin : Wherein it differs from *Mechoacan*, which, in other respects, it much resembles. He adds, it has more virtue taken in Substance than in any other manner; which is common to this and other Purgatives.

**BUBO**, in Medicine, a Tumor arising on the Glands of the Groin and Armpits, with Inflammation and Pain; owing to the overflowing of the Blood in those Glands, mix'd with some peccant Humour. There are two Kinds of *Bubo's*, the one call'd *Benign*, or Mild, the other *Malignant*. Malignant, are divided into *Pestilential* and *Venereal* : Pestilential *Bubo's* arise on a

[1] Lucius Mummius (ca. 150 BC), a Roman statesman and general.

Pestilential Fever, &c. Venereal *Bubo's* are the Product of impure Embraces; and frequently the Forerunner of the Pox. When a *Bubo* is encompass'd with a Circle of several Colours, 'tis a Sign it is Pestilential, and generally Mortal. The Word comes from the *Greek* βουβων, *Inguen*; the usual Place of such Tumors.

**BUBONOCELE**, a Tumor arising in the Groin; occaison'd by the Descent of the Epiploon or Intestines. 'Tis a Species of Hernia or Rupture; tho Chirurgeons call it an Incomplete one; and is common to Women as well as Men. The Word comes from the Greek βουβων, *Inguen*, and κηλη, Tumor.

**BULIMY**, Boulimia, a Disease, occasioning a disorderly and ravenous Appetite; call'd so *Appetitus Caninus*. In the Philosophical Transactions, we have an Account of a Person affected with a *Bulimy*, insomuch that he wou'd eat up an ordinary Leg of Veal at a common Meal, and feed on Sow-thistles, &c. cur'd by giving up several Worms, of the Length and Thickness of a Tobacco-Pipe. The Word comes the *Greek* βους, *bos*, and λιμος, Hunger; as if the Patient had an Appetite sufficient to eat an Ox.

**BURN**, in a Medical Sense, a Solution of the Continuity of a Part of the Body by the Impression of Fire : or a Mark remaining in the Thing burnt. Of Burns, Physicians make several Degrees : The first, when there are only a few Pustules rais'd on the Skin, with a Redness, and a Separation of the *Epiderma* from the genuine Skin. The second when the Skin is burnt, dried, and shrunk, but without any Crust or Scab. The third is, when the Flesh, Veins, nerves, &c. are shrunk and form a Scab. *Lusitanus*[1] recommends an Unguent, made of the Ashes of Lawrel leaves burnt, with Hog's Fat dropp'd on 'em, for *Burn*; or, on occasion, the Unguent *Populeum*, with Vine Leaves laid over it.

*Panarole*[2] observes, that Clay laid on a *Burn* abates the Pain; and the Brewers in Holland, use a Decoction of Ivy for the Cure of *Burns*.

*Burns*, however, are not only Diseases, but in some Cases Remedies. M. *Homberg* observes, that on the Isle of *Java*, the Natives cure themselves of a Cholick, otherwise Mortal, by *burning* the Soles of their Feet; and cure themselves of a *Panaris*, by dipping their Finger in boiling Water several times. Travellers relate many other Cases of other Diseases cur'd by *burning* : And we see the Effects of it in our selves, in Horses, Hounds, Birds of Prey, &c. A kind of Moss, brought from the Indies, has been likewise us'd for Gout; apply'd, by *burning* it on the Part affected : and M. *Homberg* gives us an Instance of two Women cur'd, the one of a violent Disease in the Head and Eyes, and the other of a Disease in the Legs an Thighs, by the accidental burning of those Parts. He adds, that burning may cure in three manners; either by putting the peccant Humours into a greater Motion, and making 'em take new Routs; or by dissolving and braking their Viscidity, or by destroying the Canals which brought them in too great Quantities.

[1] This is probably Zacutus Lusitanus, born Abraham ben Samuel Zacutus (1575 – 1642), a Portuguese physician.

[2] Domenico Panaroli (1587 – 1657), an Italian physician and herbalist.

**BURNING**, or Brenning, in our antient Customs, was an infectious Disease, got in the Stews, by conversing with leud Women; suppos'd to be the same with that we now call the *Venereal Disease* : Whence that Disease is argu'd to be much more antient than the common Epocha of the Siege of *Naples*.

The chief Objection against Burning being the same with the venereal Disease, is, that the Remedies prescrib'd against the former, would be ineffectual in the latter : But, beside that it is not to be expected, the Measures of the antient Physicians should be calculated for the removing of any Malignity in the Mass of Blood or other Juices, as in the Modern Practice; inasmuch as they look'd on the Disease as merely local, and the whole of the Cure to depend on the Removal of the Symptoms : Besides this, it is matter of frequent Observations, that some Diseases grow more violent, and others more remiss in the course of time : So that the Remedies which might have avail'd so the antient *Brenning*, may now fail as to the modern Pox.

The Process for the Cure, as deliver'd by *J. Arden*[1], Chirurgeon to K. *Henry* IV. is thus. *Contra* Incendium *Virgae Virilis interius ex calore & excoriatione fiat talis syringa (i.e. injectio) lenitive. Accipe lac Mulieris masculum nutrientis & parum zacarium, Oleum Viole & Ptisaneae : quibus commixtis per Syringam infundatur.*

In an antient MS. written about the Year 1300, is a Receipt for *Brenning of the Pyntyl yat Men clepe the Apegalle*; Galle being an old Word for a running Sore. And in another MS. written 50 Years after, is a Receipt for *Burning in that Part by a Woman.* Simon Fish, a zealous Promoter of the Reformation, in his Supplication of Beggars, presented to K. *Henry* VIII. 1530, speaking of the Romish Priests, says, *They catch the* Pocks *of one Woman, and bare 'em to another; they be* burnt *with one Woman, and bar it to another : They catch the* Lepry *of one Woman, and bare it to another*. And Boord, a Priest and Physician in the same Reign, geins one of his Chapters of his Breviary of Health, thus : The 19th Chapter doth shew of the burning of an Harlotte. The same Author adds, that if a Man be burnt with an Harlot, and do meddle with another Woman within a Day, he shall burn the Woman he shall meddle withal : And as an immediate Remedy against the Burning, he recommends the washing the Pudenda two or three times with Whitewine, or else with Sack and Water. In another MS. of the Vocation of *John Bale* to the Bishoprick of *Ossory*, written by himself, he speaks of Dr. *Hugh Weston* (who was Dean of Windsor in 1556, but deprived by Cardinal *Pole* for Adultery) thus : "At this Day is leacherous Weston, who is more practis'd in the Art of Breech-burning than all the Whores of the Stews. He not long ago brent a Beggar of St. Bardolph's Parish."

**BUTTER**, in Chymistry, is us'd to express several Preparations in Chymistry, as *Butter* of Antimony, of Arsenic, of Wax, of Saturn, &c. so call'd from their Form, Consistence, &c.

[1] John Arderne (ca. 1307 o 1390), an English physician and surgeon to Richard II and Henry IV.

**CACAO**, or Cocoa, in Natural History and Commerce, a kind of Nut, about the size of a moderate Almond; the Seed or Fruit of a Tree of the same Name, growing in several Parts of the *West-Indies*; chiefly in the Provinces of *Guatimala* and *Nicaragua*, and the *Antilles* Islands. The native *Mexicans* call the *Cacao* Tree, *Cucubua guahuitl*; and the *Spaniards*, *Cacaotal*. It resembles our Cherry-Tree; but is so very delicate, and the Soil it grows in so hot, that to guard it from the Sun, they always plant it in the Shade of another Tree, call'd *Mother of Cocoa*.

The Fruit is enclos'd in a kind of Pod, of the Size and Figure of a Cucumber; except that it begins and ends in a Point. Within the Pod, which is half a Finger thick, is form'd a Tissue of white Fibres, very succulent, a little acid, and appear to appease Thirst. In the middle of these Fibres are contain'd 10, sometimes 12, and sometimes more, as far as forty, Grains or Seeds, of a Violet Colour, and dry as Acorns. Each Grain, which is cover'd with a little Bark or Rind, when stripp'd thereof, separates into five or six unequal Pieces, in the middle whereof is a Kernel or Pippin, having a tender Bud, very difficult to preserve. Of this Seed, with the Addition of *Vanille*, and some other Ingredients, the *Spaniards*, and, after their Example, the rest of *Europe*, prepare a Kind of Conserve, or Cake; which, diluted in hot Water, makes that delicious, wholesom Drink, call'd *Chocolate*.

This precious Almond, the *Spaniards* make so considerable a Trade of, that there are some make 5000 *l*. Sterling, *per Annum*, from a single Garden of *Cacoa's*. There are two kinds of *Cacoa's*; the most common, which is likewise the best, is of a dark Colour, bordering on red, and round : The other, call'd *Patlaxe*, is white, larger, thicker, and flatter; its Quality is Desiccative. Some Druggists, however, sell four Kinds; *viz*. the *great* and *little Carague*, and the *great* and *little Cacoa of the Islands* : which, however, may be probably reduc'd to the two Kinds above mention'd : It being only the Greatness and Smallness that multiples the Names and Kinds.

The *Cacao* Nuts, are esteem'd by the *Mexicans* as Anodine; and us'd, eaten raw, to assuage Pains of the Bowels. They also procure a kind of Butter or Oil from 'em, as sweet as that of Almonds, and drawn in the same manner; excellent for Burns. In some Parts of *America*, the *Cacoa* Grains are us'd by the *Indians* as Money; 12 or 14, are esteem'd equivalent to a *Spanish Real*, or 6&1/4 Sterling.

**CACHEXIA**, or Cachexy, in Medicine, an ill Habit or Disposition of Body; wherein, the Nutrition is deprav'd throughout the whole Habit, at once : frequently leading towards a Dropsy; and accompany'd with a Swelling, or Bloating of the fleshy Parts; a paleness or lividness of Complexion, &c. It ordinarily arises from a Debility, or Foulness of the *Ventricle* or *Viscera*; sometimes from an Ulcer in the Reins, in Persons that have the Stone. The external Causes are unwholesom Food, frequent Drunkeness, excessive Study, much waking, suppression of the Menses, immoderate Loss of Blood, Chronic Fevers, Obstruction, &c.

*Boerhaave* ascribes the Disorder, either to the vitiated State of the nutritious Juice, to some Disorder of the Vessels that are to receive it, or to the Defect of the Faculty that shou'd apply it. The Juice, he observes, may be deprav'd, either from the Quality of the Food; as if it be farinaceous, leguminous, fat, fibrous, sharp, aqueous, or viscous; from the want of Motion; from the Organs vitiated by too much Weakness, or too much Strength : And these, again, may be occasion'd by immoderate Secretions, and Evacuations of any Kind, the Schirrosity of some of the Viscera, or the Retention of something that should be secern'd : And hence, a Diminution of the Solids, or a Repletion of the Liquids with things that can't pass : Whence two notable ill Effects of this Evil; *viz.* a Leucophlegmatia, and an Anasarcous Dropsy. Now, according to the various Colour, Quantity, Tenacity, Acrimony, and Fluidity of the nutritious Liquor, arise various Disorders, as the Effects of the *Cachexia*; *e.g.* paleness, yellowness, lividness, greenness, blackness, or redness of the Skin; heaviness, windiness, palpitation of the Heart and Arteries, increas'd with the least Motion; crude thin Urine; spontaneously watry Sweats; and, at length, a Luecophlegmatia and Dropsy.

For the Vessels that receive the nutritious Juice, there can't well be assign'd any universal Fault; unless their too great Contractility and Laxity, and the Disorders accruing from 'em, may be admitted as such. Lastly, Nutrition is impeded and perverted, by a Defect in the Faculty that should apply it; as when the circulating Force is either too languid or too violent. The Word comes from the *Greek* καχεξια; form'd from the *Greek* κακη, *ill*, and εξις, *Disposition*. The Cachexia is more frequently call'd *Cacochymia*.

**CACHOU**, a medicinal Aromatic Drug, rank'd among the Number of Perfumes; call'd also *Terra Japonica*. Notwithstanding the great use of *Cachou*, before that of Coffee and Tea; and its being still frequently us'd by many People, especially in *France*, its Nature and Origin is yet but little known; even among the ablest Physicians : Some from its being call'd *Japon Earth*, rank it among the medicinal Earths, and pretend 'tis found on the Tops of Mountains, cover'd with the Roots of Cedars, whose Food it is : and that being wash'd in the River, and dry'd in the Sun, 'tis form'd into a kind of Paste; which brought into Europe, serves as the Basis of several Pastels, or Fucus's, call'd *Cachou*.

Others, with more Probability, range it among the Gums; and maintain it to be form'd of the inspissated Decoction of a Tree in the *East Indies*, call'd *Cachous*; growing chiefly in the Kingdom of *Cochinchina*. Lastly, others, to whose Opinion we rather incline, take it to be a factitious Composition of several other Drugs; especially the Juice of Areca, Extract of Liquorice, and *Calamus Aromaticus*, and the Bark of a Tree, call'd by the Indians *Catechu*; which may probably be the same with that above mention'd.

Be it Earth, Gum, or Composition, Cachou is of much esteem in Medicine : Among other Effects attributed to it, 'tis supposed to stop a Cough, and fortify the Stomach; besides its sweetening and perfuming the Breath, when taken in an impalpable Pouder, mix'd with Gum Tragacanth.

**CACOCHYMIA**, a deprav'd Habit of Body, consisting in its being replete with ill Humors, from various Causes; see Cachexia. When the Repletion is merely with Blood, 'tis call'd a *Plethora*. *Gorræus*[1] give the name *Cacochymia*

[1] Johannes Gorraeus, born Jean de Gorris (1505 – 1564), a French physician.

to the Abundance and Excess of any ill Humor; whether it be Bile, Pituita, &c. provided there be only one that thus offends in Quantity : *Plethora* he calls the Abundance or Excess of all the Humors together. The Word comes from the *Greek* κακος, *ill*, and κυμος, Juice.

**CADMIA**, in Pharmacy, a Mineral, whereof there are two Kinds, *viz. Natural* and *Artificial* : the *Natural Cadmia*, again, is of two Kinds; the one, containing Metallic Parts, and call'd *Cobalt*; which see : The other containing none, call'd *Calamine*, or *Lapis Calaminaris*; which see.

The *Artificial Cadmia* is prepar'd from Copper, in Furnaces; of this there are five Kinds; the first call'd *Botrytis*, as being in form of a Bunch of Grapes; the second, *Ostracitis*, as resembling a Sea-shell; the third, *Placitis*, because resembling a Crust; the fourth, *Capnitis*; and the fifth, *Calamitis*, which hangs round certain Iron Rods, wherewith the Matter of the Copper is stirr'd in the Furnace; which being shaken off, bears the Figure of a Quill, call'd in Latin, *Calamus*. The *Cadmia Botrytis* is found in the Middle of the Furnace; and *Ostrytis* at the Bottom; the *Placitis* at the Top; and the *Capnitis* at the Mouth of the Furnace.

*Cadmia* is desiccative and detersive, us'd in moist stinking Ulcers; which by means hereof are brought to *cicatrize*. The *Botrytis* and *Placitis*, are also very good in Diseases of the Eyes.

**CALAMINARUS LAPIS**, *Calamine Stone*, *Calamite*, or *Cadmia*, a kind of fossile bituminous Earth, of some use in Medicine, but of more in Foundery; being us'd to dye Copper yellow, *i.e.* to convert it into Brass. It is either of a greyish Colour, as that of *Germany* and *England*; or reddish, as that about Liege, and in some Parts of *France*; accounted the best, because yellow by Calcination.

It is dug out of Mines, usually in small Pieces; having always Eyes, sometimes Veins, of Lead usually; tho not always found in Lead Mines. We have Mines of *Calamine* at *Wrington* in *Somersetshire*. It is generally dug in barren rocky Ground; its Courses running, usually, at 6 a-Clock, as they call it, *i.e.* from East to West; sometimes at 9, and sometimes at 12; or perpendicular, which is accounted the best. When dug, it is wash'd, or *buddled*, as they call it, in a running Water, which carries off the impure and earthy Parts; leaving the Lead, *Calamine*, and other sparry Parts at bottom : They then put it in a Sieve, and shaking it well in Water, the Lead mix'd with it sinks to the bottom, the sparry Parts get to the top, and the *Calamine* lies in the middle : Thus prepar'd, they bake it in an Oven four or five Hours; the Flame being so contriv'd as to pass over, and so heat and bake the *Calamine*; stirring and turning it all the while with Iron Rakes. This done, they beat it to a Pouder; picking out of it what Stones they find; and this it is fit for use.

Besides the two *Natural Calamines*, there are Artificial ones : The best is that call'd *Pompholix*.

*Calamine* is of some medicinal Virtue, being astringent, desiccative, and detersive; much us'd for taking off Films from the Eyes of Horses, &c.

**CALAMITA**, in Pharmacy, a Term sometimes us'd for Styrax, because frequently put up in Quills.

**CALAMUS** *Aromaticus*, call'd also *Calamus Verus*, and *Calamus Amarus*, and *Acorus*; a kind of Rush, of the Thickness of a Goose's Quill, two or three Foot high, growing in the *Levant*. Its chief, and almost only use, is for Treacle: It must be chosen grey-whitish without, and reddish within; its Pulp white, and its Taste insupportably bitter.

**CALCANTHUM**, is Vitriol rubify'd. Some maintain *Calcanthum* and *Colcothar* to the same Thing : but *Pomet* is of another Sentiment, and takes *Calcanthum* to be nothing else but Vitriol.

**CALCINATION**, the Action of *calcining* any Matter; *i.e.* of reducing it into a *Calx*, or a very subtile Pouder, or even only into Ashes, by Fire; sometimes also termed *Chymical Pulverization*.

*Calcination* is the next degree of the Power of Fire beyond that of *Fusion* : For when Fusion is longer continu'd, not only the more subtile Particles of the Body it self fly off, but the Particles of Fire likewise do insinuate themselves in such Magnitude, and are so dispersed and blended throughout its whole Substance, that the Fluidity which was first caus'd by the Fire, can no longer subsist : From this Union arises a third kind of Body, which being very porous and brittle is easily reduc'd to Pouder. For the Fire having penetrated every where into the Pores of the Body, the Particles are both hinder'd from mutual contact, and divided into minute Atoms; so that they are easily reducible into the finest Pouder.

Chymists, Goldsmiths, and Founders, distinguish two Kinds of *Calcination*; the one call'd *Actual*, the other *Potential*. Actual *Calcination*, is that effected by actual Fire, of Wood, Coals, or other Fuel, rais'd to a certain Heat, according to the Nature of the Substance to be calcin'd. Potential *Calcination*, is that procur'd by potential Fire, *viz.* by Waters, Drugs, &c. which have, as it were, the Force of Fire; as Strong Waters, Corrosive Spirits, &c. Gold is calcin'd in the Fire of a Reverberatory, with Mercury, and Sal Ammoniac. See Gold. Silver with common Salt and Alkali Salt. Copper with Salt and Sulphur; Iron with Sal Ammoniac and Vinegar; Tin with Antimony, Lead and Sulphur; Mercury with Aqua fortis : This last, also, with most other Minerals, *calcines* with Fire alone, without any other Ingredients.

*Calcination Philosophical*, is when Horns, Hoofs, &c. are hung over boiling Water, or other Liquor, till they have lost their Mucilage, and are easily reducible into Pouder.

**CALCULUS**, in Medicine, the Disease of the Stone in the Bladder, or Kidneys; In the Bladder 'tis usually call'd *Lithiasis*; and in the Kidneys, *Nephritis*. The Term is pure *Latin*, and signifies, literally, a little Pebble, or Flint. Whence also the Term *Calculation*.

**CALEFACTION**, a School Term for the Action of Fire in heating a Body : 'tis us'd particularly in Philosophy and Pharmacy; where *Calefaction* is distinguish'd from *Coction*; the first being apply'd, where the thing is only heated without boiling.

**CALENTURE**, is an inflammatory Fever, frequent at Sea, attended with a Delirium; wherein the Patients imagine the Sea to be green Fields; and, if not prevented, will leap over-board : which way they are frequently lost.

**CALIDUM** *Innatum*, or Innate Heat; a Term the Antients had may vague Notions about : but Geometrical Reasoning has taught is to affix a more distinct Idea hereto : For 'tis hence we know, that this *innate Heat* is no more than the Attrition of the Parts of the Blood; occasion'd by its circulatory Motion, especially in the Arteries; wherein, being propell'd from a circular Base, towards the Apex of an hollow Cone, with a Force begin in the Heart, it meets with a double Resistance; *viz.* against the Sides of the Arteries, and against the preceding Blood.

For whereas the Blood contains in it Parts that are fitted to excite Heat, whenever they can get at liberty; that is, if the Parts inclosing them can be got asunder : and whereas the Parts inclosing such Corpuscles cannot be got asunder, unless by some Nisus of the Parts of Blood with one another, whereby the Attrition and Abrasion of the cohering Particles is produc'd; it follows, that the Heat will be so much the greater, by how much such a Nisus, and Attrition of the Parts among one another is increas'd. And with the same Resistances, (that is, the Sections of the Arteries, and the Quantity of Blood remaining the same) and an increas'd Force of the Heart, and circular Motion of the Blood, the Nisus and Attrition of the Parts of Blood amongst one another, must necessarily be increas'd; both by the preceding Blood being struck harder upon, by the Protrusion of a succeeding Blood, coming on with an increas'd Velocity; and the occasioning thereby also more frequent Strokes against the Sides of the Arteries; by which means, an increas'd Velocity of Blood increases the Heat : and consequently doe sits Heat depend upon its Circulation. From hence it appears, that at the same Distances from the Heart, the Heat of equal Quantities of Blood will be as their Velocities : and, that in the same Velocities of Blood, the Heat will be reciprocally as the Distances from the Heart.

For since, in homogeneal and simple Bodies, nothing else is requir'd to disengage the Particles exciting Heat, but a Nisus and Attrition of Parts, produc'd by the Force of the Heart; to which is always proportional to the Velocity of the Blood; and the Re-action, or Resistance of the Arteries and the antecedent Blood; it follows, that if the Resistance or Re-action is not alter'd, which it will not be at the same distance from the Heart; then the Heat of the Blood will not be alter'd, unless by an Alteration of the Impetus, or Velocity impress'd upon the Blood from the Heart : that is, as Effects are proportional to their Causes, the Heat of the Blood, at the same Distances from the Heart, will be proportional to tits Velocity. In the same manner it appears, that if the Velocities impress'd by the Heart be equal, there can be no change in the Heat of the Blood, but from a diversify'd Resistance, or Re-action of the Arteries and antecedent Blood.

But if the Resistance of the preceding Blood is proportional to its Quantity; and its Quantity is reciprocally proportional to the Distance from the Heart; (for the nearer the Blood is to the Heart, so much the greater will be its Quantity between any given Place and the Extremity of an Artery.) And therefore the Resistance of the Arteries will also be so much the greater, by how much nearer they are to the Heart : For in this case, the Resistance is proportional to the Velocity; and the Velocity of the Blood is greatest at the least Distances from the Heart. Hence the Heat of the Blood may be consider'd as a Rectangle, under the Velocity and the Distance : that is, if in two Persons the Velocity be as three, and the Distance wherein we would determine the Heat, be as much more in one as in another; that is, as two to one; the Heat of one will be six, and the other three: that is, the Heat of the first will be double that of the second. If the Distance of the first be as two, and the Velocity as four; but the Distance of the second as three, and the Velocity as one; the Heat of the first will be as eight, and of the second as three : and so the Heat of the first will be more than double the Heat of the second.

**CALIX**, in Botany, is apply'd to a Flower, whose Body or even a Part of it, is form'd in manner of a Cup of *Chalice*; as the Cup or Body of a Tulip, &c. *Calix* is more particularly us'd for that outward greenish Cover which encompasses and defends the Foliage, or Leaves of a Flower. The *Calix* is sometimes of one entire Piece; as in Pinks, &c. and in some broke into several, as in Roses, &c. The *Calix* is also call'd *Perianthium*. Saffron has no *Calix*; its Flower comes out of the Earth before its Leaves.

**CALLOSITY**, a little *Callus* form'd in any part of the Skin; or a white, solid, dry, insensible Flesh; generated by the Congestion of a dry, pituitous Excrement, covering the Circumference of an Ulcer, Wound, &c. and in the Place where good Flesh should grow. The Chirurgeon is always to take care that Ulcers close without *Callosities*.

**CALLUS**, a kind of *Nodus*, or Ligature, which joins the Extremities of a fractur'd Bone. The Formation of a *Callus* may be as follows. The Juice that feeds the Bone, running along its Fibres, becomes extravasated in the Place where those Fibres are broke : So that stopping, and gathering together round the Extremities of the Fracture, it there dries, knits, and hardens, to a Consistence like a string Glue; leaving only a little Inequality in the Place where it is form'd.

*Callus's* frequently grow so firm as to supply the Place of Bones. In the *Phil. Transact.* We have an Instance of a *Callus* supplying the Place of the *Os Humeri*; taken out, upon its being Carious, by Mr. *Fowler*; and another of a *Callus's* supplying the Place of the *Os Femoris*; and the Person as strong as ever, and walking without any Lameness, by Mr. *Sherman*.

*Callus*, is also a hard dense Knob, or Substance, rising on the Hands and Feet, &c. by much Friction and Pressure against hard Bodies.

**CALOMEL**, in Pharmacy, the Name ordinarily given to *Mercurius Dulcis*. It rather seems to have first belonged to the Æthiops Mineral; from καλος, *pulcher*, fair; and μελας, *niger*, black : for that white or pale Bodies rubb'd herewith, becomes black. But some will have it given to *Mercurius Dulcis*, from the Authority of a whimsical Chymist, who employ'd a Black in his Laboratory; whose Complexion, as well as that of the Mercury, he alluded to in the Term : the Medicine being *fair*, and the Operator *black*.

**CALVITIES**, in Medicine, Baldness, or a falling off of the Hair, without being able to grow again; the Moisture of the Head, which should feed it, being dry'd up by some Disease, by old Age, or by immoderate use of Pouder.

**CALX**, in Chymistry, is a kind of Ashes, or fine friable Pouder, which remains of Metals, Minerals, &c. after they have undergone the Violence of a Fire for a long time; and by that means have lost all their humid Parts. Or, *Calx*, is what remains of a Body after Calcination. Gold and Silver, after they have been reduc'd to a *Calx*, may be again recover'd to their former Form and Nature. *Calx of Tin*, is call'd *Putty*; of considerable use in polishing Steel Mirrors, &c. *Calx of Brass*, is call'd *Aes ustum*. *Calx of Lead*, is call'd *Ceruss*. *Calx*, literally signifies, Lime; or a Stone burnt, or calcin'd in a Kiln for that Purpose, to be us'd in the making of Mortar, &c.

**CAMPANULOUS**, or *Campaniforis*, those Plants whose Flowers resemble the Shape of a Bell; from *Campana*, a Bell.

**CAMPHOR**, or Camphire, a white, shining, transparent, odiferous, volatile Gum, or Resin, of a bitterish Taste, and very hot in the Mouth; flowing from a Tree frequent in the Island of *Borneo*, and the neighbouring mountainous Coasts of *India*, resembling a Walnut Tree. It distils from the Tree in manner of a Gum; and, 'tis said, most plentifully in the Time of Earthquakes and Storms. M. *Lemery* says, the *Camphor* is found at the Foot of the Tree; where it thickens into little Grains of different Figures and Sizes; very dry, friable, light, of a bitterish Taste, &c. These little Grains falling one another, adhere lightly together and form Masses; which being squeez'd a little by the Fingers, granulate again into small Corpuscles, like Salt.

Some Authors make two different Kinds of Camphor, according to the different Parts of the Tree where they are found : That in the Veins of the Wood, is said to be different from that which oozes out upon breaking the Bark. The Camphor, as is said, being at first red, is whiten'd either by the Sun or the Fire. In effect, we have but little of the Raw Natural Camphor among us; the Dutch take care that it comes all refin'd by Sublimation; and prepar'd to our Hands.

The Method us'd to refine it, is to lay it to sublime in subliming Pots : when the Vessel is half full, it is stopp'd, and plac'd over a gentle Fire; where only the purest Part rises at first; but, by degrees, the whole is sublim'd, except a Caput Mortuum, or earthy Part sticking at Bottom : They them melt it with a gentle Heat, and run it into Moulds to give it what Figure they please. 'Tis so volatile, and apt to evaporate in Smoke, that the Merchants ordinarily inclose it in Line-seed, that the Viscosity of that Grain may keep its Particles together.

*Camphor* has its various Uses; as in Fireworks, in making Vernish, &c. In the Courts of the Eastern Princes, 'tis burnt, together with Wax, to illumine the Night. 'Tis exceedingly inflammable, so as to burn and preserve its Flame in Water; and in burning it consumes wholly, leaving no Scorium behind : But its principal use is in Medicine. 'Tis the most efficacious Diaphoretic known; its great Subtility diffusing it self thro the Substance of the Parts, almost as soon as the warmth of the Stomach has set it in Motion. 'Tis us'd in a Caries of the Bones, a Detergent in Wounds, to resist a Gangreen, &c. When mix'd with the subtile Salts of Cantharides, it prevents their injuring the Bladder; its exquisite Fineness inabling it follow them into the fine Meanders thereof, and to sheath their Asperities.

Dr. *Quincy* observes, that *Camphor* begins to be mix'd, and that to good purpose, with Mercurials, to guard against their stimulating Properties, and to send 'em in the finest Passages, top operate by Fusion, and the bare Force of Impulse. For not only *Mercurius Dulcis* or *Calomel*, may be hereby restrain'd from manifest Operation in the Glands about the Mouth; but also the Mineral Turbith, which of it self acts very strongly by Stool and Vomit, when mix'd with *Camphor*, will be much less felt in those Respects; and will go into the farthest Circuit of Motion, and promote the cutaneous Discharge, in a more efficacious manner than any Medicine of less specifick Gravity.

M. *Lemery* endeavour'd at a Chymical Analysis of *Camphor*; but either its Parts were too fine and volatile to be carry'd to any grater degree of purity or Subtilty by any Chymical Process; or it was owing to the close Union of its Principles, which, in all appearance, must be an Oil and a volatile Salt; that they could not be separated.

*Camphor*, he observes, does not dissolve in aqueous or phlegmatic Liquors; but in sulphurous ones it does : not in Alcalines, nor even in some Acids : But in Spirit of Nitre it dissolves perfectly; and is the sole Resin that does so. This Dissolution is ordinarily called *Oil of Camphor*; and 'tis to this the medicinal Virtue of Camphor in Wounds, Gangreens, and Caries are ascrib'd. They use not to take it internally, for fear of its sharpness and corrosiveness : tho M. *Lemery* has found good Effects from two or three Drops by the Mouth, in Obstructions and Fits of the Mother : indeed, he generally mix'd it with as much oil of Amber.

*Camphor*, being boil'd in Aqua vitæ, in a close Place, till the whole be evaporated; of a lighted Torch or Candle be introduc'd, the Air in the whole Place will immediately catch Fire, and appear in Flame, without doing any Damage to the Place or the Spectators.

It has been found, in *Ceylon*, that the Root of the Tree which yields Cinnamon, yields, by Infusion, a Liquor that has a string smell of *Camphor*, and many of its Virtues : whence the Naturalists, by mistake, have suppos'd that all *Camphor* came from that Tree. There is a smell of *Camphor* in several Plants, as in *Camphoreta*, *Abrotonum*, *Rosemary*, &c.

*Artificial* Camphor is prepar'd with Sandarach, and white Vinegar distill'd, kept 20 says in Horse-dung, and afterwards expos'd a Month to the Sun to dry; at the End of which, the *Camphor* is found, in form of the Crust of a white Loaf: This is also call'd *Juniper gum, white Vernish*, and *Mastic*.

The Word *Camphor* comes from the Arabic *Capur*, or *Caphur*; which signifies the same thing.

**CANCER**, in Medicine, a hard, rugged, round, immoveable Tumor, of an Ash, Livid, or Lead Colour; incompass'd round with branch'd turgid Veins, full of black muddy Blood: so call'd, as some will have it, from the Resemblance it bears to the Crab-fish, call'd *Cancer*; or, as others say, because, like that Fish, when once it has got hold, 'tis scarce possible to drive it off. It begins without any Pain, and appears, at first, like a Chicory Pea; but grows apace, and becomes very painful.

The *Cancer* arises principally on the lax glandulous Parts, as the Breasts and Emunctories : 'Tis most frequent in Women, especially such, says *Stolterfoth*[1], as are barren, or live in Celibacy. The Reason of its appearing in the Breast more than other Parts, is, that being full of Glands, with Lymphaticks and Blood-Vessels, extravasates those Liquors; which growing, by degrees, acrimonious, form the *Cancer*.

Hence, the Masters of the Art say, that a *Cancer* is that in the Glands, which a Caries is in the Bones, and a Gangreen in the fleshy Parts. The *Cancer*, however, is sometimes found in other soft, spongy Parts of the Body; and there have been some found in the Teeth, Belly, Neck of the Matrix, Ureter, Lips, Nose, Cheeks, Abdomen, Thighs, and even the Shoulders, as *Stolterfoth* shews.

*Cancers* are divided, according to the several Stages, into Occult and Ulcerated; the first is form'd as above. Ulcerated *Cancers*, are known by their roughness and fullness of Holes, thro which oozes a filthy, stinking, glutinous Matter, frequently yellowish; by their pungent Pain, which resembles the pricking with a thousand Pins; by their blackness; the swelling of the Lips of the Ulcer; and the Veins about it, which are blackish, swell'd, various, resembling, as above, the Foot of a Cray-fish. Sometimes the Extremities of the Blood-Vessels are gnaw'd off, and the Blood issues out. In a *Cancer* of the Breast, the adjacent Flesh is sometimes so consum'd, that one may see into the Cavity of the Thorax. It occasions a slow Fever, a Loathing, oftentimes Faintings, sometimes a Dropsy, and lastly Death.

The immediate Cause of a *Cancer* seems to be a too corrosive volatile Salt, approaching to the Nature of Arsenic, form'd by the Stagnation of Humours, &c. *Stolterfoth* observes, that it has been frequently cur'd by Mercury and Salivation. A Cancer arising on the Legs, is call'd a *Lupus*; on the Face, or Nose, a *Noli me tangere*: Some take the ulcerous *Cancer* to be nothing else but an infinite Number of little Worms, which devour the Flesh by degrees. The *Cancer* is allow'd the most horrible Evil that befalls the Body : 'Tis usually cur'd while yet a small Tumor, of the bigness of a Nut, or at most of a small Egg, by Extirpation : When it seizes the Breast, or is burst into an Ulcer, Amputation takes place.

**CANKER**, is a Speck made by a sharp Humour, which gnaws the Flesh almost like a Caustic; very common to Children, in their Mouth especially. It is also a Disease incident to Trees; proceeding chiefly from the Nature of the Soil.

**CANTHARIDES**, in Medicine, a Drug much us'd for the raising of Blisters. *Cantharides* are the Principle of the Tribe of Epispasticks, or Vesicatories.

*Cantharides* are a kind of venemous Insects, with Feet and Wings, like little Flies; hence also call'd *Spanish Flies*. They are form'd of a kind of little Worm, hatch'd on Wheat, the Leaves of Poplar, &c. There are various Kinds

[1] Johann Jacob Stolterfoth (1665 – 1718), a German physician.

of *Cantharides* : the best are those which appear with different Colours, having yellow Lines running across their Wings; thick, and fresh. They are kill'd by laying then over a very strong Vinegar, which is made to boil for that purpose; after which they are dry'd, and may be preserv'd two Years.

*Cantharides* are very sharp and corrosive, abounding with a subtile, caustick, volatile Salt; whereby they become exceedingly injurious to the Bladder, so as to ulcerate it, even when apply'd externally, if suffer'd to lye too long. They are much commended in Fevers; as they raise and strengthen a low trembling Pulse, give Relief in delirious Ravings, soporiferous Symptoms, Loss of Reason, &c. (the common Symptoms of high and dangerous Fevers) reduce continual Fevers to regular and distinct Remissions; and so make way for the Bark : cleanse and open the obstructed Glands, and Lymphaticks; bring on critical Sweats, &c.

Dr. *Morgan*[1] accounts for these Effects of *Cantharides* thus : "The subtile and volatile pungent Parts of which the *Cantharides* consist, being carry'd into the Blood, and passing with the Lymph or Serum into the glandular Pipes, act there by dissolving, attenuating, and rarifying the viscid Cohesions of the Lymph; and by stimulating the nervous Coats of the Vessels throw of their stagnant Viscidities, and thus restore the Circulation and free Drain of Lymph from the Arteries to the Veins; cleanse the Expurgatory Glands, and bring on critical Sweats, and Urines. Thus, the extremely subtile, active, and pungent volatile Salts, deriv'd from the *Cantharides*, purge the Glands and Lymphaticks universally; much after the same manner as common Catharticks do the Guts." *Philosop. Princip. of Medicine*, p. 304.

*Cantharides* are seldom, if ever, to be us'd internally : In the *Philosoph. Transact.* indeed, we have Instances of their internal Application, and that with success, by Mr. *Young*, in Dropsical and other Cases; sometimes mix'd with Camphor, and sometimes without; only well wash'd down with large Draughts of Posset, Ptisan, Emulsions, or the like. The form wherein he tells us he uses to administer this fiery Insect, is that of a soft Pill, or Bolus, compos'd of *three Cantharides praepar. Troch. e Myrrha 3 semi-ounces Sem. Amei.* gr. vi. *Rob. Cynosb.* q. f. This, in stubborn Suppressions of the Menses and Lochia, in difficult Childbirth, and Retention of the Secundine, he finds does Wonders : He adds, that the Heat or Pain it occasions in the Neck of the Bladder, is much short of what he has an hundred times seen, and sometimes felt, from the Application of an Epispastick to the Back. But their principal use is in Vesicatories, to raise Blisters on the Skin; and by that means to turn off and discharge some Flux of ill Humours.

*Cantharides* take their Name from *Cantharus*, an Animal, otherwise call'd *Scarabæus venenosus. Cantharides* are sometimes apply'd to the Temples for Tooth-ach : The Farriers use them in several Diseases of Horses. They must be chosen new, dry, and whole : they won't keep above two Years, without mouldering into a Dust, of no use.

**CANTHUS**, in Chymistry, the Lip of a Vessel; or that Part of the Mouth of a Vessel, which is a little hollow'd, or depress'd, for the easy pouring off a Liquor : Hence to pour by Decantation, is to pour thro that place.

[1] Thomas Morgan (ca. 1695 – 1743), a Welsh minister and physician.

**CANULA**, or Cannula, in Chirurgery, a little Tube, or Pipe, which the Chirurgeons leave in Wounds and Ulcers, that they do not, or chuse not to heal up; because still suppurating. The *Canula* is of Gold, Silver, or Lead; and is perforated, that the Pus entering within it, may fall upon a Sponge, dipp'd in Spirit of Wine, and plac'd at the Orifice, to keep the Ulcer warm, and to prevent the external Air from entering : Some of these *Cannulæ* have Rings, whereby to keep them fast in the Wound; and others have Hole with Ribbons thro 'em, to bind 'em down. Some are round, others oval, others crooked.

There is a particular kind of these *Cannulæ*, form'd taperwise, with a Skrew fasten'd to one End, in manner of a Cock : Its use is, for the Discharge of the Water out of the Abdomen, after Tapping, in an Ascites, or Dropsy. To this End it is inserted into the Body, thro a Hole near the Navel; made with a pointed Instrument, and sometimes a Punch; and is fasten'd in its Place by a Bandage, and guarded from any Injury of the Clothes, &c. by a Case, or Cover. It has this advantage over the common Tapping; that by means thereof, the Water is drawn out when, and in what measure the Patient pleases.

There are likewise a kind of *Cannulæ* for the Application of actual Cauteries; they are made very shallow, and are, in effect, little more than Hoops; thro the Aperture whereof, the actual Cautery is convey'd; which, by this means, is kept from damaging the adjacent Parts.

**CAPILLAMENT**, literally signifies Hair; being form'd of the *Latin Capillus*, of *Capus*; *q.d.* Hair of the Head. Hence the Word is figuratively apply'd to several things, which, on account of their Length and Fineness, resemble Hairs : As, *Capillaments of the Nerves,* are the fine Fibres, or Filaments, whereof the Nerves are compos'd.

"Is not Vision perform'd chiefly by the Vibrations of this Medium, excited in the Bottom of the Eye by Rays of Light; and propagated thro the solid, pellucid, and uniform *Capillaments* of the Optic Nerves, to the Sensorium?" *Newt. Opt.* p. 328.

**CAPILLAMENTS**, in Botany, more usually call'd *Staminas*; are those small Threads, or Hairs, which grow up in the Middle of the Flower; and are headed with little Knobs, call'd *Apices*.

**CAPILLARY**, of the Latin *Capillus*, a Hair; is apply'd the several Things, to intimate their exceeding Smallness, Fineness, &c. resembling that of a Hair : As *Capillary* Vessels, *Capillary* Fracture, &c.

**CAPILLARY** *Vessels*, in Anatomy, are the least, minutest, insensible Ramifications of the Veins and Arteries; which, when cut, or broke, yield but very little Blood. The *Capillary* Vessels shou'd be conceiv'd as vastly finer than Hairs.

**CAPILLARY**, or Capillaceous Plants, are a Species of Plants, thus denominated from their Form, and manner of growing. The *Capillaries* have no principal Stalk, or Stem, with Branches, &c. shooting out of the same; but grow from the Ground, like Hairs from the Head: They bear their Seeds in little Tufts, or Prominences, on the backside of their Leaves. The principle of these, is the *Capillus Veneris*, or *Adianthum*; from which the rest take their name.

The *Capillaries* are distinguish'd into those with a undivided Leaf, as the *Hæmionitis*, and the *Phyllitis*; or with a singly divided Leaf : and these have the Leaf either cut, or jagged in, but not divided into *Pinnæ*, clear home to the main Rib; as, *Polipodium, Lonchitis, Scolopendria, Adianthum, Aerostichon Thal.* Or else divided quite home to the Rib, and hanging like *Pinnæ*; as the *Chama felix Marina*, and the *Trichomanes* : Others have the Leaf doubly divided, or at least once subdivided, the first Division being into Branches, and the second into *Pinnæ*; as the *Hemionitis Multifida*, the *Filex Mas, Filex Palustris, Filex Saxatilis.* The *Adianthum album*, and *nigram*, and others, have the Leaf trebly divided, or thrice sub-divided; first into Branches, then into little Twigs, and after this into *Pinnæ*; these are, the *Felix Scandens* of Brasil, the *Felix Florida*, or *Osmunda Regalis*; the *Felix mas Ramosa*, the *Felix Fæminæ Vulgaris*, the *Adianthum album Floridum*, and the *Drioptesis nigra*.

All the *Capillaries* are reputed of use in Medicine, especially in the making of Syrops; to which, wonderful Virtues are attributed. But, in effect, only the *Capillary of Montpelier*, *Adianthum album Monspeliense*, and that of Canada, *Adianthum album Canadense*, are regularly us'd for that Purpose : The rest only serve to counterfeit 'em.

The Antients though that the *Capillaries* were all without Seed; and some of the Moderns, particularly *Dodonæus*[1], have given into the Opinion. But *Bauhinus*[2], and other of the more accurate Observers, maintain they have all their Seed. *Caesius*[3] says, he has seen them with a Microscope : Since him, Mr. *W. Cole*[4] has observ'd 'em with still more Curiosity; he tells us, the *Capsulæ*, or Seed Vessels, are in some less by half than a small grain of common Sand, in others much less; yet some of them contain about 100 Seeds.

**CAPITAL** *Medicines*, in Pharmacy, are the great, or principal Preparations of the Shops; remarkable for the number of Ingredients, extraordinary Virtues, &c. such as *Venice Treacle, Mithridate*, &c.

**CAPITATÆ** *Plantæ*, in Botany, are such Plants whose Flowers are compos'd of many edg'd and hollow little Flowers; thus call'd by Mr. *Ray*, because their scaly Calyx (or Cup of the Flower) most usually swells out into a large and round Belly, containing within it the pappous Seed; as in *Carduus, Centaury, Knapweed, Cinera, Cirsium, Lappamai, Cijanus*, &c.

**CAPITULUM**, in Botany, the Head, or Flowering Top of any Plant; being compos'd of many Leaves and Threads, or *Stamina*, closely connected in a globous, circular, or discous Figure; as the Flowers of Bluebottles, Scabious,

[1] Rembert Dodoens (1517 – 1585), a Flemish botanist.

[2] Gaspard or Kaspar Bauhin (1560 – 1624), a Swiss botanist.

[3] Fedrico Angelo Cesi (1585 – 1630), an Italian naturalist and natural philosopher.

[4] William Cole (1626 – 1662), an English botanist.

Carduus, &c.

**CAPRE**, or Caper, the Bud, or Blossom of a Shrub of the same Name, gather'd green, e'er it expand into a Flower; dry'd in a dark Place, till wither'd, then infus'd in Vinegar; to which, at last, Salt is added; after which, it is put up in Barrels to be us'd as a Pickle, chiefly in Sauces; and sometimes also in Medicine, as being very Aperitive, and entering several Compositions in Pharmacy.

All the *Capers* throughout *Europe*, are brought from about *Toulon* in *France*; except some small salt *Capers* from *Majorca*, and a few flat ones from about *Lyons*. The Bark of the *Caper*-Tree, when dry'd, is prescrib'd by the *French* Physicians in Oppilations of the Spleen.

**CAPREOLUS**, in Botany, the Clasper, or Tendril, by which the Vines, and such-like creeping Plants, fasten themselves to those things which are design'd to support them.

**CAPREOLATÆ** *Plantæ*, are such Plants as turn, wind, and climb along the Surface of the Earth, by means of their *Capreoli*, or Tendrils; as Gourds, Melons, Cucumbers, &c.

**CAPSULA**, among the Botanists, is that part of a Fruit wherein the Seed is contain'd; as in Pears, Apples, &c. which have a little Coat, in form of a Purse, wherein the Kernels, or Pippins are inclos'd.

**CAPSULATE** *Plants*, *Capsulatæ Plantæ*, are such as have a tetrapetalous regular Flower, consisting of four distinct Petals in each Flower, and which bear their Seeds in short *Capsulæ*; by which they are distinguish'd from the *Siliquosæ*, which have their Seed in long Cases, or *Capsulæ seminales*; and all the other Branches of this Genus of Plants.

**CAPSULA**, in Chymistry, is an Earthen Vessel, in form of a Pan; wherein things are frequently plac'd, that are to undergo very violent Operations of the Fire.

**CAPUT** *Mortuum*, in Chymistry, the *Fæces* remaining of any Body, after all the volatile and humid Parts, as the Phlegm, Spirit, Salt, &c. have been extracted therefrom, by Force of Fire. What remains after Distillation, is only properly call'd *Fæces*. E'er it be *Caput Mortuum*, it must likewise have pass'd the Retort.

The *Caput Mortuum*, call'd also *Terra damnata*, is found in form of a friable, porous Matter, without Taste or Smell : 'Tis rank'd among the Chymical Elements; and suppos'd to constitute the dry, fix'd, earth, and solid Part of all mix'd Bodies.

As an Element, it is more commonly express'd by the Name Earth. 'Tis what the Chymists call a *passive Element*, or *Principle*; serving as the Basis or Support of the active ones.

The Term is sometimes more immediately restrain'd to the Remains of Vitriol, after Distillation; otherwise call'd *Calcothar Vitrioli*. The *Caput*

*Mortuum* is never pure, but there is still some active Principle remaining in it, and particularly a fix'd Salt. Thus the *Calcothar Vitrioli*, expos'd to the Air, is re-converted into Vitriol.

**CARABE**, or Karabe, yellow Amber reduc'd to Pouder.

**CARACT**, Carat, or Karat, is properly the Name of the Weight, which expresses the degree of Goodness, Title, Perfection, or Imperfection of Gold. The Coiners fix the highest Purity and Perfection of Gold at 24 *Carats*; and the several Degrees are estimated from the Divisions hereof, which are call'd *Grains*.

But 'tis observ'd that what care soever is taken in purifying Gold, to clear it from Dross, it can never be brought to 24 *Carats*; but still comes short 1/4 of a *Carat*, or a Grain : this Grain they call a *Sixteenth*; and this sixteenth they subdivided into two *Eights*; and each of those eights into two *Sixteenths*: In which Calculation, they say. Gold may be purify'd as far as the first Sixteenth of the second Eighth, but no further.

Gold of 22 *Carats*, is that which has 22 Parts of fine Gold, and two of Silver, or other Metal; or that which in refining loses 2 Parts in 24 of its Weight. The Goldsmiths generally work Gold of 22 *Carats*.

The *Carat Fine*, as above, is the 24th Part of the Goodness of a Piece of gold; the *Carat Price*, is the 24th Part of the Value of a Piece of Gold : as, if the Piece be 384, the *Carat Price* is 16 Pounds. We also sometimes say, the *Carat Weight*, which is the 24th Part of the Weight of the Piece, or 192 Grains.

*Menage*, from *Alciat*, derives the Word *Carat* from the *Greek* καρατιον, which was a kind of small Weight : But *Savot*[1], with more probability, from χαρατιον, a Tribute-Penny, or small Coin struck for that purpose. Others derive it simply from the Latin *Character*.

*Caract* is also the Weight us'd in weighing Diamonds and precious Stones; and consists of four Grains. Thus, the Great *Mongul's* Diamond is said to weight 279 *Caracts*. These Grains are somewhat less heavy than those us'd in Gold, &c. In this Sense, the Word is suppos'd to be deriv'd from the *Greek* κερατιον, A Fruit which the *Latins* call *Siliqua*, and we *Carab-bean*; each of which may weight about four Grains of Wheat : whence the Latin *Siliqua* has also been us'd for a Weight of four Grains.

**CARANNA**, is a hard, brittle, resinous Gum, brought from some Parts of the *West Indies*, as *Carthagena* and *New Spain*; of an aromatick Flavour, and us'd among us in Medicine.

**CARAWAY**, or Carway, a Medicinal Seed, produc'd from a Plant of the same Name, by Botanists call'd *Carvi Officinarum*, or *Cuminum Pratense*. The Seed or Grain of the *Carvi* or *Caraway*, is narrow longish, furrow'd on the Back, and of a brisk aromatic Taste. It is esteem'd Stomachic, and Diuretic; dispels Wind, strengthens Digestion, &c. The *English* and *Germans* make great use of it; particularly in Biskets, Comfits, and other Foods and

[1] Louis Savot (1579 – 1640), a French physician.

Confections.

**CARBUNCULATION**, is the blasting of the new-sprouted Buds of Trees or Plants, either by excessive Heat, or excessive Cold.

**CARCINOMA**, in Medicine, a Tumor, more usually call'd a *Cancer*. The Word comes from καρκινος, Cancer, and νεμιω, *depasco*, to feed upon.

**CARDAMOMUM**, Cardamums, a Medicinal Seed, of the Aromatic kind, contain'd in *Capsulae*, or Pods, brought from the *East Indies*.

The Seed is distinguish'd into three Kinds, according to the several Sizes of the Pods; *viz*. great, middle, and small : but the Taste, Smell, Colour, and Form of the Grain, is the same in all; being of a Purple Colour, angular, of a sharp biting Taste, and a strong penetrating Smell. The first kind is also call'd *Grains of Paradise*; but the last excels the rest, both in Smell, Taste, and Virtue : 'Tis this that enters the Composition of Venice Treacle.

The *Cardamums* do warm, and deterge; they strengthen the nobler Parts, dissipate Wind, and help Digestion; and are us'd in Diseases of the Brain, Stomach, and Womb.

The Plants of the *Cardamum* Family, afford something very remarkable, as to the manner of their Propagation : When ripe, their Pods fly open, and dart out their Seed upon the slight touch of the Hand. Nay, what is more, Mr. *Ray* tells us, the *Cardamum Impatiens* breaks its Pod, and emits its Seed not only if touch'd, but if only the Hand be stretch'd out, as if about to touch it : and *Johnston*[1] and *Gerrard*[2] affirm it to be true.

**CARDIAC**, in Medicine, vulgarly call'd *Cordial*, a Remedy antiently suppos'd to exert it self immediately in comforting and strengthening the Heart : but the modern Physicians rather suppose it to produce its Effect, by putting Blood into a gentle Fermentation, whereby the Springs, before decay'd, are repair'd and invigorated; and the Tone and Elasticity of the Fibres of the Vessels restor'd : the Consequence of which, is a more easy and brisk Circulation. The Word comes from the *Greek* καρδια, *Cor*; the Heart being reputed the immediate Seat of its Operation.

**CARDIALGIA**, Cardialgy, or *Cardiacus Dolor*, in Medicine, a violent Pain, felt towards the upper Orifice of the Stomach, accompany'd with a Palpitation of the Heart, Fainting, and a Propension to Vomit; better known by the Name of *Cardiac Passion*, or *Heart-burn*. 'Tis occasion'd by sharp Humours, which prick and vellicate that Orifice, and the adjoining Parts. The Word comes from the Greek καρδια, Heart, and αλγ, Pain.

*Blanchard* makes the Disease consist in a Gnawing, and Contraction of the *Par vagum*, and the intercostal Nerves implanted in the Stomach; proceeding from a pungent vellicating Matter in the Stomach it self : which, by reason of the Consent of Parts, affects the Heart; straitning and contracting it so, as sometimes to occasion swooning.

[1] This may be John Johnston (1603 – 1675), a Polish physician and naturalist.

[2] John Gerard (1545 – 1607), an English surgeon and botanist.

**CARDUUS**, in Natural History and Botany, a Name common to divers Species of Plants, in English call'd *Thistles*. The Plants of this Class most in use, are the *Carduus Benedictus*, and *Carduus Fullonum*.

*Carduus Benedictus*, is a Medicinal Plant, of the Thistle kind, chiefly us'd in Infusion, as a gentle Emetic in Fevers, and certain Nauseas. Antiently it was much in vogue, as a Cardiac, Sudorific, and Alexipharmic; and in those Qualities, was prescrib'd in Stomachic Cases : but it is now succeeded by others, less nauseous, and more effectual; tho still retain'd in some of the officinal Compositions, with those Intentions. Some distill a Water from it, which they use in cordial and sudorific Potions. Its Salt has much the same Virtues.

Carduus *Fullonum*, is also call'd the *Fuller's Weed*, or *Teazle*.

**CARICOUS** *Tumor*, is a Swelling resembling the Figure of a Fig; such, frequently, are the Piles. The Word comes from *Carica*, Fig; or from *Caria*, a Country where they are frequent, or from whence they are sometimes said to be brought.

**CARIES**, in Chirurgery, &c. a kind of Rottenness peculiar to a Bone; arising, either from a constant Afflux of vicious Humours, or from their Acrimony; or from a Bruise, Compound Fracture, Luxation, Venereal Disorders, corrosive Medicines, being stripp'd, or laid bare of their Flesh, and long expos'd to Air, &c. 'Tis a common Observation that nothing is more difficult to cure than an Ulcer, when the adjacent Bone is become *carious*. The Word in the original *Latin*, signifies *Rottenness*.

The usual Medicines in a *Caries*, are Tinctures of Euphorbium, Myrrh, and Aloes; or Pouders of the same with the Addition of Iris, Birthwort of either kind, Gentian, &c. and particularly the Pouder of Diapente. After using the Tinctures, the Pouders are apply'd on Lint, in the form of a Pledget. An Actual Caustery apply'd to the *carious* Part through a Canula, &c. is frequently found successful.

Anatomists, in dissecting of Bodies, sometimes find carious Bones particularly those of the Jaws, Legs, &c. where nothing of that Kind was suspected during the Person's Life-time; nor any Disorder felt therefrom : Whence Mr. *Cheselden*[1] conjectures, that the Cure of a carious Bone might be directly attempted, without waiting, as our Chirurgeons usually do, for an *Exfoliation*.

**CARLINE**, or Caroline, a Plant, of the Thistle kind, said to have been discover'd by an Angel to *Charlemaign*, to cure his Army of the Plague : whence its Denomination. Its Root is of service as a Diuretic and Sudorific, in all pestilential Disorders.

**CARMINATIVES**, in Medicines, are Remedies, whether Simple or Compound, us'd in a Cholic, or other flatulent Distemper; to dispel the Wind. The four *Carminative Flowers*, are those of Camomile, Melilot, Motherwort, and Dill.

[1] William Cheseldon (1688 – 1752), an English surgeon and anatomist.

The Word comes from the Latin *Carminare*, to card, cleanse, purge; tho Dr. *Quincy* makes its Origin more mysterious : he says, it comes from the Word *Carmen*, taking it in the Sense of an Invocation, or Charm; and makes it to have been a general Name for all Medicines which operated like Charms, *i.e.* in an extraordinary manner. Hence, as the most violent Pains were frequently those arising from pent-up Wind, which immediately cease upon Dispersion; the Term *Carminative* became in a peculiar Sense apply'd to Medicines which gave Relief in windy Cases, as if they cur'd by Inchantment. But this Derivation appears a little to much strain'd.

**CARPOBALSUM**, Carpobalsamum, is the Fruit of the Balm, or Balsam Tree; very much resembling, both in Figure, Size, and Colour, that of Turpentine. 'Tis much doubted, whether the *Carpobalsam* sold in the Shops be the same with that of the Antients; as not having the same Marks. The Apothecaries use to substitute *Cubebs* in lieu of it, as having the same Qualities. The Word comes from the *Greek* καρπος, Fruit, and βαλσαμος, Balm.

**CARUS**, in Medicine, a Species of Apoplexy, consisting in a profound Sleep, with a sudden Deprivation of Sensation, and Motion, and an acute Fever.

The *Carus* differs from a *Coma* in this, that the Patient in the latter, answers when interrogated; but not in the former: From a Lethargy it is distinguish'd by the Fever which attends it, which the lethargic Person finds when agitated or prick'd : From a proper Apoplexy, by the freedom of Respiration, which is always hurt in an Apoplexy : From an Epilepsy, in that there is no Motion of Froth at the Mouth in the *Carus* : From a Syncope, by the Pulse, which is high, and the Face ruddy; whereas the Pulse is low, and the Face cadaverous in the Syncope : From an hysteric Suffocation, in that the Patient hears and remembers things in the latter, not in the former.

The Cause of the *Carus* is usually referr'd to an Interruption of the Motion of the Animal Spirits; occasion'd either by their being exhausted, or obstruct'd by some cold, heavy, pituitous Humour; or by a Contusion, from some external Force. The Word comes from the Greek καρος, Drousiness, heaviness of the Head.

**CASSIA**, a medicinal Drug, in frequent use as a gentle Purgative. There are four Kinds of Cassia, alike in Properties, and nearly in Figure; being all in long black Pods; but very different, if consider'd with regard to the Trees that produce them. These Cassias are, Cassia of the *Levant*, that of *Egypt*, that of *Brasil*, and of the *Antilles* Islands.

*Cassia of the Levant*, is the Fruit of a very high Tree, whose Bark is Ash-colour'd, its Wood very solid, and its Grain close; towards the Center, the Wood is of an Ebony black, towards the Circumference, yellowish : Its Flowers round and massive; of a reddish Colour, bordering on black. When ripe, it is full of black, sweetish Pulp, divided by little woody Cells : In this Pulp are found little hard Grains, in manner of Stones, shap'd like Hearts, which are the Seed of the Tree. This *Cassia* must be chose new, in large Pods, heavy, and of a tan Colour; the Bark, when broke, fine and white within, full of a black soft Pulp of a sweetish Taste.

*Cassia of Egypt*, is like that of the *Levant*, except that the Tree is higher, and the Leaves narrower; the Fruit smaller, and the bark softer.

*Cassia of Brasil*, is the largest of all : Some of the Pods are found four or five Inches in Circumference. This Kind is not very common in the Shops.

*Cassia of the Islands*, is that now chiefly us'd; tho heretofore the popular *Cassia* was the *Levantine*. It is sent from the Antilles; where 'tis produc'd in such abundance, that the Vessels, in their home Voyages, use it as Ballast : whence it is, that we find it so often foul and dirty : The Tree that yields it resembles a Peach-Tree. Its Flowers, which are yellow, grow in Clusters; and, as they decay, leave behind them a Fruit or Pod an Inch thick, and a Foot (sometimes two) long. The Fruit, while in its growth, is green; when ripe, it becomes a dark Violet. 'Tis chosen in the same manner as that of the *Levant*.

When the Pod is entire, and the Pulp not yet take out, 'tis called *Cassia Fistula*, or *Cassia in the Cane*. For use, the Pulp is taken out, and pulp'd thro a Hair Sieve. The Apothecaries put off little of this better Kind, but what is old, and boil'd up with Sugar to make it keep.

*Cassia*, when green, is also the Flowers of the *Cassia* Tree, are comfited in the *Levant* and the *Islands*; and have almost the same Effects with the common *Cassia*, the Basis of most purgative Electuaries.

The *Tincture of Cassia*, is a slight Infusion of the Pulp with the Seed. The *Extract of Cassia*, is nothing but the Pulp separated from the Shell and the Seeds; with the Addition of a certain Quantity of Sugar to preserve it from turning sour.

**CASSIA LIGNEA**, is the Bark of a Tree much like that which bears the Cinnamon; growing promiscuously with it in the Island of *Ceylon*. The two Barks are gather'd and dry'd in the same manner; their Smell and Taste are nearly alike; they are equally sweet, poignant and agreeable; and their Colour, Form , and Thickness scarce differ at all. But the *Cassia* is the fatter, and more mucilaginous; and in chewing dissolves in the Mouth, without leaving any thing woody behind; whereas the woody Part of the Cinnamon still sticks, tho ever so well chew'd. Some Authors will have the Tree which bears Cinnamon bear the *Cassia* too; and make the only Difference between them to consist in this, that the first comes from *Ceylon*, and the latter from the Coast of *Coromandel*[1].

**CASTOREUM**, in Pharmacy, a liquid Matter, inclos'd in Bags or Purses near the Anus of the Castor or Bever; falsely taken for that Animal's Stones.

These Purses are bout the bigness of a Goose-Egg, and found indifferently in Males and Females; the Liquor inclosed, serves to give the *Castor* an Appetite, being press'd out of its Receptacles, on occasion, by the Foot : When taken off, the Matter dries and condenses, so as it may be reduced to a Pouder; by hanging in the Chimney it becomes of the Consistence of Wax. 'Tis oily, of a sharp, bitter Taste, and a strong disagreeable smell. 'Tis us'd to fortify the Head and nervous Parts, it excites the languishing Spirits, resists Poisons, and provokes the *Menses* in Women. 'Tis used in *Lethargies*,

[1] The coast of Coromandel is in south-east India in the states of Tamil Nadu and Andhra Pradesh.

*Apoplexies, Vertigo's, Tremblings, Suffocations of Women*, and other Occasions. *Bartholine*, and other Authors, ascribe to it a wonderful Property of precipitating things to the bottom of the Water.

*Castoreum* is used in the Composition of *Venice* Treacle and Mithridate, besides various other Hysterick and Cephalick Medicines. They draw an Oil from it call'd *Oil of Castor*; and it is also used, while in its liquid State, to make several Kinds of Unguents.

The *Russian* Way of curing *Castoreum*, is described in the *Philosophical Transactions* thus: "To get the Milk of the Bever's *Stones*, (the *Bags* it shou'd be) put a proper Quantity of Water, with half a Shovel full of Wood-Ashes, tie the Bags in Couples, and put them in the boiling Water for half a quarter of an Hour. Lay Birch-Bark on the Fire, and smoke the Bags well over it for an Hour, till they be well dried; hang them up for a Week or more, till perfectly dry and hard, they may then be pack'd up for Use or Exportation."

Castor *Skin*, the Fur or Skin of an amphibious Animal called *Castor* or Bever, sometimes found in *England, France, Germany*, and *Poland*, but most abundantly in the Province of *Canada* in *North-America*.

Its chief Use is in the Composition of Hats, and Furs. Beside this, in 16669, an Attempt was made to employ it in other Merchandizes; accordingly a Manufactury was settled in the *Fauxbourg S. Antoine* near *Paris*, where they made Cloths, Flannels, Stockings, &c. of Castor, with a mixture of Wool. The Manufacture flourish'd for a while, but soon decay'd, it being found by Experience that the Stuffs lost their Dye when wet, and that when dry again they were harsh, and stiff as Felts.

The Merchants distinguish three Kinds of *Castor*, the all equally the Spoils of the same Animal; these are *New Castor, Dry Castor*, and *Fat Castor* : *New Castor*, called also *Winter Castor*, and *Muscovite Castor*, because ordinarily reserv'd to send into *Muscovy*, is that taken in the Winter-Huntings. This is the best, and most esteem'd for rich Furs, as having lost none of its Hair by Moulting. *Dry Castor* or *lean Castor*, is the Result of the Summer-Huntings; when the Beast is moulted, and has lost part of its Hair : This being much inferior to the former, is little used in Furs; but mostly in Hats. *Fat Castor*, is that which has contracted a certain fat, unctuous Humour, by Sweat exhaled from the Bodies of the Savages, who have wore it for some time : This, tho better than the *dry*, is yet only used for Hats.

After the Hair is cut off the Skin to be used in Hats, the Pelt of Skin itself, is us'd in various Works, *viz.* in the covering of Mails and Trunks, in Slippers, &c.

**CATAGMATICS**, Medicines proper to solder, and unite broken Bones, by promoting the Formation of a *Callus*; see Callus and Bone. The principal *Catagmatics* are the *Armenian* Bole, Gum Tragacanth, Osteocolla, *Cyprus* Nuts, Frankincense, Aloes, and Acacia. The Word comes from the Greek καταγμα, Fracture.

**CATALEPSIS**, Catoche, or Catochis, in Medicine, a kind of Apoplexy; or a Disease, wherein the Patient is taken speechless, senseless, and fix'd in the same Posture wherein the Disease first seiz'd him; his Eyes open, without seeing, or understanding. The Word is *Greek*, καταλεψις, which signifies the same thing.

This Disease is very rare, nor is its Cause easy to assign. *Boerhaave* takes the immediate Cause to be an Immobility of the common Sensory, in the Situation of the first Access; whence an absolute Rest of the Blood in the Brain, and a Cessation of all the Functions of the Brain, as well as those depending thereon; the Muscles alone remaining in their first Tension; and Respiration, and the Pulse preserv'd, tho generally weak. It is usually preceded by a long intermitting Fever, a melancholic dry Temperature, a Suppression of the Menses, or Hem-orrhoids, great Frights, and intense, continu'd Meditation on one Object.

Upon Dissection, the Arteries and Veins of the *Cerebrum* are found very turgid, and the Blood close ramm'd in them : 'Tis frequently cur'd by copious Hemorrhages of the Nose; Sternutatories, Vomitives, and Vesicatories, are likewise apply'd to good purpose. It seldom passes into any other Disease; sometimes indeed into an Epilepsy, Convulsions, Madness, or Atrophy; but it commonly ends in Death.

**CATAPASM**, a Mixture of Pouders, either Odoriferous, as for the perfuming of Clothes; or Fortifying, and apply'd to the Stomach, Heart, or Head; or Escharrotic, for eating off dead Flesh. The Word comes from the *Greek* καταπασσειν, *to water*.

**CATAPHORA**, in Medicine, a Disease, the same with Coma. According to *Blanchard*, there is this Difference between the two, that *Cataphora* is the Genus to all Kinds of Stupors, unattended with Fevers.

**CATAPLASM**, popularly call'd *Poultice*, an external Medicine, in form of a Pulp; of a soft Consistence, like an Unguent, or Cerat; compos'd of various Liquors, Parts of Plants, Oils, Unguents, &c. according to the Variety of Intentions. Its ordinary Effects are, to assuage Pain, softer, resolve, discuss, or suppurate Matter collected in the external Parts of the Body. The ordinary Cataplasm for these Intentions, is compos'd of white Bread, Milk, Yolks, of Eggs, Saffron, and Oil of Roses. The Word comes from the *Greek* καταπλασσω, *illino*, I smear, or apply outwardly.

**CATAPUTIA**, a Medicinal Plant, commonly call'd the *lesser Spurge*. It purges with such a Violence, both upwards and downwards, that few Persons of any Credit venture to prescribe it.

**CATARACT**, in Medicine, a Suffusion of Sight, arising from a little Film, or Speck, which swimming in the aqueous Humour of the Eye, and getting before the Pupil, intercepts the Rays of Light.

The *Cataract* is suppos'd to be form'd from a Condensation of the more viscous Parts of the aqueous Humour, between the Uvea and the Crystalline : tho some take it to be a Pellicle, detach'd from the Crystalline itself; which is only an Assemblage of several little Pellicles, laid over one another.

There are two Kinds of *Cataracts*, the *Genuine* and *Spurious*; the first owing to a Humour amass'd in the Eye, coagulated and fix'd therein, and destroying its use : the latter arises from Fumes or Vapours, carry'd to the Eye by some Accident; as by a Fever, &c. The Genuine *Cataract* has several Degrees and several Names : At first the Patient sees, as it were, Clouds, Motes, Flies, &c. diffus'd over the Objects in view : Thus far the *Cataract* is call'd *Imaginary*; there being nothing yet appearing to the Eye of another Person. As the *Suffusion* increases, the Pupil begins to appear of a Sea-Green Colour; sometimes like the Air, full of Clouds; and then the *Cataract* is call'd *Water*, or *Water-fall*. When the Evil is arriv'd at its height, and the Matter sufficiently coagulated, the Patient loses all Sight; the Pupil ceases to be transparent, but becomes white, or brown, or some other Colour; which last is what we properly denominate a *Cataract*.

*Couching of Cataracts*. For the Cure of a *Cataract*, recourse is had to the Operation of Couching; which is perform'd by running a Steel Needle into the Eye, thro the Adnata, by the Edge of the Cornea, on the Side of the little Canthus, till it arrive at the Middle of the *Cataract*; then, turning the Needle round, they twist the *Cataract* about its Point, till being thus reduc'd into a little Compass, 'tis brought down beneath the Pupil, and couch'd, or lodg'd in the Bottom of the Eye, and there left : Thus, the Impediment being remov'd, the Light gets admission. To render the Operation effectual, care must be taken, that the Pellicle or Cataract be ripe, or arriv'd at its Consistence, so as it may be easily roll'd up; that its Parts be crush'd, or broke in rolling up, and lodg'd so secure, as not to rise up again by its Elasticity; and perhaps also, that it dissolve and consume at the Bottom of the Eye.

This is the popular Theory of *Cataracts*, which some modern Physicians oppose, and substitute a new one in its place : Their Opinion is, that instead of Couching, or laying a little Membrane, or Pellicle, 'tis the Crystalline it self that is thus couch'd, and lodg'd in the Bottom of the vitreous Humour. This they suppose to have been condens'd, and to have lost its Transparence; whence, instead of being an Instrument of Vision, it proves an Obstacle to it, by shutting out the Rays from the Retina. This Alteration of its Transparence, is accomplish'd with a Change of Colour; it becomes greenish; and on this account is call'd by the Greeks Glaucoma. The Glaucoma and Cataract therefore, in their Opinion, are the same Things : tho in the other Hypothesis they are very different; the first being reputed incurable, but not the latter.

The chief Reason urg'd in behalf of this latter Hypothesis, in the *French* Academy Royal, where it was propos'd, is, that after the Operation of Couching, the Person can't see without a convex Lens. Now if not more were done, than the taking away a Pellicle from before the Crystalline, it wou'd be in the same Condition as before, and wou'd make the same Refractions; nor wou'd any Lens be necessary : Whereas, supposing the Crystalline couch'd, 'tis evident the Lens will be requir'd to supply its place. To this it is answer'd, that there have been Instances of Persons who have seen, after Couching, without any Lens; at least, 'tis granted, that immediately after the Operation, several Persons have seen very distinctly : And tho Lens's soon become necessary, yet the first Moment wherein they saw without, seems to be a Proof that the Crystalline was not couch'd.

M. *de la Hire*[1], in Confirmation of the antient System, assigns this Reason

[1] Philippe de la Hire (1606 – 1656), a French astronomer and physicist.

for the Necessity of a Lens, after the Operation, *viz.* that the Vice which produc'd the Cataract is still subsisting in the aqueous Humour; which being too thick and muddy, lets too few Rays pass : a Failing to be repair'd by a Lens, which throws a greater Quantity of Rays on the Retina.

He adds some Experiments made on the Eyes of Oxen; the Result of which was, that the Crystalline could never be laid perfectly in the Bottom of the Eye, but there still stuck up, so as to stop up part of the Passage of the Rays; partly on account of its Bulk, and partly on that of its being sustain'd by the aqueous and vitreous Humour : He adds, that in the Operation of Couching, the Needle is apt to scratch the anterior Surface of the Crystalline, and open the Membrane wherewith it is invelop'd; the Consequence of which will be Wrinkles, which will render the Refractions irregular, and change the Direction of the Rays which should all meet in the same Point; so as to spoil the Representation of Objects. Lastly, 'tis insisted, that of the Crystalline be couch'd, the Patient wou'd not see at all, for want of the necessary Refractions.

M. *Antoine*[1], in the other hand, relates, that upon opening a Person whom he had couch'd on both Eyes, he found the two Crystallines actually couch'd, and lodg'd at the Bottom, between the vitreous Humour and the Uvea, where they were left by the Needle; and yet the Person saw without either : which shews both that the Operation of Couching the Crystalline is practicable, and that Vision may be peform'd without it. In effect, the vitreous and aqueous Humour, upon removing the Crystalline, may be suppos'd to run into the Cavity, to assume the Figure of its Mould, and perform the Refractions and Offices of the Crystalline; it being found, by Experiment, that the Refraction is the same in each Humour.

To shew, however, that there are Cataracts distinct from Glaucomas, M. *Littre* produc'd before the Society a Eye of a Man blind 22 Years; wherein was a distinct Cataract, or Pellicle, which clos'd the Aperture of the Pupil.

**CATARRH**, in Medicine, a Flux, or Defluxion of a serous Humour from the Glands about the Head and Throat, upon the Parts adjacent. The Word comes from the *Greek* Καταρρεω, *defluo*, I flow down.

*Catarrhs* are, generally occasion'd by a Diminution of insensible Perspiration in taking a cold; the Effect whereof is, that the Lymph, that should pass by the Skin, ouzes out upon those Glands; and being this extravasated, occasions Irritations, Coughs, and all the usual Symptoms. *Degory* deduces all Diseases from *Catarrhs*; which he looks upon as the Seminary of the most Disorders of the Body. *Etmuller* distinguishes a *hot* and a *cold Catarrh*; the first attended with unnatural Heat and Pain, and a Phlogosis of whole Body; the excreted Lymph being exceeding thin and sharp: In the *cold*, all the Symptoms are more remiss.

There is also a *suffocative Catarrh*, seated in the Larynx, and Epiglottis, which constringes; and thus, obstructing Respiration, endangers Strangling.

*Catarrhs* are cured by softning the Serosities, and augmenting Transpiration, by means of Diaphoreticks, soporiferous Medicines, and Diureticks. Smoking of Tobacco is recommended as excellent in all *catarrhal*

[1] Antoine Maitre-Jan (1650 – 1730), a French physician and surgeon.

Affections : In *obstinate Catarrhs*, recourse is sometimes had to Issues and Blisters. *Catarrhs* don't arise from the Head only, but sometimes also from other Parts of the Body; the lymphatic Vessels, wherein the Serosities are contain'd, as well as the Glands that separate them, being distributed all over the Body.

**CATECHU**, in Medicine, a sort of medicinal Earth, call'd also *Cachou*, and *Japan Earth*.

**CATHARTICS**, Purgative Medicines, or Remedies that promote Evacuation by Stool. Some use the Word *Cathartic* in a more general Sense, comprehending under it Emetics, or Vomitives; but this seems an Abuse.

*Cathartics*, in the proper Sense of the Word, are of several Kinds, *mild, moderate*, and *violent* : The first purge gently, as *Cassis, Manna, Tamarinds, Rhubarb, Sena*, &c. the second pretty briskly, as *Jallop*, and *Scamony*, &c. the third severely, as *Colacinth, Hellebore, Laureola*, &c.

*Cathartics* are likewise divided into *Chologogues, Phlegmagogues, Melanogogues*, and *Hydrogogues*; the first suppos'd to purge the Bile, the second Pituita, the third Melancholy, and the fourth Serosities. The Word comes from the *Greek* καθαιρω, *purgo*, I purge.

**CATHERETIC** Medicines, such as consume and carry off Carnosities, proud Flesh, and Excrescences arising in Wounds, &c. such are the *red Precipitate, burnt Alum, blue Vitriol, Stone*, &c. Some call these Medicines *Sarcophages*, Flesh Eaters. The Word is form'd from the *Greek* καθα, and αιρεω, *I take away, carry off.*

**CATHOLIC** Furnace, is a little Furnace, so contriv'd, as to be fit for all kinds of Operations, which do not require an intense Fire.

**CATHOLICON**, in Pharmacy, a kind of soft Electuary; so call'd, as being suppos'd universal; or a Purger of all Humours. Different Authors give different Recipes for it : That call'd *Catholicon Nicholai* is most in use; it consists of 16 Ingredients, the chief whereof are Tamarinds, Cassia, Senna, Rhubarb. It is said to be *double*, when there is a double Portion of Sena and Rhubarb. The *Catholicon for Clysters*, only differs from this, in that it has no Rhubarb, and that Honey is us'd instead of Sugar.

**CAULIFEROUS** Herbs, are such as have a true *Caulis*, Stalk, or Trunk, which a great many have not; as the *Capillaries*, &c.

**CAUSTICS**, in Medicine, &c. are such Things as have the Virtue of *Burning*, or are *Corrosive*; particularly those Medicines which by their violent Activity, and the Heat thence occasion'd, destroy the Texture of the Parts to which the are apply'd.

*Caustics* are us'd to eat off proud fungous Flesh; they also penetrate within hard callous Bodies, and liquefy the Humours; and are particularly apply'd in Abscesses and Imposthumations, to eat thro to the suppurated Matter, and give it vent.

The principal Medicines of this Class, are burnt Alum, Sponge, Cantharides, and other Vesicatories, as also Orpiment, Calx viva, Vitriol, Ashes of the Fig-Tree, the Ash, and Wine Lees; the Salt of the Lixivium, whereof Soap is made; Sublimate, Mercury, red Precipitate, &c.

*Crystals of the Moon*, and *Lapis Infernalis*, made of Silver and Spirit of Nitre, become *Caustics* by that Mixture.

Those *Caustics* which burn thro the Part, and leave a Scar, are particularly call'd *Cauteries*; tho Dr. *Quincy* confounds the two together. The Word comes from καυςικος, *urens*, of καιω, *uro*, I burn.

**CAUTERY**, in Chirurgery, a burning Medicine, or a Composition of several Things, which gnaw, burn off, eat thro, and sear the Parts; us'd, principally, in Abscesses, Imposthumations, Ulcers, and Caries of the Bones, to open a Passage for the Discharge if Ill Humours, &c.

*Cauteries* are of two Kinds, *Actual* and *Potential*. *Actual* Cauteries, are those which produce an instantaneous Effect, as Fire, or a red-hot Iron, which are apply'd in the *Fistula Lachrymalis*, after Extirpation of Cancers, Amputations of Legs, or Arms, &c. in order to stop the Hemorrhages, and produce a laudable Suppuration. The Irons us'd on these Occasions, are sometimes crooked at the Extremity, and that variously, according to the various Occasions : Whence some are called *Cultellary*, others *Punctual*, others *Olivary*, &c. M. *Homberg* assures us, that a great Part of Medicine of the People of *Java*, and other Parts of the *East Indies*, consists in Burning, or the Application of actual *Cauteries*; and that there is scarce any Disease but they will happily cure thereby.

*Potential* Cauteries, are Compositions of *Caustic* Medicines, usually of Quick-lime, Soap, and Chimney Soot.

The *Actual Cautery*, or hot Iron, is frequently apply'd for the making of Issues, in Parts where cutting is difficult.

**CELIAC** *Passion*, or *Cæliaca Passio*, in Medicine, a kind of Flux of the Belly, wherein the Food does not indeed pass perfectly crude, as in the *Lientery*, but half digested; so that the two only differ from each other, as more or less. In the *Celiac* the Food is sometimes digested, without the Chyle's being separated form the Excrements.

The Causes of the *Celiac* are either the Weakness of the Ferment of the Stomach, or the short stay the Food there makes, the Obstruction of the Lacteals, or the want of Acrity in the Bile.

The Word comes from the *Greek* κοιλια, *Venter*; whence κοιλιακος, a Person subject to such Inconveniences.

**CEMENT**, in Chymistry, is a Compound, us'd for the purifying of Gold; see Gold, and Purification. There are two kinds of Cement, Common, and Royal. The first made of Brickdust, Nitre, and Verdigrease; the second of Sal Gemmæ, and Armoniac, each one Part; two Parts of common Salt, and four of Bole : the whole reduc'd into a Paste with Urine.

**CEMENTATION**, or Cæmentation, a manner of purifying Gold, by means of Cement. 'Tis perform'd thus : Thin Plates, or *Laminæ*, are stratify'd in a Crucible with *Royal Cement*; the Crucible is cover'd up, and encompass'd with Fire for 10 or 12 Hours, till being thus calcin'd, the Salts have imbib'd and consum'd the Impurities of Gold. This Method of *Refining*, is much inferior to that by means of Antimony; in regard, the Salts sometimes leave other Metals remaining with the Gold; and besides, frequently eat away the Gold it self.

**CENTURY**, or *Centaury the lesser*, in Medicine, an Herb, chiefly noted for a Stomachic, and restoring decay'd Appetites : It is seldom prescrib'd otherwise than by Infusion or Decoction; it is an Ingredient in the *Venice* Treacle; and, as a Stomachic, it enters as one of the Ingredients in the Officinal Bitter Draught; and is for the same Purpose order'd in extemporaneous Prescriptions, with others of the same Nature, for the making of bitter Wines, &c.

A strong Decoction hereof is said to be of service, drank for some time, in Obstructions of the Menses, and also to destroy Worms; a Property attributed to most Bitters. It is often prescrib'd externally in discutient Fomentations. The Tops, or Flowers, are only us'd. The *greater Centaury* is never prescrib'd.

**CEPHALIC**, in medicine, is apply'd to any thing belonging to the Head, or its Parts. The Word is form'd of the Greek κηφαλω, *Caput*.

**CEPHALICS**, or Cephalic *Medicines*, are such as are proper for Disorders of the Head: these are generally of a volatile, spirituous, or aromatic Nature, or at least join'd with such; and are suppos'd to be of service, by the Volatility of their Particles, insinuating into the Nerves, and mixing with the Animal Spirits directly, as well as by the common Circulation.

Thus, Spirit of Lavender is suppos'd directly to act upon the Nerves of the Palate, &c. upon which account it's frequently taken dropp'd on Sugar, or Bread: and Sal Volatile, by smelling to, is suppos'd to be assistant to the Head, by its volatile Particles entering the Olfactory Nerves. As to Aromatic *Cephalics*, as the Species of Diambra, Pouder of Degutetu, Nutmeg, &c. they act chiefly by their aromatic Parts warming the nervous System, and increasing their Vibrations by which the nervous Fluid circulates more freely.

**CEPHALALGIA**, in Medicine, is understood, in the general, of any *Head-ach*; but properly signifies only a fresh one : When it becomes inveterate, 'tis call'd *Cephalia*; and, when it only possesses half the Head, *Megrim*.

**CERATE**, in Medicine, a kind of Unguent, or Liniment, made of Oil and Wax; us'd in several Diseases, especially those of the Skin. It takes its Name from the its capital Ingredient, Wax, call'd in Latin *Cera*.

Its Consistence is thicker than that of a Liniment; the last having usually two Ounces of Wax to two of Oil; but the first four of Wax to two of Oil; yet 'tis thinner than a Plaster.

There are *Cerates* of various kinds, Refrigerative, Stomachic, &c. *Cerate of*

*Sulphur, of Santal, restringent Cerate of Bricks, Divine Cerate*, &c. There is a particular one, call'd the *refrigerative Cerate of* Galen, made of white Wax and Oil of Roses Omphacin.

**CERUSSE**, a Preparation of Lead, properly call'd *White Lead*; and, by the Chymists, Calx of Lead. *Cerusse* is made of very thin *Laminæ*, or Plates of Lead, so laid, as to receive and imbibe the Fumes of Vinegar, plac'd in a Vessel over a moderate Fire. The *Laminæ* are, by means hereof, converted into a white Rust; which they gather together, and grinding it up with Water, form into little Cakes. *Cardan*[1] shews how to make it of Urine.

*Cerusse* makes a beautiful white Colour, and is much us'd by the Painters, both in Oil and Water Colours. It makes the principal Ingredient in the Fucus us'd by the Ladies for the Complexion. Taken inwardly, it is a dangerous Poison; and soon shews its Malignity on the Outside; spoiling the Breath and Teeth, and hastning Wrinkles, and the Symptoms of old Age.

The best *Cerusse*, is that of *Venice*; but this is rare : that chiefly us'd, is either *English* or *Dutch*, both of which have more Marl in 'em than White Lead; the latter, however, is the better of the two. *Fallopius*[1] speaks of a Mineral *Cerusse*, but everybody else takes it to be factitious.

The Word comes from the *Greek* κηρος, *Wax*; *Cerusse* bearing a resemblance to Wax.

**CHALASTIC** Medicines, are such as have the Faculty of softening, and relaxing the Parts; when, on account of their extraordinary Tension, or Swelling, they occasion Pain. Of this Kind are Butter, and many Oils, &c. The Word comes from the *Greek* χαλαω, I *soften*.

**CHALCITIS**, sometimes call'd *Colcothar*, is a kind of Mineral; or, as some call it, a Vitriol; reddish, like Copper; friable, not very hard, and having yellow shining Veins within.

It has the Taste of a Vitriol, melts alone in a Crucible, and dissolves very easily in watry Liquors.

There are two other Minerals, call'd *Misi*, and *Sory*, very much like the *Chalcitis*. In effect, the Antients confounded them together; and not only the *Misi* and *Sory*, but also the *Melanteria*; or rather, they imagin'd a successive Transmutation of the four Minerals, which began with *Chalcitis*, became *Misi*, then *Melanteria*, and lastly *Sory*, where it fix'd.

The Moderns make these four distinct Matters : tho the chief Difference between them, is suppos'd to lie in the different Tenuity or Grossness of their Substance. Some say, the *Misi* is form'd on the *Chalcitis*, as Verdegrease on Copper, being properly its Rust; and that *Chalcitis* is form'd in the same manner on the *Sory*.

This is certain, they are all found in Copper Mines : But the modern Druggists know little of any of them but *Chalcitis*. This is brought from *Germany* : It is very Caustic and Escharotic. Its chief use is in the Comp-

[1] This is probably Girolamo Cardan (1501 – 1576), an Italian physician and philosopher.

[2] Gabriele Falloppio (1523 – 1562), an Italian physician and anatomist.

osition of Venice Treacle : in lieu of it are frequently substituted *Calcanthum* rubefy'd, or *Copperas*, or *Calamites*.

**CHALK** is us'd in Medicine, as an Astringent, an Absorbent, and a Sweetner; and is celebrated for curing the Heartburn, beyond any thing whatsoever.

**CHALYBEAT**, in Medicine, something that partakes of the Nature of Steel, or Iron; or that is impregnated with Particles of those Metals.

*Chalybeats* act chiefly as Absorbents, and Deobstruents. Iron, M. *Lemery*, observes, is a Mixture of an oily Substance with a metallic Matter; but the Oil is the Predominant in the Mixture : and between the Parts mix'd are large Pores. Hence, Iron becomes easily dissolvable; and its Oil easily disengages it self : But when once decompounded, *i.e.* when the Oil s separated from the pure, ferruginous, or metallic Part, no Dissolvent has any Effect on that *Caput Mortuum*.

Hence appears the Absurdity of that common Practice, of calcining Iron to such a degree, as to convert it into what the Chymists call a *Crocus*, or Saffron. This Operation must of necessity take away all, or most of the oily Substance, and have left nothing but the indissoluble *Caput Mortuum*. Which Oil here separated, should properly have been separated by the Heat of the Stomach; whence, according to M. *Lemery*, it wou'd have carry'd into the Blood a new spirituous, salutary Juice : He observes also, that Iron acts as an Absorbent, from the Largeness of its Pores; and the Ease wherewith all Kinds of Salts, even gross ones, insinuate themselves therein: even scorbutic Acids are absorb'd thereby.

Further, 'tis not enough that peccant Acids enter Iron; but in entering they also expel and express that salutary Juice, which is also put in Motion, and dispos'd to be evacuated by the natural Heat. Thus is Iron doubly advantageous, both by the Oil it furnishes the Blood withal, and by the Salts it frees it from. The Action of the Particles of a *Chalybeat*, by their Elasticity, together with the *Momentum* they give the Blood by their Ponderosity, makes them not only preferable to most other Deobstruents, but also proper in other Cases; especially where there is a Viscidity of the Juices, the Blood depauperated, and where the Circulation is languid; as in most Hysteric and Hypochondriac Cases, &c.

**CHELONITES**, in Natural History, a Stone found in the Bellies of young Swallows; much esteem'd by some for the falling Sickness. The Stone takes its Name from χελιδων, *Swallow*. There is also a Stone bearing the same Name found in the *Indian* Tortoises, which is said to have the Faculty of resisting Poison. Some confound it with the *Crapaudin*, or *Toadstone*.

**CHILBLAIN**, in Medicine, a Tumor afflicting the Feet and Hands; accompany'd with an Inflammation, Pain, and sometimes an Ulcer, or Solution of Continuity. *Chilblains*, by Physicians call'd *Perniones*, are occasion'd by excessive Cold stopping the Motion of the Blood in the Capillary Arteries. The Tumor, from white, generally inclines to blueness. Petroleum laid on the Part, either prevents *Chilblains*, or cure 'em.

**CHINA**-*Root*[1], a Medicinal Root, brought from the East-Indies. It is of a ruddy brown Colour, bordering on black, without side; and white, or reddish, within. It grows chiefly in fenny Places, usually cover'd with the Sea; which, upon its withdrawing, leaves great Quantities thereof on the Shore : the best is that which is firm, ruddy, and fresh. It is esteem'd a sweetner of the Blood; and us'd as such in Decoctions, in Venereal and Scorbutick Cases.

**CHIVES**, or Chieves, a Term in Botany, which Mr. *Ray* renders in Latin *Apices*, *i.e.* the small Knobs growing on the Ends of the fine Threads, or *Stamina* of Flowers. But Dr. *Green* calls the *Stamina*, or Threads themselves, on which the Apices are fix'd, the *Chives*.

**CHLOROSIS**, in Medicine, a Disease vulgarly call'd the *Green-Sickness*, *White-Jaundice*, &c. Its usual Subjects are Girls, Maids, and Widows; or even Wives, whose Husbands are deficient, &c. It gives a pale, sallow, or livid Tincture to the Complexion, with a Circle of Violet under the Eyes. The Patient is melancholy, and uneasy; has frequently a low wandring Fever, with an unequal Pulse, Vomiting, Heaviness, Listlessness, Drousiness, Difficulty of Breathing, Longing for absurd Foods, &c.

It comes on, commonly, antecedent to, or about the Time of the Eruption of the Menses. The Stoppage of the Menses is not always the Cause of this Distemper; for they sometimes flow regularly, tho but seldom, in the Progress thereof. According to *Etmuller*, the Suppression of the Menses is rather the Effect than the Cause.

The Cure is chiefly to be attempted by Chalybeats and Bitters. In the colder Constitutions, Decoctions of *Guaiacum* are found of use.

The Word *Chlorosis* signifies Greenness, Verdure; from χλοη, *Herba*, Grass.

**CHOLAGOGUE**, a Medicine which purges the Bile downwards. The Word comes from the χολη, Bile, and αγειν, to lead. Of these some are simple, others compound; and both the one and the other distinguish'd into three Kinds, with regard to their Activity; the benign, the moderate, and the violent. Of the first kind are Manna, Cassia, Roses, Tamarinds, &c. Of the second, Sena, Rhubarb, Aloes, &c. Of the third, Jalop, Scammony, &c.

**CHOLERA-MORBUS**, a sudden overflowing of the Bile, both upwards and downwards. It is suppos'd to have its rise from the great Abundance of bilious Humours, which being very acrimonious, vellicate the membranes of the Stomach and Intestines; and by that means occasion unusual and violent Contractions. 'Tis very dangerous : Whence the *French* antiently called it *Trouffe-Galand*. It has its Name, either from the great Quantity of *Choler* it evacuates; or because the Matter is incessantly expell'd at the Intestines, which they antiently call'd *Cholades*.

Dr. *Sydenham*[2] observes, it generally attacks about the latter end of Summer; and proceeds, not unfrequently, from Surfeits : That the Cure

[1] China root is a species of plant of the genus *Smilax*.

[2] Thomas Sydenham (1624 – 1689), an English physician.

depends upon a large Quantities of Chicken-Broth, drank so as to excite Vomiting plentifully; and that the Broth is also to be injected Clysterwise : after which, he says, the Cure is to be completed by *Laudenum*, given at proper Intervals, and in proper Doses.

The Remedy in the Indies for the *Cholera Morbus*, or *Mandechin*, is to keep the Patient from drinking; and to burn the Souls of his Feet.

**CHORDAPSUS**, in Medicine, a Disease of the Intestines, otherwise call'd *Miserere mei* : Tho some say 'tis only a Species of *Miserere*. *Galen* defines it, a Humour or Inflation, of the small Intestines, which makes them appear fill'd, and stretch'd like a *Chord*. *Archigenes* makes it a kind of *Miserere*; consisting in a Tumor in a certain Place of the small Intestines, which sinks in, and gives way to the Hand when press'd. He adds, that it's exceeding dangerous, and ordinarily kills in three or four Hours, unless it comes to Suppuration; which, however, does not take away all Danger.

'Tis probable, however, that the *Chordapsus* is in reality nothing else but the *Miserere*. *Celsus* informs us, that in his Time they were the same thing. The Word comes from the *Greek* χορδα, *Chord*, and απτεσθαι, *to touch*.

**CHOREA** *Sancti Viti*, in Medicine, a Distemper which some Authors reckon as an hysterical Case; and others a Species of a *Furor Uterinus*. It is suppos'd to proceed from a Turgency and Repletion of Hot Juices, especially in the Uterine Vessels, which raises violent Motions; and that only Females are affected by it : But Dr. *Sydenham* more properly observes it to be an universal Convulsion, which sometimes continues several Weeks, nay Months, without intermission.

Those affected with this Disease, are continually in strange Motions with their Heads, Legs, and Arms; so that they are unfit to feed themselves. It differs from other Convulsions, in that the Motions are not painful, nor any of the Extremities or Parts forcibly contracted, or extended for any time. Boys and Girls are most subject to this Disease, and that from ten Years of Age to Puberty; tho the latter oftner than the former.

It sometimes precedes the first Eruption of the Menses; in which Case, proper Cathartics, with Calomel and Deobstruents, are generally us'd; otherwise, Evac-uations and Antiepileptics, as in other nervous Disorders.

It takes the Name of *Chorea Sancti Viti*, or Saint *Vitus's* Dance, from the Chapel of S. *Vitus*; because it was suppos'd to seize Persons about May, which was the Time of the Year they visited that Chapel, and to make them leap and dance about in a strange manner.

**CHRONIC**, Chronical, in Medicine, is apply'd to a slow, or inveterate Disease, which lasts a long time; as the *Gout, Hæmorrhoids, Fistula, Dropsy, Asthma*, etc. *Chronic* Diseases stand in opposition to acute Diseases, which are speedy, and hasten to a Crisis; as *Fevers, Small-Pox*, &c. Most of the *Chronical* Diseases, says Dr. *Cheyne*[1], the Infirmities of old Age, and the short Periods of the Lives of *Englishmen*, are owing to Repletion : This is evident hence, that Evacuation of one kind or another, is nine Parts in ten of

[1] George Cheyne (1671 – 1743), an English physician and philosopher.

their Remedy.

The Sources of *Chronical* Distempers, says the same Author, are, 1. Viscidity in the Juices, or the overlargeness of their constituent Particles; which not being sufficiently broken by the concoctive Powers, stop, or retard the Circulation. Or, 2. Too great abundance of sharp acrimonious Salts; whereby the Juices themselves are render'd so corrosive, as to burst or wear out the Solids. Or, 3. A Relaxation, or want of a due Force and Springiness of the Solids themselves.

An Excess in the Quantity of our Meat and Drink begets the first; the bad Condition of the same Foods the second; and both together, with want of due Exercise, the third.

**CHRYSOCOLLA**, a Mineral us'd in the soldering of Gold, &c. whence its Name. It is found in Mines of Gold, Silver, Copper, and Lead : Its Colour is various, according to that of the Matter in which it is found; yellow if among Gold, white in Silver, green in Copper, and black in Lead. The *Arabs*, and Inhabitants of *Guzuratte*[1], called it *Tincar*, or *Tincal* : In *Europe*, where 'tis found in various Places, 'tis confounded with the common Borax.

The best is that which is green, like an Emerald, found among Copper : that found among the other Metals is too much wash'd. Some reckon the *Chrysocolla* a Species of Nitre. The Physicians use it in the Cure of Wounds : Some make an Artificial *Chrysocolla*, by mixing a little of the Natural, steep'd in Water, with Wood.

The Term is form'd of the *Greek* χρυσος, *Gold*, and κολλα, *Glue*.

**CHYLE**, Chyme, in the Animal Œconomy, a whitish Juice into which the Food is immediately converted by Digestion, or, more properly, by that Branch thereof call'd *Chylification*. The Word comes from the *Greek* κυλος, *Juice*.

The *Chyle*, Dr. *Drake* observes, is nothing but a Mixture of oily and aqueous Parts of the Food, incorporated with the saline ones; which, while they yet remain mix'd with the grosser Parts in the Stomach, make a thick, whitish, partly fluid Mass, called Chyme: which, as soon as it is reduc'd to a Consistence loose enough to be obedient to the pressure and peristaltic Motion of the Stomach, is gradually thrust out at the Pylorus into the Duodenum, and denominated *Chyle*. Thus is the *Chyle* begun to be form'd in the Stomach; it is perfected in the Intestines by the Mixture of the Bile and the pancreatic Juice; and is thence receiv'd into the Lacteal Veins, which carry it to the *Receptaculum Chyli*, or *Pecquets* Reservatory : thence it passes into the Thoracic Duct, which terminates in the left Sub-clavian Vein : In this Vein, the *Chyle* first begins to mix with the Blood; into which it is afterwards converted by the Action called *Sanguification*.

The Antients suppos'd the *Chyle* was chang'd into Blood in the Liver; others of 'em in the Heart : but the Moderns, with more reason, take the Change to be effected by the Blood it self, in all the Parts of the Body. Some take *Chyle* to be the immediate Matter of Nutrition; others the Blood.

[1] The state of Gujurat in India; also known as Khambhat or Cambay.

Dr. *Lister* is of Opinion, that in the Digestion of Meat in the Stomach, there is made a Separation, or Solution of urinous Salts, no otherwise than in the rotting of Plants, or Animals: that the *Chyle* is highly impregnated with this urinous Salt; that it owes its whiteness to the Fermentation it acquires from that Mixture; That the salt *Chyle* is convey'd into the venal Blood, and with it enters the Heart; and is thence thrown out *Chyle*, as it comes in, by a continual Pulsation, into the Arteries : that as often as it enters the Emulgent Arteries, it leaves behind part of its saline Liquor, or Urine, and consequently abates of its Colour : That when sufficiently freed of its Salts, it becomes a *Lympha*; which seems to be nothing else but the Residue of the *Chyle* not yet converted into Blood; as not yet sufficiently depurated of its saline Particles.

**CHYLIFICATION**, the Formation of the *Chyle*; or the Act whereby the Food is chang'd into the *Chyle*. *Chylification* is begun by comminuting, or breaking the Aliment in the Mouth, mixing it with Saliva, and chewing it with the Teeth.

By such means, the Food is reduc'd into a kind of Pulp, which falling thro' the *Œsophagus* into the warm Stomach, mixes with the Juices thereof; and is thus diluted, begins to ferment, or putrefy, and assumes a very different form from it had before; growing either acid or rancid.

Here it mixes with a Juice separated from the Blood by the Glands of that Part, whose Excretory Ducts open into the Stomach; as also with the Remains of the former Aliment : and thus it becomes better macerated, diluted, dissolv'd, and acquires still a greater likeness to the Animal Fluids, and is called *Chyme*.

Add to this, that the fleshy Membrane of the Stomach continually contracting and pressing its Contents by its peristaltic Motion, occasions a more intimate Mixture, and by degrees works out the more fluid Parts thro' the Pylorus into the Duodenum; along the Sides whereof, and the rest of the *Instestina Tenuia*, the Lacteals are planted; into the minute Orifices whereof, the finer Parts of the Mass is receiv'd.

The Fabrick of the Stomach being consider'd, the Heat of the circumambient Parts, the Pulsations of innumerable Arteries, the great Strokes of the *Aorta* underneath, the constant Compression of the *Diaphragma* and Abdominal Muscles; it must necessarily follow, that the finer Parts of the Aliment will be first expell'd by the Stomach; and that the grosser will remain; till, by the repeated Action of the Fluids, and the Contraction and Pulsation of the Solids, they also become fine enough to go off : thus is the Stomach left empty; and by means of its muscular Coat, reduc'd to a State of Contraction, and Appetite renew'd.

Thus will even fleshy Membranes, Cartilages, &c. of Animals fed on, be squeez'd, and oblig'd to give out their Juices; and thus is a Fluid obtain'd, that shall have in some measure the same Properties with those of our Bodies.

The juice being got thro' the Pylorus into the Intestines, its Liquefaction is still promoted by its mixture with two other Dissolvents, the pancreatic Juice and the Bile; which divide and subtilize those Parts that were left too gross : and by the peristaltic Motion of the Guts it is protruded forwards. In the Passage thro' the small Intestines, the fine Part of the Mass, which we call the

Chyle, enters the Orifices of the Lacteal Veins of the first Kind, wherewith the whole Mesentery is intermix'd; which either alone, or together with the Mesariac Veins, discharge themselves into the Glands at the Basis of the Mesentery.

Then the *Chyle* is taken up by the Lacteals of the second Kind, and convey'd into Glands between the two Tendons of the Diaphragma, known heretofore under the Name of the *Lumbary* Glands, now call'd *Pecquet's Reservatory*; whence it is carry'd to the Heart by the Thoracic Duct and the Subclavian Vein; wherein it begins to be mix'd with the Blood, and to circulate, and in time become assimilated thereto.

**CHYLOSIS**, in Medicine, the Action whereby the Aliment is converted into *Chyle*, or *Chyme*, in the Stomach, &c. whether it be by a Ferment in the Stomach, or the contractile Force of the Stomach, or both.

**CHYME**, an Animal Juice, the same with that commonly called *Chyle*. Some, however, distinguish between *Chyme* and *Chyle*; restraining the Word *Chyme* to the Mass of Food, &c. while in the Stomach, e'er it be sufficiently diluted and liquify'd to pass the Pylorus into the Duodenum, and thence into the Lacteals, to be further diluted and impregnated with the pancreatic Juice; where it commences *Chyle*.

**CHYMISTRY**, or more properly Chemistry, the Art of separating the several Substances whereof mix'd Bodies are compos'd, by means of Fire; and of composing new Bodies in the Fire, by the Mixture of different Substances or Ingredients.

The great Object of *Chymistry*, is to analyse, or decompound natural Bodies; reduce them to their first Principles; discover their hidden Virtues, and demonstrate their inner Contexture, or the Centre, as they call it, wherein natural Substances occur. In a word, *Chymistry* is the Anatomy of natural Bodies, by means of Fire; which is the Definition *Hanneman*[1] gives us of the Art.

The very learned *Boerhaave* defines *Chymistry* very scientifically: "An Art whereby sensible Bodies contain'd in Vessels, or capable of being contain'd therein, are so chang'd by means of certain Instruments, and principally Fire, that their several Powers and Virtues are thereby discover'd, with a View to Philosophy, Medicine, &c."

This definition appears very prolix and circumstantial, and more like a Description than a Definition; but with all his Endeavours, he assures us, he could not frame a shorter, that would express the full Scope, Object, and Instruments of *Chymistry*, so as to distinguish It from every other Art : which is a Point all the Writers of *Chymistry* have stumbled at.

For *Chymistry* cannot justly be call'd the Art *of resolving Bodies*, as *Regius*[2], *Paracelsus*, &c. define it; since Mechanicks will also do that : Nor is the Matter mended by saying, It is the Art *of analysing Bodies by Fire*; as *Helmont* has done : nor *by Salt*, as others would have it. These Definitions

[1] Johann Ludwig Hanneman (1640 -1724), a German physicist and natural philosopher.

[2] Henricus Regius, born Henri de Roy (1598 – 1679), a Dutch physician and philosopher.

include only a Part, instead of the whole. And with as little Propriety is it term'd, The Art of *separating the Pure from the Impure*, inasmuch as it compounds as well as separates, and frequently mixes the Pure with the Impure. *Chymistry*, on this footing, appears a very extensive Art : Its Object, or the Materia Chymica, is all sensible Bodies, capable of being contain'd in Vessels; and is accordingly divided into three Kingdoms, *Fossil, Vegetable*, and *Animal.*

The Operations of *Chymistry*, include all the Changes produc'd in Bodies by natural Agents or Instruments, *viz. Decoction, Infusion, Exhalation, Calcination, Extraction, Distillation, Crystallization*, &c. The Effects, or Productions of *Chymistry*, may be reduc'd to *Magisteries, Extracts, Tinctures, Elixirs*, and *Clyssus's*. The *Instruments*, or *Agents of Chymistry*, whereby its Operations are perform'd, are *Fire, Water, Air, Earth, Menstruums*, and Instruments so call'd as *Alembics, Cucurbits, Retorts, Pelicans, Furnaces*, and *Lutes. Chymistry* is divided into *Metallurgia, Alchymia, Chymical Pharmacy*, and *Chymical Philosophy.*

*Chymistry* is an Art of very great Antiquity, and is held by some very learned Persons to have been practis'd in the Antediluvian World. *Cham*, the Son of *Noah*, is commonly held to have bean its Inventor, from whom it is suppos'd to have taken its Name. Others refer the Invention to *Tubal Cain*, whom the Scripture records as the Inventor of Instruments of Brass and Iron. This is pretty certain, that some of the highest and most difficult Things in *Chymistry*, must have been known by him; among which are the separating and purifying of Copper and Iron, the making of Brass, &c.

The first mention we find made of the Art, is in *Zozimus*, the *Panopolitan*, who lived about he Year of Christ 400. "In the Sacred Writings," says that Author, "we find certain *Genii* spoke of, who had commerce with Women. *Hermes* says as much in his Books upon Nature; and scarce any Author but has some Footsteps of this Tradition. These *Genii*, intoxicated with the Love of Women, discover'd 'em all the Secrets of Nature; and taught 'em abundance of Things unfit for 'em to know : for which reason they were banish'd from Heaven. The Book wherein their Secrets was contain'd, was call'd *Chema*; and hence the Name *Chemia*, or *Chymia*." The Text of Scripture *Zozimus* here refers to, is that passage in *Moses, The Sons of God saw the Daughters of Men, and too 'em to Wife.*

This Antediluvian Origin of *Chymistry* is confirm'd by *Tertullian*[1] : "The Angels that fell, says that Father, discover'd Gold and Silver to Men, with the Arts of working 'em, of dying Wool, &c. for which reason they were banish'd, as is related by *Enoch*." *Borrichius* looks on these Passages as authentic; but adds, that *Enoch* was mistaken, for that the Angels he speaks of were not real Angels; but the Descendants of *Seth* and *Tubal Cain*, who degenerating from their Fathers, gave themselves up to criminal Pleasures with the Women descended from *Cain*; and in the Course of their Intrigues, divulg'd the Secrets God had trusted 'em withal.

Be this as it will, *Chymistry*, no doubt, was first practis'd in *Egypt*. According to *Moses, Tubal Cain* should be the first Inventor. Profane Authors

[1] Quintus Septimius Florens Tertullianus (ca. 160 – 220), an ecclesiastical writer born in Carthage.

refer it to *Vulcan*; and some of the latest and best Criticks endeavour to shew, that *Tubal Cain* and *Vulcan* were the same; as, indeed, there is found a great resemblance between their Names. After *Tubal Cain*, the first *Chymist* we read of is *Moses*; whose Skill in *Chymistry* is incontestable, from his burning and pulverizing the Golden Calf the *Israelites* had set up, and giving it the People to drink. There is scarce a more difficult Operation in all *Chymistry*, than to make Gold potable.

*Chymistry* had the common Fate of the other Arts, at the Declension of the Eastern Empire; and lay bury'd and forgot till the Time of *Roger Bacon*[1], who retriev'd it. He was follow'd by *Lully*[2], *Ripley*[3], *Basil Valentine, Paracelsus, Van Helmont, Glauber, Boyle, Lemery, Homberg,* &c. by whom the Art has been carry'd to its present degree of Perfection.

The first *Chymists* confin'd themselves to Metals : In these latter Ages, the Bounds of *Chymistry* have been greatly enlarg'd; and Plants, Animals, Minerals &c. have been taken into it. 'Tis but of late that *Chymistry* has been apply'd to the Preparation of Medicines: *Basil Valentine*, and *Arnoldus de Villa Nova*[4], seem to have been the first that attempted it. *Paracelsus* and *Van Helmont* carry'd it to such a length, as to render Medicine almost wholly *chymical.*

Criticks are divided as to the Etymology of the Name *Chymistry* : it is usually deriv'd from the *Greek* κυμος, *Juice*; or from χεθιν, *to melt. Boerhaave*, and others, more justly derive it from the Egyptian *Chema*, or *Kema*, black; and write it *Chemia*, not *Chymia*. Others, making *Cham* the Inventor of *Chymistry*, derive the Term from his Name; supporting their Etymology on the Signification of the Word חם, *Cham*, which in *Hebrew* signifies *heat, hot, black*; all of them bearing some relation to the Operation of *Chymistry*.

*Chymistry* is also known under various other Names : It is sometimes call'd the *Hermetical Art*, from a Supposition of its being invented by *Hermes Trismegistus*[5]. Others call it, the *Egyptian Art*, from the People among whom it was first practis'd : Others the *Sacred, or Divine Art*; *Poiesis*; the Art of *making Gold*, &c. Others call it the *Spagyric* Art; *Paracelsus* the *Hyssopic* Art : others *Pyrotechnia*, &c. When the *Chymists* would express the most sublime Parts of their Art, they prefix the Arabic Particle *Al* to the Word *Chymia*, or *Chymistry*, and thus form *Alchymy*.

Some Authors observe, that *Diocletian*, after the taking of *Alexandria*, order'd all the Books of *Chymistry*, antiently wrote by the *Egyptians*, for making Gold and Silver, to be sought out and burnt; that they might not have the Power of enriching themselves by this Art, or of putting themselves, by this means, into a Condition of revolting.

[1] Roger Bacon (1214 – 1292), a Franciscan monk, philosopher and scientist.

[2] Raymond Lully, born Raymon Lull (1232 – 1315), a Spanish philosopher and theologian.

[3] George Ripley (ca. 1415 – 1490) , an English Augustinian monk and alchemist.

[4] Arnoldus de Villa Nova (1235 – 1311), a Spanish alchemist and astrologer.

[5] A mythical Egyptian sage identified with the Egyptian god Thoth and the Greek god Hermes. Trismegistus means "thrice great." The early works are attributed to an unknown Greek living in Alexandria towards the end of the first century.

Authors on the Subject of *Chymistry* are very numerous : *Borel*[1] has publish'd a Catalogue of most of 'em, under the Title of *Bibliotheca Chymica*; containing the Names of above ten thousand. *Boerhaave* is the latest, fullest, and infinitely the best; he has given both the History, Theory, and Practice, in the finest, most orderly, and scientific Way in the World. Dr. *Freind*[2] has reduc'd *Chymistry* to *Newtonianism*, and accounted for the Reasons of the Operations on Mechanical Principles.

**CHYMOSIS**, in Medicine, the Act of making or preparing *Chyme*. The Word comes from χυμος, *succus*, of χεω, *fundo*, I melt. *Chymosis* is particularly us'd for the second of the Concoctions made in the Body; being a repeated Preparation of the most impure and gross Parts of the Chyle, which being turn'd back by the Lacteals, is imbib'd by the Meseraics, and thence carry'd to the Liver, to be there elaborated, purify'd, and subtiliz'd afresh. 'Tis of this, according to *Rogers*, that the Animal Spirits are form'd.

**CHYMOSIS**, or Chemosis, is also us'd in Medicine, for an Inflammation of the Eyelids, which turns out their inside to sight.

**CICATRISIVE**, in Medicine, is apply'd to such Medicines as are very Desiccative; and on that account aid Nature to repair the Skin, and to form a *Cicatrix*, or *Eschar*. Such are *Armenian* Bole, Pouder of Tutty, the Unguent *Diapompholigus*, *desiccativum Rubrum*, &c. *Cicatrisive* Medicines are otherwise call'd *Escharotics, Epuloticks, Incarnatives, Agglutinants*, &c.

**CICATRIX**, in Medicine, &c. a little Seam, or Elevation of callous Flesh, rising on the Skin, and remaining there after the healing of a Wound, &c. ordinarily call'd a Scar, or Eschar. The *Cicatrix* is the same as to the joining of the fleshy Parts, as a *Callus* is to the Bones.

In young Infants, these Callosities, or Scars, sometimes much diminish, and oftentimes quite vanish when come to Age, as is particularly observ'd in the Pits of the Small-Pox : and, in growing, they are sometimes observ'd to change their Situation.

Some derive the Word from *quasi circa cutem* : others fetch Cicatrix from *quasi Occæcatrix*, the *Cicatrix* being only *obductio vulneris*, the covering up, or hiding of the Wound : but 'tis better deriv'd from *Caecatrix*, which has the same force; of the verb *Cæcare*, to blind.

**CICUTA**, a vegetable Poison, celebrated both among Antients and Moderns. The modern *Cicuta* is the Plant *Hemlock*; whereof there are two Kinds : the *Cicuta*, absolutely so call'd, or *Cicuta major*; and *Cicuta minor*. The first grows in Places a little moist, in the Shade, among old Ruins, or along Roads.

So many unhappy Effects have been perceiv'd from it, that its Use, internally, is by no means to be recommended : And yet some Persons boast of it as a powerful Sudorific. Externally it may be apply'd, to resolve Wens, and Hardnesses of the Spleen and Liver. It is the Base of the Plaister which

[1] Peter Borel 1620 – 1678), a French physician.

[2] John Freind (1675 – 1728), an English physician and scientist.

bears its name.

The Physicians have generally rank'd it among the cold Poisons; but later Writers, with more justness, regard it as a Dissolvent, or hot Poison. The Reasons they give, as related by *Wepfer*[1], are, that it bites the Tongue; that the Effluvia it yields are hot, and arise from a volatile Salt, and an impure Sulphur; that the Madness it occasions, as well as the other Symptoms, shew a great activity of Parts; and that if the Blood be found coagulated by it after Death, Spirit of Wine does the same.

The *lesser Cicuta* is not less dangerous than the *greater*; it is ever suppos'd more violent, as well as more hasty in its Operation.

Several persons have been render'd foolish, by eating Porridge wherein *Cicuta* has been us'd instead of Parsly. It has much such an Enmity to the Brain, as *Cantherides* have to the Bladder; and *Læpus Marinus* to the Lungs.

The *Cicuta* of the Antients, is a Secret which is now scarce possible to be discover'd : it was call'd *Cicuta Aquatica*, and was of the Umbelliferous Tribe. *Wepfer*, in an express Treatise on the Subject, will have it the *Sium Erucæ folio C.B.*

*Cicuta* is also us'd, chiefly, among the Antients, for a Juice, or Liquor, express'd from the Plant *Cicuta*. This *Cicuta* was the common Poison wherewith their State-Criminals were out to death : *Socrates* drank the *Cicuta*.

*Plato*, in his Dialogue on the Immortality of the Soul, observes that "The Executioner advis'd *Socrates* not to talk, for fear of causing the *Cicuta* to operate too slowly." M. *Petit*[2], in his *Observationes Miscellaneæ*, remarks that this Advertisement was not given by the Executioner out of Humanity, but to save the *Cicuta* : for he was only allow'd so much *per Ann.* which if he exceeded, he was to furnish at his own Expense. This Construction is confirm'd by a Passage in *Plutarch* : The Executioner who administer'd the *Cicuta* to *Phocion*, not having enough, *Phocion* gave him the Money to buy more; observing, by the way, that it was odd enough, that at *Athens* a Man must pay for every thing, even his own Death.

**CINERATION**, in Chymistry, the reduction of Wood, or any other combustible Matter into Ashes, by means of Fire. This, others call *Cenefaction.*

**CINERES** *Clavellati*, among Chymists, are the Ashes of Tartar, or the Lees of Wine burnt.

**CINERITIOUS**, a Term apply'd to Things resembling Ashes; particularly in point of Colour and Consistence. Thus, the Cortical Part of the Brain, is also call'd the *Cineritious* Part.

**CINNABAR**, or Cinoper, in Natural History, a Mineral Stone, red, heavy, and brillant; found chiefly in the Quicksilver Mines; call'd also Vermilion. Many, with good reason, esteem this the *Minium* of the Antients; tho a very

[1] Johann Jakob Wepfer (1620 – 1695), a Swiss physician and pharmacologist.

[2] Francois Parfour du Petit (1664 – 1721), a French physician and anatomist.

different thing from the modern *Minium*. The ordinary Vermilion it self, is nothing else but *Cinnabar* ground up with Spirit of Wine and Urine.

Some have imagin'd *Cinnabar* to be Dragons-Blood, gather'd, as *Pliny* and *Solinus* have it, when the Dragon and Elephant fight together : This Fable is refuted by *Dioscorides* and *Scaliger*.

*Cinnabar* is either *Native* or *Factitious*. The *Native*, or Mineral *Cinnabar*, or Vermilion, which is that abovemention'd, is found in most Places where there are Quicksilver Mines; yet, 'tis true also, that it has Mines its own : those in *Spain* are very famous; the *French* too have theirs, in *Normandy*.

It may be esteem'd as Marcassite of Quicksilver, or rather, as Quicksilver petrify'd and fix'd, by means of Sulphur, and a subterranean Heat : Chymistry being found to reduce it without much trouble or loss, to the Nature of Mercury. Each Pound of good *Cinnabar* yields fourteen Ounces of Mercury. Accordingly, the principal Property and Use of this Mineral, is to yield a most excellent Mercury; and that which the Alchymists maintain to be the best dispos'd for attaining the Transmutation of Gold.

The best Mineral *Cinnabar* is of a high Colour, brilliant, and free from the Stone. It is us'd by Physicians in Venereal Cases, and others, occasion'd by sharp Serosities. It's also esteem'd a good Cephalic, and accounted of service in Epilepsies, and other nervous Distempers : Add, that it is reckon'd of efficacy in cutaneous Cases, as the Scurvy.

*Factitious*, or Artificial *Cinnabar*, or Vermilion, is form'd of a Mixture of Mercury and Sulphur, sublimed, and this reduced into a kind of Stone. The best is of a high Colour, full of Fibres, like Needles. *The Method of preparing Factitious* Cinnabar is thus. They take three Ounces of Sulphur, and four of Quicksilver; these being well mix'd, are set on the Fire, till part of the Sulphur be consum'd, and the Pouder remain black. 'Tis then sublim'd once or twice in open Pots; at bottom of which remains the *Cinnabar*, very heavy, and streak'd with Lines, or Needles; some red, others brillant, like Silver.

This serves for the same medicinal Purposes with the *Native Cinnabar* : besides which, 'tis likewise us'd by the Farriers, to make Pills for their Horses; and by Painters, as a Colour : it being a very vivid red; but drying with some difficulty.

*Cinnabar*, or Vermilion, is render'd more beautiful by grinding it with Gum-Water and a little Saffron : those two Drugs preventing its growing black.

There is likewise a *blue Cinnabar*, made by mixing two Parts of Sulphur with three of Quicksilver, and one of Sal Ammoniac : these being sublimed, produce a beautiful blue Substance; whereas Quicksilver and Sulphur alone produce a red.

The Word comes from the *Greek* κιναβρα, *the smell of Goats*; by reason, says *Matthiolus*, in digging a kind of Mineral *Cinnabar*, it yields a string scent, that has Diggers are oblig'd to stop their Nostrils.

**CINNABAR** *of Antimony*, a Composition of Mercury, common Sulphur, and crude Antimony sublimed. It is held a Diaphoretic, and Alterative; and is us'd in Scrophulous and other chronic Cases.

**CINNAMON**, an agreeable aromatic Spice, furnish'd by the *East Indies*. *Cinnamon* is allow'd to be the Bark of a Tree, growing in the Islands of *Ceylon, Java*, and in *Malabar*.

The *Cinnamon* Tree, call'd by the Natives *Corunda Gauhah*, grows in Woods, like other Trees; and is but little regarded by 'em. It never grows high: Its Leaves resemble those of the Laurel, both as to Substance, and Colour. When they first begin to open, they are red as Scarlet; and if rubb'd between the Hands, yield an Odour more like that of Cloves than of *Cinnamon*. The fruit resembles an Acorn, or Olive; and has neither the Smell nor Taste of the Bark. When boil'd in Water, it yields an Oil, which, as it cools and hardens, becomes as firm and white as Tallow. Its Smell is agreeable, and they make Candle s of it, which are only allow'd to be burnt in the King's Palace. The Wood is of no Virtue at all.

The chief Virtue of the *Cinnamon* Tree is in its Bark; which, when green, appears to be double : its exterior Surface being grayish, and the inner of the common *Cinnamon* Colour. 'Tis then divisible into two Barks of different Colours; but these drying together, become inseparable, and pass for the same Bark; the grayish Colour changing in proportion as it dries.

When the *Cinnamon* is fresh taken from the Tree, 'tis flat, has little Taste, Smell, or Colour; but it twists or convolves, as it dries, in form of a Stick, or Cane : whence the *French* call it *Cannelle*. By thus exhaling its superfluous Humidity, it acquires a sweet brisk Smell, and a sharp pungent Taste. 'Tis said, that after the Tree has been stripp'd of its Bark, in three Years it forms a new one, which is as good as the first : but this is not very probable. Some hold, that the small Branches of the same Tree make the *Cassia*; but that must be a Mistake.

The Natives draw from the Roots of the Tree a Liquor, very much resembling *Camphor*.

*Cinnamon*, to be good, must have a brisk agreeable Taste, and a bright brown Colour. Its Qualities are, to heat and dry; to promote the Menses, to fortify the Spirits, and to help Digestion : but its chief Use, in Medicine, is as an Astringent; with which Intention it is prescribed in Diarrhæas, and Weaknesses of the Stomach.

The *Cinnamon* of the Antients was different from that of the Moderns; they distinguish'd five Kinds of Cinnamon : the *Mosylitique*; *Cinnamon of the Mountain*; *black* and *branch'd Cinnamon*; another white and spongeous; and a fifth of less value, reddish, and of a strong smell : as also a *bastard Cinnamon*, call'd *Zinziber* : this last Species was antiently in very high esteem, but is now no longer known.

They extract an Oil from *Cinnamon*, call'd its Essence, or Quintessence, which is an excellent Cardiac : the manner of preparing it, is said to be a Secret known only to the *Dutch*. The common *Cinnamon* is often adulterated with that out of which this Essence has been extracted.

*Cinnamon*, by means of Fire, furnishes Waters, Extracts, and Salts; out of which are compounded Syrups, and Pastils, call'd *Oleo Sacchara*; together with an Essence, that serves to turn all manner of Wines, white and red, into *Hypocras*.

All the *Cinnamon* consum'd in *Europe*, comes from the *Dutch*; who have got the whole Commerce thereof in their own Hands, by becoming Masters of the Isle of Ceylon, and destroying all the other Cinnamon Trees about the Kingdom of *Cochin*.

*Cinnamon* Water, is made by distilling the Bark, (first infus'd in Barley-Water) in Spirit of Wine, or Whitewine.

*Clove Cinnamon*, is also the Bark of a Tree growing in *Brasil* and *Madagascar*; where it is known under the Name of *Ravendsara*. The *Portugueze* call it *Cravo de Marenhan*. This Bark, pulveriz'd, is sometimes substituted for real *Cloves*, tho far short of 'em in respect of Quality.

Sassafras, or Saxafras, is sometimes also call'd *Cinnamon-Wood*.

*White* **CINNAMON**, which some call *Costus Corticus*, or *Corticosus*, or *Cortex Winteri*, *Winter's* Bark, from the Person's name who first brought it into *England*; is the Bark of a Tree resembling the Olive Tree, frequent in the Island of *S. Domingo, Guadeloupe*, and *Madagascar*; call'd by the Natives *Fimpi*.

The Bark, which dries like that of *Cinnamon*, is at first grayish, of a sharp biting Taste, like Pepper; and a Smell like Musk : as it dries it whitens. Some use it in lieu of Nutmeg : In Medicine, it's us'd as a Stomachic, and sometimes as an Anti-scorbutic.

The same Tree yields a Gum, call'd *Alouch*, or Bdellium, which is no disagreeable Perfume.

**CIRCULATORY**, *Circulatorium*, in Chymistry, the Vessel wherein a Fluid is put, to undergo the Process of *Circulation*. There are two Kinds of *Circulatories*, the *Diota*, or double Vessel; and the *Pelican*.

**CIRCULUS**, among Chymists, is a round Iron Instrument, us'd in cutting off the Necks of glass Vessels : which they effect thus. The Instrument being heated, is apply'd to the glass Vessel, and there kept till it grows hot : then, by a few Drops of cold Water, or a cold Blast thereon, it flies asunder. Thus they cut off the Necks of Retorts or Cucurbits.

There is another Method of doing the same, *viz*. by tying a Thread, first dipp'd in Oil of Turpentine, round the Place where the Fracture is to be; and then setting fire to the Thread. This done, some cold Water being sprinkled on the Place, the Glass will be crack'd thro' precisely where the Thread was ty'd.

**CIRRI**, in Botany, a term us'd for those fine Strings, or Hairs, by which some Plants fasten themselves, for their support; as Ivy, and the like.

**CIRSOCELE**, in Medicine, a Dilatation of the Spermatic Veins; occasion'd by a too thick, grumous Blood; call'd also *Hernia Varicosa*. The Word comes from the *Greek* κερσος, *varix*, Vein, and κηλη, *Hernia*.

**CITRON**, an agreeable Fruit, in Colour, taste, Smell, &c. resembling a Lemon; and serving, like that, to cool, and quench the Thirst : being produc'd by a Tree of the same Name, much resembling the Lemon Tree. The *Citron* is distinguish'd from the Lemon, in that it is bigger, and its Pulp firmer; its

Smell brisker, and Colour higher. It is held excellent against Poison : and *Athenæus*[1] relates an Instance of two Persons, preserv'd safe from the most dangerous Aspics, by eating a *Citron.* The Distillers, Perfumers, Confectioners, &c. procure divers things from Citrons; as Essences, Oils, Confections, Waters, &c.

**CIVET**, a kind of Perfume, bearing the Name of the Animal whence it is taken. The *Civet*, or *Civet-Cat*, is a little Animal, resembling our Cat; excepting that his Snout is m ore pointed, his Claws less dangerous, and his cry different. The Perfume this Animal produces, is form'd like a kind of Grease, or thick Scum, in an Aperture, or Bag, under his Tail. 'Tis gather'd from time to time; and still abounds, in proportion as the Animal is fed.

There is a very considerable Traffic of *Civet*, from *Bassora*[2], *Calicut*[3], and other Places, where the Animal that produces it is found. Tho, part of the Civet among us is furnish'd by the Dutch; who bring up a considerable Number of the Animals.

Before any of these Animals were seen in *Europe*, or it had been observ'd how the Perfume had been gather'd; the common Opinion, founded on the Relations of Travellers, was, that it was the Sweat of the Animal, irritated, and kindled into Rage.

To this effect, 'twas said, that the Animal was inclos'd in an Iron Cage; and after having been a long time beaten with Rods, they gather'd with a Spoon, thro' the Bars of the Cage, which the Rage and Agitation had produc'd : and that without this Precaution, the Animal would yield no Perfume at all. But Experience has taught us better; and we know, that the Perfume *Civet*, is only a thick unctuous Humour, secreted by certain Glands between the two Tunics of the Bag wherein it is amass'd, under its Tail, beneath the *Anus*.

*Civet* must be chosen new, of a good Consistence, a whitish Colour, and a strong disagreeable Smell. Besides the *Indian* and *Dutch Civet*, there is also a *Civet* from *Brasil*, or *Guinea*, like that of *India*; and an *Occidental Civet*, which bears no resemblance to it.

*Civet* is little us'd in Medicine, except in a Thickness of Hearing, from Cold; where a Grain or two being put in a little Cotton, or Wool, and the Ears stopp'd therewith, is sometimes of service. It is much us'd among Perfumers and Confectioners.

The Word *Civet* comes from the Arabic *Zibet*, or *Zebet*, Scum, Froth.

**CLAP**, in Medicine, the first Stage, or State of the Venereal Disease; call'd also a Gonorrhæa.

Dr. *Cockburn*[4], and others after him, will have the Clap to consist in an Ulceration of the Mouth of the Glands of the *Urethra* in Men, and of the *Glandula Lacunæ* in Women; occasion'd by the Insinuation of an acrimon-

[1] This is probably Athanaeus of Naucratis (ca. 200), a Greek writer and grammarian.

[2] Bassora is present-day city of Basra in south-east Iraq.

[3] Calicut is the port city, now called Kozhikode, in south-west India.

[4] William Cockburn (1669 – 1739), a Scottish physician.

ious, purulent Matter, contracted from an infected Person *in Actu Coitus*. From these Glands, issues, or gleets a sharp, corrosive Matter, accompany'd with heat of Urine, Cordee, &c. which makes what is usually term'd the first Stage of the Distemper.

A *Clap* appears sometimes sooner, and other times later, tho generally in about three or four Days after the Infection is receiv'd; and discovers it self by the running, &c. of the Penis, with Inflammation of the Glans, or Nut of the Yard.

If the Person be affected with a *Phymosis*, or *Paraphymosis*; if the running be of a thin Consistence, a yellow or green Colour, and in great Quantity, and the Testicles swell'd, 'tis usually term'd a *Gonorrhæa Virulenta*; and the *Clap* suppos'd to be in its second Stage. Some Authors think, that in this Degree, or Stage, the Infection has reach'd the Mass of Blood, and the *Vesiculæ Seminales* : others insist, that the Symptoms may be accounted for from the Running, or *Virus*, being more corrosive; and by that means irritating and inflaming the adjacent Parts.

The Cure of a *Clap* consists in proper Evacuations, as Calomel-Purgatives, Refrigerant-Emulsions, Pouders, &c. Turbeth-Emeticks, and lastly, proper Terebinths, &c. to which some add Decoctions of the *Lignum Vitae*, &c. As to Externals, they are generally comprehended under the form of Fomentations, Cataplasms, Liniments, and Lotions.

Late Authors, and especially Dr. *Cockburn*, have insisted in the Cure of a *Clap* by a particular Injection, without the use of any other Medicine. This has given a Handle to Quacks, who, by affecting to do the same by their Injections, generally check the Running, and make a confirm'd Pox.

Turbeth-Mineral, Calomel, &c. given in small Doses, and continu'd for some time, so as to take effect by way of Alteratives, have been lately much commended as to Success. Mercurial Unguents, us'd in small Quantities, so as not to raise a Salivation, is said to cure all the Stages of the Venereal Disease : This Practice is usual in *Montpelier*, &c.

Mr. *Becket*[1], in the *Philosophical Transactions*, attempts to shew, that the Disease we now call a Clap, is the same with that our Forefathers call'd a *Burning*, or *Brenning*; under which Name it was known several hundred Years before the commonly suppos'd Origin of the Venereal Disease; and that the Appellation *Brenning*, &c. was only discontinu'd as that of the *Clap* commenc'd.

In a MS as old as *Henry* IV. *Arden*, Chirurgeon to that Prince, defines Brenning to be a certain inward Heat and Excoriation of the *Urethra*; which, Mr. *Becket* observes, gives us a perfect Idea of what we now call a *Clap*. For frequent Dissections of such as have labor'd under that Disease, have made it evident, that the Urethra is excoriated by the Virulency of the Matter they receive from the infected Woman : Which Excoriation, or Ulceration, he adds, is not confin'd to the *Ostiola*, or Mouths of the mucous Glands of the *Urethra*, as has been lately imagin'd; but may equally attack any Part of the *Urethra*.

The heat, or burning which such Persons feel in making water, is a

[1] William Becket (1684 – 1738), an English surgeon.

Consequence of this Excoriation of the *Urethra*; the Salts contain'd in the Urine pricking and irritating the nervous *Fibrilæ* of the Urine, thus divested of its natural Membrane.

**CLARET**, *Clareta*, in the antient Pharmacy, was a kind of Wine impregnated with Aromatics; sometimes also called *Hippocras*, or *Vinum Hippocraticum*; because suppos'd to have been first prescrib'd by *Hippocrates*. It has its Name *Claret*, from its being clarify'd by Percolation thro' a Wine-Sack, or Bag, call'd *Hippocrates's* Sleeve.

**CLARIFICATION**, in Chymistry, the Act of clearing, or fining of Liquors from the grosser Parts. Clarification is perform'd by Ebullition, Despumation, and Colature or Filtration.

The Term is chiefly apply'd to Juices, Decoctions and Syrups, which are *clarify'd* by Filtration, or by passing 'em thro' a Strainer, after having beat them up into a Froth with the Whites of Eggs; the viscous Parts of the Eggs intangling the thick gross Particles of the Liquor, retain them in the Strainer.

Sometimes the Mixture is boil'd; by which means, the Eggs intangle the grosser Parts, and carry them up to the Top in a tough Scum; which is either taken off with a Spoon, or separated by a Flannel Bag, as before, call'd *Hippocrates's* Sleeve. Another Method is, by letting the Liquor stand in a convenient Vessel, till the grosser Particles settle.

In distill'd Waters, &c. which have a milky hue, or are turbid, it is generally effected with fine Sugar, mix'd with a small quantity of Allum; which will bear down the oily Parts, and leave the rest clear.

Many Liquors are *clarify'd* by passing them thro' a thick brown Paper; among others, Hippocras, Hydromel, &c. Fine and delicate Wines are usually *clarify'd* with Fish-Glue : The thicker Wines with Omelette, or whites of Eggs diluted in Water. Sometimes with pouring them thro' a heap of little Chips.

'Tis an Error to suppose that Fish-Glue, or Omelette, can be prejudicial to the Health; since both the one and the other fall down with the Lees, without producing any ill Effect. That which makes Wines unwholesome, is not the clarifying by these innocent means, but the Mixtures and Sophistications of the Vintners, to make 'em brisk, and bring them to life again after the Fret; which is done with Aqua vitae, Spices, Pidgeons Dung, &c.

The Antients *clarify'd* their Wines by pouring them from off the Lees, into another Barrel, thro' a Tin Strainer. Sugar is *clarify'd* with the Whites of Eggs and Sugar beat together.

**CLAVUS**, in Medicine, a Name Physicians give to a shooting Pain in the Head, commonly situate a little above the Eyes, *viz*. on the *Sinus Frontalis*; and suppos'd to resemble a boring of the Head thro' with an Auge; whence the Name. In some 'tis only in one and in others in both. 'Tis generally allow'd to be a Species of an Ague; or an intermitting Fever; its Period of coming or going, being usually regular or stated. In some 'tis Quotidian, in others Tertian.

The Cure consists in giving an Emetic a little before the Fit, and after, confirming it with a proper Quantity of the Cortex, &c. as in intermitting

Fevers: tho Bleeding and Diaphoretics sometimes effect a Cure without other Assistants.

A Pain like this, on the top of the Head, sometimes attacks hysterical Persons; which by Dr. *Sydenham* is term'd *Clavus Hystericus*. *Clavus* is also us'd in Medicine, for a Callus form'd on the Toes; popularly call'd a *Corn*.

*Clavi* arise from a too great Compression of the Cutis; which by this means hardens, and forms it self into a Knot. The Cure is by first softening 'em, as with *Emplast. de Ranis cum Mercurio*, or *Mynsicht. Galban. Crocat.* with Sal Ammoniac; and the plucking 'em up. A piece of raw Beef, apply'd in manner of a Plaister, and frequently shifted, is found to dissipate 'em in a little time.

**CLOVE**, an aromatic Fruit, bore on a Tree of the same Name; by the *Latins* also called *Caryophillum*. This Tree was antiently very common in the *Molucco* Islands; where all the *European* Nations, who traffick in Spices to the Indies, *furnish'd* themselves with what quantity of *Cloves* they requir'd. At present there are scarce any found but in the Island of *Ternate* : the *Dutch*, in order to render themselves Masters of that Merchandise, having dug up the *Clove*-Trees of *Moluccos*, and transplanted them to Ternate; so that there are none now to be had but thro' their Hands.

The Tree is very large; it only bears Fruit once in eight Years, but holds, at this rate, an hundred. Its Bark resembles that of the Olive-Tree, and its Leaves those of the Laurel : Its Fruit falling, takes root, and thus multiplies it self without any culture. 'Tis said, it will not allow any other Herb or Tree near it; its excessive heat drawing to it all the Humidity of the Soil.

When the *Clove* first begins to appear, it is of a greenish white; as it ripens it grows brown : Nor is there any Preparation necessary in order to render it such as it comes to us, but to dry it in the Sum; whatever some Authors talk of first steeping it in Sea-Water, to preserve it from Worms.

The Fruit is somewhat in the form of a Nail; whence the Term *Clove*, from the French *Clou*, Nail. Towards the Head it separates into four; the four Quarters being made angle-wise, and their Apices meeting at the top, form a kind of Crown, somewhat in the antique manner. They must be chosen dry, brittle, sharp to the Touch, well grown, of a dusky red Colour; a hot aromatic Taste, an agreeable Smell, and, if possible, with the Fust, or Button.

Their Properties are to warm and dry, to correct a fetid Breath, sharpen the Sight, dissipate Films in the Eyes, fortify the Stomach and Liver, and stop Vomiting. They are us'd in Apoplexies, Palsies, Lethargies, and other Diseases of the Brain.

Such of the Fruit as escape the Gatherers, grow and swell on the Tree, and become full of a Gum us'd in Medicine, called *Mother of Cloves*.

There is also an Oil, drawn from *Cloves* by Distillation; which, when new, is of a gilded white Colour, but reddens as it grows old : 'tis us'd in Medicine as a sovereign Remedy for the Tooth-ach, and in Compositions with the same View as the Fruit. It is also much us'd among the Perfumers.

The Natives call the Tree *Chamque*, the *Persians* and *Arabs Karumfel*, and the *Turks Kalafour*. They make several Preparations both of the Flowers and the Fruit.

**CLYSSUS**, in Chymistry, is one of the Effects, or Productions of that Art; consisting of the most efficacious Principles of any Body, extracted, purify'd, and then re-mix'd. Or, a *Clyssus* is when the several Species, or Ingredients of a Body, are prepar'd and purify'd separately, and then combin'd again. Thus, Salt, Sulphur, Oil, Spirit, and Mercury, reassembled into one Body, by long Distillation, &c. make a *Clyssus*.

*Clyssus* of Antimony, is an agreeable acid Spirit, drawn from Antimony, Nitre, and Sulphur mix'd together. There is also a *Clyssus of Vitriol*, which is a Spirit drawn by Distillation from Vitriol dissolv'd in Vinegar : this is us'd by Physicians in various Diseases, and to extract the Tincture of several Vegetables.

*Clyssus* is us'd among some Authors for a kind of *Sapa*, or Extract, made with eight Parts of the Juice of a Plant, and one of sugar, seeth'd together into the Consistency of Honey.

**CLYSTER**, in Medicine, a liquid Remedy, or Injection, introduc'd into the Intestines by the Fundament; in order to refresh them, loosen the Belly, moisten and soften the Fæces, dissipate Wind, &c.

*Clysters* are made of Bran-Water, and Milk, but more usually of Decoctions of certain Herbs; to which are added Honey, brown Sugar, sometimes Catholicon, and other Drugs. *Clysters* are either *Emollient, Carminative, Lenitive, Astringent, Laxative, Anodyne, Uterine, Antifebritic, Nourishing*, &c. *Uterine* Clysters, are Injections into the Uterus, or Womb.

*Nourishing* Clysters, are those apply'd with design to nourish Persons who cannot take in any Aliment at the Mouth. *Hiddanus* tells us, that *Auberi*, a Physician, fed a Woman of Quality six Weeks by *Clysters* compos'd of Capons Flesh, and other Fowls, boil'd to a Pulp, with Yolks of Eggs, applied twice a Day.

'Tis difficult, however, to conceive how *Clysters* should nourish; and the Case is briskly controverted in the Memoirs of the *French* Royal Academy, between M. *Littre*, who maintains the Negative, and M. *Lemery*.

The Arguments urg'd by the first, are, that the Materials of the *Clyster*, for want of the ordinary Passage, want the necessary Preparations to be converted into Nourishment; and beside that, are out of the Road for getting into the Blood : For in the first of the large Intestines, call'd the *Cæcum*, is a Valve called *Valvula Bautuni*; to oppose the passage of any Food into the small Intestines : And there are no Lacteal Veins in the large Intestines, but abundance in the small ones. But the Lacteals are the only Canals that can carry the Chyle into its Receptacle, and the Chyle the only Substance that can nourish.

To this M. *Lemery* objects, that the very great Anatomists have found Lacteals in the large Intestines, tho in small number : But tho there were none, adds he, the Meseraic Veins are indisputably distributed to these Intestines; and may easily be suppos'd to pump the most subtil Part of a Broth, and carry it into the Blood. M. *Mercy* has pass'd a Liquor immediately from the large Intestines into these Veins; besides that, the animal Machine is so porous thro'-out, that Nature seems to have intended an extraordinary way of conveying Fluids into the Blood, to be ready on extraordinary occasions. This Notion will appear incontestable, if M. *Morin's*[1] Theory of the Passage of the Urine be admitted.

*Herodotus* says, the *Egyptians* were the first who invented *Clysters*; or rather, who apply'd 'em to use. *Galen* and *Pliny* add, that they learnt the thing from a Bird of their Country, call'd *Ibis*; which they frequently observ'd to make this kind of Injection with its Beak, and afterwards to discharge it self several times. Others say, that the *Ciconea*, or Stork, first taught Men the Application of *Clysters*.

**COAGMENTATION**, is used among Chymists, for the Act of melting down a Matter, by casting in certain Pouders, and afterwards reducing the whole into a Concrete, or Solid.

**COAGULATION**, the condensing or thickening of a fluid Matter, without its losing any of the sensible Parts which occasion'd its fluidity; as we frequently see in Blood, Milk, &c.

We distinguish between that kind of thickening which is effected by the Evaporation of the fluid Parts of a Body, as in Clay, which condenses in the Sun, which we properly call *hardening*; and that effected without any loss of its Substance, which we call *coagulating*. Thus, we say, that Cold *coagulates* Blood, &c.

There is one general Term, *viz. Concretion*, which includes both *Coagulation, Condensation* and *Hardening*.

*Coagulation* is perform'd by the mixing of Salts of different Natures; as when Spirit of Vitriol is pour'd on Oil of Tartar; or when Oils are mix'd in a Mortar with saline, or aqueous Liquors, as in Nutrition.

By injecting an Acid into the Vein of an Animal, the Blood *coagulates*; which stops its Circulation, and brings immediate Death. Several Poisons have their effect by inducing a *Coagulation*.

**COBALT**, in Natural History, a kind of Natural Cadmia, out of which is drawn Bizmuth, Arsenic, and Smalt. *Cobalt* usually contains a little Silver. There are various Mines of *Cobalt*, especially in *Saxony*; some in *France* and *England*.

**COCCIFEROUS**, in Botany, such Plants, or Trees, as bear Berries.

**COCCULUS** *Indicus*, a poisonous Narcotick Berry, known mostly now to Poachers, who have got a trick of intoxicating Fish therewith, so as to take them out of the Water with their Hands; for which Reason they are called *Baccæ Piscatoriæ*, Fishers Berries.

**COCHINEAL**, or Cocheneal, a Drug us'd by the Dyers, &c. for giving red Colours, especially Crimsons, and Scarlets. It is brought from the *West Indies*: but Authors are divided as to its Nature; some taking it to be a kind of Worm, and others the Grain of a Tree. F. *Plumier*[1], the Minime, a

[1] Louis Morin (1635 – 1715), a French physician and botanist.

[1] Father Charles Plumier (1646 – 1704), a French botanist.

celebrated Botanist, has maintain'd the former Opinion, and *Pomet* the latter.

It may perhaps be said, that they are both equally distant from the truth in the Description they have given of *Cochineal*; and yet that there is both a *Cochineal* which is a Worm, and another a Grain. This Opinion is founded on the Account given by *Dampier*[1]; who gives a precise Description of each kind: If it ben't true, 'tis at least more likely than any Opinion yet propos'd. His Description of each is as follows:

"The *Cochineal Worm*, is an Insect ingender'd in a Fruit resembling a Pear: The Shrub which bears it is five or six Foot high. A-top of the Fruit grows a red Flower, which when mature falls on the Fruit; and that opening, discovers a Cleft two or three Inches in Diameter. The Fruit then appears full of little red Insects, having Wings of a surprising smallness, and which would die and rot there, if not taken out."

"The *Indians*, therefore, spreading Cloth under the Tree, shake it with Poles, till the Insects are forc'd to quit their Lodging, and fly about the Tree; which they cannot do many Moments, but tumble down dead into the Cloth; where they are left till they be entirely dry : When the Insect flies it is red; when it is fallen, black; and when dry, white; tho it afterwards changes Colour."

There are whole Plantations of the *Cochineal* Tree, or *Tonna*, as the Natives call it, about *Guatimala*, *Chepe*, and *Guexaca*, in the Kingdom of Mexico.

*Cochineal Grain*, or, as *Dampier*, calls it, *Sylvestris*, is a red Berry, growing in *America*, found in a Fruit resembling that of the *Cochineal* Tree, or *Tonna*. The first Shoots produce a yellow Flower; then comes the Fruit, which is long, and when ripe opens with a Cleft of three of four Inches. The Fruit is full of Pippins, or Grains, which fall on the least Agitation, and which the *Indians* take care to gather. Eight or ten of these Fruits may yield about an Ounce of Grain.

This Berry yields a Dye almost as beautiful as that of the Insect; and a Person may be easily deceiv'd in them : tho the first is much less esteem'd.

*Cochineal* is us'd in Medicine as an Alexipharmic, tending to promote Sweating, and also as a Cordial.

**COCTION**, a general Name for all Alterations made in Bodies, by the approach of Fire, or Heat. The greatest Secret in Chymistry is to manage the *Coction* aright; to give the Fire no advantage. There are various Species of *Coctions*; as Maturation, Friction, Elixation, Assation, Torrefaction, and Ustion; which see in the Places.

**CODIA**, in Botany, is used for the Top, or Head of any Plant; but, by way of eminence, for that of a sort of Poppy : whence the Syrup made therewith is called *Diacodium*, from δια, *cum*, with, and κωδια, *the Poppy head*.

[1] William Dampier (1651 – 1715), an English navigator, explorer and botanist.

**COELIACA**, or *Cœliac Passion*, or *Affection*, is a sort of *Diarrhæa*, or Flux of the Belly; wherein the Chyle, or nutritious part of the Food is evacuated by Stool, instead of Excrements. Authors frequently confound the *Cœliaca* with the Lientery, but they are different. There is also a Cœliac *Diabetes*, call'd *Cœliaca Urinalis*, wherein the Chyle passes off along with, or instead of Urine.

**COFFEE**, in Natural History, a Seed, or Berry, brought from *Arabia felix*; used for the making a Drink of the same Name. That from the *Levant* is most esteem'd, being greener, heavier, and appearing riper and plumper than that from *Mocha*; which is larger, lighter, and whiter. For *Coffee*-Berries, some substitute Peas, Beans, Rye, and Barley; which roasted, yield an oily Matter, resembling in Flavour, but less agreeable, as well as in much less quantity than *Coffee*.

**COFFEE** is also a Kind of Drink, prepared from these Berries; very similar in *Europe* for these 60 Years, and among the Turks for above an hundred. Its Origin is not well known; some ascribe it to the Prior of a Monastery, who being inform'd by a Goatherd, that his Cattel sometimes browsing on the Tree, would wake and caper all Night; became curious to prove its Virtue : accordingly, he first try'd it on his Monks, to prevent their sleeping at Matins.

Others, from *Schehabeddin*[1], refer the Invention of *Coffee* to the *Persians*; from whom it was learnt in the XVth Century by *Gemalledin*, Mufti of *Aden*, a City near the Mouth of the Red Sea; and who having tried its Virtues himself, and found that it dissipated the Fumes which oppress'd the Head, inspir'd Joy, open'd the Bowels, and prevented Sleep, without being incommoded by it; recommended it first to his Dervises; with which he us'd to spend the Night in prayer.

Their Example brought *Coffee* into vogue at *Aden* : The Professors of the Law, for Study, Artisans to work, Travellers to walk in the Night; in fine, every body at Aden drank *Coffee*.

Hence it pass'd to *Mecca*, where first the Devotes, then the rest of the People took it. From *Arabia felix* it pass'd to *Cairo*. In 1511, *Khaie Beg* prohibited it, from a Persuasion that it inebriated, and that it inclin'd to Things forbidden. But Sultan *Causou* immediately after took off the Prohibition, and *Coffee* advanced from *Egypt* to *Syria* and *Constantinople*.

The Dervises declaim'd against it from the *Alcoran*, which declares that Coal is not of the number of things created by God for Food. Accordingly, the Mufti order'd the Coffee-Houses to be shut; but his Successor, declaring *Coffee* not to be Coal, they were open'd again.

During the War in *Candia*, the Assemblies of the Newsmongers making too free with State-Affairs, the Grand Vizier *Cuproli* suppress'd the Coffee-Houses at *Constantinople*; which Suppression, tho still on foot, does not yet prevent the publick Use of the Liquor there.

*Thevenot*[2], the Traveller, was the first who brought it into *France*; and a

[1] Schehabeddin was an Arabian scribe in the fifteenth century.

[2] Jean de Thevenot (1633 – 1667), a French natural philosopher and botanist.

*Greek* Servant, call'd *Pasqua*, brought into *England* by Mr. *Dan. Edwards*, a *Turky* Merchant, in 1652, to make his *Coffee*, first set up the Profession of *Coffee*-Man, and introduc'd the Drink among us. Tho some say Dr. *Harvey*[1] had us'd it before.

The Word *Coffee* is originally *Arabic* : the *Turks* pronounce it *Cahueh*, and *Arabs*, *Cahouah*; which some Authors maintain to be a general Name for any thing that takes away the Appetite : others for any thing that promotes Appetite; and others, again, for any thing that gives Strength and Vigour.

The *Mahometans*, 'tis observ'd, distinguish three Kinds of *Cahouah*; the first is Wine, or any Liquor that inebriates; the second is made of the Pods that contain the *Coffee*-Berry; this they call *Sultana's Coffee*, from their having first introduc'd it, on account of its heating less than the Berry, as well as its keeping the Bowels open: the third is that made with the Berry itself; which alone is us'd in *Europe*, the *peans* who imported the Pods, call'd them the *Flower of the Coffee* Tree.

The deep brown Colour of the Liquor, occasion'd its being first call'd *Syrup of the Indian Mulberry*; under which specious Name it first gain'd ground in Europe.

The Preparation of *Coffee* consists in *roasting*, or giving it just Degree of Torrefaction, on an earthen, or metalline Plate, till it have acquir'd a brownish hue, equally deep on all Sides : 'Tis then ground in a Mill, as much as serves the present occasion. A proper quantity of Water is next boil'd, and the ground Coffee put in it. After it has boil'd sufficiently, 'tis taken from the Fire; and the Decoction having stood a while to settle and fine, they pour, or decant it into Dishes.

The Custom is to drink *Coffee* as hot as possible, with Sugar; tho the *Turks* don't trouble themselves to take off its bitterness with any Sugar : their Grandees add to each Dish a drop of Essence of Amber; others boil with it a couple of Cloves; others a little *Indian* Anise; others *Cacouleh*, or the Grain of the *Cardamum minus*. *Coffee* is one of the necessaries the *Turks* are oblig'd to furnish their Wives withal.

The ordinary Method of roasting *Coffee* among us, is in a Tin cylindrical Box, full of Holes; thro' the middle whereof runs a Spit : under this is s semicircular Hearth, wherein is a large Charcoal Fire : By help of a Jack, the Spit turns swift, and so roasts; being now and then taken up and shaken. When the Oil rises, and it's grown of a dark brown Colour, it is emptied into two Receivers, made with large Hoops, whose bottoms are Iron Plates, these shut into : There the *Coffee* is shaken, and left till almost cold; and it if look bright and oily, 'tis a Sign 'tis well done.

*Coffee* is taken with very different, nay frequently with directly opposite Intentions; some us it to prevent Sleep, others to promote Digestion, &c.

Its more real Virtues, own'd by the Physicians, consist in this; that being an excellent Dryer, it carries off Fumes and Disorders of the Head arising from too much moisture, dissipates Megrims, and absorbs Acrimonies of the Stomach, whence its use after a Debauch of strong Liquors; and hence also its

[1] William Harvey (1578 – 1657), an English physician.

use in promoting watching, by bracing the Fibres, and rendering 'em too tense for the Relaxation requir'd in Sleep.

It likewise promotes Circulation, but such best with People of a pretty corpulent Habit; being found hurtful to those who are thin, lean, dry, and of a bilious Temperament; as it dries up the Nerves, and inclines them to Tremors: 'tis said to be prejudicial likewise to those who digest too fast, where the Circulation is too quick, or where there is a spitting of Blood arising from the Mouths of any the Veins and Arteries being too open, or the Blood too thing and sharp.

The oily Matter that separates from the Coffee, and appears on its surface when roasted, and its particular Smell, which distinguishes it from Peas, Beans, Rye, &c. which some substitute in lieu of Coffee, are to be the real Indications of its Effects. If consider'd with regard to the Oils drawn by the Retort, this, as well as that. Contains volatile Principles, both saline and sulphureous.

'Tis to the Dissolution of the Salts, and the Mixture of its Sulphurs in the Blood, that its chief Faculty of promoting Watchfulness is to be attributed : Hence also its Property of promoting Digestion, of precipitating Foods, of preventing Eructations, and correcting Acrimonies of the Stomach.

Hence also that Fermentation in the Blood, serviceable to corpulent People: hence also its diuretick Virtue. By Experience 'tis found of service to drink a Glass of Water before *Coffee*, to extinguish its Sulphurs, embarrass its saline Principles, and render it nourishing.

*S. Paulli*[1], a *Danish* Physician, maintains that it enervates Men, and renders them incapable of Generation : And 'tis certain the Turks attribute the same Effects to it; and from the immoderate use hereof, account for that thinness of Inhabitants found in Provinces formerly the best peopled. But this Opinion is refuted by *Du Four*[2]. F. *Mallebranch*[3] gave the Royal Academy of Sciences an Account of a Person cur'd of an Apoplexy, by giving him several Clysters of *Coffee*.

The Tree that produces the *Coffee*, is a Kind of *Arabic* Jasmin : The Berry, when ripe, is found as hard as Horn; which gave occasion to an Opinion, that the People of the Kingdom of *Iemen* in *Arabia felix*, where it is cultivated, steep'd in boiling Water, or bak'd in a Furnace all the *Coffee* they sold abroad, to prevent its growing any where else.

'Tis said, it yields a Revenue upwards of five Millions *per Annum*. Nor will that appear any wonder, when we consider that in London alone, besides the Consumption in private Houses, some have computed three thousand *Coffee*-Houses. In the three Kingdoms are yearly expended one hundred Tonn of *Coffee*-Berries; in *England* alone seventy : which at 300 l. per Tonn, a moderate Price, amounts to 21000 l. Sterling.

**COHOBATION**, in Chymistry, a repeated Distillation of the same Matter, with the Liquor drawn from it; that Liquor being again and again return'd

[1] Simon Paulli (1603 – 1680), a Danish physician and naturalist.

[2] Philippe Sylvestre Dufour (1622 – 1687), a French coffee merchant and philosopher.

[3] Nicolas Malebranche (1638 – 1715), a French priest and theologian.

upon the Matter left at the bottom. The Design of this Operation is to open the Pores, and separate and volatize the spirituous Part. *Cohobation* is a kind of *Circulation*; only differing from it in this, that the Liquor drawn off in *Cohobation* as in common Distillation, and thrown back again; whereas in Circulation it rises and falls in the same Vessel, without ever being carried out.

**COLATURE**, in Pharmacy, the Separation of a Liquor from some Mixture, or Impurity, by percolating, or straining it thro' the narrow Pores of a Cloth, or other Matter; which will give passage to the fine, and pure Part, but intercept the grosser.

**COLD**, something devoid of Heat, or which contains in it no Particles of Fire. This Definition is agreeable to the Sentiments of most of the modern Philosophers, who make *Cold* a mere negative Term; and suppose the Thing to consists in a mere Privation, or Diminution of Heat.

Others define *Cold*, much on the same Principle, to be the State of the minute Parts of the Body, wherein they are more slowly and faintly agitated than those of the Organs of Feeling : In which Sense, Cold is a mere Term of Relation; and hence the same Body becomes liable to be perceiv'd *hot* or *cold*, as its Particles are in a greater of less degree of Motion than those of the sensible Organs.

*Heat* is suppos'd to consist in a particular Motion of the parts of the hot Body; and hence the Nature of *Cold*, which is its opposite, is easily deducible : For *Cold*, we find, extinguishes, or rather abates Heat; whence it seems to follow, that those Bodies are *cold*, which check and restrain the Motion of the Particles wherein Heat consists.

Now, there are three Kinds of Bodies which may do this, *viz.* either those whose Particles are perfectly at rest; or those whose Particles are indeed agitated, but less violently than those of the hot Body to which they are applied : or, lastly, those whose Particles have a Motion proper for exciting the Sensation of *Heat*, but move with a different Determination; so as to retain and change the Motion of the Particles of the Organ.

Hence, there arise three different Kinds of *Cold*, or *cold Bodies* : The 1st is, that the *Cold* common to all hard Bodies, which consists in the Rest of their Parts. The 2d is that which arises on plunging any Part of the Body in Water; which consists in this, that the Parts of our Præcordia being more briskly agitated than those of the Fluid, communicate Part of their Motion to it. The 3d, the *Cold* felt on collecting even warm Air with a Fan, or in blowing hot Breath out of our Mouth, with the Lips close shut; which consists in this, that the direct Motion of the Particles of Air, do in some measure change and rebate the Motion and Determination of the Parts of the Body : And hence it is, that a *cold* Body cannot cool another without heating it self. Hence also it is, that the more Parts of a frigid Body are at rest, the more must the Particles of a warm Body applied to heat 'em, lose of their Motion, and by consequence of their Heat. Thus a Marble having more quiescent Parts than Wood, which is full of Pores and Interstices, is felt *colder* than Wood. Hence also we see why Air, near Marble and other dense Bodies, feels somewhat *colder* than in other Places.

On this Principle, the two latter Kinds of *Cold* appear somewhat more than Privations : The Particles inducing the *Cold*, may be esteem'd real frigorific Corpuscles; and *Coldness* be deem'd a real Quality as well as Hotness.

These Particles do not only check the Agitation of those continually diffus'd from the inner parts of the Animal to the outer; but, having an elastick Power, bend and hang about the Filaments of the Body, pinch and squeeze them; and hence that acute pungent Sensation called *Cold*.

Dr. *Clark*[1] takes *Cold* to be owing to certain nitrous, and other saline Particles, endued with particular Figures proper to produce such Effects. Hence, Sal Ammoniac, Salt Petre, or Salt of Urine, and many other volatile and alkalizate Salts, mix'd with Water, increase its degree of cold very sensibly. Hence also that popular Observation, that *Cold* prevents Corruption; which, however, must not be admitted without an Exception : since, if a hard, porous Body have its Interstices fill'd with Water, and this be too much dilated by freezing, the Including Body will be burst. And thus it is that *Cold* proves destructive to the Parts of some Plants.

**COLIC**, in Medicine, a cruel, sever, gnawing Pain, felt in the lower Venter; so called, because the ordinary Seat of the Disorder, was antiently suppos'd to be in the Intestine *Colon*.

Physicians usually distinguish three Kinds of Colic, the *Bilious*, *Windy*, and *Nephritic*. The *bilious Colic* has its rise from certain sharp, bilious, stimulating Humours, which being diffus'd thro' the Intestines, vellicate their Fibres, and occasion a Sensation of Pain. Tho *Willis*[2] takes the Part principally affected to the Mesentery.

Dr. *Sydenham* observes, that the *bilious Colic* usually attacks about the beginning of Summer; that it's generally attended with Vomiting of bilious green Liquor; that the Patient complains of excessive Heat, great Gripings, Faintness, &c. and that if it be not soon remedy'd, it is apt to turn into the Iliac Passion.

*Baglavi*[3] notes, that if the Patient sweat much, and be much enfeebled; the Disease is apt to degenerate into a Palsy. The Cure, he says, depends on Bleeding, gentle Cathartics, and Enemas; and if it arise from a *Crapula*, an Emetic is to precede : after which, the Cure is to be compleated with proper Anodynes.

The *Wind Colic* is vagabond, never staying in any fixed Place; being produc'd by windy Vapours, which swell and distend the Intestines they are inclos'd in.

The *Nephrotic Colic* is felt particularly in the Reins, whence it has its Name; the Greek νεφρος signifying *Rein*. It usually has its rise from some Stone, or Gravel detach'd from the Kidnies, and fallen into the Pelvis. The *Pareira Brava* is said to be a Specific for Nephritic Colics.

[1] Samuel Clarke (1675 – 1729), an English philosopher.

[2] Thomas Willis (1621 – 1675), an English physician.

[3] This is probably Giorgio Baglivi, born Gjuro Baglivi (1668 – 1707), an Armenian physician and anatomist who practised in Italy.

*S. Manouchi*[1], a *Venetian* Physician at the Court of the Great Mogul, gives the following Remedy as infallible in Nephritic Cases : An Iron ring, abut an Inch and half in the Diameter, and thick in proportion, is to be heated red-hot; then, laying the Patient on his Back, the red-hot Ring is to be apply'd to his Navel, so, as that the Navel be in the Centre of the Ring : The Patient will presently feel the Pain, which will occasion him to shrink back very suddenly; the sudden Revulsion thus occasion'd in the lower Venter, will in a little time dissipate all his Pains. The same Author adds, that he can warrant the Success of the Remedy.

In *Colics* arising from Flatulencies, Carminative Waters, Oils, Aromaticks, &c. are always to be added to the Compositions : And in *Nephritic Colics*, besides Emollient Clysters, Solutions of Manna, Cremor Tartari, &c. in Whey, &c. and proper oleaginous Mixtures, are to be exhibited to relax the Fibres; after which, proper Anodynes take place.

Some, particularly *Sydenham*, mention a *Nervous Colic*, mostly incident to hysteric and hypochondriac Persons; but this appears only a Species of the *Windy Colic*. *Baglavi* recommends Camomile as an Antidote against the *Colic*, from what Cause soever it arises. Where the Disease is obstinate, much riding is of special Service.

**COLLETICS**, in Medicine, such Remedies as join, and glue together the separated Parts, or Lips of a Wound, or Ulcer; in order to re-establish 'em in their natural Union. *Colleticks* are more desiccative than Sarcotics; but less so than Epulotics. Among *Colletics* are rank'd Litharge, Aloes, Myrrh, &c. The Word comes from the *Greek* κολλητικος, something that has the Virtue of gluing together.

**COLLIQUATION**, in Pharmacy, the Action of melting together two, or more solid Substances; or rendering 'em liquid by Fusion, or Dissolution; as Wax, Mucilage, &c. by Heat; Gums, &c. by Moisture. *Colliquation* is also us'd to express such a Temperament, and Disposition of the Animal Fluids, as proceeds from a too lax Compages; whereby they flow off thro' the several Glands, and particularly thro' those of the Skin, faster than they ought; which occasions Fluxes of many Kinds, but mostly, profuse greasy, clammy Sweats. If this *Colliquation* continue, it generally terminates in an Hectic Fever, and is usually a Concomitant of one. The curative Intention in this Case, is the giving a better Consistence to the Juices by Balsamicks and Agglutinants; and the hardening of the Solids by Subastringents. Hence,

**COLLIQUATION** *Fever*, is a Fever attended with a Diarrhæa, or profuse Sweats, from too loose a Contexture of the Fluids.

**COLLYRIUM**, in Medicine, an external Remedy, particularly appropriated to Diseases of the Eyes. There are two Kinds of *Collyriums*; the one *liquid*, the other *dry*.

*Liquid Collyriums* are compos'd of Ophthalmic Pouders, or Waters; as Rose-Water, Plaintain-Water, that of Fennel, Eyebright, &c. wherein they

[1] This is probably Niccolo Manucci (ca. 1638 – 1715), an Italian physician.

dissolve Tutty, White Vitriol, or some other proper Pouder.

The *Dry*, are Troches of Rhasis, Sugar-candy, Iris, Tutty prepar'd, &c. blown into the Eye with a little Pipe.

The same Name is also given to the Unguents used for the same Purpose; as Unguent of Tutty, and several others. Lastly, the Name is given, tho imprecisely, to some liquid Medicines used against Venereal Diseases.

The Word *Collyrium* comes from the *Greek* κολλουριον; and that, according to *Martinus*[1], from κολλαν τον ρους; because it glues up, and prevents Defluxions.

**COLOPHONY**, a kind of Gum; being only a finer Turpentine, boil'd in Water till it be reduc'd into a solid Consistence. The chief Use if this Drug, is in the Cure of Venereal Ailings, Seminal Weaknesses, the Whites in Women, &c. The Apothecaries make it into Pills, which they roll in Liquorice-Powder, or cover over with Gold-Leaf, and call them *Turpentine Pills*.

It is also used by Musicians, to rub the Hairs of their Bow withal; the Effect whereof is, that the Gum cleaning the Hairs, and communicating to 'em a tenacious Quality, prevents their sliding too easily over the Strings; and promotes that trembling which forms the Sound.

*Colophony* is also an oleaginous Substance, of a yellowish Colour, dry, and friable, compos'd of the Remains of Resins of Fir, and Fir-Apples, condens'd by Coction, and harden'd by Cold. To be good, it must be shining and odoriferous; and when thrown on the Fire, render a Smoke like that of Incense.

*Pliny* says, *Colophony* took its Name from *Colophon*, a City of *Ionia*, whence it was first brought. 'Tis now frequently called *Spanish Wax*, or *Grecian Resin*; as it is brought from the one or the other of those Countries. It is found to warm, dry, soften, and agglutinate, and usually enters the Composition of Plaisters and Unguents.

*Colophony* is also used for the Remains of Turpentine distilled; or the gross Part resting at the bottom of the Vessel.

**COLOQUINTIDA**, or Colocynthis, usually call'd Bitter Apple; the Fruit of a Plant of the same Name, brought from the Levant; about the bigness of a large Orange. Its Colour is that of a golden brown : Its inside is full of Kernels, which are to be taken out before the Colocinthis be us'd. Both the Seed and Pulp are intolerably Butter. The Word comes from the *Greek* κολοκυνθη, which was given it, in regard it κοιλιαν κινος, *agitates the Belly*.

*Coloquintida* is of considerable use in Medicine, but mostly in officinal Compositions; the Violence of its Operation rendring it unsafe to be given inwardly in extemporaneous Prescriptions, except with great Caution.

It enters, as an Ingredient, in the *Confectio Hamec*, and most purging Pills; and in such Cases as require purging, is attended with great success. It is one of the most violent purgative Drugs known; inasmuch that it excoriates the Passages to that degree, as sometimes to bring away Blood, and induce a

[1] Martin Akakia (1497 – 1551), a French physician.

Superpurgation. Sometimes it is taken boil'd in Water, or Small Beer, in Obstruction of the Menses; which, in strong Constitutions, is often attended with Success. Some Women have got a trick of taking it, in the same manner, in the beginning of Pregnancy, to procure Abortion; which it often effects by the Violence of its Operation.

The Pouder of *Coloquintida* is sometimes used externally, with Aloes, &c. in Unguents, Emplaisters, &c. with remarkable Success against Worms; and some, for the same purpose, recommend the Pulp, given Clyster-wise. In the Iliac Passion, Clysters of *Coloquintida* have been found of service, after most other Medicines have fail'd.

Troches made of *Colocynth*, are called *Troches of Alhandal* : They are prepared by cutting the *Coloquintida* very small, and reducing it to a fine Pouder in a Mortar, rubb'd with Oil of sweet Almonds; adding Gum Tragacanth, and Mastic afterwards.

**COMA**, in Medicine, a sort of a sleepy Disease, otherwise called *Cataphora*; consisting in a violent propensity to sleep, whether Sleep ensue, or not.

If Sleep do ensue, the Disease is called *Coma Somnolentum*, wherein the Patient continues in a profound Sleep; and when awak'd, immediately relapses, without being able to keep open his Eyes. If he do not sleep, but is continually awak'd with frightful Dreams, 'tis called *Coma Vigil* : and here too his Eyes are shut, and he appears asleep.

The Cause of the *Coma Somnolentum*, may be any thing that prevents the Course of the Spirits; as a cold, humid temperature of the Brain; hot putrid Vapours ascending into the Head, and stopping the Canals of the Animal Spirits; narcotick Vapours, &c.

The *Coma Vigil* is supposed to arise from the Conflict, or jarring Mixture of Bile with Pituita; the one urging to sleep, the other to waking. Hence, the Patient sleeps either not at all; or, at most, but for a moment; is uneasy, starts, rises up, and sometimes throws himself on the Persons near him; his Eyes, all the time fast closed.

The Remedies for a *Coma*, are those which occasion great Evacuations; as violent Clysters, or Vomitives; Medicines that purge, and dry the Brain; and those which occasion Revulsion of Humours; as Vesicatories, Cauteries, &c. to which may be added volatile Spirits, Salts, and most Cephalicks.

**COMITIALIS** *Morbus*, an antient Term for the Epilepsy, or Falling Sickness; so call'd because if any Person was seiz'd with it in the *Roman Comitia*, the Assembly was immediately dissolv'd : this being esteem'd an evil Omen.

**COMMINUTION**, the Act of grinding, or breaking any Matter into smaller Particles. Thus, we say, the Effect of chewing, or masticating our Food, is the Comminution thereof.

**COMMOTION**, an intestine Motion, or Luctation in the Parts if any thing. In Medicine, the Term is chiefly used for a blow, or shake of the Brain. Thus, we say, a Convulsion is a Commotion of the fine medullary Fibres of the Brain. A fall occasions a *Commotion*, whence frequently arises a counterstroke on the opposite Part; which occasions sometimes a Contrafissure, and at other times a Rupture of the Vessels, and an Aposthume; by shaking the whole Mass of the Brain.

**COMPLEXION**, in Physicks, is used for the Temperature, Habitude, or natural Disposition of the Body. Some Philosophers distinguish four general and principal *Complexions* in Man, *viz.* the *sanguine Complexion*, which, according to them, answers to the Air; having the Qualities thereof, as being hot and moist. It takes its Name from *Sanguis*; because Blood is there suppos'd to be predominant.

The *phlegmatic Complexion* takes its Name from the *Pituita*, or *Phlegm*, in which it abounds, and corresponds to Water; being cold, and moist. The *bilious*, or *choleric, Complexion*, takes its Name from the Bile, or Choler : it is suppos'd of the Nature of Fire, hot and dry. Lastly, the *melancholy Complexion* partakes of the Nature of Earth, being cold and dry.

**COMPLICATION** *of Diseases*, a Mixture, or Junction of several Diseases; especially where they have any affinity to one another; as the Dropsy, Asthma, and Jaundice happening together. What perplexes the Physicians, is, when with a Fever there is a Complication of some other Disorder.

**COMPRESS**, in Chirurgery, a *Bolster* of linen Cloth, folded in several Doubles, and laid under the Bandages, to prevent a Wound from bleeding or swelling; or to retain the Medicines applied thereto. The Word comes from *Comprimere*, to press hard. *Scultetus*[1], in his *Arsenal of Chirurgery*, observes, that the Antients compos'd their *Compresses* of carded Flax, or of Feathers, sew'd between two Linens; and called them Pillows, or Plumages.

**CONCOCTION**, in Medicine, the Change which the Food undergoes in the Stomach, &c. to become Chyle. This Change consists in destroying the Texture and Cohesion of the Parts of the Food; preparing part of it for some particular Service of the animal Frame, and the rest to be carried off as Excrements, by proper Emunctories.

The Antients gave the Term *Concoction*, to what we now ordinarily call *Digestion*; from the Notion of the Food's being, as it were, *boil'd* in the Stomach; and its nutritious Juice express'd by the Heat of the adjacent Parts. They assign'd two *Concoctions*, *viz.* one in the Stomach, and a second in the small Intestines, &c. which latter they attributed to the Admixture of the Bile and pancreatick Juice.

The several *Concoctions* in the Body, with regard to the Propagation of the Species, and the Preservation of the Individual, have been since reduced to five; *Chylosis* for Chyle, *Chymosis*, for Chyme, *Hematosis* for Blood, *Pneumatosis* for Spirits, and *Spermatosis* for Seed.

**CONCRETION**, the Act whereby soft Bodies are render'd hard : Or, it is an insensible Motion of the Particles of a Fluid or soft Body, whereby they come to a Consistence.

[1] Johannes Scultetus, born Johan Schultes (1595 – 1645), a German physician.

The Word is used indifferently for *Induration, Condensation, Congelation*, and *Coagulation. Concretion* is also used for the Coalition of several little Particles into a sensible Mass, called a Concrete; by virtue of which Union, the Body acquires this in that Figure, and these or them Properties.

**CONDENSATION**, the Act whereby a Body is render'd more dense, compact, and heavy. *Condensation* consists in bringing the Parts closer to each other, and increasing their Contact : in opposition to *Rarefaction*; which renders the Body lighter and looser, by setting the Parts further asunder, and diminishing their Contact, and of consequence their Cohesion.

*Wolfius*[1], and some of the more accurate Writers, restrain the use of the Word *Condensation* to the Action of Cold : what is done by external Application, they call *Compression*.

Air easily *condenses*, either by Cold, or by Art : Water congeals, but never *condenses*; can never be brought into a less space, but will penetrate the most solid Body, even Gold, rather than lose of its bulk. A Syrup *condenses* in Ebullition.

It was found, in the Observatory of France, during the great Cold of the Year 1670, that the hardest Bodies, even Metals, Glass, and Marble it self, were sensibly *condens'd* by the Cold, and became much hasher and more brittle than before; till their former State was retrieved by the ensuing Thaw.

Water alone seems to expand by Cold; inasmuch as when congeal'd, the Ice takes up more space than the Water before. But this must be rather owing to the Intromission of some foreign Matter; as the nitrous Particles of the ambient Air, than to proper Rarefaction of the Water by the Cold.

The *Cartesians*, indeed, taking it for granted there is no Vacuum, deny any such thing as proper *Condensation*, or Rarefaction. According to them, when a Body takes up more space than it did before, its Parts are distended by the Intrusion of a subtil Matter thro' its Pores : And when its bulk, again, is reduced into less Space, this is owing to the Extrusion or Egress of that Matter thro' the same Pores; by virtue whereof, the Parts of the Body, tho not the Parts of Matter, come nearer each other. For as Extension and Matter, according to them, are the same thing; a Body can never take up more or less place, any otherwise than by the Accession or Diminution of Matter : And thus they conclude there is no Vacuum.

Now, that, in the Rarefactions of gross Bodies, their Parts are distended by the accession of Air, is frequently manifest; but this does not follow from the Plenitude of the World, but from the fluid and elastick Nature of Air; or from its Gravity and Pressure.

That there is such a thing as *Condensation*, without the Loss of any Matter, is evident from *Galileus's* Experiment : A Cock, being with a female Screw fitted to a hollow brass Ball, or Cylinder, so as a Syringe, by means of a male Screw, may be applied to it; by working the Syringe, the Air will be forc'd into the Ball, and turning the Cock, will be retain'd; insomuch, that upon the examining the Vessel by the Balance, its weight will be found increas'd. If the Cock be return'd, the Air will burst out with violence, and the Ball sink to its

[1] Christian Wolff (1679 – 1754), a German philosopher.

former weight.

From the Experiment it follows, first, that Air may be crouded into a less Volume and Bulk than it ordinarily takes up, and is therefore compressible.

2dly, That from the Recovery of its weight, just so much Air is expell'd as was injected; and that, therefore, compress'd Air returns to its primitive Expansion, if the compressing Force be removed; and has therefore an elastick Force.

3dly, That 'tis a certain Sign of Compression, if, upon opening the Orifice of a Vessel, any portion of Air be observ'd to fly out.

4thly, That since the Weight of the Vessel is increas'd by injecting Air; the aerial Mass must have a *Nisus* downwards, in Lines perpendicular to the Horizon; and is therefore heavy, and presses subject Bodies in Lines perpendicular to the Horizon; according to the Conditions of Gravity.

*Condens'd* Air, has Effects just opposite to those of rarefy'd Air; Birds, &c. appear brisker and more lively therein than in common Air, &c.

**CONDUCTOR**, a Surgeon's Instrument, which being put up into the Bladder, serves to conduct the Knife, in the Operation of cutting for the Stone.

**CONFECTION**, in Pharmacy, a kind of compound Remedy of the Consistence of a soft Electuary. There are four Electuaries, which bear the Name of *Confections*; three whereof, in the Physicians Language, are *corroborative*, and one *purgative*.

The corroborative *Confections* are those of *Alkermes*, of *Hyacinth*, and the *Anacardine* : The purgative one is the *Confection Hamech*.

The *Confection of Alkermes* has its Name from the principal Ingredient therein; which is the *Kermes*, or *Alkermes*, or Scarlet-Grain. The other Ingredients are Pearls, Musk, Cinnamon, Ambergris, Leaf Gold, Juice of Pippins, and Rose-Water. It is rank'd among the best Cardiacks, and is frequently used for the Palpitation of the Heart or Syncope; sometimes in the Small-Pox and Measles.

The *Confection of Hyacinth* has nearly the same Virtues with that of Alkermes; but, beside, is frequently used as an Astringent. It consists of near triple the Number of Drugs; whereof the precious Stone, called the *Hyacinth*, is the Base : the chief of the rest are red Coral, Bole Armoniac, *Terra Sigillata*, Myrrh, the Santals, burnt Hartshorn, Camphire, Saphire, Emerald, Topaz, and most of the Ingredients of the *Confection* of Alkermes.

The *Anacardine Confection*, now disused in *England*, is compos'd chiefly of *Anacardines*, whence the Name : the other Drugs are Long Pepper, Black Pepper, most Kinds of Myrobalans, Castoreum, &c. It is used to purge the Blood, and is proper in cold Diseases.

The *Confection Hamech* takes its Name from the of its Inventor, an *Arabian* Physician. Its Ingredients are Polypody, Myrabolans, Agaric, Senna, Tamarinds, red Roses, Manna, Colocynth, &c. It is applied as a Drastic for the purging of the grosser Humors and Viscidities; 'tis also of some reputation in Vertigoes and Cancers.

**CONFORMATION**, in Medicine, is used to express that Make and Construction of the Body which is peculiar to every Individual : Hence, a *mala Conformatio* signifies some Fault in the first Rudiments; whereby a Person comes into the World crook'd, or with some of the Viscera, or Cavities unduly proportion'd. Thus, many are subject to incurable Asthma's, from too small a Capacity of the Thorax, and the like vitious *Conformations*.

**CONGELATION**, Freezing, the Act of fixing the Fluidity of any Liquid, by Cold, or the Application of cold Bodies; in which it differs from Coagulation, which is produced by other Causes. Thus, Salt-petre *congeals* Water in Summer.

Metals and Minerals are said to be Juices *congeal'd* in the Veins of the Earth, by their intermixing with one another, or with other heterogeneous Bodies, or by the Consumption and Evaporation of their finest Parts. Rock Crystal is usually held to be nothing but Water *congeal'd* in the Mountains.

The Bites of Aspicks are mortal, by the sudden *Congelation* which they induce on the Blood, which stops its Circulation.

**CONGESTION**, in Medicine, a Mass, or Collection of Humours, crouded together, and harden'd, in any Part of the Body; and there forming preternatural Tumors. Congestion is effected by little and little; in which it differs from a Defluxion, which is more sudden.

**CONGREGATION** in Physicks, is used by Dr. *Grew*[1] for the least degree of each other, but only touch in one Point. That Author declares himself of Opinion, that the Particles of all Fluids only touch in this manner; or that their Cohesion only amounts to a Congregation.

**CONGRUITY**, in a lax Sense, is also us'd to express an Aptitude in some Bodies, to unite, or incorporate, from some similitude or fitness of their Figures: as *Incongruity* denotes an Unfitness of their Surfaces for joining together.

Thus, Quicksilver will unite with Gold, and many other Metals, but will roll off from Wood, Stone, Glass, &c. and Water, which will wet Salt and dissolve it, will slip off from Tallow without adhering to it; as also from a dusty Surface, and from the Feathers of Water-Fowl.

Two drops of Water, or of Mercury, will, on contact, immediately join and coalesce; but Oil of Tartar, pour'd upon Quicksilver, and Spirit of Wine and Oil of Turpentine on that, and Air over all, will remain in the same Vessel without any manner of Union, or Mixture with each other.

And the Cause hereof, is, that the Figures of some Bodies will not admit other Bodies near enough to be within their Spheres of Attraction whence they cannot join, and cohere; but where their Fitness of Figure will let them approach near enough to feel each others attractive Power, then they close and hold together.

[1] Nehemiah Grew (1641 – 1712), an English physiologist and microscopist.

**CONIFEROUS**, a Term applied to such Trees, Shrubs, or Herbs, as bear a squammous or scaly Fruit, of a woody Substance, and a Figure approaching to that of a Cone; in which there are many Seeds, and when they are ripe, the several Cells or Partitions in the Cone gape or open, and the Seed drops out : Of this kind are the Fir, the Pine, Beach, and the like.

**CONSERVE**, in Pharmacy and Confectionary, a dry Confect, or Form of Medicine, or Food, contrived to preserve the Flowers, herbs, Roots, Peels, or Fruits of several Simples, as near as possible to what they were when fresh gather'd; and to gibe them an agreeable Taste.

*Conserves* are made by beating up the Thing to be preserv'd with a quantity of Sugar; *viz.* a triple Quantity thereof to those which are most moist and corruptible, and a double Quantity to such as are least so.

The Physicians, under the Name of *Conserves*, commonly comprehend all Kinds of Confects of Flowers, Fruits, Roots, Seeds, Barks, &c. both liquid and dry. Thus, *e.gr.* to make *Conserve* of Roses, Rosemary Flowers, Sage Flowers, or the like; they pound 'em in a stone Mortar, and when pounded, put to 'em fine Sugar, in a Glass close stopp'd up.

For Fruits, as Currants, &c. they set 'em on the Fire to make 'em cast their Juice, then drain and strain 'em, and thicken what comes from 'em over the Fire, and add it to the Sugar.

**CONSOLIDATION**, in Medicine, the Action of uniting strongly the Fractures of broken Bones, or the Lips of a Wound, by means of *consolidating Remedies*, as they are call'd; which cleansing with a moderate heat and force, taking Corruption out of the Wounds, and preserving the Temperature of the Parts, cause the Nourishment to be fitly applied to the Part affected.

**CONSUMPTION**, *Tabes*, in Medicine, a Disease arising from a Defect of Nourishment; or, a preternatural Decay of the Body, and particularly by a gradual waste of muscular Flesh.

It is frequently attended with an Hectic Fever; and is divided by Physicians into several Kinds, according to the Variety of its Causes; as *Universal*, or *Scorbutic Consumption*, where it arises from a *Cacochymia*, or Scorbutic Habit; and a *Pulmonic Consumption*, or *Consumption of the Lungs*, where it arises from some Cause in the Lungs, properly call'd a *Phthisis*.

A *Consumption* may either be *Accidental*, *Natural*, or *Hereditary* : *Accidental*, which may arise, 1st, from Ulcers, Chalky Stones, or Polypus's in the Lungs; caused by something that obstructs the Circulation in the Pulmonary Vessels, or renders the Blood viscid; as a Suppression of any natural Evacuations. 2d, From Intemperance, occasioning either a Cacochymia, or Plethora. 3d, From Peripneumonies, Pleurisies, Asthma's, Coughs, Catarrhs, Diarrhaeas, Venereal Disorders, and Excess of Venery. 4th, From Grief, hard Study, &c.

A *Natural Consumption* may arise from the Straitness of the Thorax, or an ill Conformation of the Parts. An *Hereditary* one may be communicated from the Parents, without any other visible Cause.

A *Consumption* usually begins with flying Pains, and Stitches; Pain at the Pit of the Stomach, or in the Diaphragm; frequent Spitting, loss of Appetite, a quick Pulse, a Sweetness or Saltness in the Saliva, Heat and Flushing in the Face and Palms of the Hands after Meals, an Hectic Fever toward the Evening, Heaviness, Faintness, Night-Sweats; and where the Lungs are first disorder'd, a Cough, Catarrh, or Asthma usually precede it.

When these Symptoms are violent, 'tis confirm'd; and them comes on an Expectoration of purulent or bloody Matter, and the *Vomica Pulmonum*; at length, the Feet swell, the Expectoration stops, a Diarrhæa come son; then the *Facies Hippocratica*, and Death.

The Cure of an *Universal*, or *Muscular Consumption*, depends principally upon Removal into a proper Air, and the using of a regular nourishing Diet : the Appetite is to be excited by proper Bitters, and other Stomachics.

In a *Pulmonary Consumption*, or *Phthisis*, Balsamicks, and oleaginous Medicines are to be added.

Dr. *Wainwright*, indeed, takes the Particles of oily Medicines to be too gross and viscid to enter the small Orifices of the Lacteals; and thinks, that their Operation or Effect being confin'd to the first Passages, they are not only of no service in the Cure, but are apt to pall the Appetite, occasion Obstruction in the Mouths of the Lacteals, and Diarrhæas.

But this is contrary to common Experience : That their Particles are small enough to enter the Lacteals, is evident from the sudden relief Nephritic Persons find in violent Paroxysms of the Stone, by the Passages being relax'd soon after their Exhibition. That Diarrhæas, and blunting the Appetite, in some Constitutions, will be the Consequence of their Continuance, or Exhibition in too great Quantities, must be allow'd; but then this is either accidental to some Kinds of Constitutions, or from some Error in using 'em.

As to the Lacteals being obstructed by their use, 'tis a mere Notion, and as much unsupported by Experience as that other Hypothesis, which a late Author, Dr. *Quincy*, has been fond of asserting, *viz.* that the Use of Butter is apt to foul the Glands.

**CONTAGION**, in Infection, the communicating or transferring of a Disease from one Body to another.

*Contagion*, in some Diseases, is only effected by an immediate Contact, or Touch : as the Madness of a Dog, which is communicated by biting; and the Venom of the Pox, which is transmitted from the infected Person in the Act of Copulation. In others it is convey'd by infected Clothes; as the Itch.

In others the *Contagion* is transmitted thro' the Air to a great distance, by means of Steams or Effluvia expiring from the Sick; as in the Plague, and other pestilential Distempers : in which Case, the Air is even said to be contagious, *i.e.* full of *contagious* Particles.

**CONTINUED** Fever, is such an one as does not intermit, or go entirely off, and return again, by Fits. A *continued* Fever, may be defined the *Continuance* of an increas'd Velocity in the Circulation of the Blood, beyond what is natural to the Constitution. If this Velocity often decreases, and arises again to the same height, it is called a *Continued periodical Fever*. And if it intirely cease in the Space of a Day, or two, it is call'd an *Ephemeris*. A *Continued Fever*, then, may *remit*, or abate and increase again, alternately; but not *intermit*, which would constitute it an intermitting Fever, or Ague.

**CONTRA-INDICATION**, is an Indication which forbids that to be done which the main scope of a Disease points out. Suppose, *e.g.* in the Cure of a Disease a Vomit were judg'd proper; if the Patient be subject to a vomiting of Blood, 'tis a sufficient *Contra-Indication* as to its Exhibition.

**CONTRA-YERVA**, a Root brought from *Peru*; esteem'd an Alexiterial, and a sovereign Antidote against Poison. It is said to take its Name from Yerva; which in the *Spanish* signifies white Hellebore, a Plant, whose Juice is a violent Poison, used by the *Peruvians* to poison their Arrows withal; in which Sense, *Contra-yerva* signifies *Counter-poison*.

The Root is smaller than that of the Iris, reddish without and white within, knotty, and fibrous. To be good, it must be new, heavy, and of a dusky red Colour. In Smell it resembles Fig-leaves; its Taste is Aromatic, accompany'd with some Acrimony.

There is an Officinal Composition which takes its Name from this Root, prepar'd with the Testaceous Pouders, call'd *Lapis Contrayerva*. Both the Root and *Lapis Contrayerva* are of great efficacy in the Small Pox, Measles, Fevers, and all Cases where either a Diaphoresis or Perspiration is required; its Success being more to be depended on than the *Gascons Pouder*; which, among the more knowing, begins to lose ground.

It is agreed on, by the generality of Writers, that the *Contra-yerva* Root is on of the best Anti-epidemicks yet know. Dr. *Hodges*[1], in his Treatise of the last London Plague, has a Receipt which he says was attended with great Success, and of which this Root was one of the chief Ingredients.

There is another Kind of *Contra-yerva*, brought from *Virginia*, more ordinarily called *Viperine*, very aromatic; seldom prescribed, tho said to have the same Success against Poisons and Venoms with the *Contra-yerva* of *Peru*.

**CONTUSION**, *Bruise*, in Medicine, a Solution of Continuity, either in the Flesh or Bone, occasion'd by a Fall, a Blow, or a violent Pressure, whereby the Flesh is broke, the Skin still remaining entire; and an Effusion of Blood ensures, from several little broken Vessels, so as to discolour the Skin, tho it don't make its way thro' the Pores thereof.

Or, *Contusions* may be defin'd a particular sort of Tumors; attended with a Stagnation of the Blood in the Part affected; and, generally, with an Inflammation, Discolouration, and Pain.

*Contusions* are either *internal* or *external*. When from any external Injury, there proceeds an internal Disorder, *e.gr*. an Asthma, spitting of Blood, or the like, the *Contusion* is said to be *internal*. If only external Symptoms appear, as a Tumour, Blackness, &c. it is term'd *external*.

In case of inward *Contusions*, bleeding the Patient is necessary, and

[1] Nathaniel Hodges (1629 – 1688), an English physician.

balsamicks must be given internally, such are Spermaceti, Pouder of Rhubarb, Irish Slate, oleaginous and pectoral Medicines, &c. Externals proper for *Contusions*, are Liniments or Ointments of Marchmallows, Oil of sweet Almonds, Spirit of Wine with Camphire; proper Fomentations and strengthening Emplaisters; as that of Oxycraceum, &c. according to the Nature of the *Contusion* and Part *contus'd* requires.

**CONVULSION**, *Spasmus*, in Medicine, a continued involuntary Contraction of some Parts of the Body otherwise accustom'd to move according to the Direction of the Will. It owes its Origin to a Contraction of the Muscles of the Part, occasion'd by a too copious and violent influx of the nervous Juice : Of these may be infinite Causes in the Blood, Arteries, Meninges, Brain, Nerves, Muscles, Cranium, &c.

If the Convulsion be universal, attended with violent Motions, foaming at the Mouth, and periodical; it is usually called the Epilepsy.

The usual Evacuations and Medicines proper for the Cure of Convulsions, are Phlebotomy, Emeticks, Catharticks, Epispasticks, and proper Cephalicks; as Sal. Volat. Oleos. Spirit of Lavender, Spirit of Hartshorn, Tincture of Castor, Cinnabar of Antimony, Cassuminor Root, Valerian Root, Volatile Salt of Amber, &c. given in different forms.

In periodical universal *Convulsions*, a Salivation sometimes answers, after other Course have fail'd.

Women and Children are particularly liable to *Convulsions* : Women after Delivery; as upon a Stoppage of the *Lochia*, or a violent Extraction of the *Placenta*.

**CONVULSIVE**, in Medicine, is applied to those Motions which, naturally, should depend upon the Will; but which, by some external Cause, become involuntary.

A *Convulsive* Motion, is a Contraction made by Fits and Intervals; wherein it differs from a *Convulsion*, which is a continued Contraction. *Convulsive* Motions arise from a Disorder in the Origin of the Nerves. A *Convulsive* Tension of the Solids, is one of the principal Causes which destroy the *Æquilibrium* that should obtain between the Solids and the Fluids. *Journ. De Scav.*

Convulsive is also used for any Thing that occasions *Convulsion*, or a *Convulsive Motion*. Thus, Wounds of Nerves are said to be *Convulsive*; white Hellebore is *Convulsive*. The Cramp is a *Convulsive* Contraction of some muscular Part of the Body.

Children are very liable to *Convulsive* Disorders from various Causes; as Repletion, curdling of the Blood in the Stomach or Intestines, Worms, Dentition, &c.

**COOLERS**, in Medicine, Remedies so call'd; which may be consider'd under these two Divisions :

1st, Those which produce an immediate Sense of Cold; which are such as have their Parts in less Motion than those of the Organs of Feeling.

2dly, Such as by a particular Viscidity, or Grossness of Parts, give a greater

Consistency to the Animal Fluids than they had before; whereby they are disabled from moving so fast, and will therefore have less of that intestine Force on which their Heat depends.

Of the former Kind are Fruits, and acid Liquors; to the latter belong Cucumbers, and all Substances producing Viscidity.

**COPIVI**, Capivi, Copayba, or Cupayba, a Balm or Balsam, oozing out of Incisions made in a Tree of *Brasil*; not taken notice of but by very late Writers; at least, not under this Name.

It is of a thinner Consistence than common Turpentine, but much more fragrant and detersive. It is extremely quick in passing off by the Urine, and mightily cleaneth those Passages; by which it has obtain'd very much in Gonorrhæas, Seminal Weaknesses, the Whites, and all Obstructions, and Ulcerations of those Parts.

It is likewise a powerful Balsamick, and good in many Distempers of the Breast, especially Catarrhs, tickling Coughs, spitting of Blood, &c. In Dysenteries and Diarrhæas of long continuance, where the *Mucus* that lines the Intestines is, by the Acrimony of the Humours abraded, it is of great service in supplying its Place by its balsamick quality. It mixes intimately with the Yolk of an Egg. The Jews use it to stop the Flux of Blood after Circumcision.

**COPPEL**, Copel, or Cuppel, call'd also *Test*, a Vessel used by refiners and Essayists, to try and purify their Metals.

The *Coppel of Essay*, is a little flat Vessel, compos'd of Vine Ashes, and Bones of Sheeps Feet, calcin'd and lixiviated, to separate the Salts, which would otherwise make it crackle. At the bottom of the Vessel is a little Cavity fill'd with a kind of white Varnish, compos'd of Hartshorn or of Bones of Pike, calcin'd and diluted in Water : the Use of this Liquor is, that the Gold or Silver to be essay'd may be more conveniently lodg'd, and that the Button of the Essay may be separated the more easily.

Note, Tho Metals may be tried otherwise than by *Coppeling* : and tho the Touchstone, Graver, &c. are of some service to the Goldsmith in judging of their Purity; yet, 'tis certain, without the *Coppel* 'tis difficult, not to say impossible, to know their precise degree of Purity.

*The Refiner's Coppel*, is a large Free-stone Vessel, lined withinside with a kind of Plaister made of Ashes well lixiviated, cleans'd, dry'd, beaten and sifted. In this Kind of *Coppel*, it is that the Refiners purify their Gold and Silver, by adding Lead to it, and exposing the whole to a violent Fire.

**COPPER**, a hard, dry, heavy, ductile Metal; found in Mines, in several Parts of Europe, but most abundantly in Sweden. *Copper* is of all Metals the most ductile and malleable after Gold and Silver; and abounds much in Vitriol and Sulphur. The Chymists call it *Venus*; as supposing it to have some more immediate Relation to that Planet.

By an Analysis it appears compos'd of a Sulphur ill digested, a yellowish Mercury, and a red Salt. 'Tis found both in Dust and in Stones, each of which are first well wash'd, to separate 'em from the Earth wherewith they are mix'd. In this State 'tis call'd *Virgin Copper.*

After washing 'tis melted, and the melted Matter run into a kind of Molds, to form large Blocks, by some call'd *Salmons*, and by others *Pigs of Copper.* This is the ordinary *Copper.* To render it more pure and beautiful, they melt it again once or twice; some of its coarse earthy Parts being left at each Fusion, and a Quantity of Tin and Antimony added in each. In this State 'tis call'd *Rose Copper*, in Latin *Aes Pelosum.*

Of a Mixture of this and *Lapis Calaminaris*, is form'd Brass, which the *French* call *yellow Copper*, in contradistinction to Natural Copper, which they call *red Copper.*

*Copper* melted together with 22 or 23 Pounds of fine Tin per Quintel, makes Bell Metal. *Copper* melted with Calamine, quantity for quantity, makes Brass. *Copper* and Brass melted in equal Quantities, make what the *French* call *Bronze*, used for Figures, Statues, &c.

*Copper* turns white by an Unction of Spirit of Wine and Orpiment. *Pliny* says there is a Copper naturally white, found underneath the Silver Mines.

*The Use of Copper* is very extensive : Among other works of *Copper* may be reckon'd those of Brass, Bell Metal, Pot Metal, &c. which are all Compositions were Copper makes the prevailing Ingredient.

The Chymists call *Saffron of Copper*, or *Crocus veneris*, a Preparation of *Copper* Plates stratify'd with decrepitated Salt, in a Crucible; after having extinguished 'em in Water, and scrap'd 'em with Iron Brushes. This Saffron is very red, and is used in Emplaisters to mundify Wounds and Ulcers.

Some Chymists have pretended that the Spirit of *Venus* was a real Alkahest, capable of dissolving wholly Pearls, Corals, Crabs Eyes, &c. without any Diminution of its force; but Experience has shewn the contrary.

The Calx of Brass, called *Aes Ustum*, and sometimes also *Saffron of Venus*, is nothing but *Copper* calcin'd in a violent Fire. Verdigrease is a Rust of *Copper.*

M. *Becher*[1] observes, that the drinking of acid Liquors, even out of common Silver Plate, is very unwholesome, by reason of the Mixture of *Copper* therein; much more out of Vessels of *Copper.*

The *Indian* Physicians are said to set a great Value on Talc and yellow *Copper*; which, they say, consumes the most viscid Humours, and removes the most obstinate Obstructions.

**COPPERAS**, or Coperas, a Mineral, form'd in Copper-Mines, and which is properly a Kind of Vitriol. *Copperas* is purify'd and prepar'd in the same manner as Allum and Salt-petre, by passing thro' several Lixiviums, till it be wholly reduced to Crystal. Some make *Copperas* to be the Chalcitis of the Antients. But the more common Opinion is, that 'tis rather a Calcanthum, or Vitriol.

There is *Copperas* of *England*, of *Pisa*, of *Germany*, calcin'd, laid in Water, thence filtrated, and reduced to a Salt; whereof, as it coagulates, they form

[1] Johan Joachim Becher (1635 – 1682), a German physician and alchemist.

Cakes of 40 or 50 Pounds each : such are those brought from *Gosselar* in *Saxony*. This *Saxon Copperas*, ere it be whiten'd, is of a bluish green, clear and transparent.

The *English Copperas* is of a find green; that of *Cyprus* and *Hungary* a sky-blue, in Pieces cut like the Point of a Diamond. That of *Pisa* and *Italy* is likewise green; and the last as transparent as Glass.

*Copperas* is of considerable use in many Preparations; but especially in Dying. The Hatters also use it in their dye; and this and Galls are the Ingredients that compose writing Ink.

The ordinary *English Copperas* is made of a Kind of Stones found on the Sea-shore in *Essex*, *Hampshire*, and so Westward, ordinarily called *Gold Stones*, from their Colour: they abound much with Iron.

To prepare the *Copperas* from them, they are laid in Heaps or Beds under ground. In process of Time they swell and ferment; and, by degrees, a Humour distils out, which draining into a Cistern, and afterwards boil'd, in the boiling shoots into those Crystals we see it in. The Works at *Deptford* for making it, are known to most People. Many Chymists dissolve this, and shoot it again for the common Salt of Steel.

**COQ.** *ad Med. Consumpt.* An Abbreviation among Physicians, signifying that the Thing is to be boil'd till half of it be consum'd. *Coq. in S. R. Aq.* Implies it to be boil'd in a sufficient Quantity of Water.

**CORAL**, in Natural History, a Production of the Sea, rank'd among the Number of Marine Plants.

This Opinion, which we received from the Antients, is now so well establish'd, that all other Sentiments seem precluded. *P. Kircher*, that learned Naturalist, supposes entire Forests of it, at the bottom of the Sea; and M. *Tournefort*[1], that able Botanist, maintains that it evidently multiplies by Seed; tho neither its Flower nor Grain be known. However, the Count *de Marsigli*[2] has discover'd some Parts therein which seem to serve the Purpose of Grains and Flowers.

*Coral*, then, being establish'd a Plant, has, in that Quality, Roots, wherewith it is fasten'd to the Rock whereon it grows : these *Roots* are cover'd with a *Bark*, set with starry Pores, which traverse 'em from top to bottom. Above the Roots is the ligneous or *woody* Part of the Plant, if we may so call a Matter that rather seems to resemble Stone than Wood. It is divided into Branches like other Plants; having white Streaks therein, which seem to represent a kind of Fibres. The Extremities of the Plant are soft, and rounded into little Bowls, ordinarily divided into six Cells, fill'd with a Humour somewhat like Milk, fatty, sharp, and astringent.

Lastly, that nothing may be wanting to constitute a real Tree, these Bowls are esteem'd a kind of Pods, or *Capsulæ*, containing the Seed of the *Coral*. 'Tis even said, that in what Place, or on what Matter soever this Juice be shed, it carries Fecundity with it, and produces a Plant of *Coral* : whence it is,

[1] Joseph Pitton de Tournefort (1656 – 1708), a French botanist.

[2] Luigi Ferdinando, compte de Marsigli (1658 – 1730), an Italian soldier and naturalist.

that in the Cabinets of the Curious, we find some of it on dead Mens Skulls, Pieces of Earthen Ware, and other Kinds of solid Bodies, which Chance and the working of the Sea have thrown into some of *F. Kircher's* Forests.

*Coral*, M. *le Comte de Marsigli* observes, grows chiefly in Grottos, whose Mouth or Aperture is towards the South, and the Vault, or concave Arch nearly parallel to the Surface of the Earth. For its Growth, 'tis necessary the Sea be as quiet as a Pond : It vegetates the contrary way to all other Plants; its Foot adhering to the top of the Grotto, and its Branches extending downwards. The Foot takes the exact form of the Solid it grows to, and even covers it, like a Plate, to a certain extent; which M. *de Marsigli* thinks a Proof that its Substance was originally Fluid : And what confirms the Thought, is, that the same Substance shall sometimes line the inside of a Shell, which it could never enter but in form of a Fluid.

Upon a nice Examen of the several Parts of *Coral*, M. *de Marsigli* gathers, that all its Organism, with regard to Vegetation, consists in its Bark, or Surface; that the Tubules of the Bark filtrate a Juice which fills the Cellules, and runs along the Canals as far as the Extremities of the Branches; and that this Juice being petrify'd, both in the Cells encompassing the *Coralline* Substance, and in those of the Extremes of the Branches whose Substance is not yet form'd, makes the Plant grow both in height and bulk.

The Antients believ'd that *Coral* was soft while it continu'd in the bottom of the Water; and that it only became hard and solid by the Impression of the Air. But the Moderns are convinc'd of the contrary from Experience; and know that there was more of Imagination than Truth in the Name *Gorgonium*, which they gave to shew that *Medusa's* Head did not convert Objects into Stone, more surely than *Coral* was converted as soon as it appear'd in the Air.

There are, properly, but three Kinds of *Coral*, *red*, *white*, and *black* : The white is the rarest and most esteem'd; but 'tis the red is ordinarily used in Medicine. It must be chosen thick, smooth, and shining, and of a beautiful red, not cover'd with any tartareous Matter. There is a kind of white *Coral* pierc'd full of holes, and a black one, named *Antipathes*; appearing of a different Nature from the rest : but these are of no use.

It gives Title to an Officinal Composition, call'd *Syrup of Coral*, often prescribed by Physicians; as is the Pouder of *Coral* finely ground, and after levigated on a Marble, and made up into a proper form. But there are few except those who are fond of Medicines with Pearls in 'em that make use hereof. By means if its exceeding hardness, it is suspected to take away with it a great deal of the levigating Stone.

The Virtues attributed to *Coral* and its Preparations, are that it is Cardiac, and therefore of use in Diarrhæas, too large Fluxes of the Menstrua, and Floodings; of service in the *Fluor Albus*, and to prevent Miscarriages; beside its use in common as a Testaceous Pouder in Childrens Disease, &c.

Some also attribute to *Coral* the immediate stopping of Blood, the securing of Houses from Thunderbolts, the keeping away of evil Spirits, and the promoting of Dentition. The Chymists draw a magisterial Tincture from *Coral*, and a Salt.

'Tis added, that *Coral* appears redder wore on a Man than on a Woman;

that it become pale and livid when wore by a sick Person; and that the Changes on the Plant correspond with those in the Disease. But for these, and many more Fancies of the same kind, *Credat Judaeus Apella*. Its chief Use we know of, is in Chaplets, Beads, and other Toys.

*Artificial* **CORAL**, is made of Cinnabar well beaten; a Lay whereof is applied on a piece of Wood well dried, and polish'd, first moisten'd with Size : The whole is again polish'd; and for varnish, rubb'd over with the White of an Egg.

**CORALLINE**, or Sea Moss, a Plant found adhering to Rocks, Shells, and even to Coral. It has no Stem, but its Branches shoot immediately out of the Root. Its Use in Medicine is not very considerable : yet 'tis suppos'd of some effect to destroy Worms in Children when take in Pouder; and is also used as an Ornament in Rock-work. The best is greenish; the worst ash-colour'd, the red is not much better.

**CORDIAL**, Cardiac, in Medicine, a comfortative or refreshing Remedy, that gives a sudden Strength and Chearfulness to the Spirits, by raising them when depress'd by too much Exercise, the Consequence of some Disease, or the like Cause.

*Cordials* act by giving a Springiness and Force to the Fibres, and by some of their fine Particles directly entering the *Tubuli*, or Pores of the Nerves and fine Vessels, and so mixing directly with the Fluids.

Thus, some of the Particles of the Spirit of Lavender, when dropt in Sugar and taken, are suppos'd to enter the Nerves of the Palate directly. Spirituous Liquors, as Brandy, Cinnamon Water, &c. are suppos'd also to act immediately on the Palate; but especially on the nervous Coat of the Stomach, and not by the common Current of the Circulation : by which means they often prove an immediate *Cordial*.

In Faintings, where the Circulation of the Blood is languid, Sal Volatile Oleosum, or Spirit of Hartshorn dropt in cold Water and drank immediately, occasion a Contraction of the *Fibrillæ*, the last by its coldness, and the first by entering the small Vessels; and thus they instantly augment the Circulation, or in other Words, prove Cordial. In Officinal Compositions, the four *Cordial* Flowers are *Borrage, Bugloss, Roses* and *Violets*.

The four Cordial Waters are those of Borrage, Bugloss, Endive, and Chicory; some add those of Carduus Benedictus and Scorzonera, Scabiosa, Sorrel, &c.

**CORIANDER**, the Seed of a Plant of the same Name. Both the Taste and Smell of the Seed is very agreeable; yet both in the Plant extremely nauseous. Besides the Confections made of the *Coriander*-Seed, it is of use in Medicine as a Carminative, and a Corrective to some sorts of Catharticks. It is much us'd by the Brewers both in *England* and *Holland*, to give a Flavour to their strongest Beer. The Antients had a Notion that the Juice of *Coriander* would deprive People of their Senses, and even of Life. Some derive the Word from κορη, *apple of the Eye*, and ανδρων, *hominum*, because it is suppos'd to weaken the Sight.

**CORK**, the Bark of a Tree of the same Name, much resembling the Holm-Tree. Its Leaves are green above, and white underneath; and its Fruit a real Acorn, which seeds much more than that of the Oak. It is found in great abundance in *Spain, Italy, France*, &c.

To take off the Bark they make an Incision from top to the bottom of the Tree, and at each Extremity another round the Tree, perpendicular to the first. When stripp'd from the Tree, which does not therefore die, 'tis pil'd up in a Pond or Ditch, and loaden with heavy Stones to flatten it, and reduce it into Tables : Hence it is taken, to be dry'd; and when sufficiently dry put in Bales for Carriage. If care ben't taken to strip the Bark, it splits and peels off it self; being push'd up by another Bark from underneath.

The Bark of *Cork*, as well as the Acorn, are of some use in Medicine; being both reputed Astringents, after being burnt and pouder'd, when us'd externally; but the chief employ of the former is to put under Slippers, &c. and to stop Bottles.

The *Spaniards* burn it to make that light kind of Black we call *Spanish Black*, used by Painters.

**COURNACHINE** Pouder, a purging Pouder, call'd also *Earl of* Warwick's Pouder, and *Pulvis de Tribus*. It is composed of equal Parts of *Antimonium Diaphoreticum, Diagridium*, and *Cream of Tartar*.

**CORNICULATE** Plants, are such as after they have blown into Flower, produce many distinct and horned Pods, or Seed-Vessels, called *Siliquæ*; For, which Reason, the Plants are also denominated *siliquous Plants*. Such are the *Sedum* or *Sempervivum, Telephium, Juncus Floridus, Helleborus niger, Pæonia, Caltha Palustris, Althæa Lutea*, &c.

**CORNU** *Ammonis*, in Natural History, an extraordinary kind of Stone, which in Vinegar, Juice of Lemons, &c. has a Motion like that of an Animal. 'Tis rough, knotty, of an Ash-colour, and crooked in manner of a Ram's-horn such as those wherewith the Antients represented *Jupiter Ammon* : whence its Name.

'Tis disputed among Naturalists, whether it be a Fossil, or a *Nautilus*, or a Rock-Plant. *Camerarius*[1] maintains the first, urging that 'tis frequently dug out of the Tops of Mountains; and that 'tis seldom found near the Sea-shore.

Dr. *Woodward* asserts it a Shell, and of the Number of the Nautili, form'd in the Sea, and carried thence by the Waters of the Deluge into Countries whence 'tis dug. He argues, that if it be rarely found on the Sea-Coasts, 'tis because Shells and other Bodies fasten'd to the bottom of the Sea, as most Kinds of the *Cornua Ammonis* must be, are only to be tore thence and driven ashore by Tempests : but the most violent Tempests never move the Bottom of the Sea, as the Divers have out past doubt; so that 'tis no wonder if none of the *Cornua* be thrown up : But in the overturning of the Earth by the Deluge, these, with a thousand more Productions of the Sea, might be thrown from the bottom of the Waters to the Places where they are now

[1] Rudolf Jakob Camerarius (1665 – 1721), a German physician and botanist.

found.

The *Cornua Ammonis* are of different thicknesses and lengths; some of 'em weight about three Pounds. It is found in several Places in *Germany*. From some Experiments that have been made therewith, it's found to contain a little quantity of Gold; which sinks to the bottom upon pounding it small, and stirring it in a running Water, till all the earthly Parts were carried off.

"The Stone call'd *Cornu Ammonis* is frequent in the Clay wherein the Trochites and Entrochi are found : The largest I have is seven Inches in length, and four in circumference at the big End, and two and a half at the smaller; the Tip being broke off. Tracing its Origin, I find some of the first Buddings out of it about the bigness of a young Cock's Spur, and very much like it : I have some in raw Clay; and one growing of a white cawky Stone. They generally become at last a whitish Spar, and some milk-white, as some of the trochites are."

"There are of all intermediate Proportions between these two; tho very few of any bigness are to be found entire, but all broken and imperfect Pieces. The Texture of the Stone is thus : Some have a mossy Spar in their insides, which takes up three Parts of the Stone; then from the sharp top there grows thin flat Cells, or small Pipes of Spar set edgewise one close to the other, which shoot towards the broad End, and appear outwardly like small Ridges or Seams. There are likewise Rings running round it, tending in their growth towards the broad End, as in a Ram's Horn. Most of the lesser Stones have very little mossy Spar within 'em, and some none, with Cells coming down inwardly from the top of the Stone, resembling those in the Flowers of Coral, that terminates its Branches. And doubtless, if taken from their Beds in a seasonable time, would yield the like milky Juice." *Mr. Beaumont*[1], *ap. Philosoph. Transact.* No. 129.

**CORNU** *Cervi, Hartshorn*, in Medicine, one of the Testaceous Pouders. Among Chymists, the same Name is used for the Mouth of an Alembic.

**CORPORIFICATION**, or Corporation, in Chymistry, the Operation of recovering Spirits into the same Body, or at least into a Body nearly the same, with that which they had before their Spiritualization.

**CORPUSCLE**, in Physicks, a Diminutive of Corpus, us'd to express the minute Parts or Particles that constitute Natural Bodies. *Corpuscles* are the same with what the Antients call'd *Atoms*; and differ both from the Elementary and Hypostatical Parts of the Chymists, and the *Materia Subtilis* of the *Cartesians*. Sir *Isaac Newton* shews a Method of determining the Sizes of the *Corpuscles* whereof the Particles that compose Natural Bodies consist, from their Colours.

**CORPUSCULAR** or *Atomical Philosophy*, the Scheme or System of Physicks, whereon the Phænomenon are accounted for, from Motion, Rest, Position, Arrangement, &c. of the minute *Corpuscles*, or Atoms, where

[1] John Beaumont (ca. 1650 – 1731), an English surgeon and geologist.

Bodies are compos'd.

The *Corpuscular Philosophy,* which now flourishes under the Title of the *Mechanical Philosophy,* is exceedingly antient. *Leucippus* and *Democritus* were the first who taught it in *Greece*; from them *Epicurus* receiv'd it and improv'd it insomuch that it came at length to be denominated from him, and was call'd *Epicurean Philosophy.*

*Leucippus,* again, is said to have receiv'd it from *Mochus* a *Phoenician* Physiologist and Physician, before the Time of the *Trojan* War, and the first who philosophiz'd about Atoms : Tho *Gale*[1], who borrows all Profane Philosophy from the Sacred Philosophy in the Books of *Moses,* is of Opinion he might take the Hint from the *Mosaic* History of the Formation of Man out of the Dust of the Earth.

Indeed, *Casaubon*[2] takes Μωκον, or Μωχον, to be the Name of a *Tyrian,* who among his own Countrymen was called משה *Mosche,* or according to the Method of writing which then obtain'd, *Moses* : whence 'tis conjectur'd that the *Mosche,* or *Moschus* of the *Tyrians,* was, in effect, the *Moses* of the *Hebrews.*

This appears to be the Sentiment of *Selden*[3], *Arcerius*[4], &c. But the Opinion of *Bochart*[5] is the more probable, who from *Posidonius* and others, takes *Mochus* for an Inhabitant of *Sidon,* and his Philosophy to be nothing else but a Physiological or Natural History of the Creation.

After *Epicurus,* the *Corpuscular Philosophy* gave way to the *Peripatetic,* which became the popular System. Thus, in lieu of Atoms, were introduc'd Specific and Substantial Forms, Qualities, Sympathies, &c. which amus'd the World till *Gassendus, Charleton*[6], *des Cartes*[7], *Boyle, Newton,* and others, retriev'd the old *Corpuscularian* Hypothesis; which is now become the Basis of the Mechanical, and Experimental Philosophy.

Mr. *Boyle* reduces the Principles of the *Corpuscular* Philosophy to the four following Heads : 1st, That there is but one Catholick, or Universal Matter, which is an extended, impenetrable, and divisible Substance, common to all Bodies, and capable of all Forms.

This Sir *I. Newton* finely improves on : "All Things consider'd, "*says that great Author*, "it appears probable to me, that God, in the Beginning, created Matter in solid, hard, impenetrable, moveable Particles; of such Sizes and Figures, and with such other Properties, as most conduced to the End for which he form'd 'em : And that these primitive Particles, being Solids, are incomparably harder than any of the sensible porous Bodies compounded of 'em; even so hard as never to wear or break in pieces : no other Power being able to divide what God made one in the first Creation. While these *Corpuscles* remain entire, they may compose Bodies of one and the same

[1] This is probably Thomas Gale (1636 – 1702), an English scholar and antiquarian.

[2] Isaac Casaubon (1559 – 1614), a French scholar and philologist.

[3] John Selden (1584 – 1654), an English scholar and philosopher.

[4] Johannes Arcerius (ca. 1566 –1604), a Dutch scholar.

[5] Samuel Bochart (1599 – 1667), a French pastor and scholar.

[6] This is probably Walter Charleton (1619 – 1707), an English physician and writer.

[7] René Descartes (1596 – 1650), a French philosopher and mathematician.

Nature and Texture in all Ages : but should they wear away, or break in pieces, the Nature of things depending on 'em wou'd be changed : Water and Earth, compos'd of old worn Particles, and Fragments of Particles, wou'd not be of the same Nature and Texture now, with Water and Earth compos'd of entire Particles at the Beginning. And therefore, that Nature may be lasting, the Changes of *Corporeal* Things are to be plac'd only in the various Separations and new Associations of these permanent *Corpuscles.*" *Opticks.*

2d, That this Matter, in order to form the vast Variety of Natural Bodies, must have Motion, in some or all its assignable Parts; and that this Motion was given to Matter by God the Creator of all things: and has all manner of Directions and Tendencies. "These *Corpuscles,*" says Sir *I. Newton*, "have not only a *Vis Inertiæ*, accompanied with such passive Laws of Motion as naturally result from that Force; but also are moved by certain active Principles; such as that of Gravity, and that which causes Fermentation, and the Cohesion of Bodies."

3d, That Matter must also be actually divided into Parts, and each of these primitive Particles, Fragments, or Atoms of Matter, must have its proper Magnitude, Figure, and Shape.

4th, That these differently siz'd and shap'd Particles, have different Orders, Positions, Situations, and Postures; from whence all the Variety of Compound Bodies arises.

**CORRECTION**, in Pharmacy, the Preparation of a Medicine, in order to moderate and qualify the too great Violence of its Action; as when Glass of Antimony is calcin'd with a little Salt-petre; or, to prevent its giving the Gripes, when Salt of Tartar is dissolv'd in an Infusion of Senna.

**CORRECTORS**, in Medicine, such Ingredients in a Composition as guard against, or abate the Force of others.

Thus, the Lixivious Salts, prevent the grievous Vellications of Resinous Purges, by dividing their Particles, and preventing their Adhesions to the intestinal Membranes, whereby they sometimes occasion intolerable Gripings : And thus Spices, and carminative Seeds also, assist in the easier Operation of some Cathartics, by dissipating Collections of Wind.

In the making a Medicine, likewise, such Things are called *Correctors*, as destroy or diminish a Quality in it that could not otherwise dispens'd with : Thus, Turpentine may be called the *Corrector* of Quicksilver, by destroying its Fluxility, and making it thereby capable of Mixture : and thus rectified Spirit of Wine breaks off the Points of some Acids, so as to make them become safe and good Remedies, which before were destructive.

**CORROBORATIVE**, in Medicine, any thing that increases Strength, or gives a new Force. The Word is likewise frequently apply'd to such Medicines as are of use in particular Weaknesses; as the *Fluor Albus*, Gonorrhæa, &c. All Cardiacs are *Corroborative.*

**CORROSION**, the Action of corroding, or gnawing away, by little and little, the Continuity of the Parts of Bodies. Thus, Acids corrode most Natural Bodies; and Arsenic only kills, because it corrodes the Bowels with its sharp pointed Particles.

*Corrosion* is used both in Chymistry, Medicine, and Natural Philosophy; where it stands for a particular Species of Dissolution, either by an Acid, or a saline Menstruum. What *Corrosion* has peculiar to it, is, that 'tis mostly design'd for the Resolution of Bodies the most strongly compacted, as Bones and Metals; so that the Menstruums imploy'd require an uncommon Moment, or Force.

Now the *Corrosive* Liquors, whether acid or urinous, are nothing by Salts dissolv'd in a little Phlegm : Therefore, these being solid, and consequently containing a considerable quantity of Matter, do both attract one another the more, and are also more attracted by the Particles of the Body, which is to be dissolv'd. And as their Attractions at equal Distances are proportional to their Bulks, *cæteris paribus*; so when the more solid Bodies are put into saline Menstruums, the Attraction is stronger than other Solutions; and thus Motion, which is always proportional to the Attraction, more violent.

Hence we easily conceive how they should drive those Salts, like so many Darts, into the Pores of the Bodies, and open and loosen the Cohesion of them, tho ever so firm. Again, we know, the more minute the Particles of the Menstruum are, the sooner they penetrate, and with the greater Force : The Motion produc'd by Attraction, being always greatest in the least Corpuscles, next to nothing in the large ones.

Add to this another advantage gain'd by this minuteness of the Particles, *viz.* that they approach nearer the Body to be dissolv'd; without which, the attractive Force wou'd be insensible. Hence, those very Salts, which dissolv'd in Water will hardly touch Metals, if once turn'd into acid Spirits, easily penetrate : For in Distillation, not only a greater Quantity of Water remains, but the saline Bodies are so minutely broken, and divided by the Fire, as to make them more readily capable of being mov'd by an attractive Force; and therefore such a distill'd Menstruum is much more efficacious than any Solution of Salt made with Water.

**CORTEX** *Peruvianus*, call'd also *Quinquina, Kinkinna, Quina-quina, Pulvis Patrum*, and popularly the *Jesuit's Bark*; is the Bark of a Tree growing in the *West-Indies*, called by the *Spaniards Palo de Cassenturas*, q.d. *Fever-Wood*; by reason of its extraordinary Virtue in removing all Kinds of intermitting Fevers and Agues. The Bark, while on the Tree, is streak'd, of a whitish yellow with-outside, and a pale tan-colour within.

The *Indians* commonly call it the *Fuddling Tree*, from the Property it has of intoxicating Fishes, when either its Wood or Bark is beaten, and steep'd in the Water where they are.

The Tree that yields this noble Specific, is only found in *Peru*; in the Province of *San Francesco de Quitto*, or *Quinto*, near the City of *Loxe* : tho some say 'tis also found in that of *Potosi*; and F. *Labat*[1], in the Island of *Guadeloupa*.

'Tis about 70 Years since this noble Febrifuge was first known in *England*. It was first introduc'd into use by the Cardinal *de Lugo*[1]; whence, in *France*, it

[1] Jean-Baptiste Labat (1663 – 1738), a French Dominican missionary and botanist.

was first called from the Name of that Cardinal. Afterwards it became known by the Name of the *Jesuit's Pouder*, and the *Jesuit's Bark*; because sold by the Jesuits, to whom that Cardinal, who had been of their Society, left great Quantities of it.

When first introduc'd, it is said to have been sold for about eight Shillings Sterl. the Dose; which great Price, with a little Effects found from it, by reason of their Ignorance of the manner or preparing and prescribing it, occasion'd its being disus'd, till about the Year 1706, that Dr. *Talbot*[2], an *English* Physician, brought it into vogue again, by the great Number of Cures wrought about the Court and City of *Paris*, with this Pouder, prepar'd after his manner; the Secret whereof was soon after made publick by the Munificence of *Louis* XIV who rewarded *Talbot* for the Communication.

The *Quinquina* is sold either in Bark or in Pouder : those who buy it in the Bark must chuse it very dry and compact; such as has never been moisten'd, and which is not too easily reduc'd into Pouder by breaking. The small, fine, blackish Barks, chagrin'd without and reddish within, of a bitter disagreeable Taste, are the most esteem'd. For the Pouder, it must be well sifted, and care be taken it be bought of Persons that may be trusted; it being very easy to sophisticate it, and difficult to find it out.

The *Cortex* is a Bitter, Absorbent, and Astringent or Styptic : From its bitterness, M. *Reneaume*[3] observes, it becomes fit to soften sour acrimonious Juices; for a sour and a bitter make a sweet. Again, as an Absorbent it blunts the Points of Acids, and prevents their Action; and of consequence keeps up the Fluidity of the Juices, which Acids would coagulate. As a Styptic, it must have earthy Parts to absorb Serosities, by which the Parts before moisten'd and relax'd, will contract themselves : and by this means, the *Cortex* augments the Spring and Tension of the Fibres. As a Bitter it heats; and it facilitates Perspiration, by heating, and augmenting the Fluidity of the Juices. On these Properties it is that its Medicinal Uses are ascertain'd.

But its chief use is in curing of Agues, and intermitting Fevers; it being us'd for these Purposes in all Ages, and most Constitutions. Dr. *Cockburn* says, it produces this Effect better than any other Medicine of the same Intention, in the Ration of 365 to 1. It is usual to give a gentle Emetic of *Ipecacuanha* before the Exhibition of the *Cortex* : by thus preparing the Passages, the *Cortex* has not only more Success, but also is not subject to cause these Indispositions, *viz.* swelling in the Belly, Nausea's, &c. which often arise when neglected.

The *Cortex* must never be exhibited in the Paroxysm of an Ague, or intermitting Fever; but given in such a Quantity at times between the Paroxysms, as to prevent a Return of the Fit.

The *Cortex* exhibited in continual Fevers is dangerous; and care must be taken, that the Remission of a continual Fever be not mistaken for its Intermission : When there is a Remission, it usually happens indifferently at any time; whereas an Intermission happens at particular times.

[1] John de Lugo (1583 – 1660) , a Spanish Jesuit.

[2] This is probably Robert Talbor (1643 – 1681), an English physician.

[3] Michel-Louis Reneaume (1675 – 1739), alias Reneaume de La Garanne, a French physician.

The *Cortex* is given several ways, *viz.* in Pouder, in forms of Electuary, Bolus's, Infusions, Tinctures, &c. The *Arcana Taboriana* is about two Ounces of the *Cortex* in Pouder, digested in Sand-heat, with about a Quart of red Wine : After Digestion, the Wine must be pour'd off, and two or three Ounces given every three or four Hours between the Paroxysms, till the Intention is answer'd. If the Bark take downward, Venice Treacle, Diascordium, Conserve of Roses, Terra Japonica, Doses of Laudanum, &c. must be added to its Preparations. Where there happens to be an Obstruction of the Menses from the Exhibition of the *Cortex*, or to prevent it, it is advisable to add to its Preparations the Black Hellebore, Æthiop's Mineral, Cinnabar, &c. The *Cortex* is often us'd for young Children in Agues, by way of Clyster; and also applied to the Wrists, and Soles of the Feet, wrought up into a stiff Mass, with Turpentine, Venice Treacle, &c. which usually answers the Purpose.

Dr. *Helvetius*[1], Physician to the King of *France* about 20 Years ago, wrote a Book entirely upon the Subject of curing Agues by giving the *Cortex* clysterwise : In which he pretends, that this is more safe, and no less certain than the *Cortex* given internally.

Dr. *Cockburn*, in his Treatise of *Sea Diseases*, asserts the contrary; and proves that the *Cortex* given inwardly is as safe, and by much more certain and expeditious; and shews that we know how to remedy all the Inconveniences the *Cortex* may occasion.

Dr. *Sydenham*, and after him M. *Reneaume*, and others, have prescrib'd it with Success in Melancholic and Hysteric Affections, commonly call'd *Vapours*.

**CORTEX** *Winteranus*, or *Winteri*, the Bark of a Tree brought from the Streights of *Magellan*, by Captain *Winter*, in his voyage with Sir *Francis Drake* : *Clusius*[2] calls the Tree *Magellanica Aromatica Arbor*. The Bark is Aromatic, and found of good use at Sea against Scurvy : half a Dram of it, boil'd with other carminative Seeds, sweats, and relieves scorbutic Patients. It has also prov'd an Antidote against a poisonous sort of Seal, call'd a Sea Lion, frequent in those Parts. The Bark sold in the Shops under the Name of *Cortex Winteranus*, or Wild Cinnamon, Dr. *Sloane*[3] observes, is not the true *Cortex Winteranus*; they grow on different Trees, and in different Countries, and their Appearance is very different; yet are they so like in Taste, that he thinks they may be used as Succedaneums to each other.

**CORYMBIFEROUS** *Plants*, are distinguish'd into such as have a radiate Flower, as the *Flos Solis, Calendula*, &c. and such as have a naked Flower, as the *Abrotanum Feminina, Eupatorium, Artemisia*; to which are added the *Corymbiferous Affines*, or those a-kin hereunto such as *Scabious, Dipsaus, Carduus*, and the like.

**CORYMBUS**, in the general, signifies the Top, or Summit of any thing; but among the antient Botanists was particularly used to express the Bunches or

[1] Jean-Adrien Helvetius (1662 – 1727), born Jean-Adrien Schweitzer, a Dutch physician.

[2] Carolus Clusius (1526 – 1609), born Charles de l'Ecluse, a Dutch physician and botanist.

[3] Hans Sloane (1660 – 1753), an English physician and botanist.

Clusters of Ivy, Berries, &c.

Some also call the Top of the Stalk of a Plant, when so subdivided and adorn'd with Flowers or Fruits, as to make a round spherical Figure, by this Name; as the Tops of Leeks, Onions, and the like : and others confound the Word with *Umbella*, which expresseth the flowry Tops of such Plants as have their Branches and Flowers spread round, into the Form of what the Women now call an Umberella.

But among the modern Botanists, *Corymbus* is chiefly used for a compound discous Flower, whose Seeds are not Pappous, or do not fly away in Down : Such are the Flowers of Daisies, common Marigold, &c. Mr. *Ray*, therefore, makes one Genus of Plants to be such as have a compound discous Flower, but without any downy Wings to carry off their Seeds; as the *Corymbiferous*.

**CORYZA**, in Medicine, a *running at the Nose*; or a Defluxion of sharp Humours from the Glands of the Head, arising upon a diminution of Perspiration, or catching of Cold. Proper Evacuations, as Bleeding, Epispasticks, Sternutatories, &c. are usual in this Case.

**COSMETIC**, a Term in Physick, used for any Medicine, Preparation, or Means used to beautify and embellish the Face, and preserve or improve the Complexion; as Ceruss, and the whole Tribe of Fucus's, Washes, Cold Creams, Lip-Salves, &c. The *Indians* use the Water of green Cacao-Nuts as a grand *Cosmetic*, which wonderfully improves the Complexion.

**COSTIVENESS**, in Medicine, a preternatural Detention of the Excrements, with an unusual Hardness or Dryness thereof; and, thence, a difficulty of discharging 'em. This is the opposite to Diarrhæa, or Losseness.

In the *Philosophical Transactions*, we have an uncommon Instance of *Costiveness* by Mr. *Sherman*[1] : the Patient, one *Thomas Philips*, for several Years, never went to Stool in less than 19 or 20 Weeks : He generally eat and drank as well as his Neighbours; and did all the while the Office of a laboring Man : yet was not any of the other Evacuations sensibly greater than in other People. He died of it at 23 Years old.

In *Costiveness* the usual Remedies are gentle Preparations of Senna, lenitive Electuaries, Cream of Tartar, laxative Clysters, &c.

**COSTUS** *Arabicus*, the Root of a Tree resembling Eldar, brought from *Arabia*; whence its Name. Its chief use in Medicine, is to enter the Composition of *Venice* Treacle. The best is heavy, of a cineritious Colour withoutside, a reddish within, difficult to break, of a strong Smell, and an aromatic Taste. This Root was formerly call'd *Costus Verus*, and was divided into two Kinds, the *sweet* and the *bitter Costus*; both of which are now uncommon. M. *Charas*[2], and others, are of Opinion there is but one kind of *Costus*, which proves more or less sweet or bitter, according to the Soil where it is fed.

[1] This may be Bezaleel Sherman, an English surgeon in the early eighteenth century.

[2] Moïse Charas (1618 – 1698), a French physician and chemist.

**COSTUS** *Indicus*, an American Root, called also *Costus Blavo, Costus Corticosus, Costus Corticus, White Cinnamon*, and *Winter's Bark.* The Islands of *Madagascar* in *Africa*, of *Domingo* and *Guadaloupa* in *America*, are the Places where the most and best is found.

**COUNTER-POISON**, an Antidote, or Remedy, which prevents the Effect of Poison. Of this Kind are Treacle, Mithridate, and Orvietan. *Counter-poisons* are either *general* or *specific* : General *Counter-poisons* are Angelica, Rice, Carduus Benedictus, the Vincetoxicum, Dittany, Scorzonera, Citrons, Bezoar, Hartshorn, &c. The Specificks are those that follow; Citron-Bark, *v.g.* is a *Counter-poison* to Nux Vomica; *Venice* Treacle to the Bite of a Viper; Oil of Scorpion, to the Bite of Scorpions; Oil of Pine-Apples, to Orpiment; Gentian, to the Cicuta, &c.

*Vander Linden*[1], in his Treatise *de Venenis*, says, that in every putrid Indisposition, whether arising from the Bite of venomous Beasts, or from an Aclali form'd by Putrefaction, Vinegar drank is sovereign, either simple or distill'd; either with Honey inform of Oximel, or with Sea-Onion.

**CRABS-EYES**, *Oculi Cancrorum*, or *Lapides Cancrorum*, in Natural History and Medicine, are little, white, round Stones, ordinarily flat; so call'd, because taken out of the Craw-fish, or River Lobster : and tho bearing no great resemblance to Eyes, yet resembling them more than any other Part. They are much used in Medicine, as a powerful Alcali, or Absorbent.

The most able Naturalists imagine 'em form'd in the Brain of the Animal. *Van Helmont* first found 'em in the Region of the Stomach : M. *Geoffroy* the younger has observ'd the manner of their Formation much more accurately.

Those of the Rivers divest themselves every Year in *June* of the Bones wherewith they are cover'd and arm'd; a Membrane wherewith the Inside of those Scales is lin'd, takes their Place, and hardens, by degrees, into a new Scale.

Indeed, 'tis much less wonder an Animal should discharge it self of its Skin, or Covering; than that it should discharge it self of its Stomach, as the Craw-fish does; and even, as M. *Geoffroy* thinks, of its Intestines too. The exterior Membranes of those *Viscera* taking their place.

There is room to believe, that as they putrify and dissolve, they serve for Food to the Animal; during the Time of the Reformation, the old Stomach is the first Food the new one digests.

'Tis only in this time that the Stones are found, called *Crabs-Eyes*: They begin to be form'd when the antient Stomach is destroy'd; and are afterwards wrap'd up in the new one, where they decrease by degrees till they disappear entirely.

**CRASIS**, in the Animal Œconomy, a Due Temperament or Constitution of the Blood; wherein the several Principles, *viz.* Salt and Oil, whereof it is composed, are found in their jut Proportion and Purity : in contradistinction to a *Discrasy*, which consists in an improper Union of the Principles, or in an unnatural State of some thereof. The chief Discrasies the Blood is susceptible

[1] Johannes Antonides van der Linden (1609 – 1664), a Dutch physician and anatomist.

if, whence flow most of the Diseases of the Body, are *Coagulation, Dissolution*, an Excess of Oil, or Salt. The Word is *Greek*, κρασις, signifying Mixture, Temperament.

**CRASSEMENTUM**, a Term used by some Anatomists, for the Cruor of the Blood; or that Part which, upon standing to cool and separate, forms the Coagulum : In opposition to the Serum, or Whey, wherein it swims.

**CREAM** *of Tartar*, in Pharmacy, a Preparation of Tartar, otherwise called *Crystal of Tartar.*

It is made by boiling Tartar in Water till it be dissolved, and passing the Dissolution thro' a Straining Bag : Half the Liquor being evaporated, the Remainder is set in a cool Place; where it shoots into Crystals, Part of it swimming a-top, in form of *Cream.* This latter is properly the *Cream of Tartar*, the rest *Crystal of Tartar*, both of the same Nature and Use.

It is reputed a great Sweetner of the Blood; for which some take it in Whey or Water gruel in the Spring-time, to the Quantity of Half an Ounce every Morning, for three or four Weeks.

Its operation is by Stool; and, by its saline Particles, pretty much also by Urine. It's generally mix'd with lenitive Electuaries, and other gentle Catharticks, in Nephritic and Antivenereal Cases, where it often proves serviceable.

**CREPITATION**, that Noise which some Salts make over the Fire in Calcination; call'd also Detonation.

**CRIBATION**, in Pharmacy, a Separation of the finer Parts of a Medicine, whether dry, or humid, from the grosser; the latter by means of a Pulping Stove, the former by a fine Searce.

**CRINONES**, in Medicine, a sort of Worms, sometimes found under the Skin, in Children; resembling short thick Hairs, or Bristles. They are also called *Comedones*, from the Latin *Comedere*, to eat; by reason they prey on the Substance of the Child or consume its Nourishment.

**CRISIS**, in Medicine, a Change, or Turn in acute Diseases; wherein the Morbifick Matter is so alter'd, as determines the Patient either for Recovery or Death. The Cause of such Change is owing to the remaining vital Force's being irritated by the Matter of the Disease so or so condition'd; *i.e.* fit either to be evacuated, or translated, or to kill.

If the Matter be dispos'd for Evacuation or Translation, but is not Salubrious, it produces a Change call'd a *Critical Perturbation*, or *Imperfect Crisis*. If the Change becomes sensible, they are call'd *Critical Symptoms*, or *Signs of a Crisis*, either future or present.

The Symptoms of the *Crisis* are frequently confounded with those arising from the Causes of the Disease, the Disease it self, or the Matter of the Disease; whence the most unhappy consequences.

The Differences between these critical Symptoms and morbifick ones, are, that the first proceed from the vital Powers prevailing over the Force of the

Disease; but the latter from the Disease's prevailing over the vital Faculty : that the first are preceded by a manifest Concoction, but the latter are form'd even in Crudities : that the former happen about the *critical Times*, but the latter at all Times of the Disease, chiefly during its Increase.

*The principal Symptoms of an approaching Crisis*, are, after Digestion, and about the critical Time, a sudden Stupor, Drousiness, Waking, Delirium, Anxiety, Dyspnoea, Grief, Redness, Titillation, Pricking, Heaviness, Darkness, Light, spontaneous Tears, Nausea, Heat, Thirst, trembling of the lower Lip, &c.

**CRITICAL** Days, Symptoms, &c. are certain Days, and Symptoms, usually arising on the Course of acute Diseases, as Fevers, Small Pox, &c. which indicate the Patient's State, and determine him either to recover or grow worse. The Crises have been frequently observ'd to happen on the 7th, 14th, or 20th Day; whence those have been denominated Critical Days. The Word comes from the *Greek* κρινω, *judico*, I judge.

*For the Theory of Crises*, it may be observ'd, that the Concoction of any morbifick Matter, and the Humour to be secern'd, is nothing else but a Change thereof into such a due Magnitude, or Smallness, as it may be carried by the circulating Blood along the Canals, and excern'd by Vessels destin'd for that Purpose. But if the morbifick Matter cannot be reduc'd to such a Magnitude or Smallness as may correspond to the Orifices of the Secretory Vessels; then either an Abscess or a Hemorrhage will follow, if a Crisis be begun; for which Reason, Abscesses, &c. are accounted less perfect Crises. But, that the morbifick Matter may be reduc'd to a due Magnitude, or Smallness, and its wish'd-for Discharge, there is requir'd a considerable Time, if the Quantity of Matter is large; that is, if the Distemper be great and severe : And since there are a great many Causes, and those very constant, which may occasion the Blood, and offending Humours therein, to be of a different Fluidity in the Inhabitants of different Climates; it is impossible but that different Spaces of Time should be requir'd for the finishing Concoction : which makc sit impossible to determine the critical Days in one Climate, from what they are found to be in another.

The Causes of real *Critical Days*, that is, such on which happens the last Concoction of the morbifick Matter, which is always attended with its Expulsion, are all those Things which occasion the Humours to become of such a certain Magnitude or Minuteness, and of a greater or lesser Cohesion; but with any given Power, Bodies unequally large, or unequally cohering, cannot be concocted in an equal Time : Wherefore, it is to be found by the Observations made by all nations among themselves, which are the usual Causes and Conditions of those Diseases, which require a certain Number of Days to finish such a Concoction in.

**CROCI**, among Botanists, the Apices, or small Knobs on the Tops of Flowers.

**CROCUS**, in Chymistry, is a Name given to several different Preparations; from their red or saffron Colour.

*Crocus Martis*, is a Preparation of Iron; and is of two Kinds, viz. *Crocus Martis aperiens*, and *Crocus Martis astringens*.

*Crocus Martis aperiens, opening Saffron of Mars*, is a Preparation of Iron Plates, made by first washing them, then exposing them to the Dew, till they have contracted a Rust; which Rust is scraped off, and the Plates exposed for more.

Others prepare it by calcining Iron Filings, with an equal Weight of Sulphur. Others by clapping a Bar of Iron, red, or rather white hot, between two Rolls of Brimstone; in which Case, the Iron melts, and runs down into a Vessel of Water below : which some call *Mars cum Sulphure præparatus*. Others have other Preparations.

*Crocus Martis astringens*, binding Saffron of Iron, is a Preparation of Iron Filings; wherein they are deprived of their more saline Parts, by washing them five or six times in string Vinegar, and calcining them five or six Hours.

*Crocus Metallorum*, a Kind of impure, opake, Glass of Antimony, of a liver Colour; hence frequently called Liver of Antimony; made by firing equal Parts of Pouder of Antimony and Salt-petre, well mixed in an Iron Mortar, covered with a Tile. This is kindled by dropping in a Coal of Fire, upon which a great Detonation ensue; and the Mortar is struck, to make the Matter fall to the bottom. The shining Part is the *Crocus*, or Liver, which is to be separated from the Dross, and reserved for use. Its chief use is in making *Vinum Emeticum*, or *Benedictum*, by infusing an Ounce or two of the Crocus poudered in a Quart of Wine for 24 hours.

**CROWS-BILL**, an Instrument us'd by Chirurgeons, in their Operations; especially for the drawing Bullets and other foreign Bodies out of Wounds. It has its Name from its Figure.

**CRUDE**, something that has not pass'd the Fire, or has not had the degree of *Coction*, *i.e.* of Heat, requisite to prepare it for eating, or some other Purpose.

*Crude* or Raw Silk is that which has not been put in boiling Water, to unwind it from off the Cod; nor boil'd in Water and Soap, to fit it for dying.

In Chymistry, they call *Crude Antimony* that which comes immediately from the Mines, without any Preparation. In Medicine, *Crude Humours* are those which want of that Preparation and Elaboration which they ordinarily receive from Digestion.

The Retainers to the Doctrine of Trituration, hold that the *Crudity* of the Humours only consists in this; that they are not broke and communicated so much as they should be by the ordinary Action of the Stomach.

**CRUDITY**, in Medicine, the State of a Disease, wherein the morbifick Matter is of such Bulk, Figure, Cohesion, Mobility, or Inactivity, as denominates it *crude*, *i.e.* as creates or increases the Disease.

That State of the Disease, wherein the *crude* Matter is changed, and render'd less peccant, and laudable, is call'd Digestion, Concoction, or Maturation.

A *Crudity* is discover'd, 1st, from the Disease's containing its degree of Strength, or increasing. 2nd, From a disorderly Exercise of the Functions. 4th, But chiefly from a Fault in the Quantity or Quality of the Humours; both those still circulating, and those secreted, and evacuated : as of Sweat, Tears,

Mucus of the Nose, Saliva, Sputum, the Bile, Urine, Ichor, Pus, Blood, Menses, Loches, Milk, Aphthae, &c.

**CRYSTAL**, in Natural History a Kind of Mineral; or rather, a transparent Stone, white, like a Diamond, but much inferior therein in Lustre and Hardness; used for Vases, Urns, Mirrors, &c.

The Antients were but little acquainted with the Nature of *Crystal*: *Pliny* speaks of it as harden'd, petrified Water, which was the popular Opinion of those Days; but Experience has shewn us the contrary : for by a Chymical Analysis, instead of resolving into Water, it yields nothing but a Calx, Earth, and Salts.

For the Places where 'tis found, *Pliny* adds, that he has seen it dug from off the highest and roughest Rocks of the *Alps*; whence, doubtless, its Name of *Rock-Crystal*. 'Tis sometimes also found in Brooks and Rivers, but not form'd there; only wash'd down thither from off the Mountains by the violent Rains. Several Mountains of *Europe*, and some of *Asia*, produce Rock-Crystal : If we may believe the *French* Relation of *Madagascar*, that Island yields more than all the World besides.

Its Perfection consists in its Lustre and Transparency; that with Straws, Dust, Clouds, &c is little valued. It is frequently Hexagonal; the Edges inimitably fine and accurate.

*Crystal* is of some use in Medicine, being an Astringent; and as such used in Diarrhæas and Dysenteries : 'Tis also used to increase the Milk of Nurses; and, further, is esteem'd a good Antidote against Arsenic.

The Word comes from the *Greek* κρυϛαλλος, *Glacies*; form'd of κρυος, *frigus*, and ϛελλομαι, *concresco*, because of its resembling Ice.

*The Formation of Crystal*, is deliver'd by F. *Francisco Lana*[1] in the *Philosophical Transactions*, to this Effect : "In the *Val Sabbia* I observ'd a specious round of a Meadow, some Parts whereof were bare of all Herbs; wherein, and no where else thereabouts, *Crystals* are generated : all Sexangular; both Points terminating in a pyramidal Figure, likewise Sexangular. The Country People told me, They were produc'd from the Dews; because, forsooth, being gather'd over night, there would others arise, only in a serene and dewy Sky. But having observ'd that there was no mark of any Mine thereabout, I concluded it might be a plenty of Nitrous Streams; which at the same time might hinder the Vegetation on those Places, and coagulate the Dew falling thereon : For Nitre is not only the natural Coagulum of Water, as is manifest in artificial Glaciations, but ever retains the abovesaid Sexangular Figure; which, by the way, may be the Cause of the Sexangular Figure of Snow."

"Since Crystals are only found in those narrow Places, 'tis probable, thence are rais'd the Exhalations that concrete the Dew : after the same manner as the Vapour or Exhalation of Lead coagulates Quicksilver."

*Rohault*[2] shews, that *Crystal*, Diamond, &c. must have been originally

[1] Francisco Lana (1631 – 1687), an Italian Jesuit and natural philosopher.

[2] Jacques Rohault (1618 – 1672), a French natural philosopher and mathematician.

liquid, from their Figure, which is such as Drops of Water of the same Size must necessarily have; and such as Globules of Meal or Flower, heap'd up and compress'd by their own weight, might have : For as each Crystal is encompass'd and closed round with six others; so it becomes modell'd into a hexangular Body, consisting of equal and square Sides.

*Boerhaave* takes *Crystal* to be the proper Matter, or Basis of all Gems or Precious Stones, which assume this or that Colour, &c. from the different Admixture of Mineral and Metalline Fumes, with the primitive *Crystalline* Matter.

*Crystal* is also used for a factitious Body, cast in the Glass-Houses; called also *Crystal-Glass*. It is, in effect, a Glass; but carried, in the Melting, and in the Matter whereof it is compos'd; tho it comes far short of the Whiteness and Vivacity of the Natural *Crystal*. The best Artificial *Crystals* are those made at *Mouran* near *Venice*; call'd *Venice Crystals*.

**CRYSTALS**, in Chymistry, express Salts, or other Matters, shot, or congeal'd in manner of Crystal.

**CRYSTAL**, or *Cream of Tartar*, is that Drug purify'd and dissolv'd, and again coagulated in form of Crystals. The *Cream* and *Crystals* were antiently suppos'd to be different; but are now found the same Thing.

To prepare it, they boil Tartar in Water, skim it, and strain it; when cool, there are form'd little white, shining *Crystals* at the Edges, as also a Pellicle, or Cream swimming a-top.

*Crystal of Tartar* is esteem'd Purgative, and Aperitive; proper in Hydropical and Asthmatical Cases, and Intermittent Fevers.

Crystal *of Tartar chalybeated*, is when 'tis impregnated with the most dissoluble Parts of Iron. Crystal *of Tartar emetic*, is when 'tis charg'd with the sulphureous Parts of Antimony, to render it vomitive.

**CRYSTAL** *Mineral*, call'd also *Mineral Anodyne*, and *Sal Prunella*, is Salt-petre prepar'd with Sulphur; thus : Put half a Pound of Salt-petre in a Crucible, and set that in a Furnace; and when the Salt-petre is in Fusion, add, at several times, two Drachms of Flower of Sulphur.

After the Flame is over, invert the Crucible in a flat Pewter Bason, that the Salt may shoot. This is esteem'd good against the Squinancy, whence its Name of *Sal Prunella*; *Pruna*, or *Prunella*, expressing that Disease.

**CRYSTALS** *of Silver*, or *of Luna*, is Silver, penetrated and reduced into the form of Salts, by the pointed Acids of Spirit of Nitre. 'Tis used for making Eschars, by applying it to any Part : 'tis also of use internally, in Dropsies, and Diseases of the Brain.

**CRYSTALS** *of Mars*, call'd also *Salt*, or *Vitriol of Mars*; is Iron reduced into Salts by an acid Liquor; used in Diseases arising from Obstructions.

**CRYSTALS** *of Venus*, call'd also *Vitriol of Venus*; is Copper reduced into the form of Vitriol by the Spirit of Nitre; very caustick, and used to cut off proud Flesh.

**CRYSTALLI**, among Physicians, are Pustules dispers'd all over the Body; white, and of the bigness of a Lupine.

**CRYSTALLINE HUMOUR**, is a thick, compact Humour of the Eye, in manner of a flattish convex Lens, situate in the middle of the Eye; serving to make that Refraction of the Rays of Light, necessary to have 'em meet in the Retina, and form an Image thereon, whereby Vision may be perform'd.

'Tis the Configuration of the *Crystalline* that occasions Persons to be either *Myopes*, or *Presbytae*, *i.e.* to be either long or short-sighted.

The *Crystalline* being of two Consistences; outwardly, like a Gelly; but toward the Centre as hard as Salt : Hence, some Authors think that its Figure may be varied; which Variations they suppose to be effected by the *Ligamentum Ciliare*. Hence Dr. *Grew*, and others, ascribe to the Ciliary Ligament a Power of making the *Crystalline* more convex, as well as of moving it to or from the Retina : Accordingly, by the Laws of Opticks, something of this Kind is absolutely necessary to distinct Vision : For, as the Rays from distant Objects diverge less than those from nigh ones; either the *Crystalline Humour* must be capable of being made more convex, or more flat; or else there must be an Elongation of the Eye, or of the Distance between that and the *Retina*.

The *Crystalline Humour*, when dried, appears to consist of a vast Number of thin, spherical Laminæ, or Scales, lying over one another: *Leewenhoeck* reckons there may be 2000 of 'em in one *Crystalline*; each of these, he says, he has discover'd to consist of a single Fibre, or fine Thread wound up in a stupendous manner, this way and that; so as to run several Courses, and meet in as many Centres : and yet not interfere nor cross in any Place.

**CRYSTALLIZATION**, in Chymistry, a Kind of Congelation, befalling Salts, both *essential*, *fix'd*, and *volatile*; when, being set free from the greatest Part of their Humidity, they are left to harden, dry, and shoot into *Crystals*.

The ordinary Method of *Crystallization*, is perform'd by dissolving the saline Body in Water, filtering it, and letting it evaporate, till a Film appears at the top; and lastly, letting it stand to shoot.

This Shooting is accounted for, on Sir *I. Newton's* Principles, from that attractive Force which is in all Bodies, and particularly in Salt, by reason of its Solidity; whereby, when the Menstruum or Fluid in which such Particles float, is sated enough, or evaporated, (which brings it to the same) so that the saline Particles are within each other's attractive Powers, and can draw one another more than they are drawn by the Fluid, they will turn into *Crystals*.

This is peculiar to Salts, that let them be ever so much divided, and reduc'd into minute Particles; yet, when they are form'd into *Crystals*, they each of them reassume their proper Shapes : so that one might as easily divest and deprive 'em of their Saltness, as their Figure.

This being an immutable and perpetual Law, by knowing the Figure of the *Crystals*, we may understand what the Texture of the Particles ought to be, which can form those Crystals : and, on the other hand, by knowing the Textures of the Particles, may be determin'd the Figures of the *Crystals*.

For, since the Figures of the most simple Parts remain always the same, it is evident that the Figures they run into, when compounded and united, must be uniform, and constant : and since the Force of Attraction may be stronger on one side of a Particle than on another; there will constantly be a greater Accretion of Salts upon those Sides which attract more strongly : from which it may easily be demonstrated, that the Figure of the least Particles, is entirely different from that which appears in the Crystal.

**CUBEBS**, in Pharmacy, a Fruit brought from the Island of *Java*, in Grains resembling Pepper, both in form and size; whence some call it *Wild Pepper*. 'Tis said, the Natives of the Place boil it ere they allow it to be exported, to prevent its being sown in other Countries. *Cubebs* fortify the Stomach, Brain, and other Viscera; and enter as an Ingredient in several Officinal Compositions.

**CUCULLATE** *Flowers*, among Botanists, are such as resemble a *Cucullus*, or Monk's Hood, or Helmet.

**CUCUPHA**, an antient Form of Medicine; being a Cap, or Cover for the Head, with Cephalic Spices quilted therein; wore in many nervous Distempers, and particularly such as more immediately affect the Head : as against Catarrhs, Defluxions, &c. It is now almost out of use.

**CUCURBITACEOUS** *Plants*, a Kind of Plants, so called from their resemblance to the Gourd, call'd by the Latins *Cucurbita*, which is the Head of this Family. The Pumpion, Mushroom, Melon, &c. are of the *Cucurbitaceous* Kind. Plants of the *Cucurbitaceous* Kind, send out their Branches every way; which are soft, and generally set with *Urillæ*, by means whereof they cling to the Bodies that are near 'em.

Their Flowers are either Sterile, or Fertile : The last knit, and yield fleshy Fruits of various Figures; containing within 'em several flat Seed placed in three or four Lodges, or even a greater Number. These Seeds have usually a white sweetish Kernel; the greatest part of 'em being of those call'd *Frigidæ Majores*, or greater Cold Seeds.

**CUCURBIT**, in Chymistry, an Earthen, or Glass vessel, call'd also *Body*; wherein are put the Matters to be distill'd. It is sometimes also made of Tin, and sometimes of Brass, tinn'd. When a Distillation is to be made, they fit on to it a glass Head, with an Aperture, and a Neck proportional.

**CUCURBITULA**, in Chirurgery, a Cupping-Glass, or Instrument used in the Operation of Cupping.

**CULINARY**, an Epithet frequently added to Fire; determining it to be a common Fire, excited in Wood, Coals, or other ordinary Fuel : In contraindication to Solar Fire, or that rais'd by the Action of a Burning-Glass; to Central Fire; to Animal Fire; &c.

*Culinary Fire*, according to *Boerhaave*, consists of a Portion of pure Elementary, or Solar Fire, attracted by the oily, or sulphureous Parts of the Fuel, with such Velocity, as that it moves the same, agitates and whirls 'em violently about, and by degrees breaks and attenuates them; renders 'em volatile, and disperses 'em in Air.

The Effect of Air upon the Fire, is to make, as it were, a Vault around it, and by that means, restrain and keep it in, determine it upon the Sulphur, and thus prevent its too hasty Dissipation.

The Word is form'd from the Latin *Culina*, Kitchen; this being the chief place of such Fires.

**CULMIFEROUS**, in Botany, a Term applied to such Plants as have a smooth-jointed Stalk, usually hollow; the Stalk wrap'd about, at each Joint, with single, narrow, sharp-pointed Leaves; and the Seeds contain'd in chaffy Husks. *Culmiferous Plants* are divided into two Kinds; those with a *greater* and those with a *smaller* Seed. Those with a larger Seed are called *Frumentaceous*, or *Cereales*; and are again divided into *Spicatæ*, as Wheat, Rye, Spelt, Barley, Rice, Pease, &c. and *Paniculatæ* or *Jubatæ*, as Oats, Scordium, Milium, and Maise.

**CULMUS**, is properly the Stem of Stalk of Corn, or Grass; which in other Plants is call'd *Caulis*. Hence, *Culmiferous Plants*, are such as have a smooth-jointed Stalk, and usually hollow; and at each Joint the Stalk is wrap'd about with single, narrow, long, sharp-pointed Leaves, and their Seeds are contain'd in chaffy Husks.

**CUMMIN**, the Grain of a Plant of the same Name, much like that if Fennel; growing abundantly in the Isle of *Malta*, where 'tis sown and cultivated after the manner of Corn. The *French* frequently call it *Anis aigre*, sharp or sour Anis.

'Tis us'd with Success in the Vertigo, Wind-Colics, Tympanies, &c. 'Tis esteem'd excellent to retrieve the Natural Heat in Horses, Bulls, &c. The Pidgeons are exceedingly fond of it; when some make use of it to people their Dove-houses, incorporating it with an Earth naturally saline, or some other Earth that has imbib'd Urine.

This Seed, as well as the common Anis, yields, by Expression, a kind of Oil, esteem'd sovereign in Rheumatisms; provided it be us'd with Precaution, and in small Quantities.

**CYCLISCUS**, from κυκλος, *Circulus*; an Instrument in form of an Half-Moon; used by the Surgeons to scrape away Rottenness.

**CYPHI**, a Term in the *Arabian* Pharmacy, signifying a kind of strengthening Perfume. *Mithridates*[1] gives the Appellation *Cyphi* to the Troches wherewith the *Egyptian* Priests us'd to sweeten their Gods, to make 'em grant what they requested. He used the same in the Composition of Mithridate, on account of their efficacy against Poisons, Defluxions, &c. The *Cyphi* are compos'd of Raisins, or dry'd Grapes, Turpentine, Myrrh, Bdellium, Spica Nardi, Cassia Lignea, Aspalathum, Saffron , &c. temper'd into a Mass with Honey and a little Wine.

[1] Mithridates VI (ca. 134 – 63 BC), king of Pontus, in northern Turkey on the Black Sea.

**CYPRESS**, *Cupressus*, in Natural History, a precious sort of Wood, the Product of a Tree of the same Name; frequent in the Island of *Cyprus*. The Fruit of this Tree, call'd *Cones*, is us'd in astringent Decoctions, for Hernia's, Hemorrhages, &c. It is very compact, and heavy; and its Smell as agreeable as that of Santal. It scarce ever rots, decays, or is worm-eaten, no more than Cedar, or Ebony : For which Reason, the Antients used it to make the Statues of their Gods. In *Candia*, and particularly about Mount *Ida*, the Plant is said to rise spontaneously, wherever the Earth is a little dug; but is exceeding difficult to raise by Art.

**DACROIDES**, in Medicine, a Term applied to Ulcers, which are continually yielding any putrid Matter. The Word is form'd from δακρυον, Tear, and οιδος, Form; denoting the Ulcers to weep or shed somewhat like Tears.

**DAMNATA** *Terra*, in Chymistry, is the same with *Caput Mortuum*, that is, all the Earthy Part, or Mass, remaining at the Bottom of the Retort, &c. after all the other Principles have been drawn out of the Body by Fire.

**DATE**, *Dactyl*, the Fruit of the Palm-Tree. This Fruit is gather'd in Autumn, ere ripe; and bears a near resemblance to our Bullace; being of a green Colour, very sharp and astringent. When ripe, it becomes ruddy, having a hard, longish Stone, cloven at Bottom, encompass'd with a thin white Pellicle or Skin. The Bark or Covering of the *Date*, call'd by the Ancients *Elate* or *Spata*, when the Fruit is in Flower, is various; having as many Changes of Colour as the Fig has : Some black, some white, some brown, some again are round like Apples, and very big. Ordinarily they are oblong, fleshy, yellow, somewhat bigger than the Thumb's End, and very agreeable to the Taste. Some are no bigger than a Chich-Pea, and others as big as a Pomegranate. The best are those, call'd *Royal-Dates*. There is also another Sort, call'd *Carjotes*, which are very good.

*Dates* are principally used in Medicine : Their Qualities are, to soften the Asperities of the Gullet, to strengthen the Child in the Womb, to assuage all immoderate Fluxes of the Belly, and to ease Disorders of the Reins and Bladder. Their bad Property is, that they digest difficultly, cause Pains in the Head, and produce a thick melancholic Blood. These Effects arise from the Principles they contain, which are a moderate Share of Oil, and a deal of Phlegm, and Essential Salt. The Oil and Phlegm render them moistening and nutritious, good against Acrimonies of the Breast, to assuage Coughs, &c. And the Phlegm and Salt render them detersive and astringent, and good against Diseases of the Throat. For the rest; they are an heavy Food, full of an Earthy Juice, and occasion Obstructions in the Viscera; for which Reason, People who live of Dates become Scorbutic, and lose their Teeth betimes.

Our *Dates* are brought us from *Egypt, Syria, Africa*, and the *Indies*. They never come to full Maturity in *Italy*, or the most Southern Parts of *Spain*. And yet there are tolerable Dates in *Provence*; only they don't keep, but breed Worms. Those from *Persia* exceed all others in Largeness, Colour, and Taste. The Word is form'd of *Dacte*, and that of *Dactylus*, Finger; as being round and oblong, resembling a Finger's End.

**DEATH**, *Mors*, is generally consider'd as the Separation of the Soul from the Body, in which Sense it stands opposed to *Life*, which consists of the Union thereof.

The Physicians generally define *Death* by a total Stoppage of the Circulation of the Blood; and a Cessation of the animal, vital, &c. Functions consequent thereon; As, Respiration, Sensation, &c.

An animal Body, by the Actions inseparable from Life, undergoes a continual Change. Its smallest Fibres become rigid, its Minute Vessels grow into solid Fibres no longer pervious to the Fluids, its greater Vessels grow hard and narrow, and every Thing becomes contracted, closed, and bound up; whence the Dryness, Immobility, and Extenuation observed in old Age. By such Means the Offices of the minuter Vessels are destroy'd, the Humours stagnate, harden, and at length coalesce with the Solids. Thus are the subtilest Fluids in the Body, intercepted and lost, the Concoction weaken'd, and the Reparation prevented; only the coarser Juices continue to run slowly thro' the greater Vessels, to the Preservation of Life, after the animal Functions are destroy'd. At length, in the Process of these Changes, *Death* it self becomes inevitable, as the necessary Consequence of Life.

But 'tis rare, that Life is thus long protracted, or that *Death* succeeds merely from the Decays and Impairments of old Age. Diseases, a long and horrid Train, cut the Work short.

**DECANTATION**, in Chymistry, &c. the Act of pouring out a Liquor from off the Fæces, &c. by gently inclining the Lip or Canthus of the Vessel; whence the Word is derived.

**DECIDUOUS**, in the general, expresses something apt and ready to fall : Thus Botanists say, in some Plants the *Perianthium* or *Calyx* is *deciduous* with the Flower, that is, falls off from the Plant with it; in others not.

**DECOCTION**, the Act of Boiling one, or more Plants, or other Drugs, to extract the Juice out of the same for some medicinal Purpose. *Decoctions* of Guaiac, and Sarsaparilla, are the common Drink in certain Diseases.

Monsr. *Boulduc* assures us from his own Experience, that the Infusions of Vegetable Purgatives act better and produce better Effects, than their *Decoctions*; which he attributes to this, that the purest and most active Principles of those Bodies are dissipated and evaporated by Heat. *Memoires de l'Academie Royal des Sciences*, An. 1710.

**DECOMPOSITION**, in Chymistry and Pharmacy, the same Thing with Analysis, or Resolution, *viz.* the Reduction of a Body into the Principles, or component Parts it consists of.

*Decomposition*, is sometimes taken for any Sort of Resolution, or Separation of Parts : In Propriety, however, Decomposition is a Process of an Artist, in order to a Separation of the Heterogeneities, or Impurities from any Matter.

Tradition, founded on repeated Experiments, is a much surer Way of arriving at the Knowledge of the Properties of a Plant, than any chymical *Analysis*, or *Decomposition* of its Principles.

**DECORTICATION**, the Peeling, or Unhusking of Roots, Seeds, Fruits, Branches, &c or the Freeing, of them from their Barks, Rinds, Husks, or Shells.

**DECREPITATION**, in Chymistry, a Drying, and Calcining of Salt over the Fire, continued till such Time as it ceases to crackle. The Term is also applied to the Noise, or Crackling of the Salt during the Operation. The Design of this

Operation is to free the Salt of its superfluous Moisture. But the Salt is hereby rendred soporous, and apt to imbate Moisture, that unless it be kept very close, it soon moistens again.

**DEFECATE**, a Term applied to some body that is purged, and clear'd of Feces, or Impurities. Distillations, and other Chymical Operations are intended to separate the most pure, and subtile Parts from the Feces, or Lees. Spirit of Wine well *defecate*, easily evaporates.

**DEFENSITIVE**, in Medicine, and Chirurgery, a Bandage, Plaster, or the like, used in the Cure of Wound, to moderate the Violence of the Pain, the Flux of Blood, and the Access, and Impression of the external Air. The Cauterization perform'd, the Wound is cover'd with Lint, and the Eye with a *Defensitive*, and a Triangular Compress. For the first dressing of the Entorse, Mr. *Dionis*[1] used a little *Defensitive* made of the White of an Egg, *Oleum Rosatum*, and Alumn-Powder.

**DEFLAGRATION**, in Chymistry, the Inkindling, or setting Fire to a Salt, a Mineral, or other Matter, mix'd for that Purpose with a sulphureous one, in order to purify it; As is done in the Preparing of *Æthiops* Mineral, *Sal Prunellæ*, &c. The Word is form'd of the Latin *de*, and *flagrare*, to burn.

**DEFLUXION**, a Falling, or Flowing of a Humour on any Part of the Body; as of Rheum on the Trachea, and Oesophagus in a Catarrh. Defluxions *on the Lungs* are very dangerous. Defluxions *on the Eyes* produce a Weakness of Sight, and frequently Blindness. The Word is form'd from the Latin *Defluo*, I flow down, the Humours falling upon some Part, where they are gather'd together.

**DEGLUTITION**, in Medicine, the Act of swallowing the Food. *Deglutition* is perform'd, in the first place, by means of the Tongue, driving the Aliment into the *Oesophagus*, or Gullet; and then, by the Contraction of the Sphincter, and the fleshy Fibres of the same *Oesophagus*, which lessening the Bore, or Aperture thereof, protrude the Contents downwards into the Stomach. *Deglutition* succeeds *Mastication*, and is followed by Concoction.

**DEGREE**, in Medicine, denotes a certain pitch or intenseness of the elementary Qualities. The *Degrees* usually allowed are four, answering to the Number of the peripatetic Elements. In the School Philosophy, the same Qualities are divided into eight: the last or highest Degree of Intention is called *ut octo*. We say a thing is Cold in the second *Degree*, Pepper is hot in the third *Degree*. Fire is held hot in the eighth *Degree*, and dry in the fourth *Degree*.

**DEGREE**, in Chymistry, is understood of the State or Intensity of the Fire, or Heat. Chymists distinguish four *Degrees* of Fire, or Heat: the *first*, is two or three Coals. The *second*, that of four or five Coals, or rather so much as sufficient to warm a Vessel sensibly; yet so, that the hand may be held on it a

[1] Pierre Dionis (1643 – 1718), a French surgeon and anatomist.

considerable time. The *third Degree,* is when there is a Fire capable of boiling a Vessel of five or six Pints of Water. The *fourth,* is when there is Fire enough for a Furnace. These Degrees, however, are all varied according to the different circumstances of Operations, Furnaces, Vessels, Subjects, &c.

**DEJECTION**, in Medicine, properly signifies the Act of *Ejecting*, or Evacuating the Excrements, by means of the Peristaltic Motion of the Guts; In which Sense it comes nearly to the Signification of *Excretion*. But the Term is also, and that more ordinarily, applied to the Excrements themselves, thus evacuated; in which Sense it is of the same import with *Stool*. Viscid, glutinous, or, as they call them, *unguinous Dejections*, frequent in Scorbutic Diseases, indicate a Colliquation of the Solids of the Body.

**DELIQUIUM**, in Medicine, or *Deliquium Animi*, a swooning, or fainting away; call'd also Syncope, Lipothymia, Lipopsychia, Ecthlipsis, and Asphyxea. *Deliquium*, is also used in some Authors for a Distillation by Force of Fire.

*Deliquium*, in Chymistry, is a Dissolution, or melting of a Salt, or *Calx*, by suspending it in a moist Cellar. Thus Salt of *Tartar*, or any fix'd *Alcali*, in a Cellar, or other cool moist Place, and an open Vessel, resolves, or runs into a Kind of Water, call'd by the Chymists, Oil of Tartar *per Deliquium*.

**DELIRIUM**, *Doating*, in Medicine, a Symptom, frequently befalling in Fevers, caused by internal Inflammations, Wounds, &c. whereby the Mind is disorder'd to a Degree of Folly.

*Deliriums* also frequently arise from immoderate Losses of Blood, whereby the Brain is too much weaken'd; from the Stings of venomous Beasts; from the Seed, or Menses, retain'd in the Womb; from the Rotting of a gangreen'd Member, &c. A Disorder in the Diaphragm commonly produces a *Delirium*.

Some derive the Word from *De* and *Lira*, which among the Ancients signified, Furrows drawn in right Lines; Whence, *delirare, a recto aberrare*.

There are various Species and Degrees of *Deliriums*. In some, the Patient is fierce, and outrageous; In others, more mild, and easy, offering no Violence to any body, but only indulging idle, ridiculous Discourse; Some laugh and sing; others cry, and are sullen, &c.

**DENSITY**, that Property, or Habitude of Bodies, whereby they contain such a Quantity of Matter, under such a Bulk. Accordingly, a Body that contains more Matter than another, under the same Bulk, is said to be *denser* than the other. Density stands in Opposition to *Rarity*. Hence, since the Mass is proportional to the Gravity, a denser Body is specifically heavier than a *rarer*; and a specifically heavier is *denser* than a specifically lighter.

The *Densities*, and Bulks of Bodies, are the two great Points, whereon all Mechanicks, or Laws of Motion turn : 'tis an Axiom, that Bodies of the same *Density* contain equal Masses, under equal Bulks. If the Bulks of the two Bodies be equal, their *Densities* are as their Masses: Consequently, the *Densities* of equal Bodies, are as their Gravities. If two Bodies have the same *Density*, their Masses as are their Bulks : And hence, the Gravities of Bodies of the same *Density*, are in the *Ratio* of their Bulks. The Masses of two Bodies are in a *Ratio* compounded of their *Densities* and Bulks; consequently, their Gravities are in the same *Ratio*: And if their Masses, or Gravities be equal, their *Densities* are reciprocally as their Bulks. The *Densities* of any two Bodies are in a *Ratio* compounded of the direct *Ratio* of their Masses, and the reciprocal one of their Bulks.

The Peripateticks define *Density*, a secondary Quality, whereby a Body is full of it self; its Parts cohering without any Interstice. So that the Form of *Density* consists in the immediate Coherence of Parts. Hence *Porphyry*[1] in his Predicaments defines a *dense* Body, that whose Parts are placed so near each other, that no other Body can come between them; as Gold. The efficient Cause of *Density* they usually attribute to cold : *Scaliger*, and some others, attribute it to Moisture. Many of the Moderns take the Smallness of the Parts of Bodies, to contribute much to their *Density*; as by this means the Pores are left the smaller. Tho' 'tis added, that the *Density* of Bodies does not only depend on the Smallness of the Pores, but also on their Fewness; Far are we from having any Body absolutely *dense*, in the Sense of the Ancients : Gold it self, the *densest*, and heaviest of all natural Bodies, Sir *Is. Newton* observes, does contain a great deal more Pore, or Vacuity, than Substance.

The *Densities* of Liquids are also compared together by immerging a Solid into them; for if a Solid lighter than the Liquids to be compared together, be immersed successively into different Liquids, the immersed Parts will be inversely as the *Densities* of the Liquids; for, because the same Solid is made Use of, the Portions of the different Liquors, which in every Case would fill the Space taken up by the immersed Parts, are of the same Weight; therefore the Bulks of those Portions, that is the immersed Parts themselves are inversely as the Densities.

The Density *of the Air*, is a Property that has much imploy'd the later Philosophers, since their Discovery of the *Torricellian*[2] Experiment, and the Air-Pump.

'Tis demonstrated, that in the same Vessel, or even in Vessels communicating with each other, at the same Distance from the Centre, the Air has every where the same *Density*. The *Density of the Air* always increases in Proportion to the Compression, or the compressing Powers.

And hence, the lower Air is always *denser* than the upper : Yet the *Density* of the lower Air is not proportional to the Weight of the Atmosphere, by reason of Heat and Cold, which make notable Alterations as to Rarity, and *Density*. If the Air be rendred *denser*, the Weight of Bodies therein is diminish'd; and if rarer, increased; by reason Bodies lose more in heavier than in lighter *Medium's*.

And hence, if the *Density of the Air* be sensibly alter'd, Bodies equally heavy in a lighter Air, if their specific Gravities be considerable different, will have their *Equilibrium* taken away in a *denser* Air, and the specifically heavier will preponderate; which is the Foundation of the *Manoscope*, an Instrument for measuring the Alterations in the Density of the Air.

[1] Porphyry of Tyre (ca. 233 – 209), a Phoenician philosopher.

[2] Evangelista Torricelli (1608 – 1647), an Italian scientist and mathematician.

**DENTALIS** *Lapis*, or *Dentalium*, is Kind of Shell, which the Apothecaries pulverize, and use in several Medicaments, as an excellent *Alcali*. The genuine *Dentalis*, described by Mr. *Tournefort*, is of a tubular, or Conical Form, about 3 Inches long; of a shining, greenish white; hollow; light, and divided lengthwise by Parallel Lines, running from Top to Bottom. It is about the Thickness of a Feather, and bears some Resemblance to a Dog's Tooth.

'Tis very scarce; and therefore in lieu of it, they usually substitute a Shell of divers Colours found among the Sand when the Sea is withdrawn; but not channel'd, or fluted like the *Dentalis*.

D. *Lister*, in the *Philosoph. Transact.* Makes mention of two Species of *Dentalia*; the first commonly enough found about the Island of *Guernsey*, &c. being a long, slender, round Pipe, a little bending, and tapering, and hollow at both Ends; whence it is also call'd, *the Dog-like-tooth* : The other properly call'd *Entalium*, longer, and thicker than the former; and besides, streak'd with Ridges; whence the *Italian* Term *Intaglia*.

**DENTED** *Verge*, among Botanists, is applied to such Leaves of Plants as are notched, or jagged about the Edge, or Brim; whereof some are *fine dented*; others *large*, or *deep dented*, *i.e.* cut into the Leaf.

**DENTRIFRICE**, in Medicine, Tooth-Powder; a Remedy to rub the Teeth withal, in order to cleanse, or fasten them.

There are *Dentifrices* of divers Kinds, and Forms : Some in Form of a Powder, composed of Corals, Pumice-Stone, Sale, Alumn, Egg-Shells, Lobsters, Harts-Horn, Cuttle-Bone, Tartar vitriolated, &c. Others in Form of an Electuary, or Opiate, consisting of the same Powders, mix'd up with Honey.

There are others, prepar'd with Roots boil'd with Alum, and dried in the Oven. Others in Form of a Liquor, drawn by Distillation from drying Herbs, and astringent Medicines.

The *Dutch* hold Butter the best *Dentifrice*, to keep the Teeth white and sound; And the *Spaniards*, Urine.

**DEOBSTRUENTS** are such Medicines as open Obstructions. It must be observ'd, however, that there is something further intimated by *Deobstruent*, than by *Detergent*: For a Medicine may be *deobstruent*, that is not in the strictest Sense *detergent*; as, in Effect, are most made of metalline Substances; such as Steel, and Mercury; which obtain this Appellation from their Acting by their natural Weight, whereby they increase the *Momentum* of their circulating Fluid, and make it strike against the secretory Outlet with great Force; because the *Momenta*, or *Vis Percussionis* of all Projectiles, of which Kind is a circulating Fluid, is as their Solidities, supposing their Velocities are equal. The more therefore the Animal Fluids are saturated with dense, and solid Particles, with the greater Force they distend the Vessels, and more easily break through, where the Structure favours their Escape; and upon that Account are Medicines, which add to these Qualities in the Fluids, call'd *Deobstruents*.

**DEOPPILATIVE**, a Remedy proper to soften, resolve and remove Obstructions. *Deoppilatives* are the same with what we otherwise call *Deobstruents*.

**DEPHLEGMATED**, in Chymistry, an Epithet applied to Spirits that are well clear'd of Water, or Phlegm. To effect which, they *rectify* them, *i.e.* distil them over and over, till they be left quite pure.

**DEPHLEGMATION**, in Chymistry, is the Act of purifying, or clearing a Fluid of its Phlegm, or Water. This is perform'd by distilling the Spirit, or other Fluid, over and over; by which means, the spirituous Part all rises, and leaves the Phlegm, or Water behind. When the Spirit is thus disengag'd of all its Phlegm, or, at least, as much as it can be, it's call'd, a *dephlegmated Spirit*.

**DEPILATORY**, or Depilative, in Medicine, a Plaster, or Medicine, applied on any Hairy Place, in order to bring off the Hair. The Word is form'd of the Particle *De*, and *Pilus*, Hair. *Depilatories* are principally composed of Orpiment, which is a very caustic, and even a dangerous Mineral. For hairs growing on the Fore-head of a young Girl, I prescribed the following *Dropax*, or *Depilative Liniment, Degori*.

**DEPURATION**, in Pharmacy, the same as *Clarification*, or *Purification, viz.* the purging a Body of all the Lees, Fæces, and other crass, coarse, and excrementitious Parts adhering therein. Fermentation serves to *depurate* Liquors : Syrups, Juices, &c. are *depurated* by passing them through the *Manica Hippocratis*, or Straining-Bag.

**DERIVATION**, in Medicine, the diverting a Humour, which flows on some noble Part, and drawing it to some other neighbouring Part, where it is less dangerous. Thus, in Defluxions upon the Eyes , or Teeth, they apply a Blister behind the Neck to draw the Matter thither : And in a Squinancy, they prescribe Bleeding in the *Ranulæ*, or Veins under the Throat, to *divert* the Humour from falling on the Throat.

**DESPUMATION**, is the Clarification of any Liquor, by throwing up its Foulness in a Froth, and taking that off.

**DESQUAMATION** expresses the cleansing carious bones, which flake off like Scales.

**DESSICATIVE**, in Medicine, Chirurgery, and Pharmacy, a Remedy that has the Virtue of drying up superfluous Moisture; used to skin over old Sores, &c. A Dessicative Unguent, &c. Pimprenella, &c. is held very detersive, dessicative, and vulnerary.

**DETERGENT**, in Medicine, is applied to Remedies that cleanse, mundify, and carry off viscid, and glutinous Humours adhering to Bodies. The Plant, call'd *Harts-Horn*, *deterges*, and consolidates Wounds. *Rhaponticum* is aperitive, and good against the Gravel and Stone; It also *deterges*, and expels Poyson.

*Detergents* are not only softening, and adhesive, but also by a peculiar Activity, or Disposition to Motion, joyn'd with a suitable Configuration of Parts, are apt to abrade, and carry along with them such Particles as they lay hold on in their Passage. All Medicines of this Intention are supposed to cleanse, and heal, that is, incarnate, or fill up with new Flesh all Ulcerations, and Foulnesses, occasioned thereby, whether internal, or external.

To do this, in all internal Cases especially, the Medicine must be supposed to maintain its primary Properties, until it arrives at the Place of Action, and there it does what entitles it to the Appellation of a *Detergent*, and a *Vulnerary*, first by its adhesive Quality, which consists in the comparative Largeness of Surface, and Flexibility of its component Parts : For by this it very readily falls into Contact with, and adheres to the Slough of ulcerous Exudations, which by their loose Situation are easily carried along with the Medicine, and when such Matter is so carried away, which is the cleansing, and *deterging* Part, what was instrumental in this Office, will afterwards stick to, and adhere with the cutaneous Filaments, until by their Addition, and the Protrusion of proper Nourishment *ab interno* to the same Place, the Waste is made up, that is, the Ulcer is healed.

After the same Manner is the Operation of such Substances to be accounted for in external Applications. By the Warmth of their Parts they rarify, and by their adhesive Quality, they joyn with, and take off along with them, in every dressing, what is thrown upon the Place to which they are applied, until a more convenient Matter is brought thither by the circulating Juices, which it assists in adhering to, and incarnating the eroded Cavities. Only this may be taken Notice of, that internally, whatsoever of this Kind is mixed with Animal Fluids, by the known Laws of Circulation, they will be first separated, and left behind. For all those Parts, which are specifically heaviest, will move nearest the Axis of the Canals, because their Moments are the greatest, and will carry them as near as can be in streight Lines; but the lighter Parts will always be jostled in the Sides, where they soonest meet with Outlets to get quite off, or are struck into such Cavities, we are here speaking of, in which they adhere, and make Part of the Substance.

This is understood of the milder Degree of *Detergents*; and it is easy to conceive from hence, how an Increase of those Qualities of Activity and Adhesion conjointly, may make a Medicine arise to the greatest Efficacy in this respect. And it is upon this Foot, that all those Medicines operate, which are given to cleanse Obstructions, or Foulnesses in any of the *Viscera*, or Passages; and which may be increased in Efficacy so far, as to fetch off even the Membranes, and Capillary Vessels.

**DETERSIVE**, in Medicine, the same with *Detergent*. A Clyster is a *detersive* Medicine, which cleanses the lower Venter. *Detersive* Unguents are usually call'd *Mondificatives*. The Leaves, and Summets of the Straw-berry are *detersive*, and astringent.

**DETONATION**, or Fulmination, in Chymistry, the Noise which Minerals make when they begin to heat in Crucibles; by the volatile Parts rushing out with Impetuosity, and the Humidity escaping. The Word is form'd of *de*, and *tono*, I thunder.

*Detonation* is much the same with *Decrepitation*, only its Action more forcible, and the Noise greater. Thus, *Aurum fulminans* heated, &c. goes off with a violent Crack, *i.e.* makes a great *Detonation*. *Detonation* takes away the impure, volatile Sulphur from Bodies.

In the Chymical Sense, *Detonation* is the Act, or Operation of expelling the impure, volatile, and sulphureous Parts out of Bodies, and leaving behind the fix'd, and internal Parts. It is perform'd by means of Salt-petre, &c.

**DEW**, *Ros*, a thin, light, insensible Mist, or Rain, falling while the Sun is below the Horizon. Naturalists usually rank *Dews* among the Number of Meteors of the watery Kind. Some define it a Vapour liquefied, and let fall in Drops. Others a Vapour having a like Relation to Frost, as Rain has to Snow, &c.

To us, *Dew* appears only to differ from Rain, as more, and less. Its Origin, and Matter, no doubt, is from the Vapour, and Exhalation of the Earth and Water, rais'd, as shewn under the Article Vapour. The thin *Vesiculæ*, whereof Vapours consist, being once detach'd from their Bodies, we all know, keep rising in the Atmosphere, till they arrive at such a Stage of the Air, as is of the same specific Gravity with themselves : Then their Rise is stopp'd. Now, as 'tis the Warmth, or Fire, that, dilating the Parts of Water, forms the *Vesiculæ* specifically lighter than Air, and capable of ascending therein; So when that Heat declines, or is lost, as by the Approach, or Contiguity of any colder Body, the *Vesiculæ* condense, become heavier, and descend. In the Day-time, therefore, the Sun warming the Atmosphere by a continual Influx of his Rays, the Vapours once rais'd, continue their Progress, as meeting with nothing to increase their Gravity, till such Time as they are got far out of the Reach of the reflected Warmth of the Earth, in the middle Region of the Atmosphere. Here condensing, they form *Clouds*, from which arise *Rain*, as shewn under Clouds and Rain.

But when the Sun is below the Horizon, the Case is somewhat different : For the Atmosphere then cooling, the Vapours rais'd by the Warmth of the Earth, and out of the Rays of the Sun, lodg'd therein the preceding Day, begin to condense a-pace, as soon as they are got out of the Air, spending their Stock of Fire and Heat on the cold, moist Air they pass through. Their Ascent, therefore, becomes short; and by that Time they are got a few Fathoms high, being exhausted of Fire, and restor'd to the natural Dimensions and Gravity of their constituent Water; they precipitate, and fall back again in little Spherules, or Drops, as shewn of *Rain*.

From these Principles the other Phænomena of *Dews* are easily accounted for. Hence, *e.gr.* it is, that *Dews* are more copious in the Spring, than in the other Seasons; there being then a greater Stock of Vapour in Readiness, through the small Expence thereof in the Winters Cold and Frost, than at other Times. Hence, what *Pliny* relates of *Egypt*, that it abounds in *Dews* throughout all the Heats of Summer; For the Air there being to hot to constipate the Vapours in the Day-time, they never gather into Clouds, and hence they have no Rain; But we know, that in Climates where the Days are excessively hot, the Nights are remarkably cold; So that the Vapours raised after Sunset, are readily condensed into *Dews*. Or, perhaps, that notable Coldness is rather the Effect, than the Cause of the Quantity of *Dews*. For a deal of Vapour being raised by the great Heat of the Earth, and the Stock of Fire spent on it in the Day-time, the Influx of such a Quantity of cold Moisture must greatly chill the Air.

*May*-Dew whitens Linen and Wax : The *Dew* of Autumn is converted into a white Frost. Out of *Dew* putrified by the Sun, arise a divers Insects, which change a-pace out of one Species into another : what remains is converted into a fine, white Salt, with Angles like those of Salt-petre, after a Number of Evaporations, Calcinations, and Fixations.

There is a Spirit drawn from *May-Dew*, which has wonderful Virtues attributed to it. The Method of gathering, and preparing it, is prescribed by *Hanneman*, Physician at *Kiel*. 'Tis to be gather'd in clean linen Cloths, exposed to the Sun in close Vials; then distill'd, and the Spirit thrown upon the *Caput Mortuum*; this is to be repeated till the Earth unite with the Spirit, and become a liquid; which happens about the 7th or 8th Cohobation, or Distillation. By such means you gain a very red, odoriferous Spirit. *Stolterforth*, a Physician of the *Lubec*, thinks *May-Dew* may be gather'd in Glass-Plates, especially in still Weather, and before Sun-rise. And *Etmuller* is of the same Sentiment. It might likewise be gather'd with a Glass-Funnel, exposed to the Air, having a crooked Neck to bring the *Dew* into a Vial in a Chamber. See *Philos. Transact. 1665. May. Hoffman*[1], and others. 'Tis apparently from the Preparation of this *Dew*, that the Brothers of the *Rosy-Cross* took their Denomination.

In the *Philosoph. Transact.* We have an Account of a very extraordinary Kind of *Dew*. For a good Part of the Winter 1695, says the Bishop of *Cloyne*, there fell in many Parts of the Provinces of *Munster*, and *Leimster*; a Kind of thick *Dew*, which the Country-People call'd *Butter*, from its Consistency and Colour; being soft, clammy, and of a dark yellow. It fell always in the Night, and chiefly in low, moorish Places, on the Top of the Grass, and oft on the Thatch of Cabbins. 'Twas seldom observ'd in the same Place twice. It commonly lay on the Earth a fortnight without changing Colour, but then dried, and turn'd black. It fell in Lumps; and had a strong Smell like that of Graves. Mr. *R. Vans*, in the same *Transactions*, gives an Account of the like at the same Time, in *Limeric*, and *Tiperary*; adding that if one rubb'd it with the Hand it melted; but laying it by the Fire, it dried, and grew hard.

**DIABETES**, in Medicine, a hasty, and profuse Evacuation of the Drink by the Urinary Passages; accompanied with an ardent Thirst, and a Leanness of the whole Body. The Drink thus discharged, is usually a little alter'd from what it was when taken down, and turn'd chilous, and milky; but sometimes not at all.

The *Diabetes* seems owing to a too great Laxity of the Fibres of the Arteries of the Kidneys; or to great Quantity of sharp Salts in the Blood, which dissolve the Mass of Blood, or disunite the Parts thereof; So that the Serosity is easily separated from the same.

According to Dr. *Quincy*, the Evident, and most common Cause of the *Diabetes* is the too great Use of spirituous Liquors, wherewith the *Serum* becomes so impregnated, that it will not attract, and joyn with the Cruor, or

[1] Friedrich Hoffmann (1660 – 1742), a German physician and iatrochemist.

Globules of the Blood, but runs off through the Kidneys sweet, or insipid.

There is another Kind of *Diabetes*, wherein the Person affected renders a great deal more by Urine, than he drinks, nay, sometimes more than he both eats and drinks. Some Physicians attribute this excessive Quantity of Liquor to the Air he respires, which, they suppose, becomes converted into Water; Or, at least, the Water in the Air respired is here absorbed, and collected. But others, with more Probability, attribute it to a Colliquation of the Blood, fat, and even the solid Parts of the Body.

The Word *Diabetes* is derived from the Greek διαβαινειν, *to pass quick*.

**DIABOTANUM**, in Pharmacy, and Chirurgery, a Plaster, wherewith Wens, &c. are resolved and discuss'd. The *Diabotanum* is sovereign for the *Hydatides*.

**DIABROSIS**, in Medicine, a Solution of the Continuity of a Part, caused by sharp, corrosive Humors gnawing, and devouring the same. The Word is *Greek*, compounded of δια, *per*, through, and βρωσκειν, *to eat*.

**DIACALCITEOS**, in Chirurgery, and Pharmacy, a Plaster applied after the Amputation of a Cancer. The *Emplastrum Diacalciteos* is composed of Oil, *Axungia*, and *Chalcitis*; from the last of which Drugs it derives its Name.

**DIACARYON**, or *Dianucum*, in Pharmacy. *Galen* is said to have prepar'd his *Diacaryon*, with the Juice of Walnuts, mix'd with as much Honey as sufficed to render it an agreeable Composition. The Word is form'd from καρυα, *Walnut*.

**DIACARTAMI**, in Pharmacy, an Electuary composed of Turbith, Manna, Scammony, Hermodactyls, and other Purgatives; with the Addition of the Medullæ, or Seed of the *Carthamus*, which gives it the Denomination. *Diacartami* chiefly purges *pituita*. It is prescribed in Diseases of the Brain; and is frequently mix'd in Medicines along with other Purgatives.

**DIACHYLON**, in Pharmacy, a Name given to divers Plasters, on Account of the Mucilages mix'd therein, which are viscid Juices, call'd by the *Greeks* χυλοι; drawn from certain Plants.

*White*, or *Simple Diachylon*, is compounded of common Oil, Litharge of Gold, and Mucilages, drawn from the Root of the *Althæa*, and the Seeds of the Line, and Fenigreck. It is proper to soften , digest, ripen, and resolve.

The *Diachylon*, call'd *Direatum*, has for its Basis the common *white Diachylon*, with a Pound of which, an Ounce of Powder of *Iris* is mix'd. This Plaster digests, incides, and ripens with more Force than the *simple Diachylon*.

There is also the *Great* Diachylon, *Diachylon magnum*, composed of Litharge of Gold, Oils of Iris, Camomile, and Aneth, Turpentine, Resin of the Pine, yellow Wax, and Mucilage of Line, and Fenigreck, with new Figs, Raisins of *Damascus*, *Icthyocolla*, Juices of Iris, *Squillæ*, and Hyssop. This *Diachylon* softens Schirrus's, and resolves, and dissipates Tumors. 'Tis call'd, *the Great*, not only on Account of its extraordinary Virtues, but also because compounded of a greater Number of Ingredients, than the rest.

The *Diachylon Gummatum*, is the *great Diachylon*, with the Addition of Gum Ammoniac, *Galbanum*, and *Sagapenum*, dissolv'd with Wine, and boil'd to a Consistence of Honey. This Plaster is the most powerful of all for digesting, ripening, and resolving.

**DIACODIUM**, in Pharmacy, a Medicine prepared from Poppies Heads. There are two Kinds: *Simple*, and *Compound*. The Word is form'd from the *Greek* δια, *per*, and κωδεια, Poppies Head.

*Simple* Diacodium, is a Kind of Opiate, made of the Juice express'd from the Heads of Poppies, both white, and black; and made up with the *Sapa*, or Sugar. It is prescribed to soften sharp, serous Humours, to appease Coughs, and to provoke Sleep. This Preparation was of great Use among the Ancients; but is now laid a-side, sine it has been found, that the Syrup of white Poppies, which is what we now call *Diacodium*, produces the same Effect.

*Compound* Diacodium is made of the simple, with the Addition of the Troches of Ramich, *Hypocistis*, Myrrh, Saffron, and Balaustes. It is good to stop, and soften Catarrhs, Hemorrhoids, and Fluxes of the Belly.

**DIACYDONITES**, in Pharmacy, is applied to Things, and Remedies, wherein Quinces are an Ingredient : Thus the Confection *Diacydonites* is a Confection of Quinces, or wherein Quinces have a Share. The Word comes from δια, and κυδωνιον, *Quince*.

**DIAGNOSTIC**, in Medicine, a Term applied to those Signs, or Symptoms, which indicate, or discover the present State of a Disease, its Nature, and Cause. The Physicians have *Diagnostic*, and *Prognostic* Signs; the first with regard to the present State of the Disease, and the Patient; and the second to the future. The Word is compounded of the *Greek* δια, *per*, through, or by; and γινωσκω, I *know*.

**DIAGRYDIUM**, in Pharmacy, is prepar'd Scammony. The Word *Diagrydium* is form'd, by Corruption, from δακρυδιον, *little Tear*.

The Preparation is ordinarily perform'd by boiling the Scammony in a Quince. Others make it receive the Fumes of lighted Sulphur, whence it is call'd, *Sulphurated*, *Diagrydium sulphuratum*. Some incorporate it with a Quantity of Spirit of *Vitriol rosat*. Sufficiently to make a Sort of Liquid past, which is afterwards set to dry in the Sun, or by a gentle Fire. And this Preparation they call *Diagrydium Rosatum*.

The End of all these Preparations is to correct the Scammony; But many more are of Opinion, it has nothing that needs Correction, and that it may be used in its natural State.

**DIALTHÆA**, in Pharmacy, an Unguent thus call'd from its *Basis*, which is the Root of the *Althæa*. It consists of Mucilages drawn from that Root, and from the Seeds of Line, *Squillae*, and Fennigreek. The other Ingredients are common Oil, yellow Wax, Resin, Turpentine, *Galbanum*, and Ivy-Gum. It is esteem'd proper to soften, and resolve; asswages Pains of the Side, softens

Callus's, and strengthens the Nerves. 'Tis applied, by rubbing it on the Parts affected.

**DIAMARGARITON**, in Pharmacy, a Medicine denominated from Pearls, call'd in Latin *Margarite*; which are a principal Ingredient therein. There are two Kinds : The *Hot* and the *Cold*.

The *Hot Diamargariton*, is a Powder composed of Pearls, Pellitory, Ginger, Nutmeg, Cinnamon, and divers other hot Ingredients. It is reputed Hysteric, strengthens the Womb, promotes the *Menses*, and assists in Digestion.

*Cold Diamargariton*, is a solid Electuary, composed of Pearls ground-fine, and white Sugar dissolved in Rose-Water, or Buglos, and boil'd to a Consistence. It strengthens the Stomach, moderates the too abundant Acids, stops the spitting of Blood, and Looseness of the Belly.

*Compound Cold Diamargariton*, is a Powder made of Pearls, red Roses, Flowers of Nenuphar, and Violet, *Lignum Aloes*, red and Citron Santal, Tormentil Root, Seeds of Melons, Endive, &c. It is applied to give Vigour, facilitate Respiration, and resist the Malignity of Humours.

**DIAMORUM**, a Composition in Pharmacy, either *Simple* or *Compound*. The Word is form'd from *Morus*, Mulberry.

*Simple* Diamorum, is the common Syrup of Mulberries, made of Mulberry-Juice, and Sugar. It is good against Diseases of the Throat, and to stop Dysenteries. There is also a sort of *Simple Diamorum* made of Mulberry Juice and Honey, call'd also *Mulberry Rob*.

*Compound* Diamorum is made with Mulberry Juice, Sapa, Verjuice, Myrrh, and Saffron. It is used to deterge Phlegm from the Stomach, and Breast, and ease Respiration.

**DIANA'S TREE**, *Arbor Dianæ*, a very curious Phænomenon in Chymistry, being the just Figure of a Tree, with Branches, Leaves, Fruit, &c. shooting up in a Diffusion of Silver in an Acid Spirit.

There are divers Manners of procuring *Diana's Tree*; but most of them exceeding tedious , except the following one of Monsr. *Homberg*, which may be done in a Quarter of an Hours time. Take four Drachms of Filings of fine Silver, with which make an Amalgama, without Heat, with two Drams of Quicksilver. Dissolve the Solution into 3 Gallons of common Water; stir it about a while to mingle it well together; and then keep it in a Glass Vessel well stopp'd.

When you make the Experiment, take about an Ounce of it, and put it in a small Viol, wherein likewise put the Quantity of a small Pea of the ordinary *Amalgama* of Gold, or Silver; which should be as soft as Butter; and set the Viol at rest for 2 or 3 Minutes. Immediately after this you will see several small Threads, or Filaments, arising perpendicularly from the little Bulb of the newly put in *Amalgama*, which will sensibly grow, and thrust out, on the Sides, small Branches in Form of a Tree. The Bulb, or Ball of the *Amalgama* will grow hard, and be like a Pellet of white Earth; and the little Tree f the Colour of bright Silver.

The Form of this Metalline Tree may be varied almost at Pleasure. The stronger you make the first described Water, the thicker will the little Tree be in Branches, and the sooner form'd. The same Author shews, how divers other Kinds of Trees may be produced by Crystallization, and Digestion.

**DIANUCUM**, in Pharmacy, a Kind of Rob, made of the Juice of green Walnuts, and Sugar, boil'd together by a moderate Fire, to the Consistence of Honey. It is good to strengthen the Stomach, promote Sweat, and resist Poison. The Word is form'd from *Nux, Nucis*, Nut.

**DIAPALMA**, in Pharmacy, a Desiccative, or drying Plaster, denominated from the Wood of the Palm-Tree, whereof the Spatula is made, that is to stir it while boiling. It is composed of common Oil, Hogs-fat, and Litharge of Gold. It is good to dry, resolve, deterge, and cicatrize : And is the Plaster most used for Wounds, and Ulcers.

**DIAPASMA**, a common Name for all Perfumes applied on the Body, of what Form soever they be, whether Powders, Essences, Pomatum's, or the like. The Word comes from the *Greek* διαπασσειν, *to water*.

**DIAPEDESIS**, in Medicine, an Eruption, or oozing of Blood through the Coats of the Veins, or Arteries; occasioned either by the Bloods becoming too much dissolved, or attenuated; or by the Pores of the vessels becoming too patent, and open. There are some able Physicians who deny there can be any such a Tenuity of Blood, as that it shall exude thro' the Vessels, without any Apperture made therein. The Word is compounded of δια, *through*; and πεδαω, *I leap*.

**DIAPENTE**, is also used in Pharmacy, for a Compound of five several Drugs or Ingredients. The Word is form'd of δια, and πεντε, *five*.

**DIAPHOENIC**, in Pharmacy, a soft Purgative Electuary, thus call'd from the Dates, which make its *Basis*; the Palm-Tree, whose Fruit they are, being call'd by the Greeks φοινιξ. The other Ingredients are the Penides, Almonds, Turbith, Ginger, white Pepper, Mace, Cinnamon, Rice, Fennel, *Daucus*, and Honey. *Diaphœnic* purges chiefly Serosities, and excites the Menses. It is also used in Dropsies, Lethargies, Apoplexies, and Palsies.

**DIAPHORESIS**, in Medicine, includes all Discharges made through the Skin; but chiefly that by insensible Perspiration, and Sweat.

**DIAPHORETIC**, in Medicine is applied to Remedies that promote the Expulsion of Humours by insensible Perspiration. *Diaphoretic* is much of the same Import as Sudorific : Except that the latter promote sensible, and the former insensible Perspiration. Their only Difference, therefore, is in the Degree of Action.

**DIAPRUNUM**, in Pharmacy, a soft, purgative Electuary, thus call'd from the Pulp of *Damascus* Prunes, which is its Base. *Diaprunum* is either *Simple*, or *Compound*,

*Simple* Diaprunum consists of the Pulp aforementioned, with *Cassia*,

Tamarinds, Rhubarb, red Roses, Violet Seeds, Santals both red and Citron, Scrapings of Ivory, Liquorice Juice, and the four cold Seeds. It is good to prepare, and soften the Humours.

*Compound*, or *Solutive* Diaprunum, is only the Simple, with the Addition of half an Ounce of Scammony to every Pound of the Electuary, to render it more purgative.

**DIARRHÆA**, in Medicine, a *Looseness*, or Flux of the Belly; or a profuse Evacuation of liquid Excrements by Stool. The Word, in the general, is used for any Kind of *Flux* of the Belly; but properly for that wherein the Humour, or Excrement flows out either pure, or mix'd; with, or without Pain, in a fluid State. The Word is form'd of the *Greek* δια, *through*, and ρεειν, *to flow*.

*Diarrhæa's* are of divers Kinds, according to the Diversity of the Excrements : Some being bilious; some serous; some pituitous; and some purulent. The Purulent always arises from some Abscess open'd in the Body; the rest either from morbid Humours irritating the Intestines, and expressing the Juices out of the adjacent Parts; or from a Laxness of the Intestinal Fibres; or an extraordinary Fermentation in the Blood, whereby it discharges its Excrements into the Intestines. There are also *Diarrhæa's* arising from unwholesome Foods, ad Stoppage of the other Excretions, particularly perspiration.

It is a standing Observation, that such as perspire but little, are ever subject to a *Diarrhæa*; and on the contrary, People who perspire much, are commonly bound. *Baglivi* mentions *Diarrhæa's* as one usual great Effect of Grief; as likewise of immoderate Anger; without which a Fever would be Produced.

In the Cure of *Diarrhæa's*, from whatever Cause they arise, the Stomach must be corroborated, and Sudorificks to be mix'd with Absorbents. The Patient to drink sparingly. Quince and Wine burnt with Aromaticks is good. *Wainwright* observes, that a Flannel Shirt contributes much to the Cure of an habitual *Diarrhæa*.

*Stolterforth*, a Physician of *Lubeck*, relates, that a Mechanic of that City had a continual *Diarrhæa* from 30, to the Age of 65 Years, which always gave him 5 or 6 Stools a Day, yet he was in good health all the while, having a good Appetite, and sufficient Strength and Vigour. But in his 65th Year taking some astringent Medicine, he stopp'd his Flux; upon which he was immediately seiz'd with a violent Pain in the Kidneys, Difficulty of Breathing, Loss of Digestion; He gave up his Food as he took it, grew cold at the Extremes of the Body, swell'd in the Thighs, had an insupportable Thirst, and more Appetite, and urined, with much Difficulty, a thin watery Humour, destitute of all Sulphur.

**DIARRHODON**, in Pharmacy, a name given to divers Compositions, wherein red Roses are an Ingredient.

*Diarrhodon Abbatis*, is a Cordial Powder, denominated from the Abbot who invented it. It consists of red Roses; red and Citron Santals, *Lignum Aloes*, Cinnamon, Rhapontic, Spikenard, Ivory, Harts-horn, Saffron, Mastic, Pearls, Ambergris, Musk, &c. It is used to strengthen the Heart, Stomach, and Liver, to assist in Digestion, and prevent Vomiting.

There are also *Trochisci of Diarrhodon*, composed of red Roses, Scrapings of Ivory, the Santals, Liquorice, Mastic, Saffron, Camphor, and Rose-Water. They are good to fortify the Heart, Stomach, and Liver, and to stop Dissenteries, and other Fluxes of the Belly.

*Pillulæ Diarrhodon* are composed of Aloes, *Trochisci Diarrhodon*, Wormwood Leaves, Mastic, and Rock-Salt. They purge, then fortify the Stomach, promote Digestion, and prevent a stinking Breath.

**DIARY** *Fever*, is a Fever of one Day.

**DIASCORDIUM**, in Pharmacy, a Kind of Electuary, or Opiate, first described by *Fracastorius*, and denominated from *Scordium*, which is an Ingredient therein. It is used against malignant Fevers, the Plague, Worms, the Colic, to provoke Sleep, and resist Putrefaction.

The other Ingredients are red Roses, Bole, Storax, Cinnamon, *Cassia Lignea*, *Dittany*, Tormentille Roots, Bistort, Gentian, *Galbanum*, Amber, *Terra Sigillata*, *Opium*, Long Pepper, Ginger, *Mel Rosatum*, and Malmsey.

**DIASEBESTEN**, in Pharmacy, a soft, purgative Electuary, whereof *Sebestes* are the Basis. The other Ingredients are Prunes, Tamarinds, Juices of Iris, *Anguria*, and *Mercurialis*, *Penidia*, *simple Diaprunum*, Violet Seed, the four cold Seeds, and *Diagrydium*. It is good in intermitting, and continued Fevers, appeases Thirst, promotes Sleep, and expels the morbid Humors by Urine.

**DIASENNA**, in Pharmacy, a soft, purgative Electuary, thus call'd from Senna, which is its Base. *Diasenna* eases and comforts the melancholic, and Splenetic; and is good against all Diseases arising from an *Atrabilis*.

The other Ingredients are Sugar Candy, Cinnamon, *Lapis Lazuli*, Silk, Cloves, *Galanga Minor*, black Pepper, *Nardus Indicus*, Seed of the *Basilica*, Leaves of Cloves, Cardamomum, Saffron, Ginger, Zedoary, Rosemary Flowers, Long Pepper, *Lapis Armenius*, and Honey.

**DIATESSARON**, in Pharmacy, a Sort of Treacle, thus call'd because consisting of four Ingredients, which are Roots of *Aristolochia*, and Gentian, Laurel-berries, and Myrrh. The Word is *Greek*, and signifies a Composition of four Drugs. It is also call'd *Theriaca Pauperum*, because made at a very easy Expense, and in a short Time. It is good against Stingings of venomous Beasts, Epilepsies, Convulsions, Colicks, to strengthen the Stomach, and promote the Menses.

**DIATRAGACANTH**, in Pharmacy, is applied to certain Powders, whereof Gum Adraganth is the Base. There are two Kinds, *Cold* and *Hot*.

Powder of *Cold Diatragacanth* is composed of the Gums Adraganth and Arabic, Liquorice, Starch, white Poppy Seed, and the four great cold Seeds. It is good to thicken, and soften the too sharp, and subtile ferrous Humours falling on the Breast, to assuage Coughs, and promote Spitting.

Powder of *Hot Diatragacanth* is composed of Gum Adraganth, Cinnamon, Hyssop, Almonds, Lin-Seed, and Fennegreek, Liquorice, Juice of Liquorice, and Ginger. It is good against Asthma's, to promote Expectoration, strength the Stomach, and assist Digestion.

**DICTAMNUM**, *Dittany*, a Medicinal Plant, much valued among the Ancients, and particularly applauded by their Poets. It was esteemed a Specific for Wounds of Arrows, which it drew out with wonderful Ease, and according to them, only grew in the Island of Crete, and even only in a little obscure Corner thereof; whence its Appellation *Dictamnus Creticus*. At present we scarce know whether there be any Remains thereof in that Island.

The modern *Dictamnus*, call'd also *White Dittany*, or *Fraxinella*, from its Leaves, which resemble those of the Ash, call'd by the Latins *Fraxinus*, is scarce in less Esteem than that of the Ancients. Its Root, wherein all its Virtue is lodged, is about the thickness of a Finger, and is frequently divided into a Number of little Branches; its Colour is white, its Taste bitter, its Smell string, somewhat like that of a He-goat, its Stem is about two Foot high, reddish, and full of Leaves; at the Top of the Stem is a Flower not unlike a *Spica*, or Ear; in the Middle of the Flower is a Pistil with five little Pieces wherein the Seed is contain'd, which is black, shining, and oval. The Root is excellent against the Bite of venomous Beasts, as also against Worms, the Colicks, &c. It must be chosen white, both Inside and Outside, not fibrous, and well cleaned.

There are several other Kinds of *Dittany*, but all of less Value : As the *Bastard Dittany*, whose Leaves are much less; the *Wild Dittany*, which neither bears Flowers, nor Fruit.

The Ancients have a Tradition, that the wounded Deer first discover'd the Virtue of the *Dictamnus Creticus*, which being eaten, presently drew out the Arrows sticking in 'em. Thus *Pliny* Lib. VIII. C. 27. And the like Account we have from *Cicero de Natur. Deor.* Lib. II. *Virgil. Aeneid.* Lib. XII. V. 412. *Tertull. de Paenit.* C. XI. Tho' *Cicero*, more prudent and reserved than *Pliny*, is contented to speak of it as by hear-say. *Aristotle* Lib. *de Mirabilib. Auscult.* Relates it of the Roe-buck. *Pliny* says expressly, that the Juice of this Plant taken inwardly, expels Arrows, and cures Wounds made with other Arms : He adds, that it stops Suppurations, provokes the Menses, and Delivery, and is good in Frictions and Fumigations.

**DIÆRESIS**, *Section, Dissection*, in Chirurgery, an Operation serving to divide, and separate the Parts whose Union and Continuity were an Obstacle to the Cure; or which were joyn'd, and conglutinated contrary to the Order of Nature. There are four manners of performing the *Diæresis* : *viz.* by Cutting, Pricking, Tearing, Drawing, and Burning. The Word in its original *Greek* Διαιρεσις, signifies Division.

**DIÆRESIS**, Διαιρεσις, is also used in Medicine for the Eating out, or Consuming of the Vessels, or Canals of an Animal Body : when, from some cutting, or corroding Cause certain Passages are made, which naturally ought not to have been, or certain natural Passages are dilated beyond ordinary; So that the Juices which should have been contain'd therein, extravasate, or run over.

**DIET**, in Medicine, &c. a spare Regimen or Course of living, out of regard to Health. *Diet* is a sovereign Remedy against all Diseases arising from Repletion. *Diet* is founded on this, that Nature ought not to be busied, and distracted in the Concocting of Food, but left wholly to her Work of digesting, and expelling the morbific Matter.

The Word is form'd from the *Greek* διαιτα, which signifies *Regimen*, or *Rule of Life*, prescribed by Physicians. And as the Physicians usually order a spare, scanty Modicum, less than is usually taken in; *Diet* has pass'd into a Name for this Retrenchement, or Diminution of the ordinary Quantity of Food, whether it be by Advice of a Physician, or by a Person's own Choice : Provided it be to remove, or prevent some Disorder.

Dr. *Cheyne* shews, how one may supply the Place of Medicines by *Diet* : Any one, says he, may lose a Pound of Blood, take a Purge, or a Sweat, by dropping the great Meal, or Abstaining from Animal Food, and strong Liquors for four or five Days, in Chronical Cases, as effectually as by opening a Vein, swallowing a Dose of Pills, or taking a Sudorific *Bolus*.

He advises therefore all Gentlemen of a sedentary Life, and of learned Professions, to use as much Abstinence as possibly they can, consistently with the Preservation of their Strength, and Freedom of Spirits. This they ought to have recourse to, assoon as they find any Heaviness, Inquietudes, restless Nights, or Aversion to Application : Either by lessening one half their usually Quantity of Animal Food, and strong Liquors, till such Time as they regain their wonted Freedom, and Indolence; Or by living a due Time wholly on *Vegetable Diets*, as Sago, Rice, Pudding, and the like, and drinking only Wine and Water. *Essay on Health*, &c.

**DIGESTER**, or *Digestor*, an Artificial Means, or Instrument, serving to digest, or dissolve Meats out of the Stomach, by a Way analogous to that of Animal Digestion.

Mr. *Leigh*[1], in the *Philosoph. Transact.* gives us an Artificial *Digestor* to illustrate the Natural one : It is prepared from Spirit of Sulphur, Spirit of Hartshorn, the Chyle of a Dog, and its *Saliva*. A Piece of Veal, Mutton, Beef, or the like, of a Bigness of a Nut, being put in a Dram of this Preparation, and set on a Digesting Furnace two Hours, drew from the Flesh a Juice, that had the Colour and Taste of Chyle, and left the Meat light dry, and insipid. Dr. *Havers*[2] prepares a *Digestor* of Oil of Turpentine, mix'd with Oil of Vitriol; in which, raw Flesh, and Crumbs of Bread being put, and the whole committed for four Hours to digest in *Balneo Mariæ*, the Meat is found dissolv'd, and the whole together forms a thickish Pulp : Hence, those Authors, each of 'em, conclude the Food in the Stomach to be *digested* by some such *Menstruum's*.

But the most noted *Digestor* is *Papin's*[3] *Digestor*, the Effect whereof bears a much more near Resemblance to the Operation of the Stomach. It is a Sort of Vessel, wherein Meat being put, together with so much Water as serves exactly to fill it, a Lid is screw'd close on, so as to admit of no external Air. Then, by the Application of two, or three lighted Char-Coals, or even a single

[1] This may be Charles Leigh (1662 - 1701), an English physician and naturalist.

[2] Clopton Havers (1657 – 1702), an English physician.

[3] Denis Papin (1647 – 1712), a French physicist.

small Lamp-flame, the Meat is in a few Minutes (six or eight) reduced into a perfect Pulp, or rather Liquor. By a little Increase of the Fire, or the Addition of a few Minutes in time, the hardest Bones themselves are brought into a Pulp, or Gelly.

The Effect is accounted for from the strict Closure of the Engine, which excluding the Intervention, or Escape of Air, the Succussions occasion'd by the Expansions, and Oscillations of Air included in the Flesh, are equable and strong, and so resolve the whole into one seemingly homogeneous Body, and mix the aqueous, saline, oleous, and other Particles, so strongly together, as scarce to be separable; but, while hot, to appear one Liquor, and when cold a Gelly, of a Strength proportionate to the Quantity of Flesh, or Bones dissolved in the Water.

This Experiment seems to hold a close Analogy with the Operation of the Stomach. For tho' the Stomach do not ordinarily dissolve, either so strongly, or so quick; yet in Proportion to its Heat and Constriction, Dr. *Drake* takes it to do the same Thing : Thereby breaking and resolving into small, the Bodies which it included, so mix'd, inter Minima, with its Humours. These, thus reduce into a Fluor, and intimately mix'd with the Liquids of the Drink, and the Juices of the stomach, compose that lactescent Liquor, call'd *Chyle*, or *Chyme*.

**DIGESTION**, in Medicine, call'd also Concoction, that Change of the Food taken in the Mouth, which it undergoes in the Stomach, in order to afford fit Matter to compose or distend an Animal, till it arrives at its destined Bulk,; and to repair the Loss of those Particles, which the Body, in its natural State, necessarily undergoes. The Operation of *Digestion* succeeds to *Mastication*, and *Deglutition*. It includes *Chylification*, and is succeeded by *Sanguification*, and *Nutrition*.

The Cause, Manner, and means of *Digestion*, have been infinitely controverted : It would be endless to enter into all the Systems, and Hypotheses, that have been fram'd by Philosophers, and Physicians, to account for this important Operation. Some contend, that it is done by a Kind of Elixation, or boiling of the solid, and grosser Parts of the Food, in the liquid, by the Heat of the Stomach, and the adjacent Parts, the Liver, Spleen, &c.

Others by *Attrition*; as if the Stomach by those repeated Motions, which are the Effects of Respiration, rubb'd, or ground off the minuter Particles from the grosser Matter; and agitating, and driving the rest against each other, attenuated, and dissolv'd them. Others think the Bilious Juice; Others the Spirits, &c. chiefly concern'd in the Affair.

Others will have the Food dissolved by a *Menstruum*, or *Dissolvent* : But these are greatly divided as to the Nature, and Origin of this *Menstruum*; Some supposing it an *Acid*, furnish'd by the Glands of the Stomach; Others a *Nitro-aereous* Spirit, which by penetrating the Mass of Food, breaks the Connexion of the most solid Parts; And others, a Saline Juice, which divide, and volatize the Parts of the Food.

Others again suppose *Digestion* to be perform'd by means of a *Ferment*, or *Leaven*; which, mixing with the Aliment, excites an intestine Motion in the Parts thereof, by whose mutual Fractions, and Collisions, the Parts are attenuated, and dissolved.

But these, too, differ in their Opinions of this *Ferment*; Some taking it to be the Remains of the Food last digested, which by its Continuance in the Stomach, has contracted an Acid Quality, which constitutes it a *Ferment* : Others take the *Ferment*, or Principles of Fermentation to be contain'd in the Aliment it self; which when inclosed in the Stomach, and heated thereby, being put in Motion, enters on its Office of Fermentation : But these, too, are divided; Some taking it to be the spirituous Part; and some the Air in Foods.

Others suppose this Ferment supplied by the Glands of the Stomach : And lastly, others contend for the *Saliva*, and make that the Ferment serving principally for the *Digestion* of the Food.

All these Systems are now reduced to three principal Ones; which we still find explain'd, and defended in the several Writings on that Subject ; The first holding *Digestion* to be perform'd by *Fermentation*; The second by *Trituration*; And the third by *Fermentation* and *Trituration* together.

The *first* Opinion was for a long Time the only one. The Retainers hereto hold, that the Food, after it is receiv'd into the Stomach, is there impregnated with certain menstruous Juices, which being assisted by the natural Hear of the Stomach, raises a Fermentation in the Foods, which dissolves, attenuates, and converts them into Chyle.

This was the System of the Ancients; who, tho' they only express themselves in general Terms, as dissolving, softening, subduing, Concretion, Qualities, &c. yet seem to have had the Notion of what we call *Fermentation*. Thus *Empedocles* and *Hippocrates* teach, that *Digestion* is perform'd by a Putrefaction of the Foods, after the like manner as the same *Empedocles* holds Water to be converted by Putrefaction into Wine. *Hippocrates*, and *Aristotle* use the Term Concoction, which we likewise find in *Erotian*, *Plutarch*, and *Actuarius*, to express the manner of Fruits ripening, the Must's changing into Wine, and Past's rising. *Hippocrates* expressly names *Effervescence*, and *Fermentation*, *de vetere Medicina*, C. 5. And *Galen* likewise, *L. de Consuetudine*, C. 2. And in another Place he asserts, that a certain Serosity of the Stomach concurs with the Bile and Spirits to effect *Digestion*. To say nothing of *Cicero*, who, according to the prevailing Opinion of his Time, attributes *Digestion* to the Heat of the Stomach. *Lib.* II. *de Nat. Deor.*

The Juices, or Ferments of the Stomach, to whose Action *Digestion* is supposed owing, are, the Saliva, Bile, and Pancreatic Juice. This is so true, that in certain voracious Animals, which eat, and *digest* fast, particularly Wolves, Ostriches, and Porcupines, the Bile discharges itself immediately into the Cavity of the Stomach; And we have observed a Disposition analogous thereto in a Man that been a great Eater.

There are only three Marks to know the Fermentation of Dough and Must by : First, In that the Dough rises, and swells; and the Must boils, and rarifies. Secondly, in that the Bread and Wine made by these Fermentations, have different Tastes and Qualities from those the Flower and Must had before. Thirdly, In that the Bread, and Wine, by Distillation, yield Principles that differ in those respects from those drawn from Flower and Must. Now, all these Characters are found in the Change made in the Food by *Digestion*.

Against this system it is objected by Mr. *Hecquet*[1], and others, that in every 24 Hours there is prepared a Pound of Saliva, half a Pound of Bile, and at least two Ounces of Pancreatic Juice; to which is to be added that Stomachic-Liquor, resembling Saliva; the whole amounting to about 2 Pounds, or 13824 Grains of Ferment. Now, say they, it is allowed by the Chymists, that one Grain of Ferment is sufficient for 803 Grains of Matter to be fermented; consequently 2 Pounds of Ferment would suffice for 1200 Pounds of Food : Whereas a Man ordinarily does not take above 4 Pounds in a Day.

Now, this, they say, is an Argument, that Fermentation is not the only, or principal Intention of these Juices; since, if it had, they would have been better proportioned to the Occasion. And, further, it furnishes an Objection, since such a Quantity of saline, menstruous Humour, having so little Business to employ it in fermenting the Food, must act on the Stomach, corrode and destroy the fine Membrane it is line withal, and to other Mischief.

But to this it is answered, 1. That, according to Mr. *Hecquet* himself, the Faculty of fermenting only belongs to the Salts, and that, by his own Computation, half a Pound of Bile, only contains 30 Grains of Salt; and a Pound of Saliva, with two Ounces of Pancreatic Juice, and the Stomach-Liquor, contain but 14 Grains of more : So that the Ferment of the Stomach produced each Day, only amounts to about 44 Grains, which were scarce enough for 2 Pounds of Food. But Mr. *Hecquet* diminishes the Quantity of these Salts too much, which *Verheyen*[2], and others make a deal more. To which is to be added the volatile Salt, mix'd with the Phlegm and Spirits.

2. It is not true, that there is always required a Grain, and only a Grain of Leaven for 800 Grains of Matter. Experience contradicts this Rule. In some Fermentations there is no need of any Leaven at all, and in others a deal less. As to the Ferment's acting on the membranes of the Stomach; 'tis certain, it does act on, and vellicate the same when there is not Food to employ it; and this it is, that occasions the Sensation of Hunger. But as fast as they are corroded, they are repair'd again by the Nourishment proper to them. The Stomach is sometimes gnawed, and incommoded by the Menstruum; but ordinarily it is preserv'd by a viscid Matter, wherewith its inner Coat is lined.

Another Objection against this Doctrine, is, that the Chyle yields no inflammable Spirit; which it should were it the Effect of Fermentation : But Monsr. *Astruc*[3] answers, that all Fermentations don't produce any such Spirit : That of Dough, for Instance, affords none, nor that of rotten Fruits, nor of Acids, or pure Alcali's. The inflammable Spirit, in Effect, requires a fine attenuated Sulphur, which is not found in all Fermentations.

The *second* System was invented, or at least renewed in the repent Age; and has been maintain'd with a deal of Zeal, and Vicacity, as is commonly the Case in any Thing that has the Appearance of Novelty. Those who espouse this Opinion, contend, that 'tis a mere continual Attrition, or Grinding, that breaks, attenuates, and reduces the Food, and with the Addition of a proper Fluid, forms it into that whitish Substance, call'd Chyle; much as Corn is

[1] Philippe Hecquet (1664 – 1737), a French physician.

[2] Philippe Verheyen (1646 – 1710), a Dutch surgeon and anatomist.

[3] Jean Astruc (1684 – 1766), a French physician.

ground between the Stones of a Mill. Which Opinion seems to be confirm'd by something observ'd in Birds : Their Gizzard, or Crop, is composed of two strong, solid, compact Muscles, which rubbing against each other, and being assisted by little angular Stones, or Grains of Sand swallow'd by the Birds, break and grind the dry Food those Animals live on : And when the Sand is grown smooth, they cast them off with their other Excrements, and swallow fresh ones.

This Sentiment is thus explain'd by an able Assertor thereof, Mr. *Hecquet*, in his Treatise of *Digestion*. Every thing in the Body is Vessel, consequently, every thing therein is hollow. Every thing therein lives, after its Manner; consequently, every thing is in Motion; Animal Life being nothing but Motion; and consequently all the Vessels are in Motion. Now, the Parts of the Body that are to move, will move towards those Sides, where they find the least Resistance. But the Place of the least Resistance in Tubes is the Cavity; consequently, the Motion of the Parts of the Vessels is towards their Axes. The Parts of Vessels that are to move, are the Parietes, or Sides, because flexible, and elastic; and this Motion can only be effected by an Approximation of those Parts: Consequently, the Motion of the Vessels consists in an Approximation of their Parietes; It is, therefore, a Sort of Contraction, Pression, or Coarction : Hence, as all the Parts of the Body are only Vessels, they all undergo a Systole, Pression, or Contraction. Further, all these Vessels contain Juices in their Cavities; And, therefore, all the Juices, or Liquids in the Body are continually compress'd.

This Pression is the Action of an Elastic Force; consequently the Pression will be such as is the Force; and, therefore, alternative : Consequently, it is a Pulse or Palpitation; and therefore the Juices are continually beaten. Now, these Juices are exceedingly divisible; and consequently are continually attenuated, and divided : And a Division effected by a Pulsation, or Beating, is a *Trituration*; and consequently, the Juices in the Body are continually triturated, or ground. The reason why the compressive Force should be alternative, is, that the Membranes, which compose the Vessels, consist of two Plans, or Series of Fibres; the one longitudinal, and the other circular, cutting the longitudinal at right Angles : The Longitudinal are tendinous, and Elastic; the Circular are muscular, or motive, like Sphincters, which compress. The Circular are over the Longitudinal, and embrace, or gird them round. The former, we have already observed, are Elastic; and their Elasticity opposes the Compression of the latter. From this Operation, or Resistance, arise a reciprocal Action and Reaction, which is the alternative grinding Force required.

To such as account for *Digestion* from a Ferment, these Philosophers object, that *Digestion* is a Dissolution; that to prepare the Mattes from this Dissolution, they must be soften'd; that the proper Effects of acid Ferments, is, to gnaw, or tear the hardest Matters, and to harden the softer, to thicken the fluid, fix the fat, and coagulate the milky : Consequently, that an acid Ferment should rather impede, than promote *Digestion*. Add, that beside the Force to grind the Juices, and the Vessels to compress them, there are likewise Liquors to dilute, and temper them, *viz*. the Saliva, and Stomach-Liquor. And Mineral Matters, which the Stomach-Liquor cannot dissolve, are found to be worn, and polish'd after having stay'd some time in the Stomach.

Now polishing is the Effect of Triture, or grinding, not of corroding. Accordingly we find Pelotoons, or Balls of Hairs, or Threads in the Stomach of Cattel, very smooth, and shining, and far from any Marks of Corrosion.

The Authors of Trituration require three Things for Digestion to proceed : A Liquor, to wet and dilute the Food, which they find in he Saliva, and Stomach-Liquor: A Vessel, which is the Stomach : And a Moving Power to grind, which they imagine to have found in the Muscles of the Stomach, Diaphragm, and Abdomen. The moving Force in the Muscles of the Stomach they maintain to be equivalent to a Weight of 248235 Pounds; and the Force of the Stomach alone, to a Weight of 12951 Pounds : A Power more than equal to that of one the ablest Mill-stones.

*Borelli*, on the footing of the *Equilibrium* of Fluids, has demonstrated, that the Force of the Flexor of the lost Articulation of the Thumb is equal to 3720 Pounds : Whence *Pitcairn*[1] deduces, that the Force of the Fibres of the Stomach is equal to 12951, and that of the Diaphragm, and Muscles of the lower Ventor, to 248235 Pounds. His Way of Estimating is this : The Flexor only weights 122 Grains, and yet may sustain 3720 Pounds : Consequently, the Fibres of the Stomach weight 8 Ounces, and the Diaphragm with the Muscles of the lower Ventor, weighting together 8223 Grains, have the Force abovemention'd. But this Argumentation seems founded on a Mistake; for 'tis not in Virtue of its Weight of 122 Grains, that the Flexor Muscle is equivalent to 3720 Pounds : Besides that it would follow hence, that the heavier the Muscles of the Stomach, Diaphragm, an Abdomen, are, the more Force they would have, and consequently the more easy, and expedite would the *Digestion* be : which is false.

The Patrons of this System compare the Brain to the Arbor, or Screw of a Press, the Heart to a Piston, the Lungs to Bellows, the Mouth to a Mill-stone or Pestle, the Stomach to a Press, and the Intestines to a Receiver or Vat. They contend, that *Castellus*[2], a Physician of *Messina*, was the first of the Moderns, who expressly espoused the System of Ferments, and that he was followed by *Van Helmont* and *Willis*.

But even among the Partisans of Trituration are not perfectly agreed among themselves : *Pitcairn* will have it perform'd by a total Contraction of the Stomach : And Mr. *Hecquet*, by a successive, peristaltic, or vermicular Contraction.

*Astruc*, in his Treatise, *de la Cause de la Digestion*, refutes this System of Trituration at length. He makes a strong Opposition to the *Calculus*, which raises the moving Force of the Stomach, &c. so very high. The Contraction of the Fibres of the Stomach, to compress the Food, he shews, cannot exceed three Ounces; and 'tis even *gratis* that he allows so much : That of the Diaphragm, and Abdomen, he computes at about 4 Pounds. He observes, that *Pitcairn*, surprized, in all Probability, with what he had asserted of this Force, durst not pursue the Proportion wherein his *Calculus* was founded, an according to which, one of the Forces would be found equivalent to 117088 Pounds, and other to 250734; which together make 367822 Pounds. The

[1] Archibald Pitcairn (1652 – 1713), a Scottish physician.

[2] Pietro Castelli (1574 – 1662), an Italian physician and botanist.

Diaphragm in its Motion has two Forces; the one direct, which is that, whereby its muscles draw from the Centre to the Circumference : the other lateral, whereby it rests, or presses on the Stomach; The latter very small in Comparison of the former.

Now, what has deceiv'd *Mess. Pitcairn* and *Hecquet*, is, their taking the direct for the lateral Force; the Contraction of Fibres for their Pressure on the Stomach. And the same Oversight they are guilty of in the Muscles of the Abdomen, whose pressure against the Abdomen is only lateral. Add, that there are voracious Animals without any Diaphragm at all; as Fishes, which respire through their Gills : and others that have only a single Membrane; as Birds, in whom the Muscles of the lower Venter are very small, and feeble, and in a Situation that incapacitates them from acting at all on the Stomach.

The Membranes of the Stomach being very soft, and having only a slender Motion, seem very unfit for the Office of a Mill-stone. 'Tis true, in certain Fowls the Stomach consists of a close, compact, fleshy Muscle exceeding strong, so as to break little Stones, and Bits of Glass. But to this it is urge, that it is no Digestion, which in these Animals is effected in the Intestines. And the Structure of our Stomach compared with the Gizzard, or Crop of granivorous Birds, does, on the contrary, furnish a very cogent Argument against Trituration. The Gizzard is provided on the Out-side with four fleshy Muscles, the Tendons whereof meet in two opposite Points : The Inside is lined with a hard, thick, cartilaginous Membrane; especially in the Places where the Tendons meet. By this Mechanism Nature plainly intimates the Office of the Gizzard to be the Grinding of the Grain by the Friction of its Parietes, or Sides : Whereas, the Membrane in the Stomach of a Man is exceedingly thin and fine, furnish'd with a few fleshy Fibres, cover'd with a tender, sensible Kind of Down; and the Stomach it self is of a great Capacity. And the Stomach in rapacious Birds, who devour huge Pieces of raw Flesh without chewing, is a still finer Membrane. Lastly, on the System of Trituration there seems no accounting for Hunger, Nausea's, Indigestions, Crudities, &c.

In the System of Trituration it seems impossible to explain, why certain Things easy to grind, *e.gr.* Cabbage Flowers, cannot be digested in certain Stomachs, which yet find no Difficulty in digesting more hard, and solid Meats, as Beef, and Mutton : Whereas, the Difference of Dissolvents gives a natural, and easy Solution. Hydropic People continue to digest, notwithstanding the Fibres of the Stomach, as well as the rest of the Body, are extremely relax'd through the Abundance of Humour. And the total, prompt Change of Nature induced in Foods can be the Effect of nothing else but Fermentation; which even discovers it self by Belches, &c. while it goes on.

The Iron, Needles, Pins, &c. sometimes found undissolved in the Stomach, are no Objection to the System of Fermentation; it being notorious, that no Dissolvent dissolves all Bodies. In Birds, which feed on Grain, the Fermentation is manifest, first, in the Crop where the Grain is prepar'd for *Digestion*, by being macerated in a Liquor like Saliva; and afterwards in the Gizzard, where the *Digestion* is perfected by a Dissolvent pour'd into it by a conglomerate Gland. But the Thing is still more apparent in Ruminating Animals, which are provided with four Stomachs; the two first whereof, tho' form'd of a nervous Membrane, make but little Alteration in the Aliment, for

Want of a Ferment, or *Menstruum*; So that it returns to be chew'd again; and only becomes well *digested* in the fourth Stomach, whither a Dissolvent is pour'd from a conglomerate Gland.

The Partisans of the *third* Opinion allow it incontestable, that there are Acids in the Stomach, which mix with the Foods, and act in them; and hold likewise, that their Action is aided, and promoted by the Motion of the Systole, and Diastole of the *Viscera* : They add, that the Acids produce a Fermentation; and the Oscillatory Motion of the *Viscera* a Trituration; and that this *Digestion* is the Effect of Fermentation and Trituration at the same Time.

Be it as it will with each of the three Systems; thus much we may venture to lay down from 'em all, as the real Process of *Digestion* : The End of this Operation being to prepare the Foods, so as they may serve for Nutrition; those Foods must be consider'd from the Time the Man takes them in, till being converted into Chyle, they mix with the Blood, which conveys them into all Parts of the Body. The Foods then we take, are either crude, as Oisters, Fruits, certain Pulse, &c. or dress'd, as Flesh, and Fish, which are roasted, boil'd, fried, &c. and season'd a thousand divers Ways with Salt, Pepper, and other Spices, Vinegar, Wine, &c. to heighten and enrich the Taste as much as to assist *Digestion*.

Further, there are some Foods we swallow without chewing, as Liquids; and others, which we break and comminute by chewing, as Bread, Flesh, &c. 'Tis of these last we shall here speak, as undergoing more Preparations, and more Changes to fit them for Food, than the others.

The Food, then, is first broke, and divided by the Teeth, and, at the same Time, moisten'd with a Liquor supplied by the Salival Glands, and thus form'd into a Kind of Paste. Thus prepar'd, it is pass'd through the *Oesophagus* into the Stomach, there to ferment.

This Fermentation is caused, 1. By the Salival Juice, which is a Ferment, and has the same Effect on the Aliment, that Leaven, or Barm has on Paste. 2. By the Heat of the Stomach, *Viscera* of the Abdomen, and even Excrements; which here has nearly the same Effect on Foods, as the Dunghill has on Matters laid by the Chymists to *digest* therein. 3. By the Remains on Foods left adhering in the *Rugæ*, or Folds of the Stomach, and there turn'd sour, and acrimonious. 4. By the Compression of the Muscles of the Abdomen, and Diaphragm. 5. By the Liquor which the repeated Compression of those Muscles occasions to drip from the Glands of the Stomach. 6. According to the Sentiment of some modern Physicians, by the Air itself, which being mix'd, and embarrass'd in the Aliments, dilates by the Heat of the Stomach, and separates the Parts of the Foods. These causes all contribute to attenuate, and divide the Food, so as to convert them into a cineritious Matter, call'd *Chyle*.

From the Stomach the Chyle descends into the Duodenum, where it is further perfected by the Pancreatic Juice, and the Bile, which thin it, precipitate its grosser Parts, and render it more fluid. The Chyle thus perfected and attenuated, enters the Lacteal Veins, which convey it into the Receptacle, where it is further diluted by the Lympha, which is brought hither in Abundance. Hence it rises into the Thoracic Duct, and enters the Subclavian Vein; where being taken up by the ascending Cava, it is pour'd into the right Ventricle of the Heart.

The Chyle thus mixing with the Blood, embarasses the Globule thereof, and thus abates its Motion : And hence that Inclination to go to sleep after Meals. But, by Degrees, the Blood communicates its Motion to the Chyle; and by its volatile, and exalted Parts, together with the Saline and Nitrous Parts of the Air, subtilizes, and gives it its last Perfection. Then the *Digestion* is finish'd : and the Foods being by so many Changes render'd the immediate Matter of Nutrition, are carried by the Blood into all Parts of the Body, to repair, and fill the Vacancies of such as are continually dissipating, and exhaling; or even to add new ones.

As to the grosser Parts of the Foods separated from the Chyle, by the Bile and Pancreatic Juice, they assume the Colour of the Excrements from the Bile; and that rank Smell, they derive from the coarser Sulphurs thereof. These Sulphurs, and Salts of the Excrements, serve, after they have passed through the Intestines, and are arrived at the last, which is the *Rectum*, to vellicate the Muscles thereof, and dispose 'em to relax, and thus to apprize Nature of a Necessity to discharge.

The Separation of the Urine from the Blood, may be esteem'd a Part of perfect *Digestion*; the Design of such Separation being to render the Blood more pure and balsamic, and of Consequence more fit for Nutrition; which the Salts the Urine abounds withal, greatly prevented. This Separation is thus perform'd : The Branches of the emulgent Arteries, which terminate in the Glands, whereof the Substance of the Kidneys is composed, carry the Blood thither; where a Serosity is separated from the Blood, by means of the Pores in the Glands of the Kidneys; those Pores representing the Hole sin a Sieve, which only let pass such Things as are of a less Diameter than themselves. This Serosity, call'd Urine, is discharged hence into several little Tubes, which joyning into a Kind of Pyramids, yield their Humour into the *Pelvis*, whence it runs through the Ureters into the Bladder.

**DIGESTION**, in Chymistry, is a Preparation of Plants, Minerals, Metals, and other Bodies beaten, or ground, by putting 'em in a Vessel, and heating them gradually over a gentle Fire, like the Heat of an Animal Body.

*Digestion* is a previous Kind of Disposition to a perfect Dissolution of a Body, made by means of Fire, or fiery Particles, beating and loosening the Pores of the Body, and attenuating the Parts of the Fluids, that their Connexion with the harder Matter may be more easily, and perfectly dissolved. *Bohnius*[1] seems to describe it pretty adequately by an insensible Action and Reaction of the Particles of a Mass, moving together by some subtile, ambient Fluid, to which it was exposed for *Digestion*. By calling *Digestion* a reciprocal Action, their Motion is intimated, by means whereof they are torn from the contiguous Ones; and in a Word, differently modified : So that the Motion ended, the digested Mass, differs either wholly, or in Part, from the same Mass before *Digestion*; sometimes in Colour, sometimes in Smell, sometimes in Transparency, sometimes in Taste, sometimes in Consistence, and other Affections. That *Digestion* is effected by Motion, is evident from tan Observation of Dr. *Grew*; who bringing a Mixture of Salt of

[1] Johann Bohn (1640 – 1718), a German physician and anatomist.

Tartar, and Oil of Turpentine, several Days Journey with him in a Coach to London, found it had undergone a more intimate Motion, than if it had been exposed to a long *Digestion*.

*Digestion* is ordinarily confounded with *Maceration*; but the two Things differ, in that there is Heat required to *Digestion*; whereas *Maceration* is done in the Cold.

*Digestion* is usually perform'd with the Addition of some *Menstruum* suitable to the Matter; Thus, Roses and Poppies Heads are put to *digest* in Oil, or Water, to make Unguents, or Syrups; Calcined Lead, and Ceruss, are *digested* in distill'd Vinegar, to make the Magistery thereof, or the *Sal Saturni*. Hence Dr. *Quincy* defines *Digestion* to be the Solution of Bodies, made by *Menstruum's*, with the Assistance of Fire.

To conceive the Nature of Chymical *Digestion*, it may be necessary to shew, how the Particles of Bodes can by this Process be diffused every Way, and sustain'd in the *Menstruum*; which deserves the more to be accounted for, because those solid Particles have not the same specific Gravity, as the Liquors have in which they swim. Tho' the Nature of a perfectly fluid Body be such, as that the Particle, which constitute it, do very readily give Way upon the smallest Impulse, and recede from one another; yet there is found in most Liquors some Degree of Tenacity; and from hence arise such a Cohesion of Parts, as cannot be broken without some Force. And tho' indeed this Force of Cohesion in Liquors seems to be but little, or none at all, when compared with what we experience in Solids, yet we find, it can make some Resistance. And as the Force in Liquors is either stronger or weaker, so it produces a Variety of Effects, differing more or less from the Phænomena, which would naturally flow from a perfect Fluid; So that, tho' by the Laws of Hydrostaticks, every Corpuscle, how subtil soever, if put into a Fluid, which is specifically lighter, must necessarily sink to the Bottom; yet we find some heavy Bodies, such as Gold, &c. when reduced into thin Plates, will be sustained in Spirit of Wine. This Force, therefore, of Tenacity, which resists the Motion of Bodies in a Fluid, is proportional to the Number of Parts, which are to be separated, or to the Surface of the Body, which we would have move in the Fluid.

Hence it is, that since the Surface of a Body may be enlarged, without altering any Thing if its Gravity, the Resistance of a Fluid may be augmented, as to equal the Force of Gravity, which carries the Body downwards. And a Body, tho' specifically heavier than a Fluid, in which it is immersed, may be very well sustained in that Fluid, provided it be reduced into very small Particles; because the Gravity of a Body thus reduced into small Particles, decreases in a much greater Proportion, than the Surface does, or, which is proportional to it, the Tenacity of the Fluid : So that at length the Resistance arising from its Tenacity, will be equal to the Gravity of the Particle, and so hinder its Descent. And, therefore, both in Solution, and *Digestion*, it is a general Rule, that if the Gravity of a Body be to the Tenacity of the Fluid, as P to I; and if the Body be then subdivided, so that the Diameters of the Parts be to that of the whole, as I to P; the Resistance which the Particles will meet with in their Descent, will be equal to their Gravity : for since their Weight is I/P3, but their Surface I/P2, the Gravity will be to the Resistance as P/P3, to I/P2, or as I to I. So that by this we may understand, how the Corpuscles of

Metals swim in *Menstruum's*, which are specifically lighter, as Gold in the Spirit of Nitre, which is drawn off from Bezoar Mineral, tho' the Gravity of Gold be 15 times greater. And in the same manner we may understand, how Corpuscles specifically heavier, are suspended in any other *Menstruum*. And it is for the same Reason, that such as are lighter, cannot rise up to the Surface : for the Pressure of Fluids being equal every Way, the superior Parts act reciprocally on the inferior; so that the same Force, which keeps the heavy Particles from sinking, will not permit those which are lighter, to ascend.

The Use of *Digestion*, in Pharmacy, is, to extract the Particles, which are more volatile, by a certain *Menstruum*, and to mix them intimately with it. To this End a gentle Fire is commonly used, that the Corpuscles, which are most volatile, may separate, as it were of their own Accord : for a fierce Fire forces out the Fæces, as well as the finer Particles; and it does not abate the Strength of the Liquor, it will not fail of spoiling its Clearness.

*Digestion*, in Chirurgery, is applied to Imposthumes, or Abscesses; and expresses their Disposition to ripen, and come to Suppuration. Tumors arising on the Parotides of Children, are of easy *Digestion* : They ripen in a little Time.

*Digestion* is also used for *Maturation*, or that State of a Disease, wherein the morbific Matter is so changed in Bulk, Figure, Cohesion, Mobility, &c. by the Use of proper Medicines, or even by the Force of Nature, as to be less noxious and hurtful, and consequently to abate the Violence of the Distemper.

The Greeks call it πεπασμος. The Matter of the Disease so far digested, as to become next a-kin to salubrious, or healthy Matter, is said to be *resolved*.

**DIGESTIVE**. The ancient Philosophers admitted a Digestive Faculty, or Quality in the Body; as not knowing how otherwise to account for the Act of Digestion.

*Digestive* is also used in Medicine for such Remedies as strengthen, and increase the Tone of the Stomach, and assist in the Digestion of Foods. To this Class belong all *Stomachicks*, and *Strengtheners*, or Corroborants.

*Digestive*, in Chirurgery, is a Sort of Unguent, Plaster, or the like, that ripens, and prepares the Matter of Wounds, &c. for Suppuration. It is usually composed of Turpentine, Yolk of Eggs, Oil of *Hypericum*, *Unguentum Basilicum*, and Tincture of Aloes. The Wound must be dress'd the first Day with a *Digestive*, to bring it to Suppuration.

**DIGITATED**, among Botanists, is applied to the Leaf of a Plant, which is either composed of many simple Leaves set together upon one Foot-Stalk, as in the Cinque-foil, Vetches, &c. or else when there are many deep Gashes, or Cuts in the Leaf, as in those of Straw-berries, Hops, &c.

**DILATATION**, in Medicine, &c. is the laying open any Orifice, or the Lips of a Wound wider; or the Extension of any Vessel : whence *Dilatorium*.

**DILUTE**. To *dilute* a Body, is to render it liquid; or, if it were liquid before, to render it more so, by the Addition of a thinner thereto.

Those Things thus added, are call'd *Diluents*, or *Dilutors*; such are common Wheys, Ptisans, and Juleps, which in respect of the Blood in a State of Viscidity are thinner, and therefore are said to thin, or dilute it.

Flower must be well *diluted*, to make it into Paste. Oker is *diluted* with Oil, to paint Beams, Doors, &c.

**DIOPTRA**, among Surgeons, is an Instrument whereby one may see into the Matrix, and inspect any Ulcers therein, call'd also *Speculum Matricis*, and Dilatatorium.

**DIPHRYGES**, in Pharmacy, the *Scoria*, Sediment, or Calx of melted Copper gather'd in the Furnace, when the Metal is run out. The Word is from the Greek δις, *twice*, and φρυγειν, *to roast*.

*Dioscorides* makes three Kinds of *Diphryges* : One call'd Natural, tho' made of a Kind of Clay, or Bole dried in the Sun : That made of Marcasite, or Pyrites burnt; and that of the Faeces of Copper. It is moderately sharp, and astringent, and is reputed good for Ulcers that cicatrize with Difficulty.

**DISCOUS** *Flower*. Botanists reckon on two Kinds of Plants with a *Discous Flower* : 1. Such as have the Flower compounded, and the Seed pappous, but the Leaves and Stalks not milky when broken. 2. The *Corymbiferous* Plants, whose Flowers are compounded into a Discous Figure, but their Seeds are not pappous. Of the former Kind, are the Flea-Banes, Ragweeds, Groundsels, &c. and of the latter, are Daisies, Chamomile, Tansy, Wormwood, &c.

**DISCUTIENTS**, or Discussives, in Medicine, are Remedies proper to open the Pores, and evacuate the redundant Humours of the Body, by insensible Perspiration; or to discharge Flatulencies, Swellings, &c. by shaking, jumbling, &c. *Discutients* are the same with what we otherwise call *Diaphoreticks*, and *Resolvents*.

**DISEASE**, in Medicine, that State of a living Body, wherein it is prevented the Exercise of any of its Functions, whether Vital, Natural, or Animal : Or, *Disease* is an Indisposition, contrary to Nature, whereby the Action of some Part is immediately injured.

An ingenious Author of a late *Latin* Treatise, *de Purgatione*, holds the Essence of a Disease to consist in a Want of that Equilibrium between the solid, and fluid Parts, which is necessary to the Maintenance of Health.

Of all Animals, Man is subject to the most *Diseases*; and of them, the studious and speculative are most exposed thereto. Other animals have their *Diseases*; but they are in small Number : Nor are Plants without them; tho' there Maladies scarce exceed half a score.

Several Authors have given us very compendious Theories of Diseases; reducing 'em all to some one general Disaffection : Thus, *du Broue* deduces all the Diseases of the human Frame from the *Scorbutus*; *Musgrave*[1] from the *Arthritis*; and Dr. *Woodward* from the *Bile* : Others imagine them

[1] William Musgrave (1655 – 1721), an English physician.

the Effects of a *Pocky Virus*, which has lurk'd in the Seed ever since the Sin of Adam : *Helmont*, and *Serreinus* the *Dane*, take 'em to depend on some extraneous *Ferment*, form'd in, or out of us. Lastly, it appearing from the Observations of *Pliny, Kircher, Langius*, and *Bononio*, that there are little Worms in feverish Blood, Pustules, Carbo's, and the Itch; divers Physicians have took Occasion to suspect, that all the *Diseases* arise from Worms.

A *Disease* is well describ'd to be a deprav'd, and disorderly State of the solid, and fluid Parts, whereby all, or some of the Functions either of the Body, or Mind, or both, are either abolish'd, or impair'd.

For some *Diseases* only impair the Use of the Part, as the *Ophthalmia, Gout*, &c. Others destroy it entirely; as the *Gutta serena, Palsy*, &c. Some affect the whole Body, as the *Fever, Apoplexy, Epilepsy*, &c. Others only impair a Part, as the *Asthma, Colic, Dropsy*, &c. Some only affect the Body, as the *Palsy*; Others disturb the Mind, as *Melancholy, Delirium*, &c. lastly, others affect both the Body and Mind, as the *Mania, Phrenzy, Pains*, &c.

As the Actions, or Conditions of the Body, so also the *Diseases*, or Defects thereof, may be reduced to three general Heads: *viz*. 1. *Diseases of the Solid Parts* : 2. *Those of the fluid Parts*: And 3. *Diseases compounded of both*.

A Popular *Syllabus* of *Diseases* may be given, as follows : The Solid Parts, *i.e.* the Bones and Flesh may be disorder'd five Ways : *viz*. Render'd turgid, by *Tumors*; Cut, with *Wounds*; Corroded by *Ulcers*, or *Carie's*; Removed out of their Places, as in *Hernia's, Descents*, and *Dislocations*; Or *discontinued* by *Fractures*, and *Contusions*.

*Diseases* of the Fluids are either in the Mass of the *Blood*, or the *Spirits* : Those of the Blood are reducible to two Kinds; those that thicken, and inspissate, or which amounts to the same, retard its Motion and those which attenuate, and dissolve, and of Consequence accelerate it.

To this latter Kind belong *Fevers*, and feverish Affections alone : All other *Diseases* of he Blood belong to the former.

In too thick a State of Blood, its Principles are too crass, and its Molecules too big, whence a *Lentor*, lazy Motion, and even Stoppage, particularly in the sinous Passages of the Glands : Hence *Obstructions, Inflammations, Schirrhus's, Sarcoma's, Verrucæ, Pustules, Oedemata, Impetigines*, and other *Tumors*, and *Congestions* both in the *Viscera*, and *Habit* of the Body : And hence, again, *Drowsiness, Melancholy, Hypochondriacal* Affections, &c. If this thick Blood be too much replete with sharp acid Salts, it will destroy the Texture of the Parts, and break out in Ulcers, as in *Phthysical, Scrophulous, Scorbutic*, and *Venereal* Diseases, *Gangrenes, Carbo's, Cancers*, and other Erosive Tumors, according to the Quality and Degree of Saltness and Acrimony. And from the same Source arise *Cephalgia's, Cardialgia's, Colicks, Gouts, Rheumatisms, Pleurisies*, &c. which by abrading the solid Substance, frequently emaciate the Body.

The *Diseases* of the Animal Spirits, arise either, 1. From an Intermission, or Retardation of their Motion; or a Diminution of Quantity; or, 2. From a Disorder in their Organism, or Quality.

To the first Class are reduced the *Catalepsis, Apoplexy, Coma, Carus, Palsy, Stupor, Tremor*, &c. To the second, belong the *Mania, Phrenzy, Delirium, Foolishness, Melancholy, Vertigo, Spasms, Epilepsy, Hysteric*

*Affections, Horror,* &c. Add, that as all *Diseases* of the Blood arise from external Causes, viz. some one ore more of the Non-Naturals, as Food, Air, Evacuation, &c. so those of the *Spirits* generally proceed from Disorders of the Blood.

Lastly, the *Diseases* of the Fluids, whether those in the Blood, or Spirits, are seldom confin'd long thereto; but presently come to disturb, and impede some of the Functions affected to the solid Parts; and at last corrupt the Substance of the Solids themselves. Hence *Compound Diseases*; which are infinitely various.

But the learned *Boerhaave* furnishes us a much more accurate, and scientifical Division of Diseases. Diseases of the Solids, he considers, either as of the simple, and Similar Parts; Or of the Organical.

I. *Similar Diseases*, are 1. Those of the last, and smallest Fibres; which are reducible to too great *Tension*, and *Laxness*, too great *Strength*, or *Weakness*, and a *Solution of their Continuity.*

2. Those of the *Membranes*, which being only Assemblages of Fibres just mention'd, are subject to the same Disorders.

3. Those of the last, and *smallest Canals*, which are formed of such Membranes.

4. Of the *Membranes* composed of such Canals.

5. Of *Canals* composed of such Membranes, which are all the greater Vessels of the Body.

6. Of the *solid Parts*, which are composed of Canals compress'd, and grown together, so as to be void of Humour to distend 'em; Or Canals growing into one consistent Part, the Humour hardening together with eh Vessel that contain'd it.

Lastly, Supposing these Parts all found, *Diseases* may befal them with respect to their Structure, from a Vice, or vicious Application of the Matter of Nutrition.

II. *Organical Diseases*. An Organical Part consisting of the several simple Parts abovemention'd, and fitted to perform any Office by means of some Humour contain'd in it; may be considered, either in it self, as a solid Part, or with respect to the Humour it contains : In the first View, *Organical Diseases* are reducible to four Classes.

1. *Disorders* in the *Figure*, and the Circumstances thereof, as Roughness, Solidity, Cavity, &c. To this belong the αναγομεσις, when one Vessel opens into another; the Διαπυδησις, when a Rupture is made; and Διαιρεσις, when a Breach is occasion'd by Corrosion; the εμφραξις, which is a total Obstruction of the Cavity, by a viscous, grumous Matter; the γενοχεσια, or Narrowness of the Passage; the θλιψις, or Compression of the Sides of the Cavity; συμφυσις, when the Sides are quite close up; and συνιζησις, when the Vessel is so emptied, that the Sides falling together, the Cavity is lost.

2. In the *Number*, where 'tis either deficient or redundant : But the Parts seldom err in this respect, so as to occasion a *Disease*.

3. In *Magnitude*; to which belong *Nodes, Exostoses*, and *Callus's*.

4. In the *Situation*, and *Connexion*; as when the *Ligaments* are too long, or

too short, when broke, or deprav'd; also *Distortions, Luxations, Subluxations, Herniæ,* or Ruptures in the Groin, Scrotum, Bladder; *Procidentiae* of the Womb, Bladder, and Rectum; Disorders of the Tendons, and Muscles, particularly their flying out of their Places; the Relaxation, or Rupture of the Membraneous Ligament that should retain 'em.

Lastly, there is a *Disease* common both to *Similar*, and *Organical* Parts, call'd *Solution of Continuity.*

Diseases *of the Fluids,* considering those Fluids simply and in themselves, may be reduced to Disorders in respect of Quantity, and Quality : But considering them as contain'd in Solids, they may err, too, in Place and Proportion.

As to the second, such Quality of the Humours, as disturbs the Animal Functions, is call'd *Cacochymia.* Now, this is either in the Fluids consider'd in themselves, their own Parts, and Composition; Or consider'd as they concur towards constituting some Part of the Body.

If the Morbid Quality be consider'd in the Particles of the Humour, it must either consists in an Augmentation of *Bulk,* whence the *Emphraxis, Atrophy, Symphysis,* and *Synezesis*; or in the Diminution thereof, as in the *Diapnoe,* and *Ceneangeia* : Or an Increase of *Solidity,* whence too great an *Attenuation*; or a Decay thereof, whence a *Lentor, Stagnation,* and *Cohesion*: Or in the *Figure,* as when of Spherical it becomes Angular, and consequently, with respect to the Part 'tis applied to, sharp; whence *Acrimonies,* both acid, alcaline, muriatic, ammoniac, saponaceous, vitriolic, &c. and *Oleosities* : Or in *Rigidity,* and *Flexibility* : Or in *Elasticity* : or in *Cohesion,* and Divisibility.

Again, all the Juices consider'd together, the principal Disorders they are subject to, are too great *Fluidity,* or Tenacity : too much *Velocity* in their Vessels, or too little.

Lastly, considering the Fluids as contain'd in the Solids, there arise divers *Diseases* merely from their changing of Place; which may be reduced to two Classes, *viz.* the grosser Humours *intruding* themselves into the finer Canals; and the Humours *extravasating,* or getting out among the solid Parts; whence *Inflammation, Pustules, Dropsy, Spungeous Membranes* of the Head, Breast, Abdomen, and Uterus; and *Emphysema's.*

And, that the Humours collected, and stagnating among the Parts, grow *putrid, purulent, ichorous, erosive,* and *sharp*; and thus destroy the tender Stamina, or Solids; whence *Sinus's, Fistula's, Ulcers, Gangrenes, Sphacelus's, Cancers,* and the like.

These are the prime Differences of the *Diseases* of the Body; and from these arise most of the rest : So that they may be regarded, not only as *Diseases,* but as the Causes of *Diseases.*

There is another Division of *Diseases,* in Use among Physicians, taken from certain external Accidents, which are common to a great many different *Diseases* : which Distinction, too, has its Uses; tho' they generally run it too far. *Diseases,* then, are distinguish'd,

1. With respect to their Cause, into *Idiopathy, Sympathy, Protopathy, Deuteropathy, Hereditary, Connate,* and *Acquired.*

2. With respect to their Subject, into *Diseases* of *old Age, Children, Adults,*

*Men, Women, Maids, Pregnant, Parturient, Endemical, Epidemical,* &c.

3. With respect to *Duration*, into *most acute*, which terminates in four Days; *Acute*, in twenty, and *Chronical*, which are all those of longer Continuance.

4. With respect to *Seasons*, into *Vernal, Autumnal, Continued*, and *Intermitting*.

5. With respect to their *Effects*, into *Benign, Malignant, Curable, Incurable, Mortal*, and *Contagious*.

And 6. With respect to their *State*, into *Beginning, Progress, State, Declension*, and *End*.

*Diseases of Plants*. Monsr. *Tournefort*, in an express Dissertation on this Subject, in the *Memoirs de l'Academie des Sciences*, refers all *Diseases* of Plants to the following Causes :

1. The too great Abundance of the Nutritious Juice.

2. The Defect, or Want of this Juice.

3. Some ill Qualities it acquires.

4. Its unequal Distribution in different Parts of the Plant.

And 5. External Accidents.

The *Diseases* principly observed by our Gardeners, are,

1. *Barrenness*, when the Tree, tho' outwardly fresh and healthy, bears no Blossoms; or if it does, they fall; or if they set, the Fruit drops e're it come to Maturity.

2. *Blasting of the Buds*, occasion'd by a Frost happening when the Leaves and Blossoms are wet. By this means the Pores are shut, and the vital Juice suffocated; when, if the Sun breaks out on a sudden, they turn yellow, with round fiery Specks growing on them; whence frequently proceed Tumours like Warts, which rotting, grow full of Maggots. Mr. *Mortimer* adds, that the Want of Rain at Blossoming Time, often occasions the Dropping off of the Blossoms for Want of Sap; he, therefore, recommends the watering 'em.

3. *Consumption*, proceeding from a Want of Sustenance, through the Failure of the nourishing Juices; or from Obstructions of the Veins, and Roots; or ill Digestion, and Secretion of Humours, &c.

4. The *Moss*; an Account of which, see under the Article Moss. See also Parasite.

5. The *Jaundice*, which, tho' it does not hinder the Tree from appearing sound, yet when it begins to sprout, the Leaves become of a whitish green, and as they grow bigger, turn yellow. It frequently arises from external Causes, as the Mildew; but chiefly from a stony, or chalky Soil, impregnated with an acid Salt.

6. *Mildew*, a Kind of Epidemical *Disease*, most frequent and fatal in the Spring Season. It is properly a corrosive, and nipping Dew, proceeding from pent up Vapours now exhaled, and returned back on the tender opening Buds, which infects 'em by its Acrimony, and obstructs the Circulation of the nutritive Juices. By which means the Leaves being to fade, and wither, and both the Blossoms and Fruit are much prejudiced.

7. A *thick Fog*, or too abundant Dew, *Agricola* assures us, occasions the same *Disease* as the Mildew, only in a less Degree.

8. *Falling of the Leaves*, which happens when the Trees sprouting too soon, are either surpriz'd by excessive Heat, or Cold.

9. *Uredo*, or *Scorching*, of which there are two Kinds; the first happening upon the Fall of a subtil Dew, or small Rain, immediately followed by the piercing Beams of the Sun, which suddenly closes the Pores before dilated, and burns up the Leaves : The second happening from the like Fervour in the internal Parts of the Tree, *viz.* in the Pith; occasion'd by some inner Failing. *Agricola* imputes it to the Fault of the Gardeners, who in transplanting Trees, frequently cut off the lesser Filaments, and Roots, as also the greater Roots, without covering the Wounds with Wax, or the like.

10. *Scurf*, or *Leprosy*, a *Disease* chiefly of the Bark, caused by too great Dilation of the Pores, whereby too much perspirable Matter transuding it, hangs and hardens on the Bark, which by this means chaps, and cracks, and thus a Sort of Lepra is form'd, Perspiration obstructed, &c. Add, that this scurfy Skin proves a Harbour for Vermine, which live both in the Bark and Tree.

11. The *Worm*, a little Animal generated in the corrupted Substance of the Bark, Blossoms, Fruit-Leaves, Pith, and Roots. Mr. *Gentil* mentions another Kind, call'd *Cock-chaffers*, which sick to the Roots of young tender Trees, and Bark, and kill them. There is a third Sort, call'd *Breezes*, or Gad-flies, which gnaw the Roots. The Worm is a very frequent *Disease*; whereby young hopeful Trees are all of a sudden brought to languish, and decay.

12. *Rotten Roots*, occasion'd chiefly by their being planted too deep. This *Disease* is incurable.

13. *Blights*.

**DISPENSATION**, in Pharmacy, the Disposition, and Arrangement of several Medicines, either simple or compound, all weigh'd in their proper Doses, or Quantities; in order to be employ'd in the making a Composition.

**DISSIMILAR LEAVES**, are the two first Leaves of any Plant at its first shooting out of the Ground. They are thus call'd, because they usually are of different Form from the common Leaves of the grown Plant. These Dr. *Grew* observes to be nothing but the very Lobes of the Seed expanded, and thus advanced. Their Use is for Protection of the Plume; which, being young and reader, is thus guarded on each Side, and has also some Rain, and Dew gradually convey'd down to it by this means.

**DISSIPATION**, in Physicks, an insensible Loss, or Consumption of the minute Parts of a Body; or, properly the Flux whereby they fly off, and are lost. Thus, we don't say *Dissipation*, but Loss of Blood, in speaking of the Blood lost at a Wound, or in any other sensible Manner : On the contrary, we say with Mr. *Lemery*, the *Dissipation* of the Spirits is in greater Abundance than that of the solid Parts, consequently the Reparation thereof must be more frequent and copious.

**DISSOLVENT**, something that dissolves, *i.e.* divides, and reduces a Body into its smallest Parts. Thus, *Aqua Regia* is the Dissolvent of Gold; *Aqua fortis* of Silver, and other Metals; Water, of Salts, and Gums; Spirit of Wine, of Resins; Spirit of Vinegar, of Pearls, Coral, &c. *Dissolvents* are usually call'd by the Chymists *Menstruums*.

Sea-Salt is found the proper *Dissolvent* of Gold : This, in almost any Form, whether as a Fluid, or a Solid, as a Spirit, does the Business : Accordingly, this is the *Basis*, or fundamental Ingredient of *Aqua Regia*.

So Nitre is the proper *Dissolvent* of Silver; and has that Effect, in whatsoever Form applied: and Accordingly is the *Basis* of *Aqua fortis*. Spirit of Nitre added to that of Sea-Salt, makes it *dissolve* Gold the better : But Spirit of Sea-Salt added to Spirit of Nitre, disables it from having any Effect on Silver.

Mr. *Homberg*, however, in the Memoirs of the *French* Academy, furnishes an Instance of a *Dissolution* of Silver, made by the *Dissolvent* of Gold. An *Aqua Regia* may be composed of Spirit of Salt, and Spirit of Nitre, only in such small Quantity each, that they may float separately in a third Liquor, and not meet often enough to unite, at least not in any Quantity. This Water may be made so weak, as not to *dissolve* Gold, but only extract a slight yellow Tincture from it, that scarce takes off any thing of the Weight of the Metal : Nor will it dissolve Silver; as being too weak : So that both Metals are safe from it. But this *Aqua Regia*, after it has *dissolved* Gold as far as it can do, that is, after it has extracted a yellowish Tincture from it, is in a Condition to *dissolve* Silver.

This Phænomenon Mr. *Homberg* accounts for hence : That Spirit of Salt, whether alone, or joyn'd with Spirit of Nitre, being employ'd in keeping those few Particles of Gold dissolved; will not meddle with the Silver : Which by this means receiving the Impression of the greater Quantity of Spirit of Nitre alone, is *dissolved* thereby. But the Experiment cannot be inverted, *i.e. Aqua Regia* cannot begin with *dissolving* Silver lightly first, and afterwards *dissolve* Gold; by reason Spirit of Nitre does not hinder Spirit of Salt from acting on Gold; as Spirit of Salt does Spirit of Nitre from acting on Silver.

**DISSOLUTION**, in Physicks, a Discontinuation, or *Analysis* of the Structure of a mixt Body; whereby, what was one, and contiguous, is divided into little Parts, either homogeneous, or heterogeneous.

*Dissolution*, then, is a general Name for all Reductions of concrete Bodies into their smallest Parts, without any regard either to Solidity, or Fluidity : Tho' in the usual Acceptation of the Word among Authors, it is restrained to the Reduction of solid Bodies into a State of Fluidity; which is more properly expressed by *Solution*, as a Branch of *Dissolution*.

According to the opinion of Fr. *Tertius de Lanis*[1], now confirm'd by that of the Learned *Boerhaave*, in his Chymistry, the Power, or Faculty of *Dissolving*, is lodged in Fire alone.

Other Fluids, commonly supposed *Dissolvents*, only produce their Effect

[1] Francisco Tertius de Lanis, or Francesco Lana Terzi (1631 – 1687), an Italian mathematician and naturalist.

by means of the fiery *Spiculi* they abound withal. Even Air, which is judg'd a powerful *Menstruum*, owes all its Force to the Rays of Light diffused therein.

Sir *Isaac Newton* accounts for all *Dissolutions*, and the several Phaenomena thereof, from the great Principle of *Attraction*; And, in Effect, the Phaenomenon of *Dissolution* furnish a great Part of the Arguments and Considerations whereby he proves the Reality of that Principle.

A Specimen of that great Author's Way of Philosophizing on the Subject of *Dissolution* take as follows : When Salt of Tartar *dissolves* by lying in a moist Place, is not this done by an Attraction between the Particles of the Salt of Tartar, and those of the Water, which float in the Air in Form of Vapour? And why does not common Salt, or Salt-petre, or Vitriol do the like; but for Want of such an Attraction. And when *Aqua fortis*, or Spirit of Vitriol, pour'd on Steel-filings, *dissolves* the Filings, with a great Heat, and Ebullition; is not this Heat and Ebullition effected by the violent Motion of the Parts? And does not that Motion argue, that the acid Parts of the Liquor rush towards the Parts of the Metal with Violence, and run forcibly into its Pores; till getting between the outmost Particles, and the main Mass of Metal, they loosen 'em therefrom, and set 'em at Liberty to float off into the Water?

When a Solution of Iron in *Aqua fortis* dissolves *Lapis Calaminaris*, and let go the Iron; Or a Solution of Copper *dissolves* Iron immersed in, and lets go Copper; Or a Solution of Mercury in *Aqua fortis* pour'd on Iron, Copper, Tin, or Lead, *dissolves* the Metal, and lets go the Mercury; does not this argue, that the acid Particles of the *Aqua fortis* are attracted more strongly by the *Lapis Calaminaris*, than by the Iron; by Iron than by Copper; by Copper than by Silver; and by Iron, Copper, Tin, and Lead, than by Mercury? And is it not for the same reason, that iron requires more *Aqua fortis* to *dissolve* it, than Copper; and Copper more than the other Metals; And that of all Metals Iron is *dissolved* most easily, and is most apt to rust; and next after Iron, Copper?

When *Aqua fortis* dissolves Silver, and not Gold; and *Aqua Regia* dissolves Gold, and not Silver; may it not be said, that *Aqua fortis* is subtile enough to penetrate the Pores of Gold as well as of Silver, but wants the attractive Force to give it Entrance; and the same of *Aqua Regia*, and Silver? And when Metals are dissolved in acid *Menstruums*, and the Acids in Conjunction with the Metal, act after a different Manner; So as that the Taste of the Compound is milder than that of the Simples, and sometimes a sweet one; is it not because the Acids adhere to the Metallic Particles, and thereby lose much of their Activity? And if the Acid be in too small a Proportion to make the Compound dissoluble in Water; will it not, by adhering strongly to the Metal, become unactive, and lose its Taste; and the Compound become a tasteless Earth? For such Things as are not dissoluble by the Moisture of the Tongue, are insipid. *Newt. Opt. in Calce.*

Monsr. *Geoffroy* furnishes some curious Experiments on *Cold Dissolutions*, in the *Memoires de l'Academie Royale des Sciences*; which have been translated in the *Philosophical Transactions* : 'Tis nothing surprising, that a simple *Dissolution* should be cold; that common Water, for Instance, wherein Sea-Salt, or *Sal-Ammoniac*, or Vitriol, has been cast, should become the colder, by the Mixture of such Salts; It being obvious, that the Salts, being of themselves destitute of Motion, and coming to share that which the Fluidity gives the Water, must diminish it, when they become intimately mix'd therewith by Dissolution; And it is generally agreed among Philosophers, that Heat is a Motion, and Cold a Cessation, or at least a Diminution of Motion.

Yet, notwithstanding this general Principle; 'tis no great Wonder all *Dissolutions* are not Cold, as those are of all volatile Alcalies in common Water; But that some are Hot, as those of all fix'd Alcalies. The Difference may be accounted for hence, that all fix'd Alcalies having been calcined by a vehement Fire, they have been imprison'd, and retain'd in their Pores some of the Particles thereof.

But it is surprizing, that *Dissolutions* accompanied with Fermentation, *i.e.* where the Matters boil, and swell, and that with a great Noise, should be cold, and make the Thermometer fall, when immerged therein.

This Coldness, with so considerable an Augmentation of Motion, is somewhat extraordinary. But this is not all : For, of these cold Fermentations, there are some that emit hot Vapours. Thus it is, with a Mixture of Oil of Vitriol, and *Sal Ammoniac*; the first Thermometer being plunged in the Mixture, and another a little higher, to receive only the Fumes thereof; the first Thermometer is seen to fall very hastily, through the Coldness of Fermentation, and the latter to rise through the Heat of the Vapours. Monsr. *Geoffroy* adds an Experiment, shewing that cold Water is render'd still colder for a few Moments, by throwing a large Quantity of live Coals therein.

**DISSOLUTION**, in Chymistry, Pharmacy, &c. the Reduction of a compact, hard, or solid Body into a fluid State, by the action of some fluid *Menstruum*, or *Dissolvent*.

Dr. *Quincy* gives us a Mechanical Account of Dissolution, in the Instance of Salt *dissolved* in Water, which is the most simple Operation that falls under this Head. This Motion he ascribes to that attractive Force, which is so very extensive in Natural Philosophy, that there is no Kind of Matter, but what is under its Influence. It may be observed, that the Corpuscles of Salts, which are the most simple of any, are withal very minute, and for their Bulk very solid, and, therefore, exert a very strong attractive Force, which, *cæteris paribus*, is proportional to the Quantity of Matter. Hence it comes to pass, that the Particles of Water are more strongly attracted by the saline Particles, than they are by one another : The Particles of Water, therefore, cohering but loosely and being easily moveable, approach the Corpuscles of Salts, and run, as it were, into their Embraces; and the Motion of them is quicker, or slower, according to their less, or greater Distances; the attractive Force in all Bodies being strongest, at the Point of Contact.

Therefore, if Salt be thrown into the middle of a Dish full of Water, we shall find the aqueous Particles, which are in the middle of the Dish, sharp, and pungent to the Taste; but the Water upon the Sides of the Vessel almost insipid; so that, when such a Motion once arises, the aqueous Particles are carried with the same Force towards the Salts; and the Moment of them is to be estimated from the *Ratio* of their Weight, and Celerity, conjunctly. By the Force of this Impulse, they open to themselves a Passage into the Pores of the Salts, which are very numerous; and at length break, and divided their Texture, that all Cohesion of their Parts is destroyed : hereupon, being separated, and removed to a convenient Distance from one another, they are dispersed, and float here and their about the Water.

**DISSOLUTION** of the Blood, is an Affection of that Humour, directly opposite to Coagulation. The *Dissolution* is such a Comminution of the fibrous Parts of the Blood, as indisposes it for that Separation of the *Crassamentum* from the serous Part, which always ensues. in healthy Blood on its cooling out of the Body. This *Dissolution* is frequently the Consequence of malignant, and pestilential Fevers, and shews it self in *Petechiæ*, or Purple Spots; also of certain Poisons, particularly the Bites of venomous Beasts, &c.

**DISTICHIASIS**, in Medicine, a Disorder of the Eye-lids, wherein, instead of one, they have two rows of Cilia, or Hairs. In the *Distichiasis*, over the common, and natural Hairs, there grows another extraordinary Row, which frequently eradicates, and tears up the former, and pricking the Membrane, immediately investing the Eye, occasions Pain, and draws Defluxions upon it. 'Tis cur'd, by plucking up the second Row of Hairs with Nippers, and burning the Pores, out of which they issued. The Word is form'd of δις, *twice*, and ϛιχος, or ϛοιχος, *Order, Rank*.

**DISTILLATION**, or Destillation, in Chymistry, and Pharmacy, the Art, or Act of separating or drawing off the spirituous, aqueous, oleaginous, or saline Parts of a mix'd Body from the grosser, and more terrestrial Parts, by means of Fire; and collecting, and condensing them again by Cold.

The Use of *Distillation* is very great; it being by means hereof, that Waters, Spirits, Essences, and Extracts are chiefly made. *Distillation* is usually perform'd by means of Fire rais'd to a greater, or lesser Degree, as Circumstance least require.

The Fire is either applied immediately to the Vessels wherein the Matters are to be *distilled*; or it is applied mediately, by means of Water, Sand, Iron-filings, &c. These different Methods of applying the Fire, are call'd *Baths, Balnei*; *Balneum Mariæ*, or *Maris, Balneum Arenosum*, &c. They are also call'd Heats; as *Sand-heat, Water-heat*, &c.

*Distillation* is two-fold, 1. *Per Ascensum*, by *Ascent*; when the Matter to be *distill'd* is above the Fire, and the Spirit, or other Principle, is raised from it. 2. *Per Descentum*, by *Descent*; when the Matter which is to be *distill'd* is below the Fire, and the Vapour drawn from it, precipitated to the Bottom of the Vessel. Distillation *by Ascent*, is either *Right*, or *Oblique*.

*Right* Distillation, is perform'd with a common Alembick, or Cucurbite, wherein the Liquor is rais'd, and descends again, in Form of Drops, into a Receiver : And is chiefly us'd when the Texture if the Body is such as allows of an easy Ascent, as in Vegetables.

*Oblique* Distillation, is perform'd side-ways, and in crooked Vessels, as Retorts. Its Use is for such Bodies as consist of heavier Particles, and which cannot be raised without a strong Impulse, nor even by the strongest so high as the Top of the Alembick; of which Kind are almost all Minerals, and Metals.

Distillation *by Descent*, is where he Fire is apply'd on the Top, and all around the Vessel, whose Orifice is at the Bottom; and consequently, the Vapour not being able to rise upwards, it is forc'd to precipitate, and *distil* down to the Bottom.

There is a second Kind of *Distillation by Descent*, call'd *Per Deliquium*; which is a Natural Liquifying, or Resolving of Salts into a Liquor, by means of Moisture.

In the Resolution of Simples, an excellent Method to preserve their Virtues, is, in lieu of Fire, or any other foreign Heat, which might alter, or destroy these Virtues, to make Use of the Heat of a Dunghill made of putrified Herbs of the same Kind with those to be *distilled*.

The Process, and Measures of *Distillation*, are very different, according to the different Subjects to be *distill'd*.

*Acid Spirits* are usually drawn in the Reverberatory Furnace, and with a vehement Fire : *Ponderous Woods*, as Guaiacum, Box, Amber, &c. are *distill'd* in a Retort, after the same Manner. In these, first comes a little Phlegm, and then, the Fire increasing, the Spirits fly out in white Clouds. When they cease to come, the Matter in the Receiver is filtrated through a Tunnel, which lets pass the Spirits, leaving a black fetid Oil behind.

*Odoriferous Plants*, as Balm, Wormwood, Sage, Hyssop, &c. are *distill'd* by the Cucurbite, or *Vesica*; first pouring a strong Decoction of the same Plant hot, upon the Plant it self bruis'd, and letting the whole digest in a close Vessel two Days. Then about half the Water, or Spirit is drawn away by *Distillation*; and what remains, being press'd, filtrated, and evaporated to the Consistence of Honey, is the *Extract* of the Plant. Lastly, drying what remain'd in the Cloth after Expression, and burning it, they make a *Lixivium* of its Ashes; which being filtrated, and evaporated to Dryness, what remains is the fix'd Salt of the Plant.

*Plants not odoriferous*, are generally manag'd thus : The Plant being pounded, and two Thirds of the Alembic, or Retort fill'd with it, they pour a good Quantity of the express'd Juice of the same Plant upon it, so as the bruis'd Matter may float therein, without sticking any where to the Vessel. Then they draw off about half as much Water, as there was Juice, which is the *distill'd* Water of the Plant. What remains, being press'd in a Cloth, and the Juice settled, they filtrate, and evaporate it to two Thirds, and setting it in a cool Place, the *Essential Salt* shoots into Crystals.

There is also a Method of Distilling *Cold*; which is thus perform'd : They take, for Instance, 4 Pounds of Flowers, more or less, and put 'em in 3 or 4 Pints of Water, and the whole in a Capital, which they lute exactly; then they place the Alembick in a Vessel half fill'd with Ice, beaten and salted, as if they meant to freeze the Water; then sit on a Receiver, and lute it well; The wetting a linnen Cloth in hot Water, they cover the Capital therewith, repeating this several times: by which means the finest Parts are raised from the Flowers. But Care must be taken, that all the superfluous Water have been first emptied out of the Capital.

Dr. *Beal*[1], in the *Philosophical Transactions*, mentions an extraordinary Kind of *Cold Distillations*, *viz.* made by Frost and cold Air : His Thermometer

[1] This might be John Beale (ca. 1608 – 1683), an English clergyman and natural philosopher.

being exposed out of Doors, during the severe Frosts of 1665; fine clear Drops, like Dew, ascended to the Top of the Tube, which afterwards, in time, re-descended into the Stem, and fill'd the Space of half an Inch; which, tho' the Spirit of Wine it self was tinged very deep, yet this second Spirit was clearer and brighter than any Crystal. The like he did by Exposing his Thermometer to the hot Air in the middle of Summer. And hence takes Occasion to recommend a further Prosecution of this *Psychrotechnia.*

The Ascent of Fluids, we are taught by Philosophy, is effected two Ways : 1. On Account of their Specific Gravity; and 2. By Impulse.

The first Way of *Elevation* is manifest from this *Lemma, viz.* That Particles of Bodies which swim in any Fluid, if they are specifically lighter, must be born upwards by that Fluid. Hence, as *distilled* Liquors are carried upwards thro' the Air, it is to be inquired, how they come to be specifically lighter than Air.

Now, a Fluid will be specifically lighter than another, when, under a larger Surface, it has an equal, or a less Gravity : According to this Proportion, the Bulk of the Fluid ought to be increased in *Distillation*; and how easily, by the Help of Fire, it may be increased, or, which is the same Thing, rarefied, will appear from what we have said under the Articles Rarefaction, Heat, &c.

It is known by Computation, that the Proportion of the specific Gravity of Water to that of Air, is something more than 800 to 1. Since, therefore, similar Spheres, or Solids, are as the Cubes of their Diameters, and the specific Gravity decreases reciprocally, in the very same Proportion, as the Cubes of their Diameters increase : In order to make a Particle of Water lighter than a Particle of Air, no more is necessary than to rarefy it, till its Diameter becomes ten times greater, which in this Case is but a very small Degree of Rarefaction : for the Cube of the Diameter in a Particle so rarefied is 1000. If the Diameter be made 11 times greater, the Cube will be 1331; and if twelve, 1728. So that Water, when rarefied but 12 Degrees, will be above double lighter than Air. And if the Rarefaction be carried on farther, it may easily be collected from the Increase of the Numbers, that a Particle of Water may be render'd almost infinitely lighter than Air. Now, the elevation of Bodies equally fluid, and heavy, is always proportionable to their different Aptitude to be rarefied; that is, they ascend quicker, upon the Application of any Force, the more susceptible they are of Rarefaction : but in Bodies, whose Aptitude to rarefy is equal, the Time of Ascent is to be determined by their specific Gravity.

But 'tis not only specific Gravity that serves to elevate Bodies in *Distillation,* but an external Impulse may also cause their Ascent : The Impulse, we have here to do with, comes from the Fire, whose Particles, tho' extremely small and light, yet may raise Bodies much heavier than themselves, by acting upon them with a certain Degree of Force : For since the Moment of a Body, or that Force, by which it acts upon another, is in a compound *Ratio* of the Quantity of Matter, and Celerity; the Celerity may be so increased, as to give a sufficient Force to the Body, tho' the Quantity of Matter in it be ever so small. Let some heavy Body, therefore, be supposed to descend, with no other Moment than what it receives from its own Gravity; in this Case, then, the Air, which is much lighter, may be moved with such Celerity, as not only to sustain that Body, but to mount it up higher; and the more rapid the *Impetus* of the Air is, or the Surface of the Body more diffused, the higher and swifter will the Elevation be.

So Fire, tho' it be a Body of the minutest Size, may be moved with that Rapidity, as to acquire, the communicate what Force can be desired towards removing any Obstacles. When, therefore, the Moment of Fire is augmented in the manner explain'd, so as to exceed the Force of the *distill'd* Body, it will remove it from its former Situation; or what is here the same Thing, because the Direction of its Motion tends upwards, will carry it up. And thus, Particles specifically heavier than the Air contain'd in the Retort, as those of acid Spirits are, ascend by a more violent Impulse of the Fire us'd in *Distillation.*

Another Thing, to be noted is, That the same Quantity of Matter is elevated so much the easier, in Proportion, as the Surface is enlarged; for the more this is diffused, the more Particles of Fire it receives : having, therefore, this united Force to drive it up, it more easily ascends; so that, by the same Degree of Fire, Bodies will not equally arise, tho' they are equally heavy, if there be that Difference in their Surfaces, already supposed.

The Air also has no small Share in the Business of Impulse; for being rarefied by the Fire, it is not only impelled upwards it self, but carries other Particles up with it : and it may be learned by many very familiar Experiments, what *Impetus* Bodies so rarefied exert. Whosoever, therefore, well considers these three Things, *viz.* Specific Levity; an Impelling Force; and the Extent of Surface; and what may be effected by them, and how many Ways, and in what Proportions all of them may be changed, will very easily account for all the variety, which is found in the several Processes of *Distillation.*

**DISTORTION**, in Medicine. *Distortio Oris*, or *Distortion of the Mouth*, is a Contraction, or Shortening of one Side of the Mouth, occasion'd by a Convulsion, or a Palsy of the Muscles of one Side the Face. The *Greeks* call this Disorder σπασμος κυνικος.

When the *Distortion* arises from a Convulsion, it is on the same Side with the Convulsion, the Force of the convulsed Part being superior to that of the sound Part : On the contrary, when it arise from a Palsy, it is on the opposite Side, the paralytic Part being here surmounted by the sound.

In a *Distortion of the Mouth* the Patient can only spit on one Side; and if you make him laugh, or oblige him to pronounce the Letter O, you will easily perceive, that he only moves one Side of his Mouth.

There is also a *Distortion of the Eye*, call'd *Squinting*, or *Strabismus.*

**DISTRACTION**, in Medicine, the Act of pulling a Fibre, Membrane, or the like, beyond its natural Extent; and what is capable of this Enlargement, is said to be distractable.

**DIURESIS**, from δια, *per*, through, and ρεω, *fluo*, to flow; is us'd to express that Separation which is made of the Urine by the Kidneys : whence Diuretic.

**DIURETICKS**, in Medicine, are such Remedies as provoke, or promote the Discharge of Urine. Such as Water drank plentifully, white Wine drank in a

Morning; Alcali Salts of all Kinds; Sea-Salt, *Sal Gemmæ*, Nitre, Borax, Alumn, Tartar, Ammoniac, Whey, sour Milk, Lemmon Juice, &c.

Aqueous Liquors are generally *Diuretic*, especially of mix'd with Salt, and drunk cold. Fermented Liquors are the least *Diuretic* of all. And the less as they are the fatter. Sharp thin sour Wines, *Rhenish*, &c. as also acid Spirits of Vinegar, Salt, Sulphur, Alumn, Vitriol, &c. Asparagus, bitter Almonds, Smallage, Eryngium, Eupatorium, Sassafrass, &c. do the same.

**DORSIFEROUS**, or Dorsiparous Plants, are those of the Capillary Kind; which are without Stem, and bear their Seeds on the Backside of their Leaves.

**DOSE**, in Pharmacy, &c. the Quantity of any Medicine to be taken at one Time : Or the Weight, or Measure of the several Ingredients in a medicinal Comp-osition. The Word is form'd from the Greek δοσις, which signifies the same Thing. A Secret in Physic is nothing, unless the *Dose* be known. Authors, and Dispensatories, that describe the same Remedy, frequently the *Dose* is different; which occasions a great Difference in its Effect.

**DOUBLE** *Vessel*, in Chymistry, is when the Neck of one Bolt-Head, or Matrass, is put, and well luted into the Neck of another. It is also call'd a Pellican.

**DRACHM**, is also a Weight, us'd by our Physicians; containing just sixty Grains; or 3 Scruples; or the 8th Part of an Ounce. In Averdupois Weight, the Drachm is an 8th Part of an Ounce.

**DRACUNCULI**, in Medicine, a Disease in Children, wherein they feel a vehement Itching; supposed to arise from little Worms, call'd *Dracunculi*, generated from a viscid Humour under the Skin, about the Back, Shoulders, and Arms.

Children seiz'd with the *Dracunculi*, become hectic, and scarce receive any Nourishment at all, tho' they eat plentifully.

The Disease, however, is not so peculiar to Children, but that grown Persons have been sometimes affected with it. The Emperor *Henry* V is said, to have died of it; having had it from his Birth.

The Women in *Poland* cure their Children of the *Dracunculi*, after the following Manner : The Child is wash'd and bathed in hot Water, wherein a Quantity of crum'd Bread, and a handful of Ashes have been cast. The Water being pour'd off, and the Bread gather'd into a Mass; when they come to break it again the next Day, they find in it an infinite Quantity of fine Hairs, which some call *Dog's Hairs*, and others, *Worms*; and 'tis those Hairs, or Worms, are supposed to be the Cause of the Disease.

After thus bathing the Children, they rub their Shoulders, and Arms, with Flower steep'd in Vinegar, or Honey; upon which immediately arises on the Skin a great Number of Tubercles, like Poppy-Seeds; supposed to be the Heads of Worms. These they scrape off as fast as they appear; otherwise they withdraw beneath the Skin again. The Operation is repeated till such Time as no more Tubercles arise.

The *Dracunculi* is a Disease little known in *England*. The Editors of the

*Leipsic* Acts, speaking of it, in the Tome for the Month of *October* 1682, call the Bodies, which put forth at the Pores after bathing, thick hairs, *Corpuscula Pilorum crassiorum instar densa & spissa*, and not *fine slender Hair*, as *Degori* calls 'em. They add, that these little Corpuscles are hence call'd *Crinones*; and by reason of their devouring the Food, which should nourish the Children, *Comedones*.

*Velchius*, in a curious Dissertation on the Subject, call's 'em *Capillary Worms. Exercitatio de Vermibus Capillaribus Infantum.*

As to the Nature and Figure of these little Bodies, the same Editors observe, that the Microscope has put it past doubt, they are real living Animals, of an ash Colour, having two long Horns, two large round Eyes, and a long Tail terminated with a Tuft of Hair; that 'tis difficult to draw them out whole, by scrapping the Child's Body, in that being very soft, the least rubbing bruises 'em, and breaks 'em.

**DRAGON'S BLOOD**. *Sanguis Draconis*, call'd also *Lapathum rubrum*, in Medicine.

The Ancients had a Notion, that the *Dragon* fighting with the Elephant, suck'd all its Blood through its Eyes and Ears; that the Elephant falling down dead, crush'd the *Dragon*; and that from their Blood, thus mix'd on the Ground, arose what they call'd *Dragon's Blood*, which they held in high Esteem. This is the Account given by *Solinus, Pliny, Isidore*, and others after them; but this Combat is mere Fable, invented by the Merchants. *Avicenna*, and *Serapion* likewise give the Appellation Dragon's Blood to Cinnabar.

But the genuine *Dragon's Blood* is the Juice, or Resin of a large Tree, call'd *Draco, Dragon*, growing in *Africa*, and *America*. The Resin is of a dark red, and easily dissolves when brought towards the Fire : if cast into the Fire, it flames : But dissolves with much Difficulty in any Liquor.

It is a good Astringent; and is us'd in Hæmorrhage's, and Dysenteries, to fasten the Teeth, and strengthen the Gums.

There is also a counterfeit *Dragon's Blood*, made of the Gum of the Cherry, or Almond-Tree, dissolved, and boil'd in a Tincture of *Brazil* Wood; but this is of no Use, except for outward Diseases of Horses.

It derives its Name *Dragon's Blood* from the Redness of its Colour, and gives its Name *Dragon* to the Tree that yields it. Some Botanists talk of the Figure of a *Dragon*, finely represented under the Rind of the Fruit of the Tree. But this is a mere Fiction.

**DROPAX**, in Pharmacy, an external Medicine, in Form of a Plaster, us'd to take off the Hairs from any Part. The Word is form'd from the *Greek* δρεπειν, *to pluck, to tear*.

The *Dropax* is of two Kinds, *Simple*, and *Compound*. The *Simple* is made of an Ounce of dry Pitch, and two Drachms of Oil. The *Compound* is made with Pitch, Wax, Colophony, common Bitumen, *Sulphur vivum*, Pepper, Euphorbium, Cantharides, and Castor. There are also other Ways of making it.

It was anciently much in Use to warm the Parts, to draw the Blood and Spirits to them, and to cure Atrophies. It was applied hot on the Part affected, after first shaving it; and was pull'd off again 'ere quite cold, then heated a-fresh, and applied again; and the Operation thus repeated, till the Part were render'd very red.

**DROPS**, in Medicine, a liquid Medicine, whose Dose is estimated by a certain Number of *Drops*.

A little Lowness of Spirits, says Dr. *Cheyne*, speaking of the softer Sex under Fits of the Vapours, &c. requires *Drops* which pass readily down under the Notion of Physic : *Drops* beget Drams, and Drams, beget more Drams, till they come to be without Weight, and without Measure. Higher, and more sever Fits, begot by these, bring forth farther Necessity upon Necessity of *Drops*, Drams, and Gills, till at last, &c. *Essay on Health*.

*English* Drops, or *Volatile English* Drops, or *Guttæ Anglicanæ*, is a Liquor drawn by Fire from a great Number of Ingredients, and found a powerful Remedy against Coagulations of the Blood, Obstructions, Apoplexies, malignant Fevers, Small-pox, &c.

Its Inventor was Dr. *Goddard*[1], a Physician of *London*. King *Charles* II had much ado to purchase the Secret of him, tho' he offer'd him 5000 Pounds for the same. However, he prevail'd at length; but the Physician look'd on it as a Favour done the Prince, to impart it to him on such Terms. Hence it is, that the Remedy took the Name of *Guttæ Anglicanæ*.

**DROPSY**, Hydrops, in Medicine, a Disease occasion'd by a praetor-natural Collection of Serum, or Water, in some Part of the Body; Or a too great Proportion thereof in the Blood. The Word is derived from the *Greek* υδωρ, *Water*, and οψς, *Facies*, Face.

The *Dropsy* acquires different Names from the different Parts it afflicts, or the different Parts the Waters are collected in. That of the Abdomen, or lower Belly, call'd simply and absolutely *Dropsy*, is particularly denominated *Ascites* : That of the whole Habit of the Body, *Anasarca*, or *Leucophlegmatia*: That of the Head, *Hydrocephalus* : That of the Scrotum, *Hydrocele*.

There is also a Species of this Disease cause, instead of Water, by a Collection of Wind, call'd *Tympanites*, and by *Hippocrates*, the *Dry Dropsy*.

There are also *Dropsies of the Breast, Pericardium, Uterus, Ovaries*, &c.

The Causes of *Dropsies*, in general, are whatever may obstruct the serous Part of the Blood, so as to make it stagnate in the Vessels; Or burst the Vessels themselves, so as to let the Blood out among the Membranes; Or weaken, and relax the Tone of the Vessels; Or thin the Blood, and make it watery; or lessen Perspiration.

These Causes are various, *viz*. sometimes acute Diseases, schirrous Tumors of any of the more noble Viscera, excessive Evacuations, particularly Hæmorrhages, hard Drinking, &c.

The *Ascites*, or *Water-Dropsy* of the Abdomen, is the most usual Case, and what we particularly call the *Dropsy* : Its Symptoms are Tumors, first of the

[1] Jonathan Goddard (1617 – 1675), an English physician.

Feet and Legs, and afterwards of the Abdomen, which keep continually growing; and if the Belly be struck, or shook, there is heard a Quashing of Water. Add to this three other Attendants, *viz. a Dyspnæa*; intense thirst; and sparing Urine : with which may be number'd Heaviness, Listlesness, Costiveness, a light Fever, and an Emaciation of the Body.

The Curative Indications are two, viz. The Evacuation of the Water; and the Strengthening of the Blood, and Viscera. The first is effected by strong Purgatives, particularly *Elaterium*,, and *Crocus Metallorum*. For such as are too weak to bear Purgatives, Dr. *Sydenham* recommends Emeticks, whereof the best are those of Lixivial Salts. *Etmuller* prefers Diureticks to either Kind. Along with the Evacuants are to be used Stomachicks, especially *Absynthium*, *Marrhubium*, &c.

Where other means fail for Evacuating the Water, Recourse is had to the Paracentæsis, or Operation of Tapping.

*Mayerne*[1] recommends *Mercurius dulcis*, and Nitre, and Ants Eggs, for the promoting of Urine, and draining the Tumour. As for the Viscera, they are restored by Chalybeats, and Strengtheners.

*Baglivi* notes, that in a *Dropsy* arising from a morbid Liver, there is always a vehement dry Cough : which is never observed in the Species. *Tycho Brahe*[2] observes, that Hydropic Patients usually die about full Moon. *Wainwright* extols an Infusion of Green Tea in *Rhenish* Wine; as also Briony Juice, as excellent in this Disease.

**DULCIFYING**, the Sweetening of any Thing : a Tem used in Physick, for rendering a Fluid less acid, and rough, either by taking away its Salts, or breaking their Points, or covering 'em with something smooth, and soft.

**DYSENTERY**, or Dyssentery, in Medicine, a bloody *Diarrhæa*; or a Flux of Blood by Stool; attended with Pains and Griping.

The Word *Dysentery* is form'd from the *Greek* δυς, *difficulty*, and εντερον, *Intestine*; and properly signifies that Kind of Flux of the Belly, characterized by the Frequency of Stools, or Dejections, mix'd with Blood, and accompanied with Gripes : The Fever, Ulcer, &c. which attend it, are not essential to the Disease; tho' many, both of the Ancients and Moderns, think the Ulcer is.

The *Dysentery*, *Sydenham* observes, begins with a Chilness, and Shiverings; which is followed by a Heat; then Gripings of the Belly ensure, with mucous, or sanious Stools, which in Progress of Time are found interspers'd with Streaks of Blood, with vehement Pain.

The Stools are sometimes void of Blood; and yet, if they be frequent, and attended with Gripes, and a mucous *Colluvies*, the same Author says, it is a proper *Dysentery*.

Along with the Excrements, beside a whitish Mucosity, frequently come Scrapings of the Guts, in the Form of little Skins. If pure Blood be evacuated, the Patient's Life is in great Danger.

[1] Theodore de Mayerne (1573 – 1655), a Swiss physician.

[2] Tyge Ottesen Brahe (1546 – 1601), a Danish astronomer and alchemist.

*Etmuller* makes three Kinds of *Dysenteries* : 1. When a laudable Blood is evacuated, from a mere *Plethora*, or Plenitude, without any Disorder of the Intestines; as in the *Hemorrhoidal Flux*. 2. When a thin, watery Blood is evacuated, call'd the Hepatic Flux, tho' really arising from the Hemorrhoidal Vessels.

The third Kind, which is that we properly call Dysentery, is, when Blood is cast out mix'd with a purulent Matter in the Excrements.

This is either *benign*, i.e. without a Fever, and not contagious; Or *malignant*, which is attended with a pestilential Fever; and frequently ravages whole Cities, and Provinces : Happening most commonly in Armies. In the last Stage, a Sort of Caruncles are frequently ejected along with the purulent Matter, which are difficult to be accounted for, unless from an Excoriation, and Ulceration of the Intestines. Sometimes the Intestines are even gangreen'd.

The next Cause of the *Dysentery*, as assign'd by some Physicians, is a serous, or other morbid Humour, mix'd with the Mass of Blood; the Consequence of which is a too great Fermentation in the Blood, and a Dissolution of its Parts, which are thus render'd too liquid. The second Cause is a Vellication, and Irritation of the nervous Fibres of the Intestines, occasion'd by sharp, acid Humours separated from the Blood; which occasion the Spiral Fibres, that produce the Peristaltic Motion of the Guts, to move too fast, and thus to expel the Matters to hastily out of the Intestines. The Mediate Cause, in the Physicians Language, is some foreign Body adhering strongly to the Intestines, and by its sharp Points, vellicating the nervous Fibres of the Intestines, and at length ulcerating 'em. The Remote Causes are any Thing that corrupts the Mass of Blood, as viscid, and crude, sharp Juices; ill Foods; Autumnal Fruits; Grapes; new Wine drunk in Excess; Poisons; violent Medicines; Waters convey'd through leaden Pipes; Rainy Weather in the Spring, with a dry Winter, and a hot Summer, and Autumn.

The Seat of the Disease is in the Intestines, either the big, or the small, or both: When the Disease is in the small Ones, the Gripes begin long before the Stools, and are felt about the Navel; and the Blood, and Excrements, are more blended; as being longer together. When the larger Intestines are seiz'd, the Pain is less vehement, and is felt lower, &c.

Purgatives have rarely any good Effect in *Dysenteries*; as increasing the Fermentation of the Blood, and irritating the Fibres of the Intestines more and more. Nor are Emeticks much better; as tending to draw the peccant Humours into the Stomach, or at least into the higher Intestines, and cause more frequent Stools.

*Ipecacuanha*, however, is excellent on this Occasion : Not so much as a Vomitory, Dr. *Friend* observes, as a Sudorific; having this Faculty, beyond all other Emeticks, that it corrects the *Dysenteric* Ferment, in Proportion as it evacuates it. In the *Philosophical Transactions* we have an express Discourse on the Subject; where it is asserted to be infallible in all *Dysenteries*, and Loosenesses, how dangerous and inveterate soever; except in Pulmonic and Hydropic Patients, whose Fluxes are Indications of approaching Death.

*Sydenham* commends Phlebotomy : But *Willis* says, no Evacuation is good: and prescribes hot Cardiacks, as Spirit of Wine a little burnt, &c.

Balsamic, and Styptic Medicines are also to be used, according to the divers Causes, and Symptoms of the Disease.

*Borre*, in a Letter to *Bartholin*, affirms, there is not better Medicament in *Dysenteries* than Rose-Water wherein Gold has been extinguish'd.

*Dotæus* relates, that he cured above an hundred Persons with Oil of sweet Almonds, mix'd with Orange Juice.

**DYSPEPSY**, in Medicine, a Difficulty, or Weakness of Digestion. The Dyspepsy may arise from the Softness of the Ferment of the Stomach, or its being sparing in Quantity; from a Relaxation of the Fibres of the Stomach; the Want of a proper Heat in the Stomach, &c. Bitters, and Sub-astringents, are its proper Remedy. The Word is form'd from the *Greek* δυς, *difficulty*, and πεπτειν, *coquere*, to concoct.

**DYSPNOEA**, in Medicine, a Difficulty of breathing. The *Dyspnœa* admits of three Degrees : A *Short-Breath*; an *Asthma*; and on *Orthophnaea*. The *Short-Breath*, is the first, and lightest degree. The *Asthma* is more violent, accompanied with a wheezing. See Asthma.

The *Orthophnæa* is the highest of all; the Patient affected therewith not being able to lye down, but oblig'd to keep erect, without which he could not respire.

The most usual Causes of *Dyspnœa* are Phlegms contain'd in the Bronchia; or the too strong Constitution of the Bronchia themselves, which prevent the easy Ingress of the Air into the Lungs.

The Word is form'd from the *Greek* δυς, *difficulty*, and πνεω, *I breathe*,

**DYSURIA**, in Medicine, a Difficulty of making Urine, accompanied with Pain, and a Sense of Heat. It is also call'd *Ardor Urinæ*, by reason the Urine seems to burn the *Urethra*, as it issues forth. The Word is form'd from the *Greek* δυς, *difficulty*, and ουρειν, *to make Urine*.

The *Dysuria* differs chiefly from the *Strangury* in this, that in the Strangury, the Urine only oozes out, as it were, Drop by Drop; whereas in the *Dysuria* it streams out without Interruption, and frequently in the proper Quantity.

The ordinary Causes of the *Dysuria*, are the Acrimony, or Sharpness of the Urine; and the Excoriation, or Exulceration of the Neck of the Bladder, or the Urinary Passage.

**EARTH**, *Terra*, in Natural Philosophy, one of the four Vulgar, or Peripatetical Elements; defined, a simple, dry and cold Substance; and as such, an Ingredient on the Composition of all Natural Bodies. It should be well observed, that the Element *Earth* is a very different Matter from the *Earth* whereon we tread : *Aristotle* having laid down *cold* and *dry* as his first Element; to give it a suitable Name, look'd among the divers Bodies, for that which should come the nearest thereto; which being *Earth*, he gave his first Element that Denomination : Tho', thus borrowing a Word, that had been used for a different Thing, occasioned a great Part of his Followers to run into an extravagant Error, and to suppose, that this habitable fossil *Earth*, was an Element.

**EARTH**, in Chymistry, is the fourth of the Chymical Elements, or Principles, into which all Bodies are resolvable by Fire. After drawing off the Spirit, Sulphur, and Phlegm, *e.gr.* of Wine, what remains in the Retort, is a tasteless, smell-less, dusty Matter, not capable either of being rais'd by Distillation, or dissolved by Solution, and called Earth, or *Terra damnata*, or *Caput Mortuum*. This *Earth* is supposed to be the Basis, or Substratum of all Bodies; and that, wherein the other Principles reside. 'Tis all that is solid, *e.gr.* in an Animal or Vegetable Body, *i.e.* all the Vascular Part; the rest being Juices.

**EARTH**, in Natural History, is a fossil, or terrestrial Matter, whereof our Globe principally consists; whose Character is to be neither dissoluble by Fire, Water, nor Air; not transparent, more fusible than Stone, and generally containing some Degree of Fatness.

Of such *Earth*, some is Simple, and Immutable; other, Compound, and Fatty. Of the first Kind is *Chalk*, *Pumice*, and *Rotten-stone*; of the Second, or Compound *Earths*, are *Boles* of all Kinds, red, white, and brown; *Fullers Earth*, the divers Kinds of *Medicinal Earth*, as the *Cretica*, *Hungarica*, *Turcica*, *Suecica*, *Lemnian Earth*, *Malta Earth*, *Terra Sigillata*, &c. To this Class are likewise referred *Argillæ*, or *Clay Earth*, form'd into Potters Ware.

These *Earths* are all resolvible into an Oil, a little Acid Salt, &c. and a Calx, which is the Basis, or the *Earth* properly so call'd.

Naturalists generally rank *Sand* as a Species of *Earth*; tho' with no great Propriety. Sands being, in Strictness, a Sort of Crystals, or little transparent Pebbles, calcinable, and by the Addition of a fix'd alkaline Salt, fusible, and convertible into Glass : And therefore properly reducible to the Class of Stones.

By means of Sand it is, that the fatty *Earth* is render'd fertile, and fit to seed Vegetables, &c. For pure *Earth* is liable to coalesce into a hard coherent Mass, as in Clay; and *Earth* thus imbodied, and as it were glued together, would be very unfit to nourish Plants. But if with such Earth, Sand, *i.e.* hard Crystals which are indissoluble in Water, and still retain their Figure, be intermix'd, they will keep the Pores of the *Earth* open, and the *Earth* it self loose and incompact, and by that Means give room for the Juices to move, ascend, &c. and for plants to be nourished thereby. Thus a Vegetable, planted either in the Sand alone, or in a the fat Glebe and *Earth* alone, receives no

Growth or Increase; but is either starved or suffocated : But mix the two, and the Mass becomes fertile. In Effect, by Means of Sand, the *Earth* is render'd in some Measure Organical; by preserving a Sort of Pores, and Interstices therein, somewhat analogous to Vessels is effected; by which the Juices of the *Earth* may be convey'd, prepared, digested, circulated, and at length excreted and thrown off into the Roots of Plants.

**EBONY**, in Natural History, a Kind of *Wood*, brought from the *Indies*, exceedingly hard and heavy, and taking a very fine Polish; and on that account, used in *Mosaic* and Inlaid Works, Toys, &c. There are divers Kinds of *Ebony*; the most usual among us are *black, red*, and *green*; all of them the Product of the Island of *Madagascar*, where the Natives call them indifferently, *Hazon Mainthis*, q.d. *black Wood*. That of St. *Maurice*, belonging to the *Dutch*, likewise furnishes Part of the *Ebonies* used in *Europe*.

Authors, and Travellers, give very different Accounts of the Tree that yields the *black Ebony* : By some of their Descriptions it should be a Sort of Palm Tree, by others a Cytisus, &c. The most authentick of them, is that of Mons. *Flacourt*, who resided many Years in *Madagascar* as Governor thereof. He assures us that it grows very high, and big; its Bark black, and its Leaves resembling those of our Myrtle, of a deep, dusky, green Colour.

*Tavernier* assures us, that the Islanders take Care to bury their Trees, when cut down, to make the blacker. F. *Plumier* mentions another *black Ebony* Tree, discovered by him at St. *Domingo*, which he calls *Spartium portulacæ foliis aculeatum Ebeni materiæ. Candia* also bears a little Shrub, known to the Botanists, under the Name of *Ebenus Cretica*.

*Pliny* and *Dioscorides* say, the best *Ebony* comes from *Ethiopia*, and the worst from *India*; but *Theophrastus* prefers that of *India*. *Black Ebony* is much preferr'd to the other Colours. The best is a jet black, free of Veins, and Rind, vary massive, astringent, and of a sharp pungent Taste.

Its Rind infused in Water, is said to purge Pituita, and cure Venereal Disorders; whence *Matthiolus* took *Guaiacum* for a Sort of Ebony. It yields an agreeable Perfume, when laid on the Coals : When green, it readily takes Fire, from the Abundance of its Fat. If rubbed against a Stone, it becomes brown. The *Indians* make Statues of their Gods, and Sceptres for their Princes, of this Wood. It was first brought to *Rome* by *Pompey*, after his subduing *Mithridates*. 'Tis now much less used among us, than antiently; since the Discovery of so many Ways of giving other hard Woods a black Colour.

As to *green Ebony*, besides *Madagascar*, and St. *Maurice*, it likewise grows in the *Antilles*, and especially in the Isle of *Tobago*. The Tree that yields it is very bushy, its Leaves smooth, and of a fine green Colour. Beneath its Bark is a white Rind about two Inches thick; all beneath which, to the very Heart, is a deep green, approaching towards a black; tho', sometimes, streaked with yellow Veins. Its Use is not confined to Mosaic Work : 'Tis likewise good in dying, as yielding a fine green Tincture. As to *red Ebony*, called also *Grenadilla*, we know little of it more than the Name.

The Cabinet makers, Inlayers, *&c.* make *Pear Tree*, and other Woods, pass for *Ebony*, by *Ebonising*, giving it the black Colour thereof. This, some do, by a few Washes of a hot decoction of Galls, and when dry, adding Writing Ink thereon, and polishing it with a stiff Brush, and a little hot Wax. Others heat, or burn their Wood black.

**EBULLITION**, in Physicks, the Act of *Boiling*; or, a vehement Agitation of the Parts of a Fluid, produced by Fire. Philosophers are disagreed about the Cause and manner of *Ebullition*. Some account for it from an Attenuation of the Particles of the Fluid, at the Bottom of the Vessel; which, by being attenuated, become lighter, and heave upwards against the super-incumbent Load : Others, from the Particles of Fire mixing with, and dilating the Particles of Fluid, and so rendering them specifically lighter : And others, not from any Attenuation, nor even Rarefaction of the Particles of the Fluid by the Action of Heat; but from a Rarefaction of the Air pent up, and intermix'd with the Fluid; which coming to expand, tends upwards against the Pressure of the less heated, less rarified Part of the Fluid.

**EBULLITION**, in Chymistry, &c., is also used for a violent intestine Motion, or Colluctation of Parts, occasion'd by the Mixture of Salts of different Names. Dr. *Harris*[1] will have it properly, and immediately, to signifie that particular Struggle, or Effervescence, arising upon the mingling together of an acid and alcalisate Liquor.

Mr. *Boyle* has an Experiment to shew, that a considerable *Ebullition* may be produced by such a Mixture without the Bodies acquiring any Heat; nay, that a Degree of Cold may be produced greater than was in either of the Bodies singly; tho' accompanied with a great Struggle, Tumult, Noise, and Froth. For having shook one Part of Oil of Vitriol, into 12 Parts of common Water, the Mixture was at first sensibly warm : Then, the Ball of a Thermometer was placed in it, till the included Spirit had gain'd the Temperature of the Mixture; but then a convenient Quantity of Volatile Salt of *Sal Armoniac*, being gradually put in to satiate the acid Spirits of the Mixture, the Spirit in the Thermometer descended above an Inch.

**ECCANTHIS**, or Eckantis, in Medicine, is a Disease of the Eyes. The *Eccanthis*, or *Eckantis*, is properly a fleshy Excrescence, in the *Canthus*, or Angle of the Eye; thus call'd from the *Greek*, εγκανθις, which signifies the same Thing.

**ECCHYMOSIS**, from εκχυω, *effundo*, to pour out, and αγμα, *Sanguis*, Blood, signifies those livid Spots, or Blotches, in the Skin, which are made by extravasated Blood : The same with *Ecchymoma*.

**ECCOPROTICKS**, in Medicine, Laxative, or loosening Remedies, which purge gently, by softening the Humours and Excrements, and fitting them for Expulsion. The Word is composed of the *Greek* Particle εκ, and κοπρος, *Excrement*.

**ECHINATE** *Seeds*, as such as are prickly and rough like the Coat of a Chestnut; or, as some say, like the Skin of a Hedge-Hog.

[1] This is probably Walter Harris (1647 – 1732), English physician to Charles II and William III.

**ECHYMOSIS**, or Ecchymosis, in Medicine, *Suffusio*, a Disease of the Eye; wherein the Blood, extravasated by some Blow, or Contusion, upon its Arrival between the Cutis, and the Flesh or Muscles, stops there, without any Appearance of a Wound. The *Echymosis* is either *simple*, or with *Abcess*. The Word is form'd of the *Greek*, εκχυμοσις, Effusions of Humours, των χυμων.

**ECLEGMA**, in Medicine, a Pectoral Remedy, of the Consistence of a thick Syrup; called also *Lohoch*, *Linctus*, and *Lambative*. There are *Eclegma's* of Poppy, others of Lentils, others of Squillæ, &c. The Intention is to heal, or ease the Lungs in Coughs, Peripneumonies, &c. and are usually composed of Oils, incorporated with Syrups.

The Word is form'd of the Greek εκ, and λειχειν, to lick; by Reason the Patient is to take it by licking it off the End of a Liquorice Stick dipt therein : To the End that being taken thus by little and little, it may remain the longer in the Passage, and moisten the Breast the better.

**ECPHRACTICKS**, in Medicine, such Remedies as have Faculty of opening, and unstopping the Vessels, through which the Humours are to pass : Or which incide, and attenuate tough, viscid Humours, and thereby promote their Discharge. The same with Apperients and Deobstruents.

The chief simple Ecphracticks, are the little Centaureum, Worm-wood, Agremony, Hyssop, Chamaedris, Bark of Tamarisk, Roots of Capers, Scolopendrium, &c.

The Word is form'd from the Greek εκφραοτειν, to free from Obstruction; of εκ, and φραοτω, obstruo, sepio.

**ECTHYMOSIS**, in Medicine, a vehement Agitation and Dilatation of the Blood; such as happens in extraordinary Emotions of Joy. The Word is form'd of εκ, *ex*, and θυος, *Animus*, Mind.

**ECTROPIUM**, in Medicine, a Disease of the Eyes, consisting in a Sort of Inversion of the lower Eye-lid, which disables it from covering its Part of the Eye. The Word is Greek, εκτροπιον

**ECTYLOTICKS**, Remedies proper to consume, and eat off Callus's, Warts, and other Excrescences, form'd on the Flesh. The Word is form'd of εκ and τυλom, *Callus*.

**EDULCORATION**, in Pharmacy, is the *dulcifying*, or *sweetening* of any Remedy, by Means of Sugar, or Syrups.

**EDULCORATION**, in Chymistry, is the *sweetening*, or purging any Thing of its Salts, &c. by repeated Lotions, or Washings in Cold Water; *e.gr.* the freeing of Precipitates of Mercury, Metals, &c. of the sharp Slats by Means whereof they had been dissolved; or which had been mingled with them, to effect a Dissolution.

**EFFERVESCENCE**, is popularly used for a light Ebullition, or a strong intestine Motion, produced in a Liquor, by the first Action of Heat, without any notable Separation of its Parts. Such a Liquor must be heated to a slight *Effervescence.*

**EFFERVESCENCE**, in Physicks, Chymistry, &c. is not applied to any Ebullitions, or Motions produced by Fire; but only to those resulting from the Mixture of Bodies of different Natures, which by their acting on one another, occasion a Heat, or at least an Agitation of Parts, resembling the Ebullition, or boiling produced by Fire.

Acids mix'd with Alkalies, *e.gr.* Oil of Tartar, and Spirit of Vitriol, produces an *Effervescence*, &c.

*Chauvin* defines *Effervescence* more scientifically, to be a violent Expulsion of the Air, out of the Pores of the Particles of one Body, by the Intrusion of the Particles of another Body mix'd therewith, into those Pores before possess'd by Air.

In Order for *Effervescence* to take Place, the Particles of the latter Body must be supposed conformable, both in Bulk and Figure to the Pores of the other; so as they may enter, and fill the same, like Wedges, : And beside, a strong Degree of Attraction between the Particles of the two Bodies, stronger than the Attraction, or Force of Cohesion, between the Particles of either of the Bodies alone.

Hence it should seem, that *Effervescence* only differs from Fermentation, in the Degree of Explosion; which in *Effervescences*, by Reason of the greater Purity and Freedom of the Acid and Alkali, is greater than in Fermentations.

Of *Effervescences*, some are *hot*, and others *cold*. Of the first Kind, are those produced by the Mixture of Oil of Tartar *per deliquium*, with Spirit of Vitriol; Quicklime with cold Water; all acid Spirits, with alkaline, or earthy Bodies; *Aqua fortis*, Spirit of Vitriol, Spirit of Nitre, *Aqua Regia*, &c. with all Metallic Bodies, Marcasites and Minerals; Coral with Lemmon, or Orange Juice; Marble with Spirit of Salt; Hartshorn, Chalk, Boars Tooth, Crabs Eyes, Mother of Pearl, and all Shells with Acids. In all which, the *Effervescences* are attended with a pretty intense Heat. Oil of Vitriol, and Oil of Turpentine, particularly, mix'd together, produce such a vehement Heat, that unless they be mix'd Drop by Drop, they are apt to burst forth into Flame, and break the Vial.

On the contrary, Silver-filings being dissolved in Spirit of Nitre, produce a cold *Effervescence*, which, instead of Heating, cools the Glass, so as to render it painful to the Sense of feeling.

This different Effect is ascribed to this, that in the former Case, the mix'd Bodies, one or both of them, abound with Sulphur; but not in the latter. Not but some attribute the Heat, usual in *Effervescences*, to the vehement Friction, and Collision of the particles against each other.

Powder'd Coral, mixt with distill'd Vinegar, produces a cold *Effervescence*, which the same Philosophers account for hence, that the Pores of the Coral being very great, it may be easily dissolved n the acid Spirit, without any great Friction, or Collision of the Parts, such as would be necessary to generate any considerate Heat.

An *Effervescence* may also be produced by the Mixture of two cold Liquors.

**EFFLORESCENCE**, a breaking out of some Humours in the Skin; as in the Measles, and the like.

**EFFLUVIUM**, a Flux, or Exhalation of minute Particles from any Body : Or an Emanation of subtle Corpuscles, from a mix'd, sensible Body, by a Kind of Motion of Transpiration.

That there are such *Effluvia*, continually emitted from all Bodies, is pretty certain : Thus, if a Body be immerged in Water, or any other humid Matter, there are little Bubbles continually transmitted therefrom to the Surface of the Water; which are supposed to be nothing else but little Particles, detach'd from the solid Body; and which, when they arrive at the Surface, emerge in Form of Bubbles. And this a Body, placed in the Receiver of an Air-Pump, is seen, as it were, in a Kind of Effervescence, by reason of the external Particles continually flowing from the same.

The School of Philosophers hold these *Effluvia* to be intentional Qualities, as they call them, and nothing substantial; but the Moderns laugh at the Notion as finding that these *Effluvia* refresh and nourish both the Animal and Vital Spirits.

Odoriferous Bodies, every Body knows, are continually emitting substantial *Effluvia*; by Means whereof it is, that they excite in us the Sense of *Smelling*. These minute *Effluvia* are sometimes perceived by the Eye, in Fumes and Vapours. Some Bodies are found to emit *Effluvia* for a great Number of Years, without any considerable Lose, either as to Bulk or Weight; as Magnets, Electrical Bodies, Ambers, divers odorous Bodies, &c. The Tenuity of whose emanant Corpuscles is incredible : Not but that the Loss they sustain by the continual Emission of *Effluvia*, may be made up to them by the Reception of other similar *Effluvia* of the same Kinds of Bodies, diffuses tho' the Air.

'Tis added, that these *Effluvia* are emitted in Manner of Radii, Rays, *in Orbem*, and that the Circumference or Bound of Activity of the Radiation, exhibits the same Figure as is that of the Radiant. This the Astronomers sufficiently prove, from the Ratio of the Refraction of the Atmosphere. For the Law of the Emission of these *Effluvia*.

That *Effluvia* may considerably operate upon, and have great Effect on Bodies within the Sphere of their Activity, is proved by Mr. *Boyle*, in an express Treatise on the *Subtility of Effluvia*; where he shews,

1. That the Number of Corpuscles, emitted by Way of *Effluvia*, is immensely great.

2. That they are of a very penetrating Nature.

3. That they move with vast Celerity, and in all Manner of Directions.

4. That there is frequently a very wonderful Congruity, or Incongruity in the Bulk and Shape of these *Effluvia* , with the Pores of the Bodies they penetrate into and act upon.

5. That in animal and organical Bodies, particularly, these *Effluvia* may excite great Motion of one Part of the Frame upon another, and thereby produce very considerable Changes in the Œconomy.

Lastly, That they have sometimes a Power of procuring Assistance in their Operations by the more Catholic Agents of the Universe, such as Gravity, Light, Magnetism, the Pressure of the Atmosphere, &c.

That *Effluvia* are emitted to very great Distances, we have a notable Proof in this : That our Wines grow turbid in the Hogshead, precisely at the same Time when the Grapes are at their Maturity in other remote Countries, whence the Wine was imported.

Beside that, Odoriferous *Effluvia* are, in many Cases, perceived at the Distance of many Leagues. Again, that the Generality of *Effluvia* retain the proper Colour, Smell, Tast, and other Properties, and Effects of the Bodies when they proceeded, ad this even after they have pass'd thro' the Ports of other solid Bodies, we have abundant Proof : Thus, magnetical *Effluvia* penetrate all, even the most solid Bodies, without any Change of their Nature, or Loss of Force.

And the same we see confirm'd in *Sympathetic Inks*, and Powders, the Sagacity of *Blood-hounds*, &c.

**ELATERIUM**, in Pharmacy, a purgative Medicine, prepared from the wild Cucumber. 'Tis made of the Juice of the Plant, by straining it thro' a Cloth, and evaporating the Moisture thereof, till it come to the Consistence of an Extract, or a Mass for Pills. *Elaterium* is a vigorous Purge, and is used in Lethargies, Palsies, and Hypochondriacal Melancholies. The Word is form'd from the *Greek*, ελαυνω, *I repel.*

**ELECTRICITY**, or Electric Force, is that Power or Property, whereby Amber, Jet, Sealing-Wax, Agar, Glass, and most Kinds of precious Stones, attract Straws, Paper, and other light Bodies to themselves. *Electricity* differs from Magnetism in this, that the latter only attracts Iron, whereas the former indifferently attracts most Kinds of Bodies; tho' the Effect is only sensible in light ones.

The *Peripateticks* hold this Power to consist in I know not what Quality, or sympathetick Power, subsisting between Amber, *e.gr.* and the Straw, and resulting from the substantial Form of each. But the later Philosophers generally agree to make it the Effect of a corporeal Effluvium, emitted from, and returning to the Electrical Body. Tho' as to the Nature of these Effluvia, and the Manner of their acting, they are greatly divided.

Some, with *Cabæus*[1], suppose actual Steams to issue out of the *Electric* Body, when agitated by Attrition; and that these discuss and repel the ambient Air, which, after it has been driven off a little Way, makes, as it were, a little Whirlwind, by the Resistance it meets withal in the remoter Air, to which these *Electric* Steams did not reach : And these Steams shrinking quickly back again to the attracting Body, do, in their Return, attract and bring along with them such light and small Bodies as they meet on their Way.

Others, with Dr. *Gilbert*[1], *Gassendus*, Sir *Kenelm Digby*[2], &c. hold, that on

[1] Nicolo Cabeo (1586 – 1650), an Italian Jesuit and mathematician.

[1] William Gilbert (1544 – 1603), an English physician and natural philosopher.

[2] Kenelm Digby (1603 – 1665), an English diplomat and natural philosopher.

rubbing, or chafing, the *Electric* Body is made to emit Rays, or Fibres, of an unctuous Nature; which coming to be condensed and cool'd by the ambient Air, do lose their Agitation, and so shrink back again into the Body from which they sallied; and by that Means carry along with them such light and small Bodies, as happen to be fasten'd, or sticking to their further Ends. *Gassendus* adds, that these unctuous Effluvia being emitted all Manner of Ways, do frequently decussate, or cross each other; and by that Means take the better hold of Straw, &c.

The *Cartesians*, not being able to imagine how so hard and brittle a Body as Glass, should emit Effluvia; attribute *Electricity* to the Globules of the first Element; which breaking out thro' the Pores, or Chinks of the Body, like little Darts or Swords, and not meeting with proper Meatus's, or Passages in the Air, return whence they came, and carry the little Bodies, whose Pores they happen to enter, and be entangled in, along with them.

Mr. *Boyle*, Mr. *Hawksbee*[1], &c. have made a Number of Experiments, to ascertain the Nature and Laws of *Electricity*; the Result whereof may be summ'd up under the following Articles.

1. That *Electrical* Bodies do not at all, or very rarely attract, except when warm'd, and thereby solicited to emit Effluvia more copiously.

Mr. *Hauksbee*, having heated a Glass Tube, of about an Inch Diameter, and 30 Inches long, by rubbing it vehemently on paper; and then applying it so several Pieces of Leaf Brass, found, that they were no sooner within the Sphere of Activity of the Effluvia emitted by the Tube, than they began to be put into very brisk and surprizing Motions; would leap toward the Tube, even at the Distance of 12 or 14 Inches; would sometimes adhere, and fasten to the Tube, settle on its Surface, and there remain quiet : and sometimes be thrown off from it with a great Force. And thus would they be alternately attracted and repell'd, for several Times successively. Sometimes, again, they would move slowly toward the Tube and the Table they were first laid on; and sometimes slide along in that Direction of the Side of the Tube, without touching it.

2. That Bodies, warm'd by Fire, don't attract so forcibly, as when heated by rubbing; tho' if they be first heated, and then rubb'd, they will attract the more strongly.

Mr. *Hauksbee* assures us, that the hotter he made the Tube by rubbing it, to the greater Distance did the attractive Force exert it self : But that this would answer, in Proportion, to any Degree of Heat excited, he will not undertake. When the Tube was render'd the hottest by the strongest Attrition, the Force of the Effluvia was render'd manifest to another Sense, namely that of feeling, being plainly perceived on the Face, or any other tender Part, making Strokes or Impulses on the Skin, much like those made by pushing a Number of limber Hairs against it.

3. That Tersion, or Wiping, is almost universally necessary, as well as Attrition, or rubbing, to produce *Electricity*; by Reason the Effluvia can more readily escape, when there is nothing to stop up , or choak the Pores.

4. That the Interposition of the finest Linnen, as Muslin, Gause, or the like,

[1] Francis Hawksbee, or Hauksbee, (1666 – 1713), an English scientist.

will totally hinder the Operation of *Electrical* Bodies.

5. The Effect is less sensible in thick and cloudy Weather. For the Air being clogg'd with Vapours and Exhalations rais'd from below, the Resistance the *Electric* Effluvia meet withal, must be greater than when the Air is free of any such Impediments. Hence, also, in all Probability, arises the Necessity of Tersion; the watery Particles being apt to run together, and condense on the Surface of the Body, and so obstruct the Passage of the Matter.

6. *Electrical* Bodies are more forcible, *cæteris paribus*, in hot Weather than in cold; in Summer than in Winter; by Reason the more vigorous Action of the Solar Rays, does more effectually shake the Parts of Bodies, and unlock the Pores, and so make Room for a more plentiful Emission of Effluvia. Beside, that in warmer Weather, the Medium being rarer, makes less Opposition to the Passage of the Effluvia.

7. The Air being exhausted out of the Tube, it loses almost all its *Electricity*: So that tho' rubb'd, and heated more vehemently, and Leaf-Gold applied nearer than usual, it scarce attracts at all. And what little Attraction remains, Mr. *Hauksbee* conjectures, may arise from the little Portion of Air remaining in the Tube : And so the Attraction may continue in Proportion to the Quantity of Air. When the Air is let into the Tube again, the attractive Power is immediately restor'd; and that before any new Attraction can be given the Tube, or e're it be removed from the Distance and Position it was in when exhausted. Mr. *Boyle*, however, found that a Piece of Amber did sensibly attract when the Air was pump'd out of the Receiver.

8. *Electrical* Bodies attract all Things indifferently, whereas the Magnet draws only Iron and Steel.

9. A large Piece of very *Electrical* Amber being suspended by a silken Thread, and one End of it rubb'd strongly on a little Cushion; the Cushion being brought nearer, towards the Amber at rest, will plainly make the Amber tend towards it, and follow it. Whence it appears that the *Electric* Body, is attracted by the other Bodies, as well as it attracts them. And that it is only by Accident that the small attracted Bodies approach to the *Electric* ones.

10. After an *Electrical* Body has been well rubb'd, there is a certain Nick of Time in which the light Body, instead of being attracted, will be actually repell'd, or driven away from the *Electrical* one, by the Effluvia going briskly out, and not returning again.

Mr. *Hauksbee* assures us, that the Pieces of Leaf Gold would be sometimes thrown off from his Tube with a great Force, even to the Distance of six or seven Inches. And thus, not only when they adhered to the Surface of the Tube, would they be thus suddenly and precipitantly driven from it; but also in their Motion of Ascent towards it.

11. A Glass Globe, being contrived to be whirled round, with its Axis parallel to the Horizon, and a Semi-circle of Wire fitted round the upper Hemisphere thereof, at the Distance of 4 or 5 Inches, with several Pieces of Woollen Thread hung thereon, of such Lengths, as that when extended in a Direction towards the Centre of the Glass, they would reach within an inch of the Circumference thereof; but when left at Liberty, hang down in a parallel Position : Upon applying the Hand, and so adding an Attrition to the former Rotation, the Threads presently began to change their Direction, and all

harmoniously pointed to the Centre of the Globe; and to put it pass Doubt, this Effect depended on the Attrition hither and thither, cou'd draw the Threads toward this or that End of the Globe, tho' they all still went uniformly converging towards some Centre, in the Axis thereof; and so form'd a Kind of Conical Surface.

The same Phænomena follow'd upon shifting the Wire, and putting it on the lower Hemisphere. Add, that upon suspending the Motion and Attrition, the Threads would continue in their strait direct Posture for the Space of four or five Minutes. And in the mean Time, if the Finger, or any other Body, were applied near the Extremity, or Points of the Threads, they would avoid and fly from the same : But if applied about an Inch Distance from the End of such Thread, the Thread would usually be attracted towards it.

**ELECTUARY**, in Pharmacy, a Form of a Medicine, composed of Powders and other Drugs, incorporated with Honey or Sugar; to be divided into Doses, like Bolus's when taken. It is thus call'd, by Reason all the Parts, or Ingredients it consist of, should be well chosen; from the *Latin* Verb *Eligere*, to chuse, whence *Electus*, chosen. Others derive it from *Lac*; and accordingly the *Greeks*, under the *Eastern* Empire, call'd it λακτοσαειον. *Scaliger* derives it from λειχω, *to lick*; and calls it in *Latin, Elinctum*.

*Vossius*[1] observes, that all the Remedies prescribed for the Sick, as well as the Confections taken by Way of Regale, were called by the *Greeks*, εκλειγματα and εκλειχτα, of the Verb λειχω, *to lick* : Whence, says he, was form'd the Latin *Electarium*, and afterwards *Electuarium*. This Opinion he proves from the Laws of *Sicily*, where it is ordain'd, that *Electuaries*, Syrups, and other Remedies, be prepared lawfully. The *Bollandists*[2], who relate this Etymology, seem to confirm it. *Act. Sanct. Mart. F. II. p.* 131.

*Electuaries* are either *soft*, or *solid*; and of each Kind, some are *Alterative*, others *Corroborative*, others *Purgative*, &c. The soft are of the Consistence of Honey, and consist of 3 Ounces of Powders to a Pound of Honey or Sugar. The solid are in Manner of *Tabellæ*, or Lozenges. The Purgative are usually of the soft Kind : But the Corroborative only admit of an Ounce and half or two Ounces. Among the soft *Electuaries* are reckon'd *Treacle, Mithridate*, the Concoction of *Hamech*, that of *Alkermes*, the *Catholicon, Diaprunum, Diaphoenic, Galens Hiera picra*, &c. Among the solid *Electuaries*, are reckon'd *Carthamum, Rose Juice, Violet Juice*, &c. Mons. *Lemery* reckons up above 120 Sorts of *Electuaries*.

**ELEMENTS**, in Physicks, the first Principles, or Ingredients of Things; whereof all Bodes are compounded; and into which they are all resolvible. *Elements* are conceiv'd as the most simple, homogeneous Parts, or Corpuscles; of an Assemblage, and Mixture whereof, all the Bodies we see, consist.

Authors generally talk very wildly and inconsistently of the *Elements*, and confound them with the *Principles* of the Things : Yet is there a great deal of

[1] Garhardus Johannes Vossius, born Gerhard Johann Voss (1577 – 1649), a Dutch Humanist theologian and classical scholar.

[2] An association of ecclesiastical scholars named after the Jesuit Jean Bolland or Bollandus.

Difference. As we find, by Experience, that all Things cannot indifferently be made of all; that Stone, for Instance, and Marble, are not convertible into Flesh, nor are fit to nourish or augment an animal Body : It seems to follow, that all the Variety of Bodies could never arise from the first simple Combination of the two Principles, Matter and Form; but only some infinitely simple Beings, or Corpuscles, which being variously intermix'd, might constitute all other Bodies.

Now those most simple of all Beings, thus form'd the first Determination and Concretion of Principles, are what the Philosophers properly call *Elements* : So that *Elements* and *Principles* have this Difference between them; that a Principle, as Matter, is a Kind of incompleat Nature; but an Element, a perfect or compleat one.

Hence it follows, that there must, of Necessity, be more *Elements* than one: Since otherwise all Things would be equally simple, and there would be no such Thing as a Compound in Nature. Most of the Antients, not aware of this, confounded *Element* with *Principle* : On this footing, the Elements are sometimes held corruptible, and sometimes incorruptible.

The Retainers to incorruptible *Elements*, mean precisely by *Element* what we mean by the first Matter. In Effect, their Elements are their Atoms, or Corpuscles, which are supposed indivisible, incorruptible, &c.

*Democritus* is held the first Author of this Tenet; which accordingly is adhered to by *Epicurus* and many of their Descendants, the *Epicurean* and *Corpuscular* Philosophers.

Among those who hold them corruptible, some will only have one, and some several. Of the former, the Principal are *Heraclitus*, who held Fire; *Anaximenes*, Air; *Thales Milesius*, Water; and *Hesiod*, Earth; as only the *Element*. *Hesiod* is follow'd by *Bernardin. Velesius*; and *Thales*, by many of the Chymists.

Among those who admit several corruptible *Elements*, the principal are the *Peripateticks*; who, after their Master *Aristotle*, contend for four Elements, *viz*. Fire, Air, Water, and Earth. *Aristotle* took the Notion from *Hippocrates*; *Hippocrates* from *Pythagoras*; and *Pythagoras* from *Ocellus Lucanus*, who seems to the first Author of the *Dogma*.

But there is still further Variety of *Elements* : For the Philosophers, not considering Matter in it self, or in the general, but only some of the Sensations it excites in us; some of them refer all to the Sense of Sight, and assert *lucid* and *obscure*, or *pellucid* and *opake*, to be the *Elements* of all Things : And others, regarding only the Sense of Touch, make *hard* and *liquid*, or *hot* and *cold*, the *Elements* of Things.

In this latter Class we are to reckon *Aristotle*; tho' his Way of Proceeding was somewhat different from the rest. For, considering the four principal Qualities that fall under the Sense of Touching, *Heat, Cold, Dryness* or *Hardness*, and *Humidity* or *Liquidity* : And observing that two of these Qualities might be one and the same Thing taken in two different Relations; and that they might be combined four Ways; he made four *Elements*; the first, *cold* and *dry*; the second, *cold* and *moist*; the third, *hot* and *moist*; and the fourth, *hot* and *dry*.

Then, to give Names to these *Elements*, he enquired in what Things these several Elements seem'd chiefly to prevail. Accordingly, taking the Earth to be the coldest, and, at the same Time, driest of all Things, he call'd the first Element *Earth*. And *Water*, being the coldest and moistest of all Things, he called his second *Element*, *Water*. Again, judging *Air* the moistest, and at the same Time hottest of all Things, his third *Element* he called *Air*. Lastly, *Fire* being the hottest and driest of all Things, his fourth *Element* he denominated *Fire*.

These Denominations gave Occasion to some, impertinently enough, to mistake his Meaning; and to take this habitable *Earth*, this potable *Water*, this *Air* we breath, and this *Fire* we burn on our Hearths, to be the four *Elements*; notwithstanding that the Word *Element* denotes a most simple Thing; whereas the Bodies just mention'd are all exceedingly compound.

The *Cartesians* only admit three *Elements*; which they pretend are all that could arise from the first Division of Matter : To explain their Origin, they suppose the whole Mass of Matter in the Universe, divided into an infinite Number of Particles of unequal Magnitudes, and of any Figure at Pleasure. These several Particles they suppose, further, to have been revolved, or whirled, in various Manners, each round its Centre; so as to become truly separate and apart.

Thus much supposed, 'tis impossible but the Angular, Eminent, and Implicated Parts of the several Particles must be broke off; and thus, tho' little before, they must continue continually to grow less till they arrive at a perfect Rotundity. By the Means we get two Kinds of determinate Matter for the two first *Elements* : The first, a fine Dust rubb'd, or broke off from the Angles of the Particles, till they are turn'd round; which is the Matter of the *first Element*, or the *Materia subtilis*. The other, the Parts themselves thus turn'd round, and smooth, which makes the *second Element*.

And, as 'tis probable some Particles of Matter may either separately, or conjunctly, still retain irregular, hooked, and intricate Forms; these constitute the *third Element*. 'Tis added, that the *Elements* are convertible into each other: For *the third Element*, by growing round, may become the *second*; and the *second*, by a continual Comminution and Subtilizing, the *first*.

Our great Sir *Isaac Newton*, considers the primary *Elements* of Bodies on the atomical Scale, thus : All Things consider'd, it seems probable, that God in the Beginning form'd Matter in solid, massive, hard, impenetrable, moveable Particles of such Sizes, and Figures, and with such other Properties, and in such Proportion to Space, as most conduced to the End for which he form'd them; and that these primitive Particles, being solids, are incomparably harder than any porous Bodies compounded of them; even so very hard as never to wear out: No ordinary Power being able to divide what God made one in the first Creation. While the Particles remain entire, they may compose Bodies of one and the same Nature and Texture in all Ages.

But should they wear away, or break in Pieces, the Nature of Things depending of them, would be changed. Water and Earth, composed of old worn Particles, and Fragments of Particles, would not be of the same Nature and Texture now, with Water and Earth composed of entire Particles in the Beginning. And, therefore, that Things may be lasting, the Changes of corporeal Things are to be placed only in the various Separations, and new

Associations and Motions of those permanent Particles: Compound Bodies being apt to break not in the midst of solid Particles, but where those Particles are laid together, and only touch in a few Points. It seems to me, likewise, that these Particles have not only a *Vis Inertiæ*, with the passive Laws of Motion resulting therefrom, but are also moved by certain active Principles; such as is Gravity, and that which causes Fermentation and Cohesion of Bodies.

**ELEMENTS**, in Chymistry, are the Principles, or component Parts of Natural Bodies, into which they are resolvable by Fire. The Effect of Chymistry is to analyze or resolve Bodies into their *Elements*. The Chymical *Elements* are divided into *Active* and *Passive*.

The Chymists are somewhat divided as to their *Elements* : The Generality of them to the Vulgar *Peripatetic Elements*; *Water*, which they call *Phlegm*; and *Earth*, which they call *Caput mortuum*; add three more, *viz. Salt, Sulphur*, and *Mercury*. *Salt*, they hold, the Principle of Taste; and *Sulphur*, of Smell and Inflammation : As to *Mercury*, which they also call *Spirit*, some hold it the Principle of Colours, but others deny it; and, in Effect, they agree in nothing, but that 'tis the most subtle and spirituous Part.

The *Elements* of Fossils are, 1. *Mercury*, as the Base; 2. *Sulphur*, as the Coagulator, or Binder. 3. *Salt*. 4. *Earth*. The Elements of Metals, are *Sulphur* and *Mercury* alone; *Mercury* as the Base, or Matter, and *Sulphur* as the Binder, or Cement. The *Elements* of Fossil Salts, are an insipid acid Spirit and Earth. The *Elements* of Earths, are an Oil, a little acid Salt, and a Calx. The *Elements* of Sulphurs are an acid Spirit, an Oil, and an Earthy or Metalline Matter. *Boerhaave*.

But, after all, it must be added, that there is no assigning any precise Number of Chymical *Elements*; some Bodies yielding more, and other less. And even these very *Elements* themselves are reducible, by a further Process, into other Elements.

Thus, by repeated Distillations of Wine, we successively get a Spirit of Wine, a vapid Water, a subacid Water, a more acid Water, Oil, bitter yellow Spirit, and a *Caput mortuum*, which is resoluble into Earth, Oil, &c. Now, are these so may several *Elements*? Add, that what they account an *Element*, now that it is separated, is very different from what it was when it existed in the mix'd; as appears hence, that upon remixing all the *Elements* a Body is resolved into, the Mixture will bear no Resemblance to the first Body.

In Effect, the *Elements* seem rather to be produced by the Fire, than separated by it. Beside, that they are convertible, or at least resolvable, into one another. Thus, Spirit of Wine is found to yield an acid, an Oil, and a Water : And Salts yield either an Acid, or an Alcali, with Phlegm.

What makes the Notion of the Chymical *Elements* still more precious, is, that a Pot-Herb, and a poisonous Herb, shall sometimes yield *Elements* perfectly alike; more so, that the same Plant analyzed at two different Times. Mons. *Homberg*, has consider'd the Difficulties charged on *Elements*, with great Attention.

The Result of Numerous Experiments made to ascertain the Matter is : That the four Principles, Salt, Oil, Water, and Earth, are always found in all

Plants, in what Manner soever analyzed : That these Principles are more or less Volatile, or fix'd according to the different Manners of Analysing : That this Difference arises, not only from the different Force of Fire, but also from the Fermentation of their mixt, preceding the Analysis : That a vehement Fire, rendering different Elements equally volatile, confounds them in the Analysis : That the Fire evaporates, and absolutely lose several Parts : And that to have the Elements as pure as may be, only Fermentation and a gentle Fire must be used.

**ELEMI**, or Elemy, in Pharmacy, a pellucid Resin, of a whitish Colour, intermix'd with yellowish Particles, which give it much of the Colour, and Consistence of Wax; of a pretty brisk, bitter, tho' not disagreeable, Tast; and a Smell like that of Fennel.

'Tis usually called *Gum Elemi*, tho' very improperly, inasmuch as it takes Fire readily enough, and dissolves in oleaginous Liquors, which are the Characters of a Resin. It flows from Incisions made in the Trunk, and large Branches of a Kind of wild Olive Tree, growing in *Ethiopia*, and *Arabia fœlix*. It is also found in the *Pouille*, a Province of the Kingdom of *Naples*.

*Pomet*, in his History, and *Lemery*, in his Treatise of Drugs, describe *Elemi* as a white Resin, bordering on green, odoriferous, and brought from *Ethiopia*, in Cakes of two or three Pounds a-piece, wrapp'd up in the Leaves of the *Indian* Cane.

It is excellent in Disease of the Head; and proper to digest, resolve, and suppurate. It is held a Kind of Natural Balsam; and sovereign in the Cure of all Kinds of Wounds.

The true *Gum Elemy* is that above describe; but there are several spurious ones, some natural, and others factitious, frequently sold for the same. The factitious, or counterfeit, is made of Rosin wash'd in Oil of Aspic; tho' the ill Smell, and white Colour, might easily discover the Deceit.

The natural Gums, obtruded from *Elemy*, are, 1st A Gum brought from the *American* Islands, in Barrels of divers Weight, cover'd up with the Leaves of a Plant unknown in *Europe*. The 2d might be taken for Rosin, but for its Smell, which is somewhat sweeter, and more aromatic. The 3d is of an Ash Colour, bordering on brown, brought over in large Pieces, very dry and friable.

*Pomet* does not take any of them for Natural; but rather supposes them to be originally *Elemy*, only impure and course, since melted down, and made up by the Fire.

**ELEOSACCHARUM**, from ελαιον, Oleum, and Saccharum, Sugar; a Mixture of Oil with Sugar, frequently added to distill'd Oils, to make them mix with aqueous Fluids for present Use.

**ELIXATION**, in Pharmacy, &c. the seething or boiling of any Medicine in a proper Liquor, gently and for a considerable time; amounting to what, in the dressing of Meats, we properly call *Stewing*. The Liquor ordinarily used in *Elixations*, is Spring or River Water : Tho' on some Occasions they use Milk, Whey, Beer or the like.

The ordinary Purpose of *Elixation*, is to extract the Virtue out of the

Medicine, and impart it to the Liquor. Tho' it is sometimes also used to free the Parts of Animals, Plants, &c. of their Crudities, as well as to soften, and make them tender; to take away From Foods, or Medicaments, any disagreeable Taste, or other ill Quality; to separate the earthy or grosser Parts, and for other Intentions.

The Word is form'd from the *Latin, lixare* to boil, or boil in water. *Decoction* is a Sort of *Elixation.*

**ELIXIR**, in Medicine, a compound Extract, Tincture, or Essence, drawn from a Mixture of several Ingredients, by infusing them in a proper Menstruum. Or it is a strong, spirituous Liquor, or Juice, to be taken inwardly; containing the purest, and most efficacious Parts of several mix'd Bodies, communicated to it by Infusion and Maceration.

Dr. *Quincy* defines it a strong Infusion in some Menstruum, whereby the Ingredients themselves are almost dissolved, and a Juice thus acquired of a thicker Consistence than an ordinary Tincture. *Boerhaave* takes an *Elixir* to be a compound Magistery, *i.e.* a compound of various Bodies, changed after the same Manner as a single Body is in a Magistery.

Spirits drawn from Vegetables, *i.e.* the strong, or spirituous Waters of Vegetables, are usually the Base of *Elixirs* and the Menstruum, or Dissolvent, whereby the Essence of the other Ingredients is drawn or separated. Spirit of Wine is the best and most commodious Menstruum of all.

The *Charletans* abuse the term *Elixir*, and apply it to Abundance of simple Extracts, or Tinctures; only to put them off at the higher Price. Some Authors, for *Elixir*, use the Word *Quintessence*.

*Menage* derives the Word from the *Arabic*, *Elixir*; properly signifying *Fraction*, by Reason *Elixirs* have the Force of breaking Diseases : Others, more naturally derive it from *Alecsiro*, an Artificial Extraction of some Essence. Others from the *Greek* ελαιον, *Oil*, and συρω, *I draw*, *q.d.* an Extract of the Oil, which is the essential Part of Mixts. Others from the *Greek* Verb, αλεξεω, *to help*, assist, by Reason of the great Succours we receive from *Elixirs*. Lastly, others from ελκω, *to draw*.

**ELIXIR** *Proprietatis*, is a Remedy first invented by *Paracelsus*. It is composed of Aloes, Myrrh, and Saffron; the Tincture, or Essence whereof, is drawn by putting them to dissolve, or digest with Spirit of Sulphur. Some add Spirit of Wine to the Spirit of Sulphur. *Crollius*[1] takes this *Elixir* to be the Balm, or Balsam of the Antients; adding, that it contains all the Virtues of the Natural Balm. It comforts and fortifies the Heart and Stomach, assists Digestion, purifies the Blood, and promotes Sweat.

**ELIXIR**, among the Alchymists, is used for the *Philosopher's Stone*, or the *Powder of Projection*; and sometimes for an Universal Medicine, which shall cure all Diseases, called by Way of Excellence, the *Grand Elixir*. These two Things, most Alchymists take to coincide; so that what will make Gold, will cure all Diseases.

[1] Oswald Croll (ca. 1560 – 1609), a German physician and alchemist.

The Notion of a *Grand Elixir* is of a long standing *Kircher* assures us, that the antient *Egyptians* had a Method of drawing an *Elixir* from the hardest and most precious Substances; which, on Account of its Subtilty and Perfection, they call'd *Heaven*. And this he takes to be that admirable, and celestial Water, capable of removing all Diseases; called also the *Stone*, and the *Philosopher's Stone*, as being drawn from precious Stones; and sometimes, by the Hermetical Denominations, *Aqua Vitæ, Vegetable Seed of Nature, Solar Soul*, &c. Oed. *Ægypt*. *Tom*. II. p. 430.

**ELLEBORE**, a Medicinal Plant. See Hellebore.

**EMBROCATION**, in Pharmacy, is the applying of Remedies, as Oils, Spirits, Decoctions, and other Liquids, by sprinkling, or even rubbing them on the Part affected; called also Irrigation. *Embrocations* are only a Kind of Lotions. The Word is form'd from the *Greek* βρεκω, *Irrigo, madeficio*, I sprinkle, wet, macerate. *Embrocations* are now little used, except in Diseases of the Head. If the Pain do not abate, make an *Embrocation* of Cows Milk, lukewarm, on the Head. Make an *Embrocation* on the Part with Unguent. Dialtheæ, or Oil of Lilly very hot.

**EMBRYO**, in Medicine, *Fœtus*; the first Beginning or Rudiments of the Body of an Animal, in its Mother's Womb, before it have received all the Dispositions of Parts, necessary to become animated: Which is supposed to happen to a Man on the 42d Day; at which time, the *Embryo* commences a perfect *Fœtus*.

The Word is derived from the *Greek*, εμβρυον, which signifies the same Thing; form'd of the Preposition εν, and βρυο, *scaturio, pullulo*, I spring out : From the manner of the first Growth of the *Embryo*, which resembles that of the first Shoos of a Plant, as being a Kind of Zoophyte, and having only a Vegetative Life.

Mons. *Dodart*[1] having an *Embryo* of 21 Days Age put in his Hands, made a nice Examen thereof; to find the Order Nature observes in the Formation of the Parts, and the first Rise of the Parts themselves.

The *Placenta*, he found, more than half of the whole; and thence concludes, that the nearer the *Embryo* is to the Moment of its Conception, the greater is the Placenta with *Respect* to the Secundines, and the *Fœtus*. Which Circumstance furnishes a Reason why Miscarriages are more dangerous than regular Deliveries; notwithstanding the *Fœtus* in the former Case is much less than in the latter. For tho' the *Embryo* have made a Way sufficient for it self, it may not for so great a *Placenta* as is to follow it.

The *Embryo* it self was only seven Lines long, from the Top of the Head to the Bottom of the *Spina dorsi*, where it terminated. The Thighs were not yet unfolded : They only appeared like two little Warts at the Bottom of the Trunk : The Arms made just the same Appearance on the Shoulders. The Head was 1/3 of the Length of the whole seven Lines : On this were seen two little black Points, which would one Day have been Eyes. The Mouth was very big; which M. *Dodart* takes for an Indication that the *Foetus* was fed by the

[1] Denis Dodart (1634 – 17107), a French physician and botanist.

Mouth. There was no Eminence for the Nose; but two little, almost imperceptible, Pits for the Nostrils.

The Painters usually make the Head 1/8 of the Height of a well proportion'd Man; and ¼ of that of a young Child : In the *Embryo* before us, the Head was thrice the Height of the Head; whence it follows, tat the younger the Embryo, the bigger the Head in Proportion to the Body. The Parts nearer the Head are also bigger in Proportion to the rest; and the Legs and Feet the smallest.

The *Embryo* was a little crooked forwards, and bore some Resemblance to the Maggot of a Silk-Worm : It weighted less than seven Grains, which is an extraordinary Lightness for a Body seven Lines long. It was so soft, that no Part of it could be touch'd without making a Change in its Form.

Upon opening it, M. *Dodart* discover'd the Heart, and the right Auricle : All the other Parts in the *Thorax,* and lower *Venter,* were only simple Lineaments, or Contours, and all Vesicular, excepting a Part on the left Side, which may be supposed to be the Spleen. There was no Appearance of any Thing on the right Side for a Liver. *Mem. de l'Acad.*

**EMBRYO** is also used by Naturalists, to express the Grain, or Seed of a Plant; or rather the Germ, or first Sprout appearing out of the Seed : By Reason the whole future Plant is supposed to be contain'd therein. Just as the whole Chick, is supposed contained in the Cicatricula, or Treddle of an Egg.

**EMETIC**, in Medicine, a Remedy that excites Vomiting; or that evacuates by Vomiting. Of these there are a great Variety; as *Ipecacuanha, Carduus Bendictus,* &c. The Word is form'd from the *Greek,* εμεω, *I vomit.*

The Use of *Ementicks* is indicated by a Foulness of the Mouth in a Morning, rifting, loathsome, gnawing of the Stomach, gradual Loss of Appetite, spontaneous Vomiting, &c.

Vomiting is rais'd by irritating the Spirits with the Presence of something loath'd; by an unusual Agitation, as Sailing, &c. by tickling the Fibres of the Jaws, and Pharynx with a Feather dipp'd in Oil; by drinking Quantities of warm Water, &c. by any Thing sharp and viscous; as the Flowers and Seeds of *Dill,* Leaves of *Cæsarum,* &c. Crocus and Glass of *Antimony*; the Flowers, and Regulus thereof; *Mercurius Vitæ, Mineral Turbith,* and *Mercury* sharpen'd with Acids.

The *Emetic* Wine, *Vinum Emeticum,* is only white Wine, wherein is infused some *Crocus Metallorum,* or Glass of Antimony.

The *Emetic Powder,* called also Powder of *Algareth,* from the Nature of its Author, is a Precipitate of Antimony, or Butter of Antimony, sweeten'd and softened by repeated Lotions.

*Emetic Tartar,* is Cream, or Crystal of Tartar, powder'd and mix'd with one fourth of *Crocus Metallorum.*

The Operation of *Emetic* Medicines is thus accounted for By Dr. *Quincy* : The Particles of the *Emetic* wedging themselves into the Orifices of the Emissaries of the Glands, placed adjacent to the Surface of the Stomach, do dilate the same; (which by some extrinsic Cause had been contracted) and after the same Manner, do dissolve (at least in some degree) the Cohesion of the stagnant morbifick Matter; rendering it more fluid, and consequently making its Resistance less.

Now the natural and constant Action of the Glands being Secretion; and the Impediment (by the Dilatation of the Orifice and the Attenuation of the Fluid) being taken away, or at least made less than the natural Momentum of the Glands; the Matter must naturally flow into the Cavity of the Stomach, till it be heaped up on such a Quantity, (which not being to be done in an Instant, must require some Time) as is sufficient by its Stimulus to vellicate, and force the Fibres of the Stomach, Abdomen, and Diaphragm, by Communication of the first with the two last, into a violent Contraction; and thereby throw all out by the Oesophagus : And this makes all quiet for a Time, till a new and sufficient Quantity be excerned from these Glands to produce the aforesaid Contraction.

Thus there happens Fits of Vomiting and Quiet alternately, till either all the morbific Matter be thrown out, or the Force of the *Emetic* be so diluted, that it is no longer able to draw out the morbific Matter from the Glands.

And the string Contraction in so many Muscles, and muscular Canals, as are at Work in the Action of Vomiting, and the violent Concussion which is produced all over the whole Body by a Power, which, by just Computation, is not inferior to 26000 *l.* Weight, may, and often does, take away the Obstruction in many other Canals, besides those which are adjacent to the Stomach and Gullet; as we plainly see, by those vast Sweats, which plentiful Fits of Vomiting occasion.

*Emetic* and Purgative Medicines differ only in this, that the Particles of the latter do not immediately vellicate the Fibres of the Stomach, dilate the Orifices, and attenuate the Matter contain'd in the Glands of the Stomach; but act gently, and assist the natural Motion of the Digestion, and so are carried down into the Guts : And how they operate there.

**EMMENAGOGUES**, in Medicine, such Remedies as promote the Menses; thus call'd from εν, in, μην, *Month*, and αγω, *duco,* I lead; by Reason their natural Periods of flowing are once a Month.

*Emmenagogues* either act by giving a greater Force to the Blood in Circulation, whereby its Momentum against the Vessels is increas'd; or by making it thinner, whereby it will more easily pass through any Outlets.

The former Intention is helped by Chalybeates, which give a greater Weight and Momentum to a languid, heavy Blood, and all other Substances of the like Gravity and Elasticity. And such is the Case of a Leuco-phlegmatic Habit, or as it is commonly called, the Green-sickness, and its Cure.

But, in the latter Case, where the blood is florid and too high; attenuating Alteratives and Detergents are the only Remedies, because fittest to render the Blood more thin, and give it such a Property, as will better carry it thro' little Apertures, destined for its Discharge into the *Uterus.*

**EMOLLIENTS**, in Medicine, and Pharmacy, Remedies used to soften, and loosen, Hardnesses, or Constructions of the Belly; or those of Tumors and Swellings. Such are mallows, *Mercurialis, Lilly Roots, Althaea, Lin-seed, Butter, Wax, Gum Ammoniac,* &c.

The Term *Emollient* is not only applied to internal Remedies, but also to other Things : A Laxative, Anodyne, and *Emollient* Clyster : An *Emollient* Emplaster, made of resolutive Unguents : An *Emollient* Cataplasm : Fresh Cherries are an *Emollient* Food; tho', when dry, they rather constringe than relax; as wanting a great Part of the Phlegm, which render'd them *Emollient.* Ripe Grapes, of Astringent, which they were before, become Laxative and *Emollient.* Hog's Grease, applied externally, is resolutive and *Emollient.*

Dr. *Quincy* defines *Emollients,* more scientifically, to be such Things as sheath and soften the Asperites of the Humours, and relax and supple the Solids at the same Time.

For it is easy to conceive how these should be both effected by the same Medicine; thus : By what Means soever, (whether in the Stomach, or any other Parts) the Juices have obtained a Sharpness, or Asperity, so as to vellicate and render uneasy the Fibres, and nervous Parts; which often happens; these Things which are smooth, soft, and yielding, cannot but wrap up their Points, and render them imperceptible; whereby they may gradually, by the proper Course of Circulation, be brought to some convenient Emunctory, without doing any Injury by the Way.

Such Sharpness of Parts, likewise, draws the Fibres into Spasms, keeps them too tense, and frequently thereby occasions Obstructions of the worst Kind.

In all such Cases, therefore, *Emollients* lubricate, and moisten the Fibres, so as to relax them into their proper Dimensions, whereupon such Disorders cease.

**EMPASMA**, in Pharmacy, a Powder thrown, or sprinkled, over the Body, to correct some ill Smell thereof, or to prevent unnecessary Sweats. The Word is form'd from the *Greek*, εμπαςειν, *to sprinkle.*

**EMPHRACTIC**, in Pharmacy, the same with *Emplastic.* The Word is form'd from the *Greek*, εμφρατιο, *I stop.*

**EMPHYSEMA**, in Medicine, a windy swelling, or bloating of the whole outer habit of the Body; like that in the Parts of divers Animals, when blown up, after they are kill'd. The Word is *Greek*, εμφυσημα, which signifies the same Thing.

The Wind, or Air, which is the Matter of the *Emphysema,* is lodged under the Cutis, and principally in the *Cellulæ Adiposæ.* Hence, the Seat of the *Emphysema,* or the Place wherein the Wind is chiefly lodg'd, is in the Adipose Cells, under the Skin, covering the Thorax : The ordinary Occasion is some Wound in the Thorax.

Mons. *Littre* accounts for it thus : When a Person is wounded in the Breast, there enters Air in at the Wound; now, it may happen, either from the Narrowness of the Wound, or the Flesh's closing again readily, or some other Cause, that the Air thus admitted, cannot readily get out again, at least not all of it : And thus Air comes to be inclosed in the Capacity of the Breast.

Now, at every Inspiration, the Lungs are to full this Capacity, by their swelling with the Air naturally received. But here they cannot swell without pressing upon the other extraneous Air : The Consequence of which is, that it obliges it to flip between the Interstices of the fleshy Fibres, and perhaps to enter the little Oscula of the minutest Veins or Lymphaticks.

Immediately, another Force come to take Place, contrary to that of Inspiration; *viz.* Expiration : In this, the Breast contracting it self, presses the extraneous Air still more than the Lungs had done in their Dilation : And the two opposite Moments or Actions conspire to the same Effect.

The Air, thus continually impell'd, will be propagated along the Passages it first open'd it self, till at length it meets and becomes collected in some Place. Now this Place will be the *Cellules* of the fat, rather than any where else, by Reason of the Thinness, and Flexibility of their Membranes; and as the Air came from within the Cavity of the Breast, it will be in the Fact that covers the Breast, under the Skin, rather than elsewhere, that the windy Tumor, or *Emphysema* will lie.

Now, such Tumor cannot be very considerable, as only form'd by the Air receiv'd in at a Wound : But if we suppose the Wound to have pierced the Substance of the Lungs, then beside Air taken in by the Wound, there will be Part of that taken by Inspiration; so much as was contain'd in the *Bronchiæ*, or *Vesiculæ*, thus perforated or open'd, escaping into the Cavity of the Breast, and driven along with the former, into the Flesh. And as a fresh Quantity of this is supplied every Moment, there will be a continual Accession, so long as the Wound of the Lungs remains open.

Hence, an Emphysema from a Wound in the Lungs, sometimes possesses the whole habit; the Air being carried to the several Parts of the Body by Circulation.

**EMPIRIC**, or Empirick, a Name attributed, of all Antiquity, to such Physicians as form'd themselves Rules, and Methods, on their own Practice and Experience; and not on any Knowledge of Natural Causes, or the Study of good Authors; and who prescribed, without enquiring into the Nature of the Disease, or the Properties and Virtues of their Medicines : depending wholly on the Authority of some general experienced Remedies.

Medicine was almost altogether in the Hands of *Empiricks*, till the time of *Hippocrates*; who first introduced Reason and the Use of Theory therein : And hence arose a new Sect, called *Theoretici*.

The Word is form'd of the *Greek*, εμπειρικος, and that of εμπειρος, *knowing, able*; but, particularly, knowing and learned by Experience. The Root being πειρα, *Essay, Trial.*

*Pliny*, and *Celsus*, make mention of the *Empiricks*, and their Professions, which the *Greeks*, and the *Latins* after them, called *Empirice*; as attributing all the Experience, and nothing to the Authority of the Masters of the Art, or the Deductions of Reason.

*Pliny* relates, that the Sect of *Empiricks* had its Rise in *Sicily* : The first who profess'd it, he says, were *Apollonius* and *Glaucias*; others say, *Acron Argentinus*. They, and their Followers, made great Opposition to the dissecting of human Bodies; particularly to that practised by *Herophilus*, and *Erasistratus* on living Bodies, of Criminals condemn'd to Death.

But the Word *Empiric* is now more odious than ever; being confounded with that of *Charletan*, or Quack, and applied to Persons who practise Physic at Random, without a proper Education, or understanding any thing of the Principles of the Art.

Indeed, 'tis possible, the Word may be abused even on this Side of the Question; for those of the Physicians attached to the Train and Method of the Schools, the Reasonings of *Hippocrates* and *Galen*, and the Statutes of the Faculty, we all know, have been ever forward to treat those who think more freely, and are less stiffly devoted to Antiquity, Custom, and the reigning Practice, or Mode, as *Empiricks, Charletans*, and *Quacks*.

**EMPLASTER**, popularly call'd Plaster, a Medicine, of a stiff, glutinous Cons-istence, composed of divers simple Ingredients, spread on Leather, or Linnen, and applied externally.

*Emplasters* are made up in a strong solid Body, that by remaining a long Time on the Part, the Medicinal Ingredients, they are chiefly composed of, may have Time enough to produce their Effects.

The Drugs, used to give a Body and Consistence to *Emplasters*, are usually Wax, Pitch, Gums, Fats, Litharge, and other Preparations of Lead.

There are *Emplasters* of divers Kinds, and used with divers Intentions : *Stomachic Emplasters; Cephalic, Styptic, Hepatic, Diaphoretic, Resolutive, Detersive, Emollient, Incarnative, Astringent, Conglutinative,* &c. *Emplasters*.

The most usual *Emplasters*, are those of *Diapalma*, and *Diachylon* : The *Emplastrum Polychreston*, the *Divinum*, the *Manus Dei*, the *Magnetic*, of *Angelus Sala*. That of *Charpi*, of *Safran*, *de Ranis*, &c.

The Word is form'd from the *Greek*, εμπλαττω, or εμπλαοσω, *to put in a Mass*, or *to do over* : By Reason the *Emplaster* is made of divers Kinds of simple Drugs, work'd up into a thick tenacious Mass; or because it covers over the Piece of Leather, or Linnen, to be applied on the Part affected.

**EMPLASTICKS**, in Pharmacy, are Salves, or Medicines, which stop up, and coagulate the Pores of the Parts they are applied on. Such are Fat's, Mucilages, Wax, the Whites of Eggs, &c. The Word is form'd from the *Greek*, εμπλασειν, *to stop up*. They are also call'd *Emphrasticks*. The Plaster is cover'd over with a very *Emplastic* Unguent, that it may stick the stronger to the Skin. *Dionis*.

**EMPROSTHOTONOS**, in Medicine, a Kind of Tonic Convulsion, where in the Head is drawn forwards, till the Chin touch the Breast. Sometimes, too, 'tis so general, that the whole Body is bent forward, and makes a Bow; and even, sometimes, a Kind of Circle, the Knees meeting the Head. The Cause of the Disorder is a Contraction of the Anterior Muscles, particularly those of the Head, call'd *Mastoides*. The Word is *Greek*, composed of εμπροθεν, *before*, and τονος, *Tension, Stiffness*, of the Verb τεινω, *to stretch*.

**EMPYEMA**, in Medicine, a Collection of Pus, or purulent Matter, in the Cavity of the Breast; discharged thither upon the bursting of some Abscess, or Ulcer, in the Lungs, or Membranes, that inclose the Breast. The *Empyema* sometimes succeeds a *Squinancy*, sometimes a *Peripneumony*, but more usually a *Pleurisy*; as being ordinarily the Effect of a *Peripneumonic* or *Pleuritic* Abscess. An *Empyema*, in Course of Time, breeds a *Phthisis*.

It usually comes 15 or 20 Days after those Diseases. Sometimes, also, 'tis generated of extravasated Blood, issued out of a bursten, broken, or putrified Vein : 'Tis distinguish'd by a Difficulty of Breathing, a dry Cough, a Heaviness about the Diaphragm, a Noise, and fluctuating of the Matter upon moving; ruddy Cheeks, hollow Eyes, the Tips of the Fingers hot, and a Swelling of the Abdomen.

The Cure is difficult, from the Difficulty of absorbing or evacuating such extravasated Matter : If Nature shews any Endeavour to throw it off by Vomiting, or Urine, or the like, she must be seconded, and assisted therein. Thus, if the Urine be purulent, administer Diureticks; if the Stools, Laxatives; if the Spitting, Expectorants, or even Emeticks; otherwise, Recourse must be had to the Paracentesis, or Tapping.

In Order to this, an Aperture must be made in the Thorax, by a proper Instrument, on the Side affected, between the *4th* and *5th*, or the *5th* and *6th* Ribs, reckoning from the lowest; and thro' this, the Pus must be slowly drawn.

There is also a Kind of *Spurious*, or *Bastard Empyema*, proceeding from a pituitous, or serous Humour, brought by some Duct, or Passage, into the Thorax; where corrupting, it degenerates into a Matter like Pus.

The Word is form'd of the *Greek*, εν, *in*, and πυον, *Pus* : The Letter *ν*, being here changed into *μ*. Which is a Thing often observed in other Languages, when the *n* happens to come, in Composition, before the Labials *b* and *p*. Witness the Latin *Embamma, Emblema, Emporium*, &c.

**EMPYREUMA**, in Chymistry, &c. *Smell or Taste of Burning*; a Quality of Change, in Bodies that have been burnt, or much scorch'd with Fire, sensible to the Taste and Smell; or, perhaps, it may be the foreign Matter impress'd, or added by the Fire, and remaining on the burnt or scorch'd Part, that gives the new offensive Smell and Taste.

The Term is chiefly used when in boiling, or distilling any Thing, it sticks and burns to the Bottom of the Vessel, or Alembic, the offensive Smell and Taste whereof are express'd by the Word *Empyreuma*. It is also used for the Heat remaining upon the Declension of a Fever.

The Word is form'd of the *Greek*, εμπυρευειν, *to inflame, kindle*.

**EMULSION**, in Medicine, a liquid, gentle Remedy, of a Colour, and Consistence, resembling Milk. The Word is form'd from the Latin, *emulgere*, to milk. *Emulsions* serve to temper, dilute, and soften Acrimonies of the Breast; to moderate the Heat of the Kidneys; soften the Sharpness of the Urine; and give the Patient Rest and Ease. It is composed of Oleaginous Seeds, Kernels, or Fruits, pounded in a Mortar, and dissolved in distill'd Waters, or light Decoctions; afterwards, express'd, or strain'd and sweeten'd with Sugar, or Syrup. The Seed of the Melon is one of the four greater cold Seeds, much used in *Emulsions* : The Seed of the great Gourd is also used in *Emulsions*, Broths, and Decoctions.

**EMUNCTORY**, in Medicine and Anatomy, a Part of the Body destined for the Separation of some Humour, judg'd useless, or even hurtful to the Animal; after it shaving circulated some Time with the Blood. The Word is form'd from the *Latin* Verb, *Emungere*, to wipe.

The Word also implies Cavity, adjoining to the Part that separates; wherein the excrementitious Humour is collected and preserved in Readiness for Evacuation.

The Kidneys, urinary Bladder and milliary Glands of the Skin, are *Emunctories* : The Parotides are not properly *Emunctories*, because destined to separate the Saliva, which is no useless, or excrementitious Humour, but necessary for the Digestion of the Food.

Some, without much Propriety, confine *Emunctory* to the Receptacle into which the secreted Excrement is discharged; as the pituitous Humour of the Brain into the Nostrils; the Cerumen into the Ears; the Excrements into the Intestines, &c. Tho' this last has not undergone any Circulation.

**ENCANTHIS**, in Medicine, a Tumor of the *Caruncula Lachrymalis*, in the great *Canthus* or Angle of the Eye. It is opposed to *Rhyas*, which is a Diminution of, or Consumption of the same Caruncle. The *Encanthis* is occasion'd by a Defluxion on that Part, or an Ulcer therein not readily enough dried. The Word is Greek, εγχανθις, form'd of the Preposition εν and χανθος, *Corner of the Eye*.

**ENCEPHALI**, in Medicine, an Epithet applied to Worms generated in the Head; where they occasion violent Pains, insomuch as sometimes to produce Distraction. The Word is compound of the Preposition εν, *in*, and κεφαλη, *Head*.

There are four Kinds of *Encephali*; those properly so call'd, which are found in the Brain : The *Narinarii*, in the Nose; *Auriculares*, in the Ears; and the *Dentales*, in the Teeth. The *Encephali*, properly thus call'd, are rare : But there are certain Diseases wherein they swarm; and we are told of pestilential Fevers that arose wholly from them.

In one of these Fevers, the Physicians having open'd the Body of the Person it had carried off, they found a little, short, red Worm in the Head. Hereupon, they tried various Medicines to find what might destroy it : But all in vain, till *Malmsey* Wine, wherein Horse Radish had been boil'd, was applied : This was no sooner thrown on the Worm than it died. The same Remedy was afterwards tried on the Sick; and it recover'd 'em almost all. The like have also been taken out by Trepanning, and the Patient recover.

**ENDEMICK**, Endimial, or Endemious Disease, (thus call'd from εν, *in*, and δημος, *Populus*, People) is any Disease which affects many People together, in the same Country; as proceeding from some Cause, peculiar to the Country where it reigns. Such are the Scurvy to the Northern Climes, intermitting Fevers in marshy Places, &c.

**ENÆOREMA**, from εναιρεω, *I lift up, or float*; expresses such Contents of the Urine, as float about in the middle, resembling a Cloud; and thence also call'd *Nubecula Hypostasis.*

**ENGASTRIMYTHUS**, Engastrimander, a Person who speaks from, or with, the Belly; without opening the Mouth; or, if open, without stirring the Lips. Thus call'd by the *Greeks*, from εν, γαςηρ, *Belly*, and μυθος, *Speech*; and by the Latins *Ventriloquus, quasi ex ventre Loquens.*

The antient Philosophers, &c. are divided on the Subject of the *Engastrimythi* : *Hippocrates* mentions it as a Disease. Others will have it a Kind of Divination, and ascribe the Origin, and first Discipline thereof, to one *Euryclus*, whom no Body knows any Thing of. Others attribute it to the Operations, or Possession, of an Evil Spirit : And others to Art, and Mechanism.

The most eminent *Engastrimythi*, were the *Pythia's*, or Priestesses of *Apollo*, who deliver'd Oracles from within without any Action of the Mouth or Lips.

St. *Chrysostom*[1] and *Oecumenius*[2], make express Mention of a Sort of Divine Men, call'd by the Greeks *Engastrimandri*, whose prophetic Bellies pronounced famous Oracles.

M. *Schottus*, Library-Keeper to the King of *Prussia*, in a Dissertation on the Apotheosis of *Homer*, maintains, that the *Engastrimythi* of the Antients, were only Poets, who, when the Priestess could not speak in Verse, supplied the Defect, by explaining, or delivering, in Verse, what *Apollo* dictated in the Cavity, or Belly, of the Bason, that stood on the sacred *Tripod.*

*Leo Allatius*[3] has an express Treatise of *Engastrimythi*, entitled, de *Engastrimytho, Syntagma.*

**ENIXUM** *Sal*, among Chymists, a Kind of Neutral Salt, being neither Acid nor Alcalious, but participating of both. Such us common Salt, Nitre, Allum, Vitriol, &c.

**ENS**, or *Ens primum*, among the Chymists, is the efficacious Part of any natural mixt Body, whether Animal, Vegetable, or Fossile; wherein, all the Qualities or Virtues of the Ingredients of the mixt, are comprehended in a little Compass.

*Paracelsus* pretends to have been able to separate the *Ens primum* from Bodies, and with it to effect prodigious Things towards the Renovation, and Restoration of Youth : But his Processes are so obscurely deliver'd, that Nobody has been induced to try 'em.

Mr. *Boyle* gives us a Process from M. *le Fevre*[4], whereby the *Ens primum*, or Essence of Balm, is easily obtain'd : He adds, that the Effects of an *Ens* of Balm, thus drawn, are no Ways inferior to those of *Paracelsus*; and instances in a special Friend of his, who, upon taking it only for a Fortnight, the Nails of his Hands and Feet fell off, and were succeeded by a Set of new ones;

[1] John Chrysostom (ca. 347 – 407), archbishop of Constantinople.

[2] Oecumenius, Bishop of Trikka in Thessaly around the end of the tenth century.

[3] Leone Allaci (ca. 1586 – 1669), Greek theologian and scholar.

[4] Nicolas Le Fevre (1615 – 1669), a French scientist.

Which convinced him so far of its Efficacy, that he left off taking it himself : But giving some of it to an old Woman of 70 Years of Age, who served in the House, it produced the *Menses* again; and that so copiously, as wonderfully to startle the Woman.

Upon giving a little of it to an old Hen, her Feathers began to moult on the sixth Day, and she grew stark naked; but ere a Fortnight was over, she had others in their Room, fairer, and better colour'd than the former.

The Relation is off enough; yet considering the Hands we have it from, and how easily the Thing is tried, 'tis much no body has yet attempted to prosecute it. The Process is thus :

Having gather'd, *e.gr.* some Balm, or other fitting Plant, at the proper Season and Time; beat it into a Pulp in a Marble Mortar, and putting it into a Bolt-Head hermetically seal'd, digest it 40 Days in a Dunghill, or other analogous Heat. This done, take out the Matter which will now be more liquid than before, and separating from it the Dregs, or grosser Parts, digest it anew in a gentle Bath; that the remaining grosser Parts may also subside : Filtrate it, and add to it the fix'd Salt, drawn from the former Dregs, dried and calcined. To the Liquor thus prepared, add equal Parts of the Liquor of good Sea-Salt well purified, and melted, and then let it run *per deliquium*. Lastly, seal up the Mixture in a Bolt-Head; and expose it to the Sun six weeks longer. At the End of which Term, the *Ens primum* of the Plant will be found swimming on the Liquor, in a liquid, transparent Form, sometimes of a green, and sometimes a reddish Colour, according to the Plant used.

**ENS** *Veneris*, or *Flower of Venus*, a chymical Preparation from Vitriol, first published by Mr. *Boyle*. It has its Name from the Particles of Copper therein, carried away from the Vitriol. It is had by subliming equal Parts of the Powder of Cyprus Vitriol (calcined till it is of a dark Colour) and of Sal Ammoniac, into the Form of yellow Flower. It is held a Specific in the Rickets, and is much commended in nervous Cases, obstinate Cachexies, Loss of Appetite, and Obstructions of all Kinds.

**ENTELECHIA**, a Greek Term, by which *Aristotle* defines the Soul; and which not occurring in any other Author, has given the Criticks and Philosophers infinite Perplexity to discover its meaning.

*Hermolaus Barbarus*[1], is even said to have consulted the Devil about it; after which, in his Paraphrase on *Themistius*, whether from the Devil or himself we know not, he renders it by *Perfectihabia*, which is not a whit the clearer.

*Cicero*, whose Interpretation should be preferable to that of any Modern, defines *Entelechia* (*Tuscul. q.* L. I. C. 1.) to be *a certain, continued, and perpetual Motion* : Whence it should appear that *Aristotle* took the Soul for a Mode of the Body; *a continuous Motion* being doubtless a Mode of Body.

The common *Peripateticks* hold *Entelechia* to signify *Act*; and under it, suppose the Form of the Compound, or Animal, to be understood : Accordingly, they define it any Act, whether Substantial or Accidental,

[1] Hermolaus Barbarus or Hermolao Barbaro (1454 – ca. 1493), an Italian scholar.

considered as capable of performing some Operation in the Body. Others of them define it to be a substantial Act, whereby a Thing is, what it is, in Substance.

Lastly, others of the *Peripateticks*, and those the latest, agree that the *Act* of *Entelechia*, whereby *Aristotle* meant to explain the Nature of the Soul, either signifies some Mode of the Body, as Motion, or nothing at all. And thus the *Peripatetic* Notion comes round to that of *Cicero*.

**ENTEROCELE**, in Medicine, a Descent of the Intestines. The *Enterocele* is a Kind of *Hernia*, or Rupture, wherein the Intestines, particularly the Ilion, fall into the Groin, or the Scrotum. The Word is form'd of the *Greek*, εντερον, *Intestine*; and κηλη, *Tumor*.

The next Cause of the *Enterocele*, is the Relaxation, or Extension, of the lower Part of the Peritoneum, wherein the Intestines are contain'd : The remote Causes are great Lifts, too violent Exercises, great Coughs, frequent Vomiting, much Crying, &c. Whence it is that Children are much subject thereto.

There are two Kinds of *Enterocele*; the *Perfect*, which happens when the Intestine falls into the Scrotum; and *Imperfect*, when it only falls into the Groin. The Remedy is chiefly by External Applications, as Trusses and Boulsters.

**ENTERO-EPIPLOCELE**, a Kind of Rupture; wherein the Intestines, and *Epiploon*, or Caul, fall together into the Scrotum; when the Appellation *Entero-epiplocele*. The Word is compounded of εντερον, *Intestine*; επιπλοον, *Caul*, and ομφαλος, *Umbilicus, Navel*.

**ENTERO-HYDROMPHALUS**, in Medicine, a Kind of *Exomphalus*, wherein, beside a displacing and bunching out of the Intestine, there is a deal of water Humours collected with it. The Word is compounded of εντερον, *Intestine*; and ομφαλος, *Umbilicus, Navel*.

**ENTEROLOGY**, from εντερος, *intestinum*, a Gut; and λογος, *Sermo*, Discourse, is properly a Treatise of the Bowels; tho' the word is generally understood to include the Contents of the three Cavities, Head, Breast, and Belly.

**ENTEROMPHALLUS**, in Medicine, a Kind of *Exomphalus*, consisting in the Intestines being out of their Place, and occasioning a Tumor. The Word is form's of the Greek εντερον, *Intestine*; and ομφαλος, *Umbilicus*.

**EPHEMERA**, in Medicine, an Epithet applied to something that only lasts one Day; particularly to a Fever, which terminates in the Compass of a Day, *i.e.* to an Access of a Fever which returns no more, called by *Galen*, εφημερος πυρετος, *Febris Ephemeris*, and also *Diaria*. The Word, and the following one, *Ephemerides*, are form'd of the Preposition επι, *de, super, apud, ob, in, praetor*, in English, of, on, at, for, in, by, near; and ημερα, *Dies*, Day.

**EPHEMERA**, or Ephemeron, in Natural History, an Animal that only lives five Hours: Within the Term whereof it is born, grows, and extends its Members, appears young, breeds Eggs, casts Seed, grows old, and dies.

*Aristotle*, who gives the first Account thereof, in his Book *de Animal*, gave it the Name εφημερον, because its Life was bounded within the Day. *Aldrovandus*[1], *Jonston*[2] and *Clusius*, furnish us Accounts of the Ephemeron; and above all, Swammerdam, in an express Work *de Ephem. Vitæ*. He calls it *Ephemera, Hemerobios*, and in Latin *Diaria*.

It must be observed, however, that e'er it assumes this Figure, it has lived three Years under that of a Worm, in a clay Cell, or Case.

It never eats from the Time of its Change to its Death; nor is it furnish'd with the Parts necessary for the Reception and Concoction of Food. Its Change seems intended merely for the Sake of Generating and Multiplying its Kind.

Its Life is summ'd up in a few Words. In the Beginning, it sheds his clay Coat; which done, and the poor little Animal thereby render'd light and agile, it spends the rest of its short Life in frisking over the Waters. During which, the Female drops her Egg on the Waters, and the Male his Sperm on them, to impregnate them. These Eggs, thus impregnated, descend to the Bottom of the Water by their own Gravity, and are hatch'd by the Warmth of the Sun into little Worms, which make themselves Cases in the Clay, and feed on the same without any Need of parental Care : Till the Time of their Change or Metempsychosis come.

**EPHEMERA**, is also applied among Botanists, to a Kind of Flowers, which open, and expand themselves at Sun-Rising, and wither and fade away again at his Setting. Such are the *Dent de lion*, vulgarly Dandelion, and divers others.

The Travellers into *Arabia* tell us of several *Ephemeron Trees*, which grow every Day, from Morn to Noon, and then disappear; tho' 'tis not known, whether they wither away entirely, or sink back into the Sands among which they grow.

**EPHILATES**, in Medicine, a Disease, by the English call'd the Night-Mare, and the *Latins* Incubus; chiefly affecting Persons asleep, when laid on their Back, and having the Stomach loaded with Food of difficult Digestion. In this State they are oppress'd, as it were, with a huge Weight on the Breast, and imagine some Spectre, or Demon, stopping their Breath.

This Disease does not arise, as was antiently imagined, from gross Vapours filling the Ventricles of the Brain : But rather from a too great Repletion of the Stomach, which hinders the Motion of the Diaphragm, and of Consequence, the Dilation of the Breast necessary for Inspiration.

*Etmuller* observes, that they are but rarely affected with this Disorder who use a laudable Diet, and sup sparingly : lying on the Side, with the Head

[1] Ulysses Aldrovandus, born Ulissi Aldrovandi (1522 – 1605), an Italian physician and naturalist.

[2] This may be John Jonston (1603 – 1675), a Polish physician and naturalist.

pretty high, generally prevents it.

The *Arabs* call it, the *Nocturnal Epilepsy*, because, when habitual, it usually degenerates into the Epilepsy, being the usual Forerunner thereof, especially in young People. In old, it frequently terminates in an Apoplexy.

*Menjoitius* accounts for its being most usual in Boys, from their being too voracious, and eating more than they can digest. *Aurelianus*[1] assures us, it has kill'd several; adding from *Silimachus*, that there was a contagious, or epidemic Incubus at *Rome*, which over-run Numbers like a Plague.

**EPICARPIUM**, in Medicine, a Kind of Remedy, usually in Form of a Cataplasm, or Plaister, consisting of sharp, penetrating Ingredients, as Garlic, or Onion, Spiders-Web, Hellebore, Camphor, Treacle, &c. applied round the Wrist, at the Beginning of the Access of a Fever, to prevent the same. The Word is form'd of the *Greek* επι, *super, on*, and καρπος, *Carpus, Wrist.*

**EPICERASTICKS**, in Medicine, are Remedies, which by their emplastic Virtue, or temperate Moisture, soften the Acrimony of an Humour, and asswage the painful Sensation of the Part irritated or afflicted ; Such are the Roots of Althæa, Mallows, Liquorice; Leaves of Lettice, Mallows, Nenuphar[2], Purslain; the Seeds of Flax, Poppy, &c. The Word is form'd of επι and χεραγνυμαι, *tempero*, I moderate, correct.

**EPIDEMIA**, or *Epidemic Disease*, is sometimes used for a catching, or contagious Disease; communicable from one to another : Such as the Plague, Pox, Scorbutus, &c. *Epidemic Disease*, however, is more properly, and usually understood of a general or spreading Disorder, as a Plague, arising from some Corruption, or Malignity in the Air, which seizes a great Number of People in a little Time.

The Word is form'd of επι and δημος, *Populus*, People; such Diseases running among all Kinds of People, of whatever Age, Sex, Quality, &c. as arising from a common or general Cause. Whence the *Latins* call them *Populares Morbi*, popular Diseases; in Opposition to those call'd *Sporadici*, which are only here and there, as arising from private, or particular Causes.

**EPILEPSY**, in Medicine, a Convulsion, either of the whole Body, or some of its Parts; attended with a Deprivation of the Senses and Understanding; and returning from Time to Time in Fits, or Paroxysms.

The Patient seized herewith, falls instantly and suddenly down; or, rather, throws and precipitates himself violently to the Ground. When down, he grinds his Teeth, foams at Mouth, and frequently shakes his Head; his Arms, Legs, Neck, back, &c. either becoming rigid, or variously distorted. And as all Parts are in a violent Contraction, there is frequently an involuntary Flux of Urine, Seed, and fecal Matter. After some Time he returns to himself; only retaining a Head Ache, Heaviness, Weariness of their Limbs, &c.

[1] Caelius Aurelianus (ca. 5th cent.), an African physician born in Numidia, which now corresponds to Algeria and parts of Tunisia.

[2] The plant known as the White Waterlilly or White Lotus (*Nymphaea alba*).

*Etmuller* more accurately distinguishes the Disease into three Degrees : The first, or lowest, is much the same with the highest degree of Vertigo.

In the second, there arise various Agitations and Gesticulations; and the Senses, both external and internal, either remaining, or being transported into a Delirium; they dance, sing, laugh, weep, talk idly, shreek, and beat their Breasts. Sometimes they remember all after the Fit is over, and sometimes nothing at all.

In the third Degree, which alone is ordinarily call'd *Epilepsy*, they lose the Use of both Reason and Sense; fall, or fling themselves down, foam, grind their Teeth, and bite their Lips, with the other Circumstances above related. Those affected with the second Degree, are usually held for *possess'd by the Devil.*

The Cause of this Disease, *Boerhaave* attributes to too much Action of the Brain, on the motory Nerves, and none on the sensitive ones. Some are pleas'd to account for it, from the Abundance of sharp Humours mixing with the animal Spirits, and giving them extraordinary and irregular Motions, and Directions; Whence arises its Distinction from a Syncope, and Apoplexy, which take way all Motion as well as Sense.

The *Epilepsy* is either *Idiopathic*, or *Sympathetic* : It is Idiopathic, when it arises merely from a Disorder of the Brain, or Spirits : And Sympathetic, when it is preceded by some other Disease which brings it on.

The *Epilepsy* sometimes hangs many Years to a Person, without much Danger: Tho' when its Paroxysms return fast, it renders the Patient more or less paralytic, delirious, or stupid. In young People there is Hopes of its going off about the Time of Puberty. *Hippocrates* observes, that when it seizes a Person after 25 Years of Age, it lasts for Life; but this does not always hold.

The Cure is very difficult : The principal *Anti-epilepticks* are, the Roots of Pæony, Leaves of the Lilly of the Valley, Seeds of Rue, Mistletoe of the Oak, or Hazle, Box-wood, Spirit of black Cherries, Spirit of human Blood, human Secundines, human Cranium, Tooth of the Sea-Horse, Castoreum, Peacocks Dung, Camphor, Salt, and Oil of Amber.

To recover a Person in a Fit, Tobacco Smoak, or that of burnt Feathers, is recommended. *Barbette*[1] above all Things directs the Flowers and Spirits of Sal Ammoniac against this Disease; *Crato*[2], native Cinnabar. *Sir John Colbatch*[3] has an express Treatise on the Mistletoe of the Oak, to shew it a Specific in this Disease. Elks Claws have long had the Reputation of the same. See each Remedy, its Pretensions, &c. under its proper Term in this Work.

M. *Poupart*[4], from a Dissection of an *Epileptic* Person, wherein, immediately under the *Dura Mater*, was found a deal of white, thick, viscid *pituita*, glued, and, as it were, incorporated with the Membrane; thinks, that this might be the Cause of the Disease; The excessive Quantity of such thick Lympha, loading the Brain, and obstructing its Motions. The first Cause, he judges, might be the Spongeousness of the *Dura Mater*, which imbibed the

[1] Paul Barbette (ca. 1620 – 1670), a Dutch physician.

[2] Johann Craft (1519 – 1585), a German physician.

[3] John Colbatch (1666 – 1729), an English physician.

[4] Francois Poupart (1616 -1708), a French surgeon and anatomist.

Serosities of the Brain.

He adds, that he knows an *Epileptic* Person, who, upon the first approach of his Disorder, rubs his Forehead with his Hand, and bends his Head as far backwards as he can, resting it against a Wall; and by that Means secures himself against the Convulsion. 'Tis probable, that by this he gives a Motion to the Lympha, and drives it from the Place which before it disturb'd.

The Word *Epilepsy* is form'd of the *Greek*, επιλαμβα-νεσται, *to surprise, grasp hold of one*, by reason the Disease seizes and overcomes the Senses, so that the Patient seems as if dead.

In *English*, it is usually call'd the *Falling Sickness*, by reason People fall down when attack'd therewith. The *Latins* call it *Comitialis Morbus*, by reason when any body was seiz'd therewith in a *Comitia*, or Assembly of the Roman People, they presently broke up the Assembly, as deeming it an unhappy Presage.

Some call it the *Morbus Sacer*, as supposing it sent by way of immediate Punishment from God. Others, the *Morbus Caducus*, others *Herculeus, Sonticus, Lues Deifica*, &c.

**EPIPHORA**, in Medicine, a Disease of the Eyes; consisting in a preternatural Defluxion of Rheum, or the Matter of Tears; accompanied, frequently, with Heat, Redness, and Twitching. *Pitcairn* calls it a Kind of Catarrh of the Glands of the Eye. The Word is *Greek*, form'd of επιφερομαι, *I am drawn*.

The internal Causes of the *Epiphora*, or Rheum in the Eyes, are a Relaxation of the Glands of the Eyes, and a too great Acrimony, or Sharpness of the serous Humour separated thereby; which fretting and vellicating the Eye, draws an unusual Quantity of Blood and Lympha thereto; by which, at length, the Cheek becomes excoriated, &c. Children are most liable to it, from the frequent Use, and straining of the Glands of the Eye in Crying.

The external Causes of the *Epiphora*, are sharp Dusts, Steams, &c. entering the Eye, and irritating the same. A too cold and sharp Air has frequently the like Effect. Children are most liable to it. An inveterate *Epiphora* frequently degenerates into a *Fistula Lachrymalis*.

The Cure of the *Epiphora*, is 1°. By causing a Revulsion, or Derivation, of the peccant Humour, to some other Part, as by Venæfection, Cupping, Blistering, or Cathartic ks. 2°. By correcting its Acrimony by proper Remedies. And, 3°. By applying Astringents externally. *Lapis Calaminaris* is much commended.

**EPIPLASMA**, the same with Cataplasm.

**EPIPLOCELE**, in Medicine, a Kind of Hernia, or Tumor, occasion'd by the Descent of the *Epiploon*, or Caul, into the Scrotum.

**EPILOMPHALUS**, in Medicine, a Species of *Exomphalus*, or Navel-Rupture; being a Tumor, or Swelling of the Part, occasion'd by the *Epiploon's* bearing too hard against it. The Word is compounded of the Greek επιπλοον, and ομφαλος.

**EPIPLOON**, in Anatomy, a fatty Membrane, spread over the Intestines, and entering even into the Sinuosities thereof; call'd also the *Omentum*, and popularly the Caul. The Word is form'd of the *Greek*, επιπλεθιν, to swim, by reason it seems to float on the Intestines.

**EPIPLOSARCOMPHALUS**, in Medicine, a Sort of Tumor, of the *Exomphalous* Kind. It is form'd of the *Epiploon*, and the Flesh. The Word is compounded of the three Greek Words, επιπλοον, *Epiploon*, σαρξ, *Flesh*, and ξμφλος, *Umbilicus*, Navel.

**EPISPASTIC**, in Medicine, a Remedy, which being externally applied, draws or attracts the Humour to the Part; call'd also an Attractive. The Word is *Greek*, form'd of επι and σπαω, *traho, I draw*.

Of *Epispasticks* there are some which act very gently, and others, with a deal of Violence. Those of the latter Kind swell, and bloat the Skin, make it Red, and even raise Blisters thereon. The principle simple *Epispasticks* are *Pellitory, Garlic, Mustard, Onions, Yeats, Goose-dung*, and that of *Pidgeons, Cantharides*, &c.

**EPITHEME**, *Epithema*, in Pharmacy, a Kind of Fomentation, or Remedy, of a liquid, spirituous Kind; applied externally upon the Regions of the Heart or Liver; to strengthen and comfort the same, or to correct some Intemperature. The Word is form'd of the *Greek*, επι, *upon*, and τιθημι, *pono*, I put.

There are two Kinds of *Epithems*; the one *Liquid*, and the other *Solid* : The *Liquid Epithem* is a Fomentation of a more spirituous Nature than the rest; the *Solid*, is a Mixture of Conserves, Treacle, Confections and Cordial Powders, generally spread on a Piece of Scarlet or Leather.

**EPITHYME**, a Medicinal Plant, of a very extraordinary Nature and Figure. Its Seed is very small, from which arise long Threads like Hairs, which soon perish, as well as the Root, unless they meet with some neighbouring Plant, both to sustain and feed them.

The *Epithyme*[1] grows indifferently on all Kinds of Herbs; and, of Consequence, the Kinds thereof are infinite; To which Writers usually attribute the particular Virtues of the Plants they grow on.

The most known of these Plants, and those most used in Medicine, are such as grow on Thyme; which are the proper *Epithymes*; and those on Flax. Three are two Kinds un the Shops; the one from *Venice*, the other from *Candia* : They have both an Aromatic Taste, but that of *Venice* is the strongest.

**EPULOTICKS**, in Medicine, dry, astringent, Remedies, proper to cicatrize, or incarnate Wounds and Ulcers. Such are the Emplasters of Ceruss, and Diapalma; the Unguent Pompholix, &c. The Word is form'd of the *Greek*, επι, *super*, and ουλη, *Cicatrix, Eschar*. Whence the Verb επουλοω, *cicatrictem, infero*.

[1] The parasitic plant called Dodder (*Cuscuta epithymum*).

**ERADICATIVE**, in Medicine. An Eradicative Cure is that which takes away the Cause, or Root of the Disease; in which Sense it stands opposed to palliative; which relives for a Term, but not going to the Cause of the Disorder, does not prevent its Return. The Word is a Compound of *e* out, and *radix*, Root.

**EROSION**, in Medicine, the Act of sharp, acid Fluids, or Humours, gnawing and tearing off Parts from the Flesh, and other Substances. Arsenic, and other Poisons, make Erosions, in the Intestines.

**ERRHINA**, Errhines, in Medicine, are Remedies taken by the Nose, to enliven the Spirits, stop Bleeding, &c. but principally to purge the Humidities of the Head. The Word is derived from εν, *in*, and ριϛ, *Nose*.

Of these, some are taken in *Powders*, as Betony, Tobacco, Marjoram, Iris, white Hellebore, *Euphorbium*, &c. Others in a *liquid* Form, made of the Juice of Marjoram, Sage, Beet, Cyclamen, Iris, &c. Others in Form of *Liniments*, incorporated with *Unguent. Rosat.*

Others, *solid*, form'd like Pyramids, to sop Bleeding at the Nose; composed of Armenian Bole, *Terra sigilllata*, Mastic, human or Hogs-blood dried, &c. Such *Errhina* as are dry, and made up in Powders, are properly call'd *Sternutatories*. The Moderns sometimes call 'em *Caput purgia*.

**ERUCTATION**, Belching, the same as Ructation.

**ERUGINOUS**, or Æruginous, some Thing partaking of, or like to the Rust of Brass, or Copper.

**ERYSIPELAS**, in Medicine, call'd also *Sacer Ignis*, and *St. Anthony's* Fire, a Disease of the Skin. Its Seat is any Part of the Body, but principally the Face : It shews it self in a ruddy Inflammation of the Part, with a little Swelling of the same; an intense Pain, and a Croud of little Pustles, which, as the Inflammation increase, grow into *Vesiculæ*. The *Erysipelas* is either simple, or attended with an Ulcer.

The Disease spreads it self a-pace; shifting from one place to another, with a Fever attending it. It attacks the Patient all at once, and chiefly when out in the Air; whence the Country people call it *blasting, Sideratio*.

Dr. *Quincy* accounts for the *Erysipelas*, from a too lazy Blood, which obstructing the Capillaries, occasions Inflammations : Others, from a too sharp and bilious Blood, which, on Account of its great Subtilty, occasions no sensible Tumor; but spreads, or diffuses it self in Length and Breadth. Its Colour, tho' red, generally inclines towards a yellow, on Account of the Mixture of Bile; and always the more of the Bile, the more dangerous the Disease.

There is another Species of *Erysipelas*, tho' less usual than the former; most commonly arising from a too copious drinking of spirituous Liquors. It begins with a Fever, after which there is an universal Eruption of Pustles, almost over the whole Body, much like those after the stinging of Nettles, and sometimes rising into *Vesiculæ*. At going off, they leave an intolerable Itching, and as often as scratch'd return again.

*Etmuller* gives it as the distinguishing Character of an *Erysipelas*, that when press'd very lightly by the Finger, there follows a white Spot, which presently after becomes red again; which does not happen in an ordinary Inflammation, unless when violently press'd. Scorbutic People are most subject to this Disease.

'Tis disputed, whether Purging be good in the *Erysipelas* : *Sydenham* recommends it the next Day after Bleeding. *Etmuller* cautions against 'em both; and recommends Diaphoreticks. Dr. *Friend* observes, that in the last Stage of an *Erysipelas* of the Head, attended with a Coma, Delirium, &c. unless Cathartick will do good, the Case is desperate. All unctuous, astringents, and cold Applications, externally, are dangerous, and sometimes make the *Erysipelas* degenerate into a Gangrene.

The Word is form'd of the *Greek*, ερυειν, *trahere*, to draw; and ρελας, *prope*, by reason it withdraws it self towards the Skin : Whence *Galen* calls it *Passio Cutis*.

**ESCHAR**, in Chirurgery, a hard Crust, or Scab, form'd on the Flesh, by means of a hot Iron, or a Caustic Medicine, or some sharp, corrosive Humour within. The Caustic Stone, or *Lapis Infernalis*, produces a round *Eschar* in the Place where it has burnt. The Word is derived from the *Greek*, εσχιρα, Crust, or Scab. Some Authors derive it from ες, and καιω, I burn; but this comes with some Difficulty, by reason καιω is wrote with a κ; and εσχιρα with a χ.

**ESCHAROTICKS**, Medicines, which being applied externally, produce Eschars, or Scabs, by burning the Flesh. Such are the Lapis Infernalis, red precipitate, &c. these are also call'd Causticks. The Word is derived from the *Greek* εσχιρα.

**ESCHYNOMENOUS** Plants, are sensitive Plants; that us, such as upon approaching 'em shrink back, and contract their Leaves.

**ESCULENTS**, are Plants or Foods, as Artichokes, Carrots, Turnips, Parsnips, Cabbages, Cauliflowers, &c.

**ESSENCE**, that which constitutes, or determines the Nature of a Thing; or which is absolutely necessary for its being what it is. In Philosophy, the *Essence* of a Thing is defined to be that whereby a Thing is distinguished from every other Thing.

The *Cartesians* hold the *Essence of Matter* to consist in Extension; and on that Principle, deny that there is any such Thing as Mere Space, or Vacuity : But the *Hypothesis* is false, as is shewn under the Articles Matter, Space, Vacuity, Plenum, &c.

*Gassendus*, and most of the Corpuscular Philosophers, hold the Essence of Matter to consist in Solidity, or Impenetrability, or Resistance, or, more adequately, in a solid Impenetrability resisting the Touch which, it must be allow'd, of all the Properties of Matter, seems to have the fairest Title.

The School Philosophers give us two Significations of the Word *Essence*;

the first denotes the whole *Essential* Perfection of a Being, and consequently its Entity, with all its intrinsic, or *Essential*, and necessary Attributes taken together. In which Sense, *Essence* may be defined to be *all that whereby a Thing is, and is what it is*. In which Case, the *Essence* of a Thing, is to the thing it self, what Humanity, *e.gr.* is to Man.

The second Signification of *Essence*, is that whereby it denotes the principal, and most intimate of all the Attributes of a Thing; or that which agrees to every such Thing, and such alone, and that always, and in such manner, as that the Mind, with all its Attention, cannot perceive any Thing prior thereto. By which, *Essence* is distinguish'd from the *Essential Attributes*, *i.e.* from such as flow from its *Essence*, or first Attribute. Thus, the *Essence* of the human Mind is commonly supposed to consist in the Power of Thinking; by reason all its other Perfections seem to pre-suppose this; but this pre-supposes none. And thus, the Powers of understanding, doubting, assenting, willing, &c. do all flow from the Power of Thinking; and cannot exit without it, tho' this may without any of them.

It must be allow'd, however, that the *Essential* Properties of a Thing do so closely cohere, nay, and inhere in the *Essence* it self, that 'tis scarce possible to distinguish the one from the other. Hence, what some urge, that setting aside all the Attributes and Properties of a thing, and what remains is its *Essence*; is a mere Chimera. For set aside, *e.gr.* from the Mind, the Powers of understanding and willing, with the rest of its Attributes : and what will there remain to call its *Essence*?

'Tis greatly disputed in the Schools, whether the *Essence* of created Things be Eternal : Or, whether the *Essences*, as well as the Existences, had their Origin in Time? The *Cartesians* hold, that the *Essences* of Things depend absolutely on the free concurring Will of God.

**ESSENCE**, in Medicine and Chymistry, is the purest and most subtle Part of a Body, extracted from the same, by means of Fire. Of these there are a great Variety, drawn from Flowers, Fruits, &c. used on Account of their agreeable Smells, Tasts, &c. by the Apothecaries, Perfumers, &c.

The principal are *Essence* of Rosemary : Of Turpentine : Of Anis : Of Cloves: Of Cinnamon; and of Citron.

The *Essences* commonly sold by Perfumers, are only the Oil of Ben, and of bitter Almonds; to which they give the Smell of certain Flowers, or Spices, as Violets, Jassemin, and Cinnamon, &c.

The *Essences* to be drunk, or mix'd with Liquors, are of a more elaborate Composition : The most usual and best, is prepared with the Spirit of Wine, Cloves, Cinnamon, Mace, Long Pepper, and Coriander : The whole being put up in a very close Vessel, is exposed to the Sun for six Weeks, or two Months, during the Day-time, and in the Night set on the Fire.

The Winter they use the Fire alone : This *Essence* being exceedingly strong; 'tis frequently used only to give a Strength to other weaker Liquors. After the same manner may the *Essences* of Amber, Musc, &c. be drawn.

The *Essences* of odoriferous Flowers, to give a fine Smell to Liquors, are drawn by laying Strata, or Lays of the Flowers, and of Sugar, alternately, in a proper Vessel, and leaving 'em to infuse in a Cellar for 24 Hours; and after that as long by the Sun; and lastly, straining or percolating the whole thro' a Sieve, without squeezing the Flowers.

**ESSENTIAL** *Oils*, are such as are really in a Plant, and drawn from it by Distillation, in an Alembic, with Water; in Contra-distinction to those made by Insolation.

**ESSENTIAL** *Salts*, are such as will crystallize in the Juice or Infusion of a Plant; in Distinction from those made by Incineration.

**ESULA**, a medicinal Root. The *Esula*, is properly the Bark of a little reddish Root, which produces green, narrow, milky Leaves. It grows chiefly in France. 'Ere they use it, 'tis infused in Vinegar : After which, they draw Extracts from it, used in the Dropsy.

**ESURINE** *Salts*, are such as are of a fretting, eating, or corroding Nature; which chiefly abound in Places near the Sea-side, and where great Quantity of Coal is burnt: As appears from the speedy rusting of Iron in such Places.

**ETHERIAL** *Oil*, a name the Chymists give to high rectified Oils, which differ little from inflammable Spirits; such are Oil of Turpentine, &c.

**EVACUANTS**, in Medicine, Remedies proper to expel, or carry off any ill, peccant, or redundant Humor in the animal Body; by the proper Ways or Emunctories. Of *Evacuants*, there are divers Kinds, distinguish'd according to the various Humours and Emunctories.

Some, *e.gr.* carry off their Matters by *Stool*, call'd *Purgatives*, or *Catharticks*. Others by *Urine*, call'd *Diureticks*. Others by *Perspiration*, call'd *Diaphoreticks*. Others by *Sweat*, call'd Sudorificks. Others by the Mouth, call'd *Vomitories*, or Emeticks. Others by the salival Glands, as *Sialigogues* : And others, lastly, by the *Menses*, as *Menagogues* and *Aristolochicks*.

**EVACUATION**, in Medicine, a Diminution of the animal Fluids, in Order to a Discharge of some morbid, or redundant Matters therein; or, only, for the Sake of thinning, attenuating, and promoting the Motion and Circulation thereof.

The Matter of a Disease, or what is prescribed by Art to remove or ease it, is Evacuated in two Ways. 1°. By the natural Emunctories, or Out-lets of the Skin; the Nostrils, Mouth, Fauces, Oesophagus, Ventricle, Intestines, Bladder, and Urethra. And 2°. By artificial Outlets, made either in the Blood Vessels; as by *Phlebotomy, Arteriotomy, Scarifications*, and *Leaches*. Or, in the Lymphatic Vessels; as by Caustick and Vesicatories. Or, lastly, in both, as by *Issues, Setons, Ulcers, Fistula's*, &c.

Hence, the first Distinction of *Evacuants* is derived from the different *Emunctories*; and the 2d, from the Diversity of Matter *evacuated* thro' them.

Most of the Chronic Diseases, the Infirmities of old Age, and the short Periods of the Lives of *Englishmen*, Dr. *Cheyne* observes, are owing to Repletion. This is evident from hence; that Evacuation of one Kind or another, is nine Parts in ten of their Remedy : For not only Cupping,

Bleeding, Blistering, Issues, Purging, Vomiting and Sweating, are manifest *Evacuations*, or Drains, to draw out what has been superfluously taken down; but even Abstinence, Exercise, Alteratives, Cordials, Bitters, &c. are but several Manes to dispose the gross Humours, to be more readily *evacuated* by insensible Perspiration.

**EVAPORATION**, in Philosophy, the Act of exhaling the Humidity of the Body; or of dissipating it in Fumes or Vapour.

Common Salt is form'd, by evaporating all the Humidity in the Salt-Water, or Brine; which Evaporation is either perform'd by the Heat of the Sun, as in the Salt-Works by the Sea-Coast, &c. or by Means of Fire, as in the Salt Springs, &c.

By the Observations of Mons. *Sedileau* it appears, that what is rais'd in Vapour, exceeds that which falls in Rain.

Tho' the *Evaporation* of Liquids is generally look'd on as an Effect of the Heat, and the Motion of the Air; yet Mons. *Gauteron*[1], in the *Memoirs de l'Academ. des Scien.* An. 1705. shews, that a quite opposite Cause may have the same Effect; and that Liquids lose a deal more of their Parts in the severest Frost, than when the Air is moderately warm. In the great Frost of the Year 1708, he found, that the greater the Cold, still the more considerable the *Evaporation*; and that Ice it self lost full as much as the warmer Liquors that did not freeze.

Dr. *Halley*[2] furnishes us with some Experiments of the Quantity, or Measure of the Evaporation of Water. The Result is contain'd in the following Articles :

1°. That Water salted to about the same Degree as Salt Water, and exposed to a Heat equal to that of a Summer's Day, did, from a circular Surface of about Eight Inches Diameter, *Evaporate* at the Rate of 6 Ounces in 24 Hours. Whence, by a Calculus, he finds, that the Thickness of the Pellicle, or Skin of Water *Evaporated* in two Hours, was the 53d Part of an Inch : But, for a round Number, he supposes it only a 60th Part; and argues thence, that if Water as warm as the Air in Summer, evaporates the Thickness of one 60th Part of an Inch in two Hours, from its whole Surface; in twelve Hours it will exhale one tenth of an Inch. Which Quantity, he observes, will be found abundantly sufficient to furnish all the Rains, Springs, Dews, &c.

In Effect, on this Principle, every 10 Square Inches of the Surface of the Water, yields in Vapour, *per diem*, a Cubic Inch of Water; and each Square Foot half a Wine Pint; every Space of 4 Foot Square, a Gallon; a Mile Square, 6914 Tons; and a Square Degree, suppose of 69 *English* Miles, will *Evaporate* 33 Million Tons.

2°. A Surface of Eight Square Inches, *Evaporated* purely by the natural Warmth of the Water without either Wind or Sun, in the Course of a whole Year, 16292 Grains of Water, or 64 Cubic Inches; consequently, the Depth of Water thus *Evaporated* in one Year amounts to 8 Inches. But this being much too little to answer the Experiments of the French, who found, that it

[1] Antione Gauteron (1670 – 1737), a French phsycian and medical writer.

[2] Edmund Halley (1656 – 1742), an English astronomer and mathematician.

rain'd 19 Inches of Water in one Year at Paris; or those of Mr. *Townley*, who found the Annual Quantity of Rain in Lancashire, above 40 Inches : He concludes, that the Sun and Wind contribute more to *Evaporation*, than any internal Heat, or Agitation of the Water.

3°. The Effect of the Wind is very considerable, on a double Account. For the same Observations shew a very odd Quality in the Vapours of Water, *viz.* that of adhering and hanging to the Surface that exhaled 'em, which they clothe, as it were, with a Fleece of vaporous Air; which once investing the Vapour, it thenceforward rises in much less Quantity. Whence, the Quantity of Water lost in 24 Hours, when the Air was very still from Winds, was very small; in proportion to what went away when there was a string Gale of Wind Abroad to dissipate the Fleece, and make Room for the Emission of Vapour : And this, even tho' the Experiment was made in a Place as close from the Wind as could be contrived.

Add, that this Fleece of Water hanging on the Surface of Waters in still Weather, is the Occasion of very strange Appearances, by the Refraction of the Vapour's differing from, and exceeding that of common Air. Whence every thing appears rais'd, as Houses like Steeples, Ships as on Land above the Water, the Land rais'd, and as it were lifted from the Sea, &c.

4°. The same Experiments shew, that the *Evaporations* in *May, June, July,* and *August*, which are nearly equal, are about three Times as great as those in the Months of *November, December, January,* and *February.*

**EVAPORATION**, in Pharmacy, an Operation by which the more aqueous and volatile Parts of Liquids are spent, or drove away in Steam; so as to leave the remaining Part stronger, or of a higher Consistence than before. *Evaporation* is properly the setting a Liquor over a gentle Heat, to carry off the most fluid and volatile Parts, without lessening the Quantity of the other Matter the Liquor is impregnate withal. *Evaporation* differs from Exhalation, in that the former is practised on moist Things, and the latter on dry.

**EVIL**, or *Kings*-Evil, in Medicine, a Disease by the Physicians call'd *Strumæ*, and *Scrophulæ*, consisting of schirrous Tumours, arising most commonly about the Neck, but sometimes also on the other glandular Parts, as the Breasts, Arm-pits, Groin, &c.

The Kings of *England* and *France*, have, of a long Time, pretended to the Privilege of Curing the *Kings-Evil* by *Touching*.

The Right, or Faculty, 'tis said by some, was originally inherent in the *French* Kings; and those of *England* only claim'd it, as an Appendage, or Appurtenant to that Crown, to which they laid a Claim. Tho' some of our own Monkish Writers set the Thing on a different Footing; and will have it to have been practised by our Kings, as early as *Edward the Confessor*; which Opinion the ingenious Mr. *Becket* has abundantly overthrown.

*Steven de Conti*, a Religious of *Corbie*, who lived in the Year 1400, and wrote a History of *France* still preserved in MS. in the Library of St. *Germains des prez*, describes the Practise of Touching for the Evil. After the King had heard Mass, a Vessel of Water was brought him, and his Majesty having put up his Prayers before the Altar, *touch'd* the diseased Part with his right Hand, and wash'd it with the Water.

*Matthew Paris*[1] will have S. *Louis* the first who practised it : Others contend, that King *Robert* was the first who was gifted this Way. 'Tis certain, we find no mention of any such Prerogative, before the Kings of the 11th Century, when that Prince reign'd.

*Polydore Virgil*[2] strains hard to prove the same Virtue in the Kings of *England*; but to little Purpose.

The Continuer of *Monstrelet*[3], observes, that *Charles* VIII touch'd several Sick Persons at Rome, and cured 'em, *dont ceux des Italies*, says he, *voyant ce Mystere ne furent onques si emerveilles.*

The same Virtue, we know not on what Grounds, is commonly attributed to a Seventh Son, born without any Daughter between : As also to the Chiefs of certain particular Families; particularly, the Eldest Person of the House of *Aumont* in *Burgundy.*

**EUPHORBIUM**, or *Euphorbia*, in Pharmacy, a Kind of Gum, brought from Africa, in little roundish Pieces, whitish when new, and yellowish when old, very sharp to the Taste, but void of Smell.

The principal Use of *Euphorbium*, is external; being a great Ingredient in divers resolutive Plasters, as well as in Tincture, and Powder for stopping of Gangrenes, cleansing of foul Ulcers, and exfoliating carious Bones.

Internally used, 'tis a Purgative, but so violent a one, that 'tis almost out of Doors, as tearing off the necessary Mucus or Covering of the Stomach and Bowels, and occasioning Dysenteries. Yet we are told the *Africans* use it very commonly; tho' they first quench its Fire in Purslain Water.

Its Powder is a violent Sternutatory, and to be used very cautiously, and never alone, but mix'd with a small Quantity of some other Powder, to guard against its intolerable Heat.

The Gum we call *Euphorbium*, is form'd of the Juice of a Tree, or rather Plant, of the same Name, pretty frequent in *Mauritania*; tho' the Species of the Tree, or Plant, has been greatly controverted. The Generality of our latest Botanists, make it a ferulaceous Plant; and Mr. Professor *Hermannus*[4] calls it the *Tithymalus Mauritanus Aphystos Angulosus & Spinosus*. Hort. *Acad. Lug. Batav.* 598.

It has no leaves; but in Lieu thereof puts forth along its Stem a Kind of long prickly Eyes, or Buds. Which Buds, it is, that yield that gummy Juice, call'd *Euphorbium Officinarum.*

Some Authors will have it, that the Gum is drawn from the Plant by Incision; others, on the contrary, say it oozes spontaneously : The Juice, we are told, is so very subtile, and penetrating, that the Person who taps the Tree, is forced to stand at a good Distance, and make the Incisions with a long Pike; otherways it gets to the Brain, and occasions dangerous Inflammations. It oozes out in great Abundance, and is gather'd in a Sheep's

[1] Matthew Paris (ca. 1200 – 1259), an English Benedictine monk.

[2] Polydore Virgil (ca. 1470 – 1555), an Italian scholer who chronicled English history.

[3] Enguerrand de Monstrelet (ca. 1400 -1453), a French scholar.

[4] Paulus Hermannus, or Paul Herman (ca. 1640 – 1695), a German botanist.

skin, wrapp'd round the Tree.

*Pliny* tells us, that the first Discovery of *Euphorbium* is attributed to Juba King of *Lybia*, who denominated it from *Euphorbius* his Physician, Brother of *Musa*, Physician to *Augustus*.

*Etmuller* assures us, that the Plant, which yielded the *Euphorbium* of the Antients, is now unknown to us; but if we go by *Pliny's* Description, the Plant call'd *Schadida Calli* in the *Hortus Malabaricus*, must be the antient *Euphorbium*. This Discovery is owing to *Commelinus*, Bourguemaister of Amsterdam, and Professor of Botany.

**EXALTATION**, Physicks, is the Act, or Operation of elevating, purifying, subtilizing, or perfecting any natural Body, its Principles and Parts; as also the Quality, or Disposition, which Bodies acquire by this Operation.

'Tis this *Exaltation* of the sulphureous Part in the Straw-berries, that gives them their agreeable, vinous Tast. A gentle and temperate Heat of the Body, *Exalts*, and disengages the most volatile Parts of our Food, and disposes 'em for Nutrition.

The Term *Exaltation*, is peculiarly affected by the Chymists and Alchymists, who imagining it to have some extraordinary Emphasis, are using it at every Turn. Most sulphureous Matters, much *Exalted*, are observed to be of a red Colour.

**EXANTHEMA**, in Medicine, an Eruption, or Efflorescence on the Skin. *Exanthemata* are of two Kinds : The one only a discolouring of the Skin; such are the Measles, the purple Spots in malignant Fevers, &c. The other are little Eminences, or *Papillae*, standing out from the Skin, not unlike Pustles, only smaller. The Word is form'd of the *Greek* εξανθεο, *Effervesco, Effloresco*, I flower, or work out.

**EXCORTICATION**, the stripping off the Cortex, or Bark, from any Thing; call'd also *Decortication*.

**EXCREMENT**, what is evacuated, or *excreted*, out of the Body of an Animal, after Digestion; being what in other Respects is superfluous and prejudicial thereto.

*Chauvin* describes *Excrement*, to be all that Matter taken in by way of Food, which cannot be assimilated; and which, of Consequence, not growing or adhering to the Body, wanders about thro' the laxer, and more patent Parts thereof, till it be ejected.

The Urine and Fæces or fecal Matter, are the *great Excrements*, expell'd from the Bladder and the Intestines by Stool, &c.

The Matter of insensible Perspiration is also an *Excrement*, and a more considerable one than either of the others.

Among *Excrements*, are likewise ordinarily rank'd divers Humours and Matters, separate from the Blood by the several Strainers, or Emunctories of the Body, tho' far from being useless; and serving divers valuable Purposes of the Oeconomy. Such are Cerumen, or Ear-wax; the Mucus of the Nose; *Lachrymæ*, or Tears; Salia, Bile, Lympha, Menses, Lochia, &c. Some hold

*Ambergrease* an *Excrement* of the Whale; others, an *Excrement* of the Sea.

All Foods have two Parts, the one Nutritious, the other *Excrementitious*.

**EXCREMENT**, is also attributed, by way of Analogy to Plants. Thus Gums, divers Juices, Balms, &c. issuing spontaneously from their respective Trees, are sometimes call'd *Excrements*.

**EXCRESCENCE**, in Chirurgery, a superfluous, or unnecessary Piece of Flesh, or other Matter, growing on certain Parts of the Bodies of Animals, contrary to, or beyond the ordinary Structure and Disposition of Nature.

Such are Wens, Warts, &c. Such also are the Woman's Horns now shewn in London; a parallel Case to which, see in the *Philosoph. Transact.* N°. 297. Natural, or customary *Excrescences*, as those of Bones, &c. are call'd by Physicians *Apophyses*.

The Word is form'd of the Latin, *ex*, and *cresco*, I grow; *q.d.* something that grows from, or out of another.

**EXCRETION**, in Medicine, the Act whereby Nature expels, or ejects out of the Body, some Humour that is useless, or even hurtful thereto. Most Crises are effected by *Excretions*; as Fluxes of Blood, and Urine, Sweats, Vomitings, Loosenesses, &c. The Word is form'd of the Latin, *excernere*, to excern, separate.

**EXÆRESIS**, or Exheresis, in Chirurgery, an Operation whereby something foreign, useless, and even pernicious, is taken from the human Body. The Word is *Greek*, εξαιρεσις, which signifies the same Thing. The *Exæresis* is perform'd two Ways : By *Extraction*, when something formed in the Body is drawn out of the same : And by *Detraction*, when something is taken away, that had been introduced into the Body from without.

**EXFOLIATION**, in Chirurgery, the sealing of a Bone; or its rising and separating in Leaves, or Laminæ. The Word is compounded of the Latin *ex* and *folium*, Leaf. Any Part of the Surface of the Cranium that has been bored, is liable to *Exfoliation*. The Use of the Cephalic Powders avails nothing for promoting the *Exfoliation*. *Dionis*. The Wound must not be stopp'd too much, but the Bone left at Liberty to recover it self, which it sometimes does, without *Exfoliating*, particularly in Children.

**EXFOLIATIVE**. An *Exfoliative* Trepan, is a Trepan proper to scrape, and at the same Time pierce, a Bone, and so to exfoliate, or raise several Leaves, or Flakes, one after another. The Use of the *Exfoliative* Tepan is very dangerous; as being apt to shake and disorder the Head.

**EXHALATION**, a Fume, or Steam, *exhaling*, or issuing from a Body, and diffusing it self in the Atmosphere. The Terms *Exhalation* and *Vapour*, are ordinarily used indifferently; but the more accurate Writers distinguish them: Appropriating the Term *Vapour* to the moist Fumes rais'd from Water, and other liquid Bodies; and *Exhalation* to the dry ones emitted from solid Bodies; as Earth, Fire, Minerals, Sulphurs, &c.

In this Sense, *Exhalations* are dry, subtile Corpuscles, or Effluvia, loosen'd from hard terrestrial Bodies, either by the Heat of the Sun, or the Agitation of the Air, or some other Cause; and emitted upwards to a certain Height of the Atmosphere, where mixing with the Vapours, they help to constitute Clouds, and return back again into Dews, Mists, Rains, &c.

Nitrous, and sulphureous *Exhalations* are the chief Matter of Thunder, Lightening, and diver other Meteors generated in the Air.

Sir *Isaac Newton* takes true and permanent Air to be form'd from the *Exhalations* rais'd from the hardest and most compact Bodies.

**EXOMPHALUS**, in Medicine, a Generical Name for divers Disorders. *Exomphalus* expresses all Kinds of Ruptures, or Tumors, happening in the *Umbilicus*, or Navel.

Authors distinguish three Kinds of *Exomphali*; the first are, Tumors, or Swellings of the solid Parts, whereof there are three Varieties, denominated from the several Parts affected, as the *Enteromphalus, Epiplomphalus*, and *Entero-epiplomphalus* : The second are, Tumors form'd by Collections, or Gatherings of Humours, of which there are four Varieties, distinguish'd by the particular Humours they are form'd of, as the *Hydromphalus, Pneumatomphalus, Sarcomphalus*, and *Varicomphalus* : The third are those compounded of both the other, *viz.* the *Enterohydromphalus*, and *Epiplosarcomphalus*.

**EXPIRATION**, in Medicine, that Motion in an Animal, whereby the Air, inspired into the Lungs, is expell'd, or thrust out of the same, and the Cavity of the Breast contracted. Respiration consists of two Alternate Motions, or Actions of the Lungs, corresponding to those of a Pair of Bellows; *Inspiration*, whereby the Air is drawn in; and *Expiration*, whereby 'tis driven out again. By Means of this Alteration, the Circulation of the Blood, and the Motions of the Heart are maintain'd.

**EXPRESSED** *Oils*, are such as are procured from Bodies, only by pressing; as the Oil of Olives, Almonds, and the like.

**EXPRESSION**, in Medicine, Chymistry, &c. the Act of Expressing, or extracting the Juices of Plants, Fruits, and other Matters, by squeezing, wringing, or pressing them in a Press. After having let the Herbs infuse their due Time, their Juice must be drawn by Expression in a Linnen Cloth, or under a Press.

**EXSICCATION**, in Chymistry, &c. the Act of drying, or evaporating the Moisture of a Thing. The Word is *Latin*, form'd of *ex*, and *siccus*, dry.

**EXSUDATION**, the Act of sweating out – in which manner Gums, Balsams, &c. are produced from Trees.

**EXTENUATION**, the Act of diminishing, or lessening, the Force of a Thing. Thus, in Medicine, we say, Fevers, Agues, long Abstinences, &c. occasion great Extenuations or Emaciations.

**EXTRACT**, in Pharmacy, the purest, and finest Part of a Vegetable, or other Body, separated from the coarser, by dissolving and digesting it with a proper Menstruum; and afterwards reduced into a thick, moist Consistence by a Distillation, or Evaporation of the Humidity of the Menstruum.

**EXTRACTING**, an artful drawing out of the Juices, Virtues, and Qualities of a natural Body. There are divers Ways of Extracting the Virtues of Vegetables, Minerals, &c. by *Pression, Infusion, Lotion, Calcination, Distillation, Cohobation*, and other Operations taught in Chymistry and Pharmacy.

**EXTRACTION**, in Pharmacy and Chymistry, an Operation whereby Essences, Tinctures, &c. are drawn from natural Bodies.

Some will have *Extraction* to signify any Solution made by Menstruums ; But, in Strictness, there is this Difference; that in *Solution* the Menstruums absorb the whole Substance of the Body, but in *Extraction* they carry off only a certain Party of it : And in this Sense, Camphire is dissolved in Spirit of Wine, but Jalap is more properly said to be *extracted*; for the Resin is only taken out by the Menstruum, the other Particles being left untouch'd.

*Extraction* does also frequently signify such an Inspissation, or thickening of a Solution, as that when a certain Quantity of the Menstruum is drawn off, reduceth the remaining Mixture to the Consistence of Honey; as in the *Extracts* of Saffron, Gentian, and the like.

*Extracts* are chiefly made from Vegetables, and require different Menstruums, according to the different Nature of the Plants; especially in Gummous Kind : For such as are mucilaginous, as *Gum Arabic*, and *Tragacanth*, &c. are not easily dissolved but in aqueous Liquors; whereas, on the other Hand, resinous Gums, as *Galbanum, Scammony*, &c. must have burning Spirits to dissolve them.

There are others again of a middle Nature, which may be dissolved in either Sort of Menstruums, tho' not so easily in one as the other.

Thus Aloes, and Rhubarb, which are sometimes resinous, are better made into *Extracts* with Spirit of Wine, than Water : But Plants, which abound less with Resin, such as Hellebore, &c. are more commodiously extracted with Water. To perform *Extraction* therefore aright, a proper Menstruum is necessary, and one which is as near a-kin as possible to the Body to be *extracted.*

**EXTRAVASATION**, in Medicine, the Act, or Motion, whereby the Blood *extravasates* it self, *i.e.* breaks out of its ordinary Vessels, the Veins and Arteries, an gathers and stagnates in some Part of the Body : The Blood that flows out of the Body, or that is drawn from it in opening a Vein, Is not properly said to be *Extravasated.* The Word is form'd of the Latin, *extra*, without, and *vas*, vessel.

The ordinary Causes of *Extravasations*, are unnatural Repletions, and Distentions of the Vessels; or Lacerations and Erosions thereof.

There is a Necessity for bleeding, to prevent the Blood's growing to such a Head as to *Extravasate. Extravasated* Blood always corrupts and turns into an Imposthume. In Wounds of the Head, particularly, bleeding is necessary, to prevent the *Extravasation* of the Blood in the Brain.

The Term is likewise used with Regard to other Humours beside the Blood, as the Lympha, Urine, &c. The Gardeners likewise use it, in speaking of Gums, Juices, &c. oozing out of their Trees either spontaneously, or at Incisions.

**EXULCERATION**, in Medicine, the Act of occasioning, or producing Ulcers. Thus, Arsenic *Exulcerates* the Intestines : Corrosive Humours *Exulcerate* the Skin. The Term is sometimes also used for an Ulcer it self; but more generally for those beginning Erosions, which wear away the Substance, and form Ulcers. *Exulcerations* in the Intestines, are Marks of Poison.

*Hares*-**EYE**, *Oculus Leprinous*, in Medicine, a Disease arising from a Contraction of the upper Eye-lid, which prevents its being able to cover its Part of the Eye. Whence the Patient is obliged to sleep with the Eye half open after the Manner of *Hares*. The Physicians call it *Lagophthalmia*, a *Greek* Word signifying the same Thing; being compounded of λαγως, *Hare*, and οφθαλμος, *Eye*.

*Goats*-**EYE**, *Oculus Caprinus*, is when there is a white Speck on the Cornea; as is seen in the *Eye* of Goats. Physicians call it *Aigis*.

**FACIES** *Hippocratica*, in Medicine, is when the Nostrils are sharp, the Eyes hollow, the Temples low, the Tips of the Ears contracted, the Fore-head, dry, and wrinkled, and the Complexion pale, or livid. The *Facies Hippocratica* is chiefly observed toward the Period of Phthises and other Consumptions. It is held a sure Prognostick of Death.

**FACTITIOUS**, signifies any Thing made by Art; in Opposition to what is the Produce of Nature. Thus Cinnabar is divided into Natural and *Factitious*. Distilled Waters are *Factitious* Liquors.

**FACULTY**, a Power, or Ability of performing an Action. The Term is much used by the antient Philosophers, and still retain'd in the Schools, to explain the Actions of natural Bodies by. Thus, to account for the Act of Digestion, they suppos'd a *Digestive Faculty* in the Stomach : To account for Motion, they imagin'd a *Motive Faculty* in the Nerves, &c. which is only a substituting of one Name of an unknown Phaenomenon for another.

Yet this Practice of attributing Effects to their respective Virtues, or *Faculties*, still obtains in divers Things, which our Philosophy has not yet afforded us a better Account of. Thus, say our Medicinal Writers, Senna and Rhubarb have a *Purgative Faculty*; Barberries an *Astringent Faculty*, &c. which amounts just to this, that Senna purges, and Barberries bind.

The Faculties or *Powers of the Soul*, are commonly reputed two, *viz*. of *Understanding* and *Willing*.

A Faculty *of an Animal Body*, is defined to be the Principle whereby the Body performs its Functions. This is usually distinguish'd with regard to the several Functions, into *Vegetative* and *Animal*.

Under the *Vegetative Faculty*, are comprehended the divers subaltern one, whereby Nutrition and generation are affected. The *Vegetative Faculty* then is divided into *Nutritive* and *Generative*; and the Nutritive is again subdivided into *Natural* and *Vital*.

To the first, belong the Functions of the lower Belly, relating to the Preparation of the Food; to the latter, the Actions of the Heart and Lungs, wherein Life is chiefly concern'd.

Others subdivide the Vegetative *Faculty* into *Attractive, Retentive, Concoctive*, and *Expulsive*.

The *Animal Faculties*, being those whereby an Animal perceives and moves, become divided into *Sensitive* and *Locomotive*.

**FÆCAL MATTER**, a Term used by Physicians, particularly the French, for the Faeces or great Excrements of a Man, *i.c.* those discharged by Stool.

The *Fæcal Matter* is become famous for a chymical Operation thereon, by Mons. *Homberg*, related at length in the *Mem. de l'Academie R. An.* 1711. He had a Notion suggested to him, that the *Fæcal Matter*, by Distillation, yielded an Oil clear as Water, without any Smell, and which had the Property of fixing Mercury into fine Silver. Upon this, to work he goes; and because he would have as laudable and promising a *Matter* as he could, hired four robust health young Fellows, whom he shut up for three Months, and agreed with them, that they should eat nothing but the finest Bread, which he supplied them withal fresh every day, and drink the best *Champain* Wine as long as they would. After a long Process, and numerous Essays on the Excrements they made, he at length got the clear, inodorous Oil; but it had not Effect at all on Mercury, which was the great Point aim'd at.

However, missing of what he expected, he fell on something he never dreamt of, *viz., a Phosphorus*. The *Caput Mortuum* of the Oil, he found to have a surprizing Property of taking Fire without any Motion, or the Application of any other Fire; insomuch, that it might deserve a Place in the first Rank of Phosphori known. The Quantity of a Pea taken out of the Matras, and laid on a Paper, or other combustible Matter, begins to smoak immediately, and sets the Paper on Fire.

**FÆCES**, or Fœces, or Feces, the Dregs, Sediment, or Impurities remaining of a mixt Body, after the purer, more volatile and fluid have been separated therefrom by Evaporation, Dissolution, Decantation, Derivation or the like. Thus we say the *Fæces of Oils*, &c. Those of Wines are properly call'd *Lees*. Those of Malt-liquors, *Grounds*.

**FÆCES** is particularly used in Medicine, &c. For the gross impure Matter found at the Bottom of the Compositions and Preparations of either Pharmacy.

**FÆCES**, in Chymistry denotes, the Lees, Refuse, Dirt, Mud, Ordures, Impurities, Excrements and heterogeneous Matters remaining in the Alembic after the Distillation of any Body. What remains in the Retort, instead of Fæces, is properly denominated *Caput Mortuum*, or *Terra damnata*.

**FALSE** *Flower*, a Flower, which does not seem to produce any Fruit; as those of the Hazle, Mulberry-Tree, &c. Or a Flower, that does not arise from any Embryo, or that does not knit; as those of the Melon, Cucumber, &c.

**FAMES** *Canina*, by the *Greeks* call'd *Cynodes Arexis, q.d.* Dog appetite, is such an insatiable Hunger, as is not to be satisfied with Eating; but continues, even when the Stomach is full. This is a Case, much talk'd of by Antients; but rarely met with amongst us. It may be supposed, to arise from sharp fretting Juices in the Stomach, which by their continual Vellications excite a Sense like that of Hunger.

**FARINA**, the Flower, or Powder of some Grain, or Pulse ground, and sifted from the Bran. The Word is pure Latin, *Farina*, form'd of *Far*, Corn, Wheat : And *Far*, according to *Guichard*, comes from the *Hebrew* בר, *bar*, signifying the same Thing.

**FARINA** *fæcundans*, among Naturalists, is a fine Dust prepar'd in the Male flowers of Plants; which being afterwards shed on the Female, does the Office of a Sperm, or Semen, by impregnating the same.

The *Farina fæcundans*, call'd also the *Male-dust*, and *Male-seed*, is form'd and secreted in the *Apices*, or Tops of the *Stamina*; where, when it becomes mature, and copious enough, bursting its Capsula, it is spilt on the Head of the *Pistil*, and thence convey'd to the *Matrix*, or *Utricle* thereof, to fæcundify the *Ova*, or female Seed, contain'd therein.

This *Dust*, in any one Plant, being view'd with a Microscope; every particle thereof appears of the same Size and Figure : But in different Plants, the Figure, Size, Colour, &c. of the Dust, is very different. Some are clear, and transparent, as Crystal; as those of the *Maple, Burrach*, and *Hemlock* : Others are white, as those of *Henbane, Balsamins* : Others are blue, as those of *Flax* : Others purple, as of some *Tulips*: Others flesh-colour'd, as some Species of *Lychnis*; and others red, as those of the *Geum*.

It may be observ'd, however, that the Colour of the *Farina* varies, in the same Species according to the Colour of the Flower; and even, sometimes, the *Farina* of the same Flower is of different Colours; as is easily observ'd in the *Caryophillus arvensis*.

The Figures of the divers Kinds of *Farinæ* are much harder to describe. The most general Figure is the Oval, more or less sharp at the Ends, with one or more Channels, or Furrows, running length-wise; so that through the Microscope they look not unlike the Stone of a Date, a grain of Wheat, a Coffee-berry, or an Olive. Such are those of Polygonatum, Bugles, Bryony, Tithimal, &c. Those of the Melilot, are Cylinders : Those of the great Consolida, represent two crystal Globules, closely fasten'd to each other : Those of the Sycamore, represent two Cylinders, plac'd a-cross : Those of Jonquille, are in form a Kidney : Those of the *Camponulæ*, Passion-flower, &c. are nearly round, but unequal in their Surfaces : Those of *Caryophyllus silvestris*, are round, and cut in Facets : Those of the *Geranium*, and some other Species, are round, with a kind of *Umbelicus*, or Indenture, as in an Apple, *Bradley* says, they are perforated quite through, like the Bead of a Necklace, which we doubt : Those of *the Caltha, Corona Solis*, &c. are little Globes, set with Prickles, &c.

Of these *Farinæ,* some are very hard; others, soft, and easily broke. They all contain a deal of sulphureous Matters, more than the other Parts; whence, they are very odorous. Those of the Lilly, are so full of Oil, that they grease the Paper they are put in, as if it had been oil'd. The *Farinæ* of most Aromatic Plants, swim in an essential Oil, or sort of liquid Turpentine : Others are involved in a dry Rosin; as these of the *Lycopodium*, or *Muscus terrestris clavatus*. C.B. Others, as those of Fumitory, are inclos'd in a little, viscid, mucilaginous Matter; and all. In effect, have something so glutinous, that they stick to any thing, that touches them : So that 'tis difficult to separate them from each other.

Some have imagin'd, that these *Farinæ* were only Particles of Wax, or Rosin : But the Contrary is easily prov'd : For they neither dissolve in Water, not Spirit, not Oils; even when assisted with Fire.

Mr. *Bradley* supposes a Magnetick Virtue lodg'd in the *Farina fæcundans*, or Male Dust; by means whereof, when deposited in the Utricle of the Female, it draws the Nourishment from the other Parts of the Plant into the Ova, or Rudiments of the Fruit, and makes them swell. The Reality of this Virtue, he argues from the same being found in Wax, which is chiefly, or wholly gather'd hence by the Bees.

Some, against the great Use of the *Farina fæcundans* in Generation, may object, that in Flowers, which hang downwards, as the Cyclamen, &c. the *Farina fæcundans* cannot be cast on the Orifice of the Pistil : To which it may be answer'd, that the Pistils of such Flowers, hanging lower than the dusty Apices which surround them, the glutinous Matter and Velvet, covering the Extremity of the Pistil, may be capable of receiving, and retaining some of the *Farina* as it falls : And without any Intromission of the *Farina*, its Lodgement on the Mouth of the Pistil, may by Virtue of its attractive Power fecundify the Seed in the Uterus.

**FASCICULUS**, in Medicine, a Term sometimes used to express a certain Quantity, or Measure of Herbs. By *Fasciculus* is meant so much, as may be held in the Arm, when bent, and rested on the Top of the Haunch. Physicians note it in Prescription by *Fasc.*

**FAT**, in an Animal Body, a white, oily, sulphurous Substance, collected in little membranous *Loculi* or Cells, in divers Parts of the Body; serving to keep the Parts warm, and to soften and temper the sharp Salts in the Mass of Blood.

The *Fat* of Animals, for the generality, is not reckon'd good Food; as being hard of Digestion, and producing a thick, viscid Chyle. But it is of good use in Medicine.

*Calves Fat* is us'd in Pomatums, and Unguents; being resolutive, and emollient. That of *Hogs* and *Boars*, has the same Qualities, and is strengthening besides. *Deers Grease* is good to fortify the Nerves, against the Rheumatism, Sciatica, Gout, and Fractures. *Hares Grease*, applied externally, promotes Digestion, and the Suppuration of Abscesses. That of *Rabbits*, is nervous, and resolutive. That of *Cocks*, and *Hens*, resolves and softens Hardnesses. That of *Geese*, has the same Qualities; and likewise abates Hemorrhoids, assuages Pains in the Ear, being applied within the same; and opens the Belly, being taken inwardly. *Eels Fat* is esteem'd good against the Hemorrhoids, and Deafness; to take away Pits of the Smallpox, and to make the Hair grow. That of the *Trout*, beside its being emollient, is good in Diseases of the Anus, and Ulcers of the Breast.

**FEBRIFUGE**, in Medicine, a specifick Remedy for the Cure of Fevers. The Word is Compounded of *Febris*, and *Fugo*, I drive away.

The Quinquina, or Jesuit's Bark, is the greatest, and surest of all the Class of *Febrifuges*. The little Centaureum is sometimes also call'd *Febrifugum*, on account of its Virtues. The *Chinese* Ginseng is particularly fam'd as a *Febrifuge*. For such as cannot take the Bark in Substance, Dr. *Fuller*[1] prescribes a *Febrifuge Enema*, made of a Decoction thereof.

The inner Bark of the Ash-tree, with a little Salt of Wormwood, taken like the *Peruvian* Bark, is said to equal or even exceed it, as a *Febrifuge*. The like is said of the Bark of the Elm near the Root. The Flowers of *Sal Armoniac* are held an excellent *Febrifuge*, especially in intermitting Fevers. Cold Water has been lately much extoll'd as a Febrifuge. Dr. *Hancock*[2] gives it the emphatical

[1] Thomas Fuller (1654 – 1734), an English physician and moralist.

[2] John Hancock (ca. 1700), rector of St. Margaret, Lothbury, and prebendary of Canterbury.

Denomination of *Febrifugium Magnum.*

Mr. *Reneaume*, in the *Hist. de l'Academ. R. de Sciences, An.* 1711. proposes a new *Febrifuge*, of his own Discovery, *viz. Galls.* From a great Number of Experiments, he has learnt, that Galls alone will frequently cure an intermitting Fever, as well as the Quinquina; over which it has some Advantages in other Things; in that it is not so bitter, does not heat, is taken in a lesser Dose, seldomer, and cheaper.

At his Motion, several other Physicians tried with Success, particularly Mr. *Homberg*; though it did not succeed so well with M. *Bulduc*, *Lemery*, and *Geoffroy*.

**FECULA**, or Fæcula, in Pharmacy, a white, mealy Substance, or Powder, which subsides, and gathers at the Bottom of Juices, or Liquors of divers Roots; as those of Briony, Arum, Iris, &c. This Substance, or Sediment, they dry in the Sun; after having pour'd off the Liquors; and it serves for divers Remedies. The Word *Fæcula* is a Diminutive of *Fæces.*

**FECULENT**, or Fæculent, is applied to the Blood, and other Humours, which abound in Fæces, or Dregs; or have not the proper and usual Degree of Purity.

**FENNEL**, or *Fennel-Seed*, in Commerce, &c. a longish, striated Seed, flat on one Side, and roundish on the other; of a sweetish Taste, not unlike that of Anis-seed; being the Produce of an umbelliferous Plant of the same Name, well known as a Pot-herb.

*Fennel* makes part of the Commerce of the Druggists and Apothecaries. 'Tis esteem'd a Carminative, and us'd like Anis-seed, to dispel Winds on the Body; and correct Senna, and the rest of the vegetable Purgatives.

There is also a strong Water, or Brandy made of the Seeds of *Fennel*, and call'd *Fennel-Water*. The Ingredients are *Fennel* Seed, Liquorice, Brandy, and white Wine, which are distill'd together; and to the Essence thereof are added Spirit of Wine, Sugar, and sweet Almonds : The whole strain'd, &c.

**FENNUGREE**, *Fænum Graecum*, or Fennigreek, a medicinal Plant, thus call'd, because antiently brought from Greece, tho' now cultivated in several Parts of Europe.

Its Stem is about a Foot high : Its Leaves small, and dispos'd somewhat like those of Trefoil. It yields a little white Flower, from whence arises a long, pointed Pod, shap'd nit unlike a Bullock's Horn.

The Grain, or Seed is inclos'd in this Pod, which bears the Name of the Plant it self, is less than Mustard Seed, very hard, and solid, of a triangular Form, and a strong disagreeable Smell; When new, 'tis of a yellow, gold Colour; but when kept, ruddy, or brown.

The Farina, or Flower of these Seeds is esteem'd good to ripen and digest; and as such, is used in Cataplasms of those Intentions; as also in emollient Clysters, Decoctions, and Cataplasms. It yields a Mucilage used in Inflammations of the Eyes and on other Occasions.

**FERMENT**, in Physicks, a Body of any Kind, which being applied to another, produces a *Fermentation* therein : Or, any thing capable of exciting an intestine Motion, in the Part of another; and of swelling, or dilating the same, by means of its more penetrating and moveable Parts, which by their Agitation divide and agitate the Particles thereof. See Fermentation.

Thus, the Acid in Leven, is a *Ferment*, which makes Bread rise, or swell. The Moisture in Hay is the *Ferment*, which heats and makes it smoak. Thus also, Rennet is the *Ferment*, that curdles and breaks Milk : Balm, or Yeast is the *Ferment*, that sets Wort a-working, &c. See Leven, &c.

The Force or Effect of a *Ferment*, arises hence, that by dissolving, and breaking the Texture or Combination of the component Parts or Principles of the Body, and giving them a new Motion; it disposes them to take a new Arrangement, or to combine again in a new manner; and so to constitute a new Species of Body. Its Effect is somewhat like that of a Person, who opening the Gates of a City, lets in the Enemy who soon raises terrible Disorders : Thus, the Bite of a mad Dog excites a slow *Fermentation* in the Blood, whereby the divers Liquors, or Matters it consists of, lose that Nexus, or Union, necessary to a State of Health; and occasion an Irregularity in the Spirits, from which arise the Horrors, and other Symptoms of the Disease.

One way of accounting for Digestion, is by supposing a certain *Ferment* or Menstruum in the Stomach, which dissolves the Food contain'd therein. But what this *Ferment* is, or whence it should be derived, is greatly disputed. Some will have it an Acid; others, alcalious; others, sulphureous; others, alcalino-sulphureous; others, muriatick, &c. as their own Fancies suggest to them.

**FERMENTATION**, an intestine Motion, or Commotion of the small, insensible Particles of a mix'd Body, arising without any apparent mechanical Cause, and producing a considerable Alteration therein. Or, it is an easy, slow, gentle Motion of the intestine Particles of a Body, arising usually from the Operation of some active, acid Matter; which rarifies and subtilizes the softer, yielding Particles thereof.

*Fermentation* differs from *Dissolution*, as the latter is the Result or Effect of the former. *Fermentation* is frequently without Dissolution, *i.e.* the *fermentative* Motion frequently does not go so far as to dissolve the Body : But Dissolution always supposed an antecedent *Fermentation*.

*Fermentation* differs from *Ebullition*, and *Effervescence* in this, that the Motion, which in the former is slow; in the two latter, is violent; and that in the former, the Motion is restrain'd to the minute Particles of the Body; but in the latter it extends to large Masses thereof. See Ebullition and Effervescence.

Indeed it must be observ'd, that Authors usually allow of divers kinds of *Fermentation*; *viz.* an *insensible* one, which is only know from its Effects; and a *sensible* one : A *violent* and a *moderate* one : A *hot*, and a *cold* one : A *natural*, and an *artificial* one.

Plants bruis'd, and left a certain Time in a close Vessel, ferment of themselves; and if let alone, the *Fermentation* will proceed to Putrefaction.

In order to *Fermentation*, 'tis necessary, the Ferment or Liquor have something acid and spirituous in it; that its Motion be tumultuous; that it tend to exalt and purify the Liquor, and produce vinous, or inflammable Spirits. These are the particular Properties and Conditions of *Fermentation*; tho' in the general, all required to effect a *Fermentation*, is a Body, or Liquor, which is not homogeneous, that is, consists of different Principles; that there be a strong Attraction between the Particles of the *Ferment*, and the Body; that the Parts of this latter be moved and agitated irregularly; and that this Motion produce some Alteration in the mixt.

*Fermentation* is one of the most obscure Processes in all Nature. The Generality of our later Philosophers allow it in great Measure a Mystery, to which there Principles will not fully reach.

Dr. *Morgan*, in his late *Philosoph. Prin. of Medicine*, attempts to account for it, on the *Newtonian* System. His Principle is, that the expansive Force of Air, rarified by the Action of Fire; or the mutual Action of Fire and Air, is the universal natural Cause of *Fermentation* and Dissolution.

To shew this, he considers, two great Powers, or Principles in Bodies; *viz.* as attractive, cohesive Power, in the small Particles of Matter, as the Principle of all Rest, Concretion, &c. And the expansive Force of heated Air; as that of *Fermentation*. On the different Proportion and Adjustment of these two opposite Forces, with respect to each other, the Constitution, Texture and Cohesion of Bodies depend.

By the attractive Forces, acting alone, the constituent Parts of compound Bodies, must be brought to their nearest and greatest Contacts, and remain there in a Degree of Firmness, and Cohesion, proportional to the Quantities of Contact.

On the other hand, by the repulsive, expansive Force, acting alone, all Bodies, even the most compact and solid, must be dissolved and diffuses into one perfectly fluid, incoherent Mass.

If both are found in the same Body, and equal in Degree, such Body must continue in its present State of Fluidity, or Cohesion; if the attractive Power prevail, the Quantity of Contact, or Degree of Cohesion will be continually increased to a certain Pitch, where it will rest : On the Contrary, if the expansive Force of the Fire and Air, included in any Body, or Mass of Matter, prevails against the attractive Power of the contiguous Parts, the Parts must necessarily recede from their Points of Contact.

And this happening thro' all the Subdivisions of which the Body of Mass is capable, every small Part must be divided and separated into other smaller Parts; and these again into others, and so on, till we come to the first constituent Particles or Atoms, which are supposed to be perfectly solid, and indivisible.

This Recess of the Parts of Bodies from their Points of Contact, and the Separation, and Division consequent thereon, is what we call Rarefaction; as, on the Contrary, the Approach of the Parts nearer to the Points of Contact, is called *Condensation*. Now from the contrary Effects of these two Forces, there necessarily arises an intestine Commotion, Collision, and natural Struggle of the Parts among themselves, *i.e.* the Parts acted on by two such opposite Forces, will fly off, and recoil, recede, and accede, in Proportion to the Strength and Energy of the opposite Powers, till one or the other prevail, either to *fix* and condense, or *dissolve* and diffuse it; which alternate Motion is what we call *Fermentation*.

If the attractive Force prevail, the most fluid Body will be consolidated, as Water into Ice. On the contrary, if the expansive Force prevail, the firmest Body will be broke, and dissolved.

*Fermentation* is a Point of the utmost Consequence in Medicine : It is one of the principal Means, or Instruments we have for altering, exalting, or calling forth the Properties and Powers of Bodies. To get an Idea of these Changes, we cannot consider it better, than in the procuring of a spirituous Liquor from Malt, by means thereof.

It is to be observ'd then, that the Malt being made as shewn under the Article Malt; and then laid to infuse or *mash* in hot Water, the rest of the Process of brewing is nothing but a raising and directing of a *Fermentation*, or intestine Motion.

How such Motion is mechanically effected, and how it brings forth such a Spirit, may be conceived from what follows; supposing the Reader acquainted with these common Properties in Hydrostaticks; *viz.*

1°. That a Body immersed in any Fluid, specifically lighter than itself, will sink; otherwise, emerge and get to the Top.

2°. That if two equal Bodies of different specifick Gravities be immersed in a Fluid, lighter than either of them, the Celerities of their Descents will be as their Gravities.

3°. That if two unequal Bodies of unequal specifick Gravities be immersed in a Fluid lighter than either, the Celerities of their Descent will be compounded of their Gravities and Dimensions together.

The same Law, by which Bodies descend, hold good in the Ascent of those specifically lighter than the Fluid.

Hence in all heterogeneous Fluids, the constituent Parts of which are not fitted to associate and cohere, so as to form what is called an uniform homogeneous Fluid, the heavier may be accounted as sold Bodies, immersed in a Fluid specifically lighter; and the lighter Parts, as such Bodies in a Fluid specifically heavier; as it may be demonstrated, that the component Parts of all Fluids, separately consider'd are solid.

This Liquor, therefore, called *Wort*, which is a Decoction of Malt, may be consider'd as such an heterogeneous Fluid, whose Parts cannot be interchang'd in their Positions, till each has obtained such an Elevation, as corresponds to its proper Gravity ; But lest this alone should fail of the Intention, by not being sufficient to break those Moleculæ and Vicidities, which entangle the spirituous Parts, and likewise to prevent their flying off at the Surface, some Portion of an already fermented Substance is mix'd with it.

This Substance, term'd *Barm* or *Yeast*, consists of a great Quantity of subtile spirituous Particles, wrapp'd up in such as are viscid. Now, when this is mix'd with such a Liquor, it cannot nut much contribute to that intestine Motion, which is occasioned by the Intercourse, and Occursions of Particles of different Gravities; as the spirituous Particles will be continually serving to get up to the Surface, and the viscid ones continually retarding such Ascent, and preventing their Escape.

So that by these two concurring Causes the Particles extracted from the Grain, will by such frequent Occursions be so comminuted, as continually to increase the more subtile and spirituous Parts, until all that can be made so by Attrition, are set loose from the their former viscid Confinements : and this appears by the Warmth of the Liquor, and the Froth drove to the Top; just at which Time, if it be thrown into the Still, it affords some Quantity of an high inflammable Spirit.

Moderate Warmth much hastens this Process, as it assists in opening the Viscidities, in which some spirituous Parts may be entangled, and unbends the Spring of the included Air, which cannot but contribute to the Rarefaction and Comminution of the whole.

The viscid Parts, which are raised to the Top, not only on account of their own Lightness, but by the continual Efforts and Occursions of the Spirit to get uppermost, both shew, when the *Ferment* is at the highest, and prevent the finer Spirits make their Escape : For if this intestine Luctus be permitted to continue too long, a great Deal will get away, and the remaining grow flat, and vapid, and raise little besides Phlegm in the Still.

The greatest Use of this Theory in Medicine, will be in teaching, what Parts of the Materia Medica are most properly brought under this Procedure; and how such intestine Motion, does in some Things, destroy their Virtues : For by some Medicines an Intention is required : In such Cases therefore, when by any adventitious Cause those Medicines get into a *Ferment*, they are destroyed, and should not be administered.

**FERULÆ**, among Chirurgeons, called also Splinters; are little Chips, of different Matter, as Woods, Barks, Fir, Leather, Paper, &c. applied to Bones, that have been disjointed, when they are set again. The Bark of the Herb Sagapene, called in Latin *Ferula*, was antiently much used on this occasion; whence this Name *Ferula* became common to all.

**FEVER**, *Febris*, in Medicine, a Disease, or rather Species, or Class of Diseases; it being an Observation of *Sydenham*, that Fevers with their Appendages, make two Thirds of all the Diseases of the Body.

This Disorder is very differently defined by Physicians, according to the different Views and Relations they consider it in. *Sydenham* defines it a strenuous Endeavour or Effort of Nature, to throw off some morbific Matter, that greatly incommodes the Body. *Etmuller*, with the same View, calls it a Motion, or Struggle of Nature, whereby with the Assistance of the Spirits, more or less alter'd, she seeks to expel what is hurtful to the animal Œconomy. *Quincy* defines it an augmented Velocity of the Blood : Others, a Fermentation of the Blood, accompanied with a quick Pulse, and excessive Heat. A *Fever*, *Boerhaave* observes, is an inseparable Companion of an Inflammation.

The Causes of *Fevers* are innumerable; and the Disease most often arises in the soundest Bodies, where there was no previous morbific Apparatus; as Cacochymia, Plethora, &c. But merely from a Change of Air, Food, or other Alteration in the Non-naturals.

The Symptoms are many : Every *Fever* arising from any internal Cause, is attended with a quick Pulse and unusual Heat, at different Times, and in different Degrees. Where these are intense, the *Fever* is *acute*; where remiss, *slow*. The Disease begins almost always with a Sense of Chilness; and in its Progress is chiefly distinguish'd by the Velocity of the Pulse : So that a too quick Contraction of the Heart, with an increased Resistance or Impulse against the Capillaries, furnishes the proper Idea of a *Fever*; and the Health of the Patient is the scope Nature chiefly aims at in the Disease.

The other attendant Symptoms are usually a laborious and disturb'd Respiration; an uniform, high colour'd Urine; a Parchedness and Dryness of the Tongue, Mouth, &c. a Clamminess of the Saliva; Thirst; Wakefulness; and Nausea against every thing but thin diluting Liquors.

From these Symptoms, Dr. *Morgan*, our latest Writer on that Subject, lays it down as a Principle, that in every *Fever*, there is a *general Obstruction, and Diminution of the glandular Secretions*; that is, a great Part of the Lymph, or Serum of the Blood, which ought to be continually drain'd off by the Glands, is, during the *Fever*, so retain'd in, and closely united to the Mass, that it circulates together with it in the Veins and Arteries. This he endeavours to prove to be the State and Condition of the Blood in the Production of a *Fever*, by accounting for all the above mentioned Phaenomena from it, as the just and adequate Effects of such a Cause. How he does it, see in his *Philos. Princ. of Med.* P 207, &c.

The general Indication of the Cure of *Fevers*, is, to restrain the Commotion of the Blood, with in the Bounds agreeable to the End, Nature had in raising it, *i.e.* neither to let it rise too high, for fear of the Consequences; nor yet keep it too low, for fear of frustrating the Endeavour of Nature. And hence the Rule, and Measure of letting more, or less Blood, or none at all.

The Cure of *Fevers*, *Boerhaave* summarily comprehends in correcting the sharp, irritating febrile Matter, dissolving the Lentor, and mitigating the Symptoms. If Nature seem to carry the *Fever* too high, it must be moderated by Abstinence, thin Diet, drinking of Water, bleeding and cooling Clysmas : If she bring it on too slowly, it must be excited by Cardiacs, Aromaticks, Volatiles, &c. The Cause removed, the Symptoms cease of course; and if the can be bore without much Danger to Life, it were best not to enter into any particular Cure thereof: If they be unreasonable, or too severe, they are each to be abated with the proper Remedies.

*Sydenham* recommends an Emetick in the Beginning of a *Fever*; or if it have been then omitted, in any other Stage thereof; especially where there is a Propensity to Vomiting : For want of this, a Diarrhæa frequently succeeds, which is exceedingly dangerous. After this, he uses a Paregorick; and the following Days, if there be no Indication to repeat the Venæfection, nor any Diarrhaea, he prescribes every other Day an Enema, till the twelfth Day, when Matters coming to a Crisis, he has Recourse to hotter Medicines, in order to promote and accelerate it. He adds, that if the Disease proceed well, and the Fermentation be laudable, there is no occasion for any Phsyick at all. About the 15th Day, if the Urine be found to separate, and give a Sediment; and the Symptoms be abated, a Cathartick is usually order'd, lest the Sediment returning into the Blood again, occasion a Relapse. Nothing cools the Patient, and abates the *Fever* so much, as a Cathartick after Venæfection.

The more acute the *Fever*, the thinner, according to *Etmuller*, must be the Diet. 'Tis no matter, if the Patient should fast for several Days running; for never did feverish Persons die of Hunger : Eating, always exasperates the Disease. Vomitories, he allows the principal Place in the Cure of all *Fevers*; but, as a Patron of the hot Regimen, assigns Sudorificks the second. Spirit of Sal Ammoniack, or its Sal Volatile, he observes is an universal Febrifuge, and rarely fails : All sugar'd Things are hurtful. *Hippocrates*, in all Fevers, prescribes Wine. Dr. *Hancock*, Water.

So long as the Urine remains crude, that is, does not give a Sediment, the Patient's Case is very dubious : But when once the Coction commences, and the Urine separates, the great Danger is over.

Among the Signs of Death, the same Author adds, there is none more certain, than a frequent blowing of the Nose, without any Discharge of Matter. A strong, equable Pulse, with Deliria, Tremors, Twitches of the Tendons, and other Symptoms, fatal in Diseases of the nervous kind, always presage well in *Fevers* : On the contrary, a quick, weak, faltering Pulse, howsoever favourable the other Symptoms may seem, infallibly proclaim Death at the Door.

It appears, by Observation, that a frequent letting of Blood, renders Persons more inclinable to *Fevers*.

There are various Kinds of *Fevers*, denominated and distinguish'd from the particular Cause that produce them; the Time they continue; their Accesses, or Returns; and their several Symptoms. The most general and genuine Division of *Fevers*, into *Essential*, and *Symptomatick*.

An *Essential* Fever, is that whose primary Cause is in the Blood it self; and which does not arise as an Effect, or Symptom from any other Disease in the Solids, or other Parts. This is, what we absolutely and properly call a *Fever*.

A *Symptomatick* Fever is that which arises as an Accident, or Symptom of some other antecedent Disorder, as an *Inflammation, Phlegmon, Erysipelas, Impostume,* small *Pox, Pleurisy,* &c. When it is peculiarly denominated *Inflammatory, Erysipelatous, Purulent,* &c.

*Essential Fevers* are generally distinguished into *Continued* and *Intermitting*. Others chuse to divide them into *Diary, Intermitting, Continent*, and *Continued*.

A *Continued* Fever is that which gives the Patient no Respite, or Intermission; but sticks to him from its first Seizure, to its final Period. This is subdivided into *Putrid* and *not putrid*.

A *Continued Fever not putrid*, is that wherein the Parts of the Blood are not so dissolved and broke, as to give Room and Occasion for the principal Parts thereof to be secreted : Or that, wherein there is not any Discharge of putrid, purulent Matter into the Blood. Of this there are two Kinds, the *Diary*, and *Synochus*; to which some add the *Hectick*.

A *Diary Fever* is that, which does not ordinarily hold beyond 24 Hours. 'Tis also called *Ephemera*, from the *Greek* ημερα, *Day*. It is the gentlest of all *Fevers*: Is frequently got by too much Exercise, or other external Accident. It is cured by Rest alone, and keeping a-bed : If it remain for several Days, it is either call'd a continued *Ephemera*, or Simple *Synochus*.

A *Hectick Fever* is a slow, durable Fever, which attenuates and emaciates the Body by insensible degrees. It is thus called from the *Greek* εξις,

Habitude, as being difficult to get rid off. It has three Stages; the first, while it consumes the Juices of the Body : The second, when it exhausts the fleshy Substance of its Humidity; And the third, when it lays hold of, and destroys the Solids themselves : In which last Stage it is reputed incurable. Its Effect is somewhat like that of a Flame; first consuming the Oil of the Lamp; then the Moisture of the Wick; and lastly the Wick it self. But this *Fever* is frequently consider'd as of the *Symptomatick*, or secundary kind, arising in *Phthises*, &c.

A *Putrid*, or *continued Putrid Fever*, is that wherein the Texture of the Blood is render'd so lax, or even dissolv'd, that its Parts or Principles separating, some of the principal are secreted, and lost. Or *Putrid Fevers* are frequently consider'd as secondary ones, arising from the Discharge of putrid, purulent Matter from some morbid Part, as an Ulcer in the Lungs, &c. *Putrid Fevers* are divided into *Simple*, and *Compound* or *Remitting*.

A *Simple continued putrid Fever*, or a *Continued Fever*, properly so called, by the Greeks call Συνοχος, is that which continues uniformly, from first to last, without any Fits pr Periods of Exasperation and Remission of Heat, and other the Symptoms.

*Willis* divides the *Putrid Fever* into four Stadia, or Stages. The *Beginning*, which is attended with a Chillness, Shivering, Weariness, Thirst, Wakefulness, Pain in the Head and Loans, Nausea, and Vomiting : The *Increase*, wherein the former Symptoms are heighten'd, with the Addition of Deliria, convulsive Motions, Foulness of the Mouth, high turbid Urine, without any laudable Sediment, or Hypostasis; the *State*, which contains the Crisis, which in this Disease is much what the Paroxysm is in Intermitters : For as that returns at certain Hours, so do the critical Motions in continued *Fevers* happen on the fourth, fifth, sixth, or seventh Day. See Crisis. The last Stage is the *Declension*, which ends either in Recovery, or Death. These *Fevers* are divided into *Burning*, and *Slow*.

*Ardent*, or *Burning Fever*, called by the *Greeks* καυσος, is a very acute *Fever*, attended with a vehement Heat, intolerable Thirst, a dry Cough, Delirium, and other violent Symptoms. It frequently kills on the third or fourth Day; rarely exceeds the seventh. It often goes off in a Hemorrhage, on the third, or fourth Day; which, if it probe to sparing, is deadly. Sometimes it goes by Stool, Vomiting, &c. and sometimes ends a Peripneumony.

To the Class of *Burning Fevers* are reducible, the *Liperia, Assodes, Elodes*, &c. The *Fever Liperia* is a burning *Fever*, wherein the Heat is very intense within side, and the same time the external Parts cold. The *Assodes* is a burning *Fever*, attended with great Inquietudes, Nauseas, Vomitings, &c. The *Elodes* is a *Fever*, wherein the Patient sweats continually.

The *Syncopal Fever* is that attended with frequent Swoonings.

The *Epeal Fever* is that wherein both Heat and Cold are felt the same Part at the same Time.

*Slow fevers* are gentle, but durable ones, which consume the Patients by degrees. They usually arise from Disorders in the Lympha, or Pituita; whence *Sylvius* calls them *Lymphatick Fevers*.

The principal of these are the Catarrhal, attended with a Catarrh, Cough, Hoarseness, &c. And the *Scorbutick Fever*, into which acute *Fevers*, and sometimes Intermittent degenerate. To this Class are reducible,

*Colliquative Fevers*, wherein the whole Body is consumed and emaciated in no long Time; the solid Parts, with the Fat, &c. melted down, and carried off by a Diarrhaea, Sweat, Urine, &c.

A *Remitting* **FEVER**, called also a *Continent*, Συνεχης, and a *compound continued Fever*, is that which continues some Time, without any gradual Increase of Heat; yet is liable to alternate Fits of Remission and Aggravation; either stated and periodical, or irregular.

Of this there are divers Kinds, denominated from the Periods of returning; as the *Remitting, Continued, Quotidian*, the *Continued Tertian, Continued Quartan*, &c. which are only a continued *Fever*, whose Accesses or severer Fits return every Day, or any other Day; or every third Day; or every fourth Day.

Some enumerate divers other more complicated continued *Fevers*; as the *double* or *triple Quotidian*, which has two or three Paroxysms every Day : *Double*, or *triple Tertian*, or *Quartan*, which have two or three every third or fourth Day : The *Semi-tertian*, by the *Greeks* called ημιτειταιος, which consists of a *Continued*, and two intermitting *Fevers* of different Kinds, *viz.* a Quotidian and Tertian. The Patient, beside a Continued Fever, has an extraordinary Fit every Day; and every other Day two.

Others divide the *Remitting*, Συνεχης, *Continent*, or *Compound Continued Fever*, into *Simple*, and *Spurious*.

The *Simple Remitter* returns regularly, and is only distinguish'd from an Intermediate, in that the feverish Heat in the Intervals of this latter is never quite extinguish'd; and that the Paroxysms don't begin with so much Chillness and Horror; and go off in a profuse Sweats.

The *Spurious Remitter* is attended with grievous Symptoms on the nervous Kind, resembling those of the Rheumatism, Colick, Pleurisy, and other inflammatory and spasmodick Diseases; beside immoderate Excretions, Vomitings, Diarrhæas, &c. Whence its Returns are uncertain, and variable.

The *Simple* rarely, if ever, kills; the *Spurious*, frequently. Sometimes it degenerates into a malignant Συνοχος.

The first is cured with the Cortex Peruv. almost as infallibly an Intermitter; the febrile Ferment being much the same in both : And the same Medicine is found almost a sure, tho' not so speedy a Remedy of the Spurious, if properly applied.

An *Intermitting* **FEVER**, or *Ague*, is that which ceases, and returns again alternately, at stated Periods. In this kind, Cold, and Heat, Shivering, and Sweating succeed each other.

The Paroxysms are attended with Sickness, Nausea's, Vomitings, Headach, Pain the Back and Loins, &c. The Paroxysms are acute, but the Disease usually more or less chronical.

No body was ever killed of an intermitting *Fever*, except in the first stage of the Paroxysm, during the Shivering, caused by the Oppression of the Spirits. When the Disease becomes of a very old standing, it sometimes degenerates into other very fatal ones.

As to the Cure, 'tis found by abundant Observations, that neither Bleeding, nor Emeticks, nor Catharticks, nor any other Remedy, administer'd during the Fit, avail anything. A just Dose of *Vinum Benedictum*, three Hours before the Paroxysm, *Morton*[1] assures us, has often cured it : *Antimonium Diaphoreticum*, a little before the Paroxysms, has the like Effect : And Salt of Wormwood is commended on the same Occasion. *Dolæus*[2] mentions *Lapis Lazali* taken in Spirit of Wine before the Fit, is admirable.

And several Bitters, as Carduus Benedictus, Gentian Root, Camomile Flowers, Pulvis Febrifugus, &c. were much valued before the Invention of the Cortex Peruv. But that bark has almost thrown them all out of use; being by the universal Consent of al Physicians allowed a Panacea, or Specifick for all intermitting *Fevers*, on all Seasons, Ages, and Constitutions.

Intermitting *Fevers* are of divers kinds, as the *Quotidian Fever*, where the Paroxysm returns every Day. *Double Quotidian*, which returns twice in twenty four Hours. *Tertian Fever*, which only returns every other Day; which again is, either Legitimate, or Spurious. The *Legitimate Tertian* only holds twelve Hours, and is followed by an absolute Intermission. The *Spurious Tertian* exceeds twelve Hours, and sometimes holds 18, or 20.

The *Double Tertian* is that which returns twice every other Day. The Word *Double Tertian* is also used, where the Fever returns every Day, like a Quotidian; only at different times of the Day; the third Fit answering to the Time of the first; the fourth to the that of the second, &c.

The *Quartan Fever* is that which only returns every fourth Day; leaving two Days Intermission between every two Fits.

The *Double Quartan* is that which has two Fits every fourth Day. The same Name is given to a *Fever*, which returns two Days successively; only leaving one Day's Intermission.

*Triple Quartan Fever* is that which has three Fits every fourth Day : Or that which returns every day like a Quotidian, only at different Seasons of the Day; the fourth Fit answering to the Time of the first; the fifth to the second, &c.

Lastly, there are some extraordinary Species of Fevers, not reducible to any of the forementioned Classes; as *Malignant, Eruptive*, and *Pestilential Fevers*.

*Malignant* **FEVERS** are those, wherein the usual, regular Symptoms do not appear (Nature being oppress'd with the Malignity of the febrile Matter) but other foreign Symptoms arise; as a Pain about the Stomach, and Præcordia; a livid Complexion, with the Face much disfigur'd, &c. Sometimes Efflorescences on the Skin, &c.

Some Authors, from microscopical Observations affirm, that in all malignant *Fevers* the Blood is so corrupted, that Swarms of little Worms are generated therein, which occasion most of the Symptoms.

[1] Richard Morton (1637 – 1698), an English physician.

[2] Johannes Dolaeus (1651 – 1707), a German physician.

In all malignant *Fevers* the Blood is too fluid. Blood-letting has here no Place: Vomitories do well at first; afterwards Sudorificks and Alexipharmachicks : Blisters are commended in the Progress of the Disease.

*Eruptive* Fevers are those, which beside the Symptoms common to all *Fevers*, have their Crises attended with cutaneous Eruptions. Such are those of the small Pox, Meazles, Petechiæ, the Purple or Scarlet Fever, and Military Fever : Their other Symptoms are, a grievous Oppression of the Breast; laborious, short Breadth, obstinate Waking; Spasms, soar Throat, Cough, &c.

*Pestilential* Fevers, are acute, contagious, and mortal Diseases. Some with have the Fever to be the Disease or Plague it self : Others only account it a Symptom of the Plague. See Plague.

*Petechial* Fever, is a malignant Fever, wherein, beside the other Symptoms, on the fourth, or more frequently the seventh Day, *Petechiæ*, or red Spots, like Fleabites, appear, chiefly on the Breast, Shoulders, and Abdomen. The Spots afterwards turn paler, then yellow, and so disappear. When they grow livid, or black, they usually prove fatal. This Fever is contagious, and often Epidemical. It is treated much as those just mentioned.

**FEWEL**, or Fuel, in Philosophy, the Pabulum of Fire, or whatever receives, and retains Fire, and is consumed, or render'd insensible thereby. Pure Fire, if left to it self, would dispose, and disappear : To preserve it, it is necessary there be some Fuel, to sustain, and keep it together.

The only proper *Fuel*, known in all Nature is Oil, commonly called Sulphur: And all Bodies, whether vegetable, fossil, or animal, are only inflammable, as they contain Oil in them.

Oil feeds and sustains Fire by virtue of its ramose, tenacious Particles, which are disposed to be put into a most vehement, rotatory Motion, before they will let each other go. But, by this rotatory Motion the Fire at length breaks and comminutes the ramose Particles of the *Fuel*; till, ceasing to cohere, they are no longer able to sustain the Fire.

In the popular Sense of the Word, *Fewel* is any Body, which contains this Pabulum, or oil, in such Quantity, as to fit them for culinary Uses.

Such 1°, Are dry, or green Vegetables; especially those abounding in Oil; as the rosinous, and balsamick Woods.

2°, Fossil Coals, whether vegetable, or animal; as being little else, but the oily Part of the Vegetable, or animal, purged of Salt, Water, &c. so that the blacker they are, the better.

3°, Fossil and bituminous Earths, as Turf , and Pea, which are a fatty Earth, dug out of the Ground.

4°, All mineral Sulphur, whether pure, or mix'd with Earth, Stone, &c.

5°, The Fat and Dung of Animals dried.

And 6°, The Productions of Chymistry, which are either Coals, or Oil, or oily Bodies; as, inflammable Spirits, produced by Fermentation, Putrifaction, &c.

**FICUS**, a kind of Wart, or Excrescence, yielding a very stinking Sanies, arising sometimes on Fractures of the Skull, but more usually about the

Fundament, and Pudenda. The Physicians more usually call it *Sarcoma*, of σαρξ, Flesh.

**FIG**, *Ficus*, a soft, sweet, delicious Fruit; the Produce of a Tree of the same Name. There are *Figs* of divers Kinds; chiefly denominated from the Colours; White, Violet, Black, Purple, Green, and Ruddy : The White are esteem'd the best : The Black and Violet are the worst. They are gather'd in Autumn, and laid on a Rack, or Hurdle, to dry in the Sun.

*Figs* contain a deal of Phlegm; a little volatile, alkali Salt, and a moderate Quantity of Oil. They are very nourishing, and soften the Asperities of the Breast, &c. And accordingly are used in Medicine, to make Gargarisms, against Disorders of the Throat and Mouth. They are also applied externally, to soften, digest, and promote Maturation.

*Figs* are dried, either by a Furnace, or the Sun. The *Latins* call them *Caricæ*, or *Ficus passæ*, when thus dried. In this Condition they are used both as Medicine and Food; being both wholesomer, and easier of Digestion, for being thus clear'd of the a deal of their aqueous and viscid Parts.

The Word is form'd of the *Latin Ficus*; and that of the *Greek* φυω, I produce; by reason the *Fig* Tree is a great Bearer, and has usually two Crops a Year.

The best *Figs* are the Produce of *Italy, Spain, Provence*, &c. The Islands of the Archipelago yield Figs in great Abundance; but they are much inferior in Goodness to those of *Europe*. The *Greeks* in those Islands cultivate them with wonderful Care, and Attention; as making the principal Food, and a considerable Part of the Riches of the Country.

They have two Kinds of *Fig* Trees, the first called *Ornos*, or the wild *Fig* Tree; the second, the domestick *Fig* Tree. The wild, called by the Latins *Caprificus*, yields successively three sorts of Fruits, called *Fornites, Cratitires*, and *Orni*; none of which are of any use as Foods; but all absolutely necessary for the ripening of those of the domestick *Fig* Tree.

The Art of Cultivating and ripening these Figs, makes a peculiar Art, by the Antients called *Caprification*; often spoke of among them in Terms of Admiration. Some of the modern Naturalists have look'd on it as a Chimera; but Mons. *Tournefort* has assured us of the Contrary, and given us that Process, as he learn'd it upon the Spot.

The Generation of the *Fig* is somewhat anomalous; the Parts subservient to the Office in other Plants; *i.e.* the Flower, not being here apparent. But the Anatomy of the Fruit helps out of the Difficulty.

**FILAMENT**, in Medicine, Anatomy, Nat. History, &c. a Term used in the same Sense with Fibre; for those fine Threads, whereof the Flesh, Nerves, Skin, Plants, Roots, &c. are composed.

**FILLET**, in Botany, is understood as those Threads usually found in the middle of Flowers; as in the Lilly, Tulip, Rose, &c.

**FILM**, a thin Skin, or Pellicle, dividing several Parts of the Flesh. In Plants, it is that thin woody Skin, which separates Seeds in the Pods, and keeps them apart.

**FILTRATION**, the Act of passing a thing thro' a Filtre; called also Percolation, and Trans-location. *Filtration* is a kind of Distillation; perform'd by straining a Liquor thro' a Cloth, Bag, Linen, or brown Paper, in order to clarify or purify it. The most commodious way of *filtrating* is by brown Paper, fasten'd over the Mouth or Aperture of a Funnel.

The Secretion of the divers Juices in the Body, from the Mass of Blood, seem to be little else but *Filtration*.

*Pitcairn*, and other late Authors, hold that the Differences of *Filtrations* don't depend on the different Configurations of Pores; but on their different Sizes or Diameters. And Springs seem to be rais'd from the Ocean by the same Principle.

There are also *Filtrations* thro' Sand, pulverized Glass, &c. Spirits of Vitriol, Salt, and Nitre, are *filtrated* thro' a Quantity of beaten Glass, in the Bottom of a Funnel.

*Filtration* is chiefly concern'd in Tinctures; as when some Portion is drawn from the Ingredients, or suspended in the Tincture, which is not necessary thereunto; but disturbs and renders the rest unpleasant, both to the Palate, and Sight.

The *Filtration* most in use, is the straining a Liquor thro' Paper, which by the Smallness of the Pores admits only the finer Parts, and keeps the rest behind.

Besides this, there is a *Filtration*, which hath much tortur'd the Philosophy of some Ages to account for, *viz.* that perform'd by the Ascent of the finer Parts of a Liquor, up a Cord, or Skain of Cotton, or such like Matter, which is contrived to drop over another Vessel, and leave the grosser behind.

Some say, that the Cause of this Ascent is, because the Liquor swells those Parts of the Filtre, that touch it by entering into the Pores of the Threads, which compose it, whereby they rise up, touch, and wet those next above them; and these again the next Threads; and so on, to the Brims of the Vessel; when , the Liquor runs over, and descends in the other Part of the Filtre, which hangs down, by its own natural Gravity.

But this Account is liable to many Objections; especially as Liquors rise, after the like manner in Glass Tubes, much above the Surface of the Liquor they are immersed in; where the Glass cannot be imagin'd thus to swell.

Others account for it, by considering every Fibre, as composed of a great Number of long, small, solid Bodies, which lie very close together; so that the Air getting in between them, loses much if its Pressure, and cannot gravitate so strongly, as it doth on the Fluid without them : The Consequence is, that the Parts of the Water between the Threads of the Filtre must be press'd upwards, and ascend till they come so high, as by their Weight to counter-balance the general Pressure on the other Parts of the Surface of the Water.

Lastly, the Retainers to Sir. *I. Newton's* Philosophy deduce the Phæno-menon from the Principle of Attraction. The Principle of this Filtration is doubtless the same with that whereby Fluids ascend up Heaps or Lumps of Ashes, Sand, &c. The same with that, whereby Water is raised in form of Vapour : The Sap rises in Vegetables; and the Blood circulates through the capillary Arteries, and the extremely minute glandular Strainers.

**FILTRE**, Filter, or Philter, in Chymistry, &c. A piece of Cloth, Linen, or Paper, or other Matter, used to *filtrate* or strain Liquors through.

The *Filtre* has the same Use and Effect, with regard to Liquids, that the Sieve or Searce has in dry Matters. *Filtres* are of two sorts : The first, simple pieces of Paper, or Cloth; through which the Liquor is pass'd without further Ceremony.

The second are twisted up like a Skain or Wick, and first wet, then squeez'd, and one End put in the Vessel that contains the Liquor to be filtrated. The other End is to be out, and hang down below the Surface of the Liquor. By means hereof, the purest Part of the Liquor distils Drop by Drop out of the vessel; leaving the coarser Part behind. This *Philtre* acts as a Syphon.

**FILTRE** is also a Charm, supposed to have a Virtue of inspiring Love. The Word is derived from the *Greek* φιλτρον, which signifies the same Thing, of φιλεω, *amo*, I love.

**FIRE**, in Physiology. The most universal and sensible Character of *Fire*; and that which best defines and distinguishes it from every other thing, is its *Heating*. *Fire*, therefore, may be defined to be whatever warms, or heats Bodies.

Again, as Heat is something, whose presence we best perceive by the Dilatation of the Air or Spirit in the Thermometer : *Fire* may be defined to be that whose Presence we perceive by the Expansion of the Air, or Spirit in the Thermometer. When it follows, that *Fire* is a Body, and a Body in Motion.

Its *Motion* is argued from its expanding the Air; which is not effected without communicating Motion thereto : And its *Corporeity* is proved by Experiment.

For pure Mercury being inclosed in a Phial with a long Neck, and kept in a gentle Heat for the space of a Year, is reduced into a Solid; and its Weight considerably increased; which Increase can arise from nothing but the Accession of *Fire*.

'Tis a Dispute of some Standing among Philosophers, Whether *Fire* be any specifick Substance, originally distinct from all other; or whether it be the Matter of other Bodies, only under certain peculiar Modifications, *i.e.* Whether *Fire* be such by its own Nature, or by Motion.

*Fire*, makes one of the vulgar, or Peripatetick Elements, defined to be hot, and dry; or, it is that Part, or Ingredient in all Bodies, which is hot in the highest Degree, and dry in an inferior one.

What the School-Philosophers add further, as to the Nature of *Fire*, is, that it is a *Simple* Body; as not including any Contrariety of Qualities; and a Body absolutely light, as tending naturally upwards : For which reason they hold its natural Place above all the other Elements, between the Extremity of our Atmosphere, and the Moon; and the Source of *Fire* supposed to reside in that Sphere, they call *Elementary Fire*.

*Fire*, according to the *Cartesians*, is an Assemblage of the more solid, earthy Particles; which swimming in the rapidly fluid Motion of the first Element, become vehemently agitated thereby; and by this intense Agitation or Motion are disposed to give the Sensation of Heat, Light, &c.

*Fire*, according to Sir *I. Newton*, is a Body heated so hot, as to emit light copiously. For what else, says the Philosopher, is a red-hot Iron, but *Fire*? And what else is a *fiery* Coal, than red-hot Wood? By which he suggests, that Bodies which are not *Fire*, may be changed and converted into Fire.

*Fire*, according to some of the latest Philosophers, is a certain Substance, or Body *sui generis*, originally such; and not producible by any Motion or Alteration of other Bodies. These Authors lay it down as a very subtile, moveable, penetrating Body; and the Cause or Instrument of Heat and Light. Some of them add, that when *Fire* enters the Eye in right Lines it produces or excites the Idea of *Light*; which rectilinear Motion they account absolutely necessary to the Idea of Light.

Whereas, to produce Heat, and the other Effects of *Fire*, such Motion is not required; but on the Contrary, an irregular, various Motion is fitter to produce the same.

The Nature of *Fire* is so wonderful, and sublime, that the Antients generally revered it as a God : Among the Moderns, we can scarce name one Point in all Philosophy of more Importance, or less understood.

*Fire*, in Effect, is the universal Instrument of all the Motion, and Action in the Universe : Without *Fire*, all Bodies would become immoveable; as in a sever Winter we actually see out Fluids become solid, for want thereof. Without *Fire*, a Man would harden into a Statue; and the very Air cohere into a firm, rigid Mass.

*Fire*, then, is the universal Cause of all Mutation, or Change; for all Mutation is by Motion; and all Motion by *Fire*.

Several Authors have labor'd to set this grand Agent in its just Light; and particularly the excellent *Boerhaave*, in a new Course of Experiments, and Lectures expressly on the Subject, *De Igne*. That Author has indeed done Wonders : The Sum of his Doctrine we shall here subjoin.

*Fire*, then, is distinguish'd into two Kinds; as it is in it self, called *Elementary*; or as it is join'd with other Bodies, called *Culinary Fire*. *Pure*, or *Elemental* Fire, is such as it exists in it self; which alone we properly call *Fire*.

*Common*, or *Culinary Fire* is that existing in ignited Bodies; or excited, by the former, in combustible Matters, the minute Particles whereof joining with those of the pure *Fire*, constitute pure Flame. This latter is improperly called *Fire*; in regard only a small Part of it is real, or pure *Fire*.

Pure *Fire*, such as collected in a Burning Glass, yields no Flame, Smoak, Ashes, or the like: Consequently, in *ignited* Bodies, that which flames, smoaks, &c. is not simply *Fire*.

The Effected, Nature, Properties, &c. of each shall be consider'd. 1. *Pure*, or *Elemental Fire* of it self, is imperceptible; and only discovers it self by certain Effects, which it produces in Bodies; which Effects are only learnt, by observing the Changes that arise in those Bodies.

The First *Effect* of *Elemental Fire* on Bodies, is *Heat*; which arises wholly from *Fire*; and in such manner as that the Measure of Heat is always the

Measure of *Fire*; and that of *Fire*, of Heat. So the Heat is inseparable from *Fire*.

The Second is, *Dilatation* in all solid Bodies; and *Rarefaction* in all Fluids.

That both these are inseparable from Heat, is evident from numerous Experiments. An iron Rod, or Bar being heated, increases in all its Dimensions; and the more so, as it is further and further heated : Upon exposing it to the Cold again, it contracts and returns successively through all the Degrees of its Dilatation, till it arrive at its first Bulk; being never two Minutes successively of the same Magnitude.

The like is observed in the heaviest of all Bodies, Gold; which, when fused, takes up more Space than before : So Mercury, the heaviest of all Fluids, we have known to ascend in a narrow Tube over the *Fire*, to above 30 times its Height.

The Laws of this Expansion. Are 1°. That the same Degree of Fire rarefies Fluids sooner, and in a greater Degree than it does Solids. Without this, the Thermometer would be of no use; since the Cavity of the Tube would then be dilated in the same Proportion, as the Fluid is rarefied. 2°. The lighter the Liquid, the more it is dilated by Fire. Thus Air, the lightest of all Fluids, expands the most; and after Air, Spirit of Wine.

The Third *Effect of Fire* on Bodies, is Motion : For *Fire*, in warming and dilating Bodies, must of Necessity move their Parts.

In Effect, all the Motion in Nature arise from *Fire* alone; and taking this away all Things become immoveable : Upon the Absence of only a certain Degree of *Fire*, all Oils, Fats, Waters, Wines, Ales, Spirits of Wine, Vegetables, Animals, &c. become hard, rigid, and inert: And the less the Degree of *Fire*, the sooner, and more violently is this Induration made.

Hence, if there were the greatest Degree of Cold, and all *Fire* were absolutely taken away, all Nature would grow into one concrete Body, solid as Gold, and hard as Diamond. But upon the Application of *Fire*, it would recover its former Mobility.

Consequently, every Diminution of Fire is attended with a proportionable Diminution of Motion : And *vice versa*.

This *Fire*, whose Effects we have been relating, needs no Air, or Pabulum to sustain or perceive it.

For, putting some Calx of Tin or Lead, in the exhausted Receiver of an Air Pump; and apply a Burning Glass, so as the focus shall fall in the Calx; the Consequence will be a vehement Dilatation of the Calx, from the Centre towards the Circumference, whereby the Receiver will be broke into a thousand Pieces. And if a Quantity of any essential aromatick Oil be pour'd in Vacuo, upon Spirit of Nitre, there will immediately arise a huge *Fire*, to the great Danger of the Bystanders.

All the above-mentioned Effects of Elemental *Fire* may be increas'd divers ways, *viz.* 1°. By Attrition, or a swift Agitation, or rubbing of one Body against another. This is apparent in Solids : A vehement Attrition of a Flint, and Steel, every Body knows, will produce Sparks. So in Fluids, Cream, by long churning to separate Butter, will grow sensibly warm; and a Barometer renders the Effect still more discernable.

In effect, all the Heat of an Animal is owing to the Agitation and Attrition of the Parts of its Juice against each other, and the Sides of the Vessel.

The more solid, hard, and elastick the Bodies this agitated are; the more Points of Contact they have; the more intense the Force whereby they are struck against each other, is; the greater their Motion; the quicker the Returns of the Strokes; and the longer continued; the greater is the Heat produced.

Thus, a piece of Spunge rubb'd lightly, and for a little while against another, acquires no sensible Heat : But a large, heavy piece of Iron briskly rubb'd against another in a cold Season (when Bodies are the densest) will presently acquire an intense Heat, sufficient to *fire* Sulphur, Gunpowder, or the like.

So a Knife whetted briskly on a dry rough Stone, shall yield Sparks of *Fire*; but if Oil, or any other fatty Matter be interposed, no sensible Heat shall arise: And the Points of two Needles rubb'd against each other so strongly, or so long, will never grow warm; as only touching in a few Points.

Hence 1°, The Globules of the Cruor, or red Blood drove by the Force of the Heart against each other, or against the Sides of the Arteries, excite more Heat than the Globules of the Serum, or any other Humor in the Animal. Hence 2°. Those Parts abounding most in these Globules thus agitated, as the Heart, Liver, and Head, will be the hottest of all others : And the denser the Blood, *cæteris paribus*, the greater the Heat, &c. 3°, The quicker the Contractions of the Heart are repeated, the greater will the Heat be.

The Second *Manner of increasing the Effect of Elemental Fire*, is by throwing a Quantity of moist or green Vegetables, cut down while full of Sap, into a large Heap, and pressing them close down : The Result of which, is, that they grow warm, hot, smoak, and break out into Flame.

The Third way is, by the Mixture of certain cold Bodies. Thus, Water and Spirit of Wine, first warm'd, grow much hotter by the Mixture : So, any of the heavy aromatick Oils, as of Cloves, Cinnamon, Sassafras, Guaiacum, &c. mix'd with Spirit of Nitre, grow exceedingly hot, and burst forth like Vulcano's. And the same may be said of Spirit of Nitre, and Steel Filings.

The like Effect may be had from dry Bodies. Thus, pure Sulphur, and Steel Filings, well ground and mix'd in equal Quantities, with Water enough to make them into a dry Paste, and laid an Hour or two any where, even under Ground, will smoak and emit Flame; and that with the greater Vehemence, as it is more strongly press'd down.

The Fourth is by *Phosphorus*, which is a kind of Magnet, prepar'd from the Parts of Animals, that imbibes and retains *Fire* for many Ages.

But, in all these manners, it does not appear, that any *Fire* is excited, or generated of what was not *Fire* before : For, if in a severe Winter's Day you rub a Plate of Gold briskly against another, they will both grow hotter and hotter by Degrees, till at length they become red hot, and at the point of melting : And yet all this time the Plates lose nothing of their Weight; but swell or grow bigger in all their Dimensions.

Hence it follow, that the Particles of the Gold are not converted by the Friction, into *Fire*; but the *Fire* existed before; and all the Effect of the Friction, &c. is to collect, or bring together a Quantity thereof before dispersed throughout the Atmosphere.

In Effect, there is no making or producing of *Fire de novo*. All we can do, is, of insensible, to render it sensible, *i.e.* to collect it out of a greater Space into a lesser; and to direct and determine it to certain Places. This is effected, as above mention'd, by Motion, Attrition, &c.

The Sun also contributes very much to the bringing of *Fire* to light, by means of his rapid Motion round his Axis; whereby the fiery Particles, every where diffused, are directed and determined in parallel Lines towards certain Places, where their Effect becomes apparent.

Whence it is that we perceive the *Fire* when the Sun is above the Horizon; but that, when he disappears, his Impulse or Pression being then taken away, the *Fire* continues dispersed at large thro' the ethereal Space.

In effect, there is not less *Fire* in our Hemisphere in the Night time, than by day; only it wants the proper Determination to make it perceived.

Another way of rendering it sensible, is, by collecting the parallel Rays into a less Compass, by means of Convex Glasses, or Concave Specula.

This Elemental *Fire* is present every where, in all Bodies, all Space, and at all Times; and that in equal Quantities : For, go where you will, to the Top of the highest Mountain, or descend into the lowest Cavern; whether the Sun shine, or not; in the coldest Winter, or the most scorching Summer; by one or other, or all of the means above mentioned may *Fire* be collected. In a Word, there is no assignable physical Point without *Fire*; no Place in Nature, where the Attrition of two Sticks will not render it sensible.

So long as *Fire* remains equably, and undetermin'd in any Place, it does not discover it self by any Effect. In the severest Weather we perceive no Influence or Effect of Fire, when, at the same time being collected and determined by Attrition, it becomes manifest.

By changing *Fire* out of its indeterminate State, and impelling it in converging Lines, its Moment is increased. Witness the Phænomena of Burning Glasses.

But, how Attrition, crude Vegetables, &c. contribute towards altering the Direction, &c. of *Fire*, does not appear.

Of this *Fire*, and the Effects thereof above mentioned, depends all Fluidity of Humours, Juices, &c. All Vegetation, Putrifaction, Fermentation, animal Heat, &c.

II. But in what manner soever, *Fire*, is collected in Bodies; upon a Cessation of the collecting Cause, it soon disappears again, unless it be supplied with a *Pabulum*, or Fuel. In which case it becomes Culinary Fire.

By *Pabulum*, or *Fuel* of *Fire*, we mean whatever receives, and retains Fire; and is consumed, or at least render'd insensible thereby.

The only *Pabulum* of *Fire*, in all Nature, is the Oil, Sulphur, or Fat of Bodies : And Bodies are only Fuel, on account of the Oil they contain.

Hence 1°, All vegetables not too moist, nor too dry, afford such a Pabulum; particularly those, which contain the greatest Quantity of Oil; as Balsamick and Resinous Woods, &c. 2°, All vegetable and animal Coals are a proper Pabulum for maintaining of *Fire*; as being only the Parts of Vegetables and

Animals, which have exhaled their Water and Salt, and retain'd the Oil alone inhering, in a black Form, in their Earth. 3°, All fossil and bituminous Earths, Turfs, &c. 5°, All Mineral Sulphur, whether pure or join'd with Earth, Stone, or Metals; as Pit-Coal, &c. 6°, The fat and Dung of Animals; and 7°, Several Productions of Chymistry; as Oils, inflammable Spirits, &c.

This *Fire*, which burns combustible Bodies, requires Air, to sustain it; which taken away, the Fire is immediately dissipated : As appears from the Exper-iments *in Vacuo*.

And yet, *Fire* does not immediately bear, or endure the Air; but always repels it : And by that means forms a kind of Vault, or aerial Furnace all round; which by its Weight, and the Pressure of the incumbent Air acts on all the Particles, or Corpuscles that would make their Way through it; and thus retains the *Fire*, and applies it to the combustible Matter.

Hence, the heavier the Air, the more vehement the *Fire* : And accordingly, in still cold Weather we observe the Fire to act with more Violence than in warm Weather.

But whether the Air retains *Fire* by its Weight alone (which Water it self would do), may be questioned : And whether its Elasticity does not contribute something thereto; as also, whether there be not some further unknown Property in Air, that has a Shape, may be doubted. Something of this kind one would suspect from hence, that all Air is not proper to maintain Flame.

This *Fire*, in burning a combustible Matter, affords a *shining Fire*, or a Flame, or both, according to the Diversity of Fuel; and frequently, Smoak, Soot and Ashes.

*Shining*, or *luminous Fire*, seems to be elemental *Fire*, attracted towards the Parts of the Sulphur, or Oil, with such Force and Velocity, as to move, and shake them very violently, whirl them about, divide, and attenuate them, and thus render them volatile, and ready to be expelled : While, in the mean time, the Air, makes its Vault all around, restrains and keeps them in, directs them to the Sulphur, and keeps them still collected in their Place or Pabulum, while the combustible Matter is diffused all around.

*Flame* seems to be nothing but a thick Sulphur agitated, as before, by Elemental *Fire*; so as the *Fire* is driven with a great Motion around the revolving Particles of the Sulphur.

*Soot*, seems to be produced, when *Fire* and Sulphur cannot break into a Flame; being but a sort of Coal, consisting of a thick Sulphur, and an attenuated Oil with Earth and Salt. See Soot.

*Smoak* seems to be the combustible Matter, when it begins to be relinquish'd by the Elemental *Fire* : For, if this Smoak be afterwards pass'd thro' a Flame, it will it self become Flame, as before. See Smoak.

Lastly *Ashes* are the Earth, an Salt; which the Fire leaves untouch'd.

*Fire* may be distinguish'd into *Shining*, and *not Shining* : For, that there is *Fire* which does not emit Light, is evident hence, that a piece of Iron taken out of the *Fire*, before it be red hot, shall yet give *Fire* to Sulphur.

*Shining Fire* again may be subdivided into two Kinds : That which *warms*, as red hot Iron; and that which does *not warm*, as that observed in putrid

Fishes, rotten Wood, &c. The Oil whereof beginning to be agitated, and attenuated, produces Light, without any Heat, so far as the Thermometer may be a Judge. Of *Shining*, and at the same time *Warming Fires*, the principal is that of the *Sun*, as it is called; tho', whether the Fire be really emitted from the Body of the Sun; or whether it be only the common, vague, universal *Fire*, determin'd by the Sun, is not easy to say. This *Fire* we more usually consider under the Denomination of *Light*. This Solar Fire, in calcining certain Bodies, makes some Addition to the Weight thereof.

Thus, Antimony exposed in the Focus of a Burning Glass, will smoak a considerable Time; and the greatest Part of it seem to evaporate in Fumes : But, if tried by the Balance, it will be found to have gain'd in Weight. And if it be again applied to the Focus of a larger Glass, it will again emit Fumes; and yet still be increased in Weight.

Beside Solar, there is likewise a *Subterraneous Fire*. This appears in digging under Ground: For the first Glebe, next to the Surface, is warm'd by the Heat of the Sun; and as you go deeper, you will find it colder; whence in hot Countries they have Conservatories of Ice at some depth under Ground : till, arriving at a certain Depth, *viz.* forty or fifty Foot, it begins to grow warmer; so as no Ice can there subsist : And at a yet greater Depth, 'tis so hot, as to take away Respiration, extinguish Candles, &c. And if the Miner will venture further, and carry a Candle along with him, he frequently sets the whole Place in a Flame, the sulphurous Fumes render'd volatile by the subterranean *Fire*, catching Flame from the Candle.

Whence it appears, that there is another Source of *Fire*, or another Sun, in the Bosom of the Earth, which gives Motion and Life to every thing growing in, or upon the Globe; and even, that the Centre of the Earth is mere *Fire* : which *Fire* is likewise argued to be perpetual from Vulcano's or burning Mountains, which have been known to cast up *Fire*, from the earliest Account of Times. There are two great Fires therefore, the Higher, or Solar; and the lower, or subterraneous; in every other respect perfectly alike.

**FIRE**, in Chymistry, is the great Instrument, by which most of the Operations of that Art are perform'd. The Kind, Degree, Direction, &c. of *Fire* are Things, the Chymist is principally to attend to. The Diversity of Fire makes a great Difference in the Result of the Experiment; so as, the same Effect, *e.gr.* Shall not arise, if an Experiment be made with the *Fire* of Spirit of Wine, and that of Pitcoal. And to this cause, Mr. *Boyle*, in his Treatise of the unexpected Failure of Experiments, attributes it, that a great many Experiments successfully tried by some, have not succeeded to others.

The *Fires* chiefly required by the Chymists, are such as yield no Faeces, or Remains; no Salt, or Smoak : And such alone are those of the Sun, and of Spirit of Wine. Those which come next in Purity, are Oils distilled per Vesicam; which lose their Earth and Salt, by their Boyling and Agitation in the Water; so that the oftener the Distillation is repeated, the purer they are render'd : After these come Turf.

Indeed, the very Manner wherein the *Fire* is blown, is found to have some Effect : Thus, *Acosta*[1], *lib.* 4. c. 5. relates, that in *Peru*, when they

[1] Jose de Acosta (1539 – 1600), a Spanish missionary in Peru.

would melt and separate their Silver from the Earth, &c. if the Fire be blown up with Bellows, the Fusion will not succeed : Nor will any other *Fire* do but that blown by the Wind raised from the Fall of some Water; so that they are forc'd to have Recourse to large Tubes laid to the Feet of Large Mountains, or Cataracts to convey the Wind generated by the Fall of Water to their Works.

The *Degree of Fire*; or the Collection and Direction of *Fire*, to the Degree proper for each operation, is almost the Whole of Chymistry: For the *Fire*, *e.gr.* requisite to melt Metals, is by no means proper for the Distillation of Spirit of Wine.

Now, the greater or less Force of *Fire* depends altogether on a greater or less Quantity thereof collected into a Focus : For, as to its Motion, it does not seem in our Power to alter it; or to make any Increase or Diminution of the Force of *Fire* on that account.

The Chymists use four principal Degrees of *Fire* in their Operations. The First is equal to the natural Heat of the human Body; or rather that of a Hen, hatching her Eggs; which is the Standard : And accordingly this first Degree is best measured by applying a Thermometer to a Hen; and some Chymists, by keeping a *Fire* continually to this Degree, by means of a Thermometer, have hatch'd Chickens.

By this Degree all their Digestions, easy Separations and Solutions, gentle Distillations, with all Fermentations and Putrifactions are perform'd.

The Second *Degree of Fire* is that which gives a Man Pain, but does not destroy, or consume the Parts : Like the Heat of a scorching Summers Sun, which chafes and inflames the Skin; and even sometimes raises Blisters.

It is used in making Separations of the more ponderous Bodies, which the first Degree is not equal to; as also in some Fixations, particularly that of Mercury, which is render'd fix'd by a gradual Introduction of such *Fire* among the Parts of the Mercury.

It makes the Serum of the Blood, and White of an Egg coalesce, and so occasions deadly Inflammations; and is too intense for any Digestion, Putrifaction, or Fermentation to be effected by it.

The Third *Degree of Fire* is that of boiling Water, which separates and destroys the Parts of Bodies. This Degree is perfectly stable; for Water, when once it boils, is at its utmost Degree of Heat, and cannot be rais'd a whit further, by any Augmentation of *Fire*, or Fuel; as was first observ'd by Mons. *Amontons*[1]. This Degree serves to attenuate, separate, fix, and perform other Operations, where the two former would not be effectual.

The Fourth *Degree* is that which melts Metals, and destroys every thing else. This Degree is too vehement to be estimated by Thermometer; that Instrument not being able to endure it; so that it is only determinable by its Effect in the Fusion of Metals : As the Heat of boiling Water cannot be increased, so neither can that of melted Metals.

This Degree is used in abundance of Operations, and particularly about Minerals, where the three preceding Degrees are insufficient. This is the last Degree known to the antient Chymists.

[1] Guillaume Amontons (1663 – 1705), a French physicist and scientific instrument maker.

The latest Chymists reckon a Fifth *Degree of Fire*, *viz.* that where by Gold is made to emit Fumes, and evaporate. This was first discover'd in the Year 1690, by Mr. *Tjchirnhausen*[1], whose Burning Glass render'd every thing, even Gold it self volatile.

Besides these five Degrees, the Chymists have several intermediate ones; all which however may be easily reduc'd to the former.

As, *the digesting Fire*, or *Venter Equi*, which is the Heat of a Dunghill. The *Balneum Mariæ, Arensum*, &c. explain'd under the Article Balneum. The *Naked*, or *Intermediate Fire*, which is the common *Fire* applied under a Vessel. The *Fire of a Lamp*, which is moderate and equal, and may be increased by the Addition of more Wick; used by Enamellers, &c. The *Wheel Fire*, which is lighted all round a Crucible, or other Vessel, to heat it all alike.

That called *by Suppression*, which is when the Vessel is not only encompass'd round, but cover'd over with Fire.

The *Reverberatory Fire*, when it is in a Furnace close a-top, by which the *Fire* is reflected back, and all around upon the Vessel. See Reverberatory. The *Melting*, or *Fusing Fire*, for the Solution and Calcination of Metals and Minerals. The *Glass-house Fire*, for the Vitrifying of the Ashes of Vegetables. And the *Olympick Fire*, which is that if the Sun collected in the Focus of a burning Mirror, &c.

To the several Degrees of *Fire* required, several Forms of Furnaces are accommodated; which see under the Article Furnace.

There are five principal ways *of altering the Degree of Fire*. For *Fire* differs

1°, According to the *Weight of the Pabulum*, or Fuel; it being a Rule, that the heavier the Fuel or combustible Matter is, the more vehement, *cæteris paribus*, is the Fire. Thus, Spirit of Wine affords a weaker and less destructive Fire than Oil; and this than Pitch, and so on; the heavier and grosser, still the fiercer.

2°, According to the *Quantity of Pabulum*.

3°, According to the *Distance of the Fire* from the Object; it being a Rule, that the Heat of the *Fire* at different Distances is reciprocally, as the Square of those Distances.

4°, By the introducing or blowing of Air into the *Fire*; it being a Rule, that the stronger the Current of Air, or Wind, provided it be not so string as to break the aerial Fornix or Vault incumbent on the *Fire*, the more is the *Fire* increas'd.

5°, According to the *Solidity*, or *Resistance* of the Medium between the Fire and the Object: For the more solid the Medium, the greater Quantity of Heat, *cæteris paribus*, does it receive from the *Fire*, and communicate to the Object.

Thus, a Vapour Bath communicates much less Heat to the Bodies distilled by it, than a Water Bath; and this, less than a Sand Bath; and this again less than a Bath of Steel Filings; for all Bodies exposed to the *Fire*, grow hot in Proportion to their specifick Gravities.

[1] Ehrenfried Walther von Tschirnhaus (1651 – 1708), a German physician and mathematician.

Thus, if a piece of Metal be put in Water, and both set over the Fire; while the Water only grows lukewarm, the Metal shall be so hot, as to be past touching : And thus, a Key in a Person's Pocket sitting near the Fire, shall frequently be very hot, while his Cloaths themselves have not any sensible Warmth. Indeed, this Rule admits of some Exceptions; for we have Oils, lighter than Water, which yet admit of triple its Degree of Heat, before they Boil.

'Tis a great Controversy in Chymistry, whether *Fire*, when applied to Bodies, only separates and dissolves them; or whether it does not also change them.

Mr. *Boyle*, in his Sceptical Chymist, we think, has abundantly proved, that *Fire* alters Bodies; and that the Parts or Elements procured form Bodies by *Fire*, did not exist such in the Bodies themselves.

Add, that *Fire* does not only separate and decompound; but it also compounds and mixes Bodies. This no body can doubt of, who knows that *Fire* in acting on many Bodies, insinuates and fixes it self among them, and so constitutes one Body together with them.

This is the Case in dissolving of Lead by *Fire*; as is evident from the Increase in Weight of the Lead : The like is observable in Salt of Tartar, which when first melted, loses somewhat of its Weight; but as it is calcined further and further, grows still heavier and heavier. In like manner, Antimony calcined by a Burning glass, receives a notable Accession of Weight.

To say no more, Phosphorus must derived its shining Matter from the fiery Particles it imbibes in the Distillation : For no body will imagine that any of that shining Matter before existed in the human Body.

**FIRE**, in Medicine and Chirurgery, is used in the same Sense with Cautery; and is distinguish'd into *Actual*, and *Potential*.

*Actual Fire* is a hot Iron. There are several Diseases, only to be cured by the Application of a *Actual Fire*; which Method of Cure is practised with great success in the *East Indies*. See Burning. *Potential Fire* is that contain'd in Caustick Medicines.

*Fire* also gives the Denomination to divers Diseases, as St. *Anthony's Fire*, by Physicians more usually called Erysipelas. St. *Anthony's Fire* is also called *Holy Fire*, or *Sacer Ignis*; and in an antient Instrument, belonging to the Hospital in the Church of St. *Anthony*, at *Marseilles*, it is called *Fire of Hell*, or *Ignis infernalis*. This Distemper made great Ravages in *France*, in the XIth and XIIth Century; and it was for the Relief of Persons labouring under it, that the religious Order of St. *Anthony* was founded, in the Year 1093, under the Pontificate of *Urban* II.

*Wild* **FIRE**, is a kind of artificial or factitious *Fire*, which burns even under Water; and that with greater Violence than out of it. It is composed of Sulphur, Naptha, Pitch, Gum, and Bitumen; and is only extinguishable by Vinegar, mix'd with Sand and Urine; or with raw Hides.

Its Motion or Tendency is said to be contrary to that of natural *Fire*, and always follows the Direction in which it is thrown; whether it be downwards, sidewise, or otherwise.

The *French* call it *Greek Fire*, or *Feu Gregeois*, because first used by the *Greeks*, about the Year 660; as is observ'd by the Jesuit *Petavius*, on the Authority of *Nicetas, Theophanes, Cedrenus*, &c.

The Inventor, according to the same Jesuit, was an Ingineer of *Heliopolis*, in *Syria*, named *Callinicus*, who first applied it in the Sea Fight commanded by *Constantine Pogonat*, against the *Sarazens*, near *Cizicus*, in the *Hellespont*; and with such Effect, that he burnt the whole Fleet therewith, wherein were thirty thousand Men.

But others will have it of a much older Date; and hold *Marcus Gracchus* the Inventor; which Opinion is supported by several Passages, both in the *Greek* and *Roman* Writers, which shew it to have been antiently used by both those Nations in their Wars.

*Constantine's* Successors used it on divers Occasions, with equal Advantage, as himself; and what is remarkable enough, is, that they were so happy as to keep the Secret of the Composition to themselves; so that no other Nation knew it in the Year 960.

*Hugh*, King of *Burgundy*, demanding Ships of the Emperor *Leo*, for the Siege of *Fresne*, desired likewise the *Greek Fire. Chorier Hist. de Dauph.*

Fa. *Daniel* gives us a good Description of the *Greek Fire*, in his account of the Siege of *Damiette*, under St. *Louis*. Every body, says the Author, was astonish'd with the *Greek Fire* which the *Turks* then prepared; and the Secret whereof is now lost. They threw it out of a kind of Mortar; and sometimes shot it with an odd sort of Cross Bow, which was strongly bent by means of a Handle, or Winch, of much greater Force than the bare Arm. That thrown with the Mortar, sometimes appear'd in the Air of the Size of a Tun, with a long Tail, and a Noise like that of Thunder. The *French* by Degrees got the Secret of extinguishing it; in which they succeeded several times.

**FISTULA**, in Medicine, A deep, winding, callous, cavernous Ulcer, with a narrow Entrance, but opening thence into a spacious Bottom; and generally yielding a sharp, virulent Matter. *Fistula's* differ from the winding Ulcers in this, that the former are callous, and the latter not.

They attack all Parts of the Body, without Exception; particularly the Anus, Foramen lachrymale, Thorax, &c. The general Cause of *Fistula's*, is some Abscess, or Ulcer, which either being inveterate, or having been ill used, comes to be callous; the Orifice being at first lined or incrustated therewith, and at length the whole Sinus.

The Cure consists, in consuming the Callus, and healing, and consolidating the Ulcer with cleansing Medicines, and Sarcoticks.

The Antients gave the Name *Fistula* to this sort of Ulcers, from the Resemblance they bear, on account of their Depth, to a *Flute*, or *Pipe*, called by the *Latins* Fistula.

**FISTULA** *in Ano*, is a Fistula form'd in the Anus, or Fundament. Of this, some Authors reckon four Kinds, *viz.* the *Cæcum Internum*, which is open outwards, but not into the Rectum : The *Cæcum Externum*, which has an Aperture into the Rectum, but none outwards : The *Compleat*, which opens both into the Anus, and the Intestine: And the *Cuniculatus*, or that with several Sinus's, which discharge themselves into one common Cavity, that the Fund, and as it were, Reservoir of them all.

Others, as *Wiseman*[1], reduces *Fistula's an Ano* to two Classes. The *first* are those arising from a Phyma : These are very painful, and difficult to cure; as entering deep amongst the *Intestines* of the *Muscles*, and forming various Cuniculi, or Sinus's; which, the more remote they are from the Anus, the worse they be, by reason they do not allow of being cut : The second, owe their Origin to an internal Hæmorrhage, or Extravasation between the Coats of the Rectum; and have a small Perforation, near the Circumference of the Anus, whence they yield a thin Sanies, or Ichor, without Pain : They in time bring on Itchings and Excoriations; and the Orifices at length become callous and are sometimes closed, and sometimes open again.

*Fistulæ*, if they do no Harm by the Copiousness of the Flux, Stench, or the like Accidents, are a Benefit to Nature, as carrying off cachectic Humours; and ought not to be cured, but kept open. The fresh, simple *Fistulæ* may be cured without Danger.

The great way is by cutting; where that may be done without Damage to the Muscle of the Anus, which might occasion an involuntary Discharge of the Excrements. Cutting is either peform'd with a Thread, or a cutting Instrument.

**FISTULA** *Lachrymalis*, is a *Fistula* in the greater Canthus of the Eye, call'd also *Aegilops Lachrymalis*.

It is a little deep callous Ulcer, in the greater Caruncle, or the Place of the Glandula Lachrymalis. It usually begins with an Abscess, call'd *Anchylops*, which in time produces an Ulcer, that afterwards degenerates into a *Fistula*. When press'd with the Finger, it yields a stinking Matter, not unlike the Yolk of an Egg; and the corrosive Humor finding, or making it self a Passage, there ensures a perpetual Oozing.

Sometimes the *Os Ethmoidis* it self is corroded, and render'd carious by it; in which Condition it is supposed to be only curable by an actual Cautery : Sometimes it becomes cancrous; and then, *Riverius*[2] directs, all Medicines to be laid aside.

The Cure of the *Fistula lachrymalis*, is wholly external and chirurgical; excepting that Evacuants and Mercurials may be given internally, as also Decoctions of the Woods. Some perforate the Os Nasi, to give room for the Matter, to be evacuated that way.

A *French* Chirurgeon named *Anel*[3], has found out a new way, *viz.* by putting a Probe and Syringe of an inconceivable Fineness, thro; the *Puncta lachrymalia* into the *Sacculus lachrymalis*.

**FISTULAR** *Flowers*, among Herbalists, are those made up on many long, hollow, small Flowers, like Pipes; all divided into large Jaggs at the end.

[1] Richard Wiseman (1625 – 1686), an English surgeon.

[2] Lazare Riviere (1589 – 1655), a French physician.

[3] Dominique Anel (1679 – 1730), a French surgeon and ophthalmologist.

**FISTULOUS**, or Fistular, is applied by the Chirurgeons to Wounds and Ulcers which degenerate into Fistula's. Care must be taken, not to leave the Seton too long in the Wound, lest it renders it callous and *fistulous*. Among Botanists, *fistulous* is understood of such Leaves of Plants, as are round and hollow within, like a Fistula, or Flute. Thus the Leaves of Onions are said to be *fistulous*.

**FIXATION**, in Chymistry, is a peculiar Preparation of Mercury, whereby it is put in a Condition to bear the Fire without evaporating; or the Hammer without flying, or separating.

The Alchymists hold, that if they had the true Secret of fixing Mercury, without the Addition of any foreign less heavy and solid Ingredient, they could make Gold, at least Silver. See Philosophers Stone.

Mons. *Homberg* has a long Process of many Months, to prepare an Oil from the fecal Matter, or human Excrements, which he imagin'd would have fix'd Mercury into Silver, but he fail'd.

The Term is likewise applied in the general to any thing that fixes, and binds together what of its own Nature is volatile; and enables it to sustain the Force of the Fire for some considerable Time.

*Geber* defines *Fixation* an Operation whereby a volatile thing, *i.e.* a thing that cannot endure the Fire, is render'd capable of enduring it. In the general, Fixation is the changing of a volatile Body into a fix'd one.

**FIXT**, or Fix'd Bodies, in the general, are such, as neither the Fire, nor any Corrosive, has such Effect on, as to reduce or resolve them into their component Elements, *i.e.* absolutely to destroy them.

*Chauvin* holds it not sufficient to denominate a Body *fixt*, that it can withstand the Fire, or any one Agent; but it should withstand all. He contends, that Fixity should not be restrain'd, as it usually is, to an Exemption from Evaporation; but from Destruction, or Resolution into primary Elements; in which sense, Gold, pretious Stones and Glass, and even Sulphur, and Mercury it self, are properly *fix'd* Bodies; for Mercury, and Sulphur retain their Nature, notwithstanding all their Evaporations.

**FIXT**, or Fix'd *Bodies*, among Chymists, are such as bear the Violence of the Fire, without evaporating. The Chymists divide all Natural Bodies into *fix'd* and *volatile*, *i.e.* such as bear the utmost Force of the Fire, without dissipating, or spending themselves in Fume; and such as do not.

Of *fix'd* Bodies, the principal are Gold, Silver, pretious Stones particularly the Diamond, Salts, &c. Of all Metals, Gold and Silver alone are *fix'd*, *i.e.* remaining a long time exposed to the most intense Flame; they alone lose nothing of their Weight.

Whence this Property shou'd arise, is difficult to say. If the Reader is not contented with the Causes enumerated under Fixity, he may add the following one from *Boerhaave*, *viz.* The Homogeneity and Equality of the Parts.

The Parts, *e.gr.* of Gold being all homogeneous and equal, will equally sustain each other, and leave equal Pores between them; through which

Pores, when fus'd, the Fire finding an easy, equal Passage, goes off, without carrying any thing of the Metal with it : Or rather, the Particles of Gold being of all others the most solid, and heavy (as appears from the Weight of that Metal) and of all others the most strongly united, or bound together (as appears from the infinite Ductility of that Metal) the Force of the Fire is not sufficient to overcome so powerful a Resistance : The Solidity of the Particles, and their Freedom from Air prevents their being rarified, or set further apart; which might lessen their specifick Gravity, and diminish their *vis cohesionis* : So that what has the chief Effect in the raising of Fumes and Vapours, *viz.* the Rarefaction, or Expansion of the Body being here precluded, the Metal maintains its natural Weight and Tendency to the Centre.

Mr. *Boyle*, the Prince of *Mirandola*[1], Mons. *Homberg*, and others, have made numerous Experiments on Gold, Silver, &c. to see how far their Fixity extended. Pure Gold, kept in an intense Heat for two Months, lost nothing sensible of its Weight. Silver, under the like Circumstances and in the like time, lost one twelfth Part of its Weight; tho' Mr. *Boyle* attributes this to the Metal not being fine and pure.

Indeed, by the great Burning Glass of Mess. *Tschirnhausen* and *Villette*[2], the most fix'd Bodies, as Gold itself, are render'd volatile, and lose of their Weight; so that there is no Body at all Nature absolutely fix'd.

**FIX'D** *Salts*. The Chymists distinguish Salts into *fix'd* and *volatile*. *Fix'd* Salts are those extracted or gain'd from Bodies by Calcination and Lotion. They are call'd *fix'd*, in that the *Fire* was not able to sublime or raise them; as those carried off in the Course of Calcination, by the Vehemence of the Fire, are called *volatile*. The Ashes of all Plants yield *fix'd* Salts. The Chymists also give the Appellation fix'd to certain of their Preparations.

**FIX'D** *Nitre* is Preparation of that Salt, by fusing it in a Crucible, and then inflaming it with throwing in a few Coals and this again and again, till no more Flame or Detonation arise : The letting it cool, they pulverize, and then dissolve it in Water, and afterwards evaporate it into a fine white Salt; which serves to draw the Tinctures out of Vegetables. This Salt, *per deliquium*, yields, what we call, the *Liquor of fix'd Nitre*.

**FIXITY**, or Fixedness, in Philosophy, the Quality of a Body, which denominates and renders it *fix'd* : Or, a Property, which enables it to endure the Fire and other violent Agents.

According to *Chauvin*, *Fixity* consists in this, that the component Principles of the Body are so closely united, or cohere so strongly, and are mix'd in such Proportion, that they cannot easily be divided either by fire, or nay other corrosive Menstruum; or their integral Parts separated, and carried off in Vapour. For a Body may be said to be *fix'd* in two respects.

First, when exposed to the Fire, or a corrosive Menstruum, its Particles are indeed separated, and the Body render'd Fluid; but without being resolved into its first Elements : The Second, when the Body sustains the active Force

[1] Giovanni Pico della Mirandola (1463 – 1494), an Italian philosopher.

[2] Francois Villete (1621 – 1698), a French microscope and telescope maker.

of the Fire, or Menstruum, without its integral Parts being carried of in Fumes. Each kind of *Fixity* is the Result of a strong or intimate Cohesion between the Particles of the mix'd.

**FIXITY**, or Fixedness, in Chymistry, is in a peculiar manner used for the Property opposite to Volatility, *i.e.* the Property whereby Bodies bear the Action of the fire, without being dissipated in Fumes. The principal Causes of Fixity, or the Qualifications that contribute most to the rendering a Body fix'd, according to Mr. *Boyle*, are

1° That its Corpuscles be singly of a certain proportionable Bulk, too big and unwieldy to be carried up by Heat, or buoyed up in the Air.

2° That they have also a proper Degree of Weight, or Solidity.

3° That thief Figure be such as unfits them for Evaporation, or flying off; some being branched, others hook'd, &c. So that being entangled with one another, they cannot easily be extricated, loosen'd, and separated.

To these may be added a fourth Circumstance, *viz.* the Nearness of the Particles, and their being contiguous in a great many Points, or a deal of their Surface, which produces a stronger Force of Attraction and Cohesion.

**FLAME**, the brightest and subtilest Part of a Fire, ascending above the Fewel in a pyramidal or conical Figure.

*Flame* seems to be the Smoak, *i.e.* the Fumes, or volatile Parts of the Fewel, greatly rarified, and at last kindled, or heated red hot. By the great Rarifaction, the Matter becomes so light, as to be rais'd with great Velocity in the Air : And by the Pressure of the incumbent atmospherical Fluid, it is kept for some time together; the Air forming a sort of Arch, or Sphere around it, that prevents its immediate Diffusion and Dissipation, and by its Contiguity and Fixation sustains and feeds the Fire of the Flame; the aqueous and earthy Parts of the Fume being naturally incapable of being ignited, are only rarified, and so impelled upwards, without *flaming*.

*Flame* is defined by Sir *I. Newton*, in his little Treatise *De Acido*, to be *Fumus Candens*, red hot Smoak. The same Author argues, Is not *Flame*, a Vapour, Fume, or Exhalation heated red hot, that is, so hot as to shine? For Bodies do not *flame* without emitting a copious Fume; and this Fume burns in the *Flame*. The *Ignis Fatuus* is a Vapour, shining without Heat; and is there not the same Difference between this Vapour, and *Flame*, as between rotten Wood, shining without Heat, and burning Coals of Fire? In distilling hot Spirits, if the Head of the Still be taken off, the Vapour which ascends, will take Fire at the *Flame* of a Candle, and turn into *Flame*. Some Bodies, heated by Motion or Fermentation, if the Heat grow intense, fume copiously; and if Heat be great enough, the Fumes will shine, and become *Flame*. Metals in Fusion do not *flame*, for want of a copious Fume. All *flaming* Bodies, as Oil, Tallow, Wax, Wood, fossil Coal, Pitch, Sulphur, &c. by burning, waste in Smoak, which at first is lucid; but at a little Distance from the Body, ceases to be so, and only continues hot. When the *Flame* is put out, the Smoak is thick, and frequently smells strongly; but in the *Flame* it loses its Smell, and according to the Nature of the Fewel, the Flame is of divers Colours. That of Sulphur, *e.gr.* is blue; that of Copper open'd with sublimate, green; that of tallow, yellow; of Camphire, white, &c.

We can find that when Gun-powder takes Fire, it goes off in a *flaming* Smoak. The manner we conceive to be this : The Charcoal and Sulphur easily take Fire, and set fire to the Nitre; by which the Spirit of Nitre, sets loose the Spirit of the Nitre, and excites a greater Fermentation, whereby the Heat is increased, and the fix'd Body of the Nitre rarified into Fume; and thus is a vehement Explosion effected. The *Flame* of Gun-powder arises from a violent Action, whereby the mixt being quickly and vehemently heated, is rarified and converted into Fume and Vapour : Which Vapour by the Violence of the Action becoming so hot as to shine, appears in the Form of *Flame*. *Newt. Opticks*, p. 318.

'Tis a remarkable Phænomenon of the *Flame* of a Candle, Torch, or the like, that in the dark it appears bigger at a Distance, than at near at hand. The reason is, that as a Distance, *e.gr.* of six Feet, the Eye can readily distinguish between the *Flame*, and the contiguous Air illuminated by it; and sees precisely where the Flame terminates : But at the Distance, *e.gr.* of thirty Foot, tho' the Angle subtended by the *Flame* be much smaller than before; yet the Eye not being able to distinguish the precise Bound of the *Flame*, takes part of the Sphere of Air illuminated by it, for the *Flame* it self.

We have several Instances of actual *Flame's* being produc'd by the Mixture of two cold Liquors. Dr. *Slare*[1] gives us a List of the Oils which burst into *Flame*, upon mixing them with compound Spirit of Nitre : Such are those of Carroways, Cloves, Sassafras, Guaiacum, Box, Camphor, Pepper, Hartshorn, Blood, &c. *Phil. Transact.* No. 213.

*Vital* **FLAME**, *Flamma*, or *Flammula Vitalis*, a fine, warm, kindled, but mild Substance, supposed by many both of the Antients and Moderns, to reside in the Hearts of Animals, as necessary to Life, or rather, as that which constitutes Life it self. To the Preservation of this *Flame*, they suppose Air as necessary as it is to the Conservation of common Flame; And hence refer the Necessity of Respiration to animal Life.

Mr. *Boyle*, by Experiments in an exhausted Receiver found, that the *Vital Flame* of Animals, if Life may be so called, survives, or outlasts the *Flame* of Spirit of Wine, or of a Wax or Tallow Candle, &c. Some Animals would remain alive and well in Vacuo, for three or four Minutes, whereas no common *Flame* would last there one Minute. The Light of Gloworms he found would presently be destroy'd by exhausting the Air; and retriev'd again upon its Re-admission.

Dr. *Quincy* can find nothing more in the Notion of Vital *Flame*, than the natural Warmth, which is the Effect of a circulating Blood; and which is always as its Velocity.

**FLATULENT**, something, that has a relation to Flatus's or Winds. Peese, and most kinds of Pulse, Onions, &c. are *flatulent* Foods.

**FLATUS**, or Flatulency, a Wind gather'd in the Bowels, or other Cavity of the Body, by Indigestion, or a gross internal Perspiration. It is discussed by warm

[1] Frederick Slare (1646 – 1727), a English physician.

Aromaticks, which rarify it enough to break away wherever Vent can be found.

**FLAX**, or Line, a Plant with a slender hollow Stem, usually about two Foot high; whose Bark consists of Fibres, or Threads, much like those of Hemp, which being dress'd and work'd in a due manner, makes that noble Commodity, *Linen Cloth. Flax* thrives best in a Soil that has long lain fallow.

To bear *Flax*, it must be well plowed, laid flat and even, and the Seed sown in a warm Season, before the Middle of *March*, or Beginning of *April*. The best Seed is that brought from the East; which, though dear, repays the Charges with Abundance. One Sowing will produce two or three Crops, before it need be renewed.

*Flax* pull'd up in the Bloom, proves whiter and stronger, than if left standing till the Seed is ripe; but then the Seed is lost.

The Preparations *Flax* must undergo, to fit it for Spinning, are *Pulling*, *Drying*, and *Swingling*.

The Seed of the *Flax* has several considerable Properties. It enter the Composition of several Medicines, and yields an Oil, by Expression, which has most of the Properties of Nut-Oil; and which is frequently used, in defect thereof in Painting, to burn in Lamps, &c. That drawn cold, is reputed good in divers Diseases.

**FLOWER**, *Flos*, is that Part of a Plant, which contains the Organs of Generation; or the Parts necessary for the Propagation of the Kind. The *Flower* is a natural Production, which precedes the Fruit, and yields the Grain or Seed.

The Structure of *Flowers* is somewhat various; though the Generality, according to *Grew*, have these three Parts in common, *viz*. The *Empalement*, The *Foliation*, and the *Attire*.

Mr. *Ray* reckons, that every perfect Flower has the *Petala, Stamina, Apices*, and *Stylus*, or *Pistil* : Such as want any of these Parts, ne deems Imperfect Flowers.

In most Plants there is a Perianthium, Calix, or Flower-Cup, of a stronger Consistence than the Flower it self, and design'd to strengthen and preserve it.

In some Flowers the two Sexes are confounded, *i.e.* the Male and Female Parts are found in the same Flower; in others, they are separated : And of these again, some are followed by Fruits, and others not : Whence, Flowers become distinguish'd into male, Female, and Hermaphrodites.

The Generality of *Flowers* are of the *Hermaphrodite* kind : Such *e.gr*. are the Lilly, Tulip, Daffodil, Rosemary, Sage, Thyme, Gernaium, Althaea, &c.

The Structure of Parts is much the same in those where the Sexes are divided : The Difference between them consists in this, that the Stamina and Apices, *i.e.* the male Parts, in these, are separated from the Pistils; being sometimes on the same stand, and sometimes on different ones.

Those, wherein the Stamina are, in regard they bear no Fruit, are called *Male*, or barren *Flowers*, and by the Botanists, *Stamineous Flowers* : Those which contain the Pistil, being succeeded with Fruit, are called *Females*, or

*Knitting*, or *Fruitful Flowers*.

Among the Plants which bear both Male and Female Parts on the same Stand, but at a distance from each other, are reckon'd, the Cucumber, Melon, Gourd, Turky Wheat, Turnsol, Wallnut, Oak, Beech, Fir, Alder, Cypress, Cedar, Juniper, Mulberry, Plantan, &c.

Those, where the Male and Female Parts of the Flowers are bore on different Stands, are some Species of Palm, the Willow, Poplar, Hemp, Mercury, Spinage, Nettles, and Hops.

Mr. *Ray* divides Flowers into *Perfect* and *Imperfect*. *Perfect Flowers* he here accounts all such as have the Petala, tho' they want the Stamina. These he subdivides into *Simple*, which are those not compos'd of other smaller ones, and which usually have but one single Style; and *Compounded*, which consist of many Flosculi, all making but one *Flower*.

*Simple Flowers* are either *Monopetalous*, which have the Body of the Flower all of one entire Leaf, though sometimes cut, or divided a little way, into many seeming Petala, or Leaves, as in Borrage, Bugloss, &c.

Or *Polypetalous*, which have distinct Petals, and those falling off singly, and not altogether, as the seeming Petala of the monopetalous *Flowers* always do.

Both those are farther divided into *Uniform* and *Difform Flowers*. The former have their Right and Left hand Parts, and the forward and backward Parts all like; but the Difform have no such Regularity; as in the *Flowers* of Sage, Dead-nettle, &c.

A Monopetalous *difform* Flower is likewise farther divided into 1° *Semi-fistular*, whose upper Part resembles a Pipe, cut off obliquely, as in the Aristolochia. 2° *Labiate* : And this either with one Lip only, as in the Acanthum and Scordium; or with two Lips, as in the far greater Part of the Labiate *Flowers*.

And here the upper Lip is sometimes turned upwards and so turns the convex Part downwards, as in the Chamæcissus, &c. but most usually the upper Lip is convex above, and turns the hollow Part down to its Fellow below, and so represents a kind of Helmet, or Monk's Hood; whence these are frequent. Such are the *Flowers* of the Lamium, and most verticillate Plants. Sometimes also the Labium is entire, and sometimes jagged or divided.

3° Corniculate, that is, such hollow Flowers, as have on their upper Part a kind of Spur or little Horn; as in the Linaria, Delphinium, &c. And the Corniculum or Calcar is always impervious at the Tip or Point.

*Compound* Flowers are 1° *Discous* or *Discoidal*, that is, whose Floculi are set together so close, thick, and even, as to make the Surface of the *Flower* plain and flat; which therefore, because of its round Form , will be like a Discus. This Disk is sometimes radiated, when there are a Row of Petals standing round in the Disk, like the Points of a Star; as in the Matricaria, Chamæmelum, &c.

2° *Planifolious*, which are compos'd of plain *Flowers*, set together in circular Rows, round the Centre, an whose Face is usually indented, notch'd, uneven, and hajjed; as the Hieracia, Sonchi, &c.

3° *Fistular*, which are compounded of many long, hollow little Flowers, like Pipes, all divided into large Jags at the Ends.

*Imperfect Flowers* are such as want the Petals, and are called likewise *Stamineous*, *Apetalous*, and *Capillacious*. Those which hang pendulous by fine Threads like the Juli, are by *Tournefort* called *Amentacious*; we call them *Cats-tails*.

Botanists furnish other Divisions and denominations of *Flowers*. *Campaniform*, or Bell-like Flowers, are those in Shape of a Bell.

*Cruciform* Flowers are those consisting of four Petals, or Leaves : The Calix also containing four Leaves; and the Pistil always producing a Fruit. Such are those of the Clove Tree, Cabbage Tree, &c.

*Infundibuliform* Flowers, are such as resemble the Figure of a Funnel, *i.e.* a broad, and ample top, and contracted in the Neck at bottom : Such is that of the Bear's Ear.

*Cucurbitaceous* Flowers, are such as resemble the Flower of the Gourd; or have the same Conformation therewith.

*Stamineous* Flowers, are such as have no Pistils, but consist wholly of Stamina's or Threads, with Apices a-top.

The Leaves placed around these Stamina, are not to be esteem'd as Petala, but a Calix; in regard they afterwards become a Capsula, or Cover, including the Seed; which is the Office of the Calix alone.

In effect, it is essential to the Leaves of *Flowers*, not to serve as a Cover to the Seeds that succeed them : And this is the only Characteristic that distinguishes the Leaves, or Petala of *Flowers* from their Calix; for, that no particular Colour of the Leaves does determine, whether the Parts in dispute be Leaves of the *Flower*, or the Calix of the *Flowers*, appears hence, that there are some Leaves of the *Flowers*, which are green like the Calix; and some Calices colour'd, like Petals.

*Leguminous* Flowers are those of Leguminous Plants. These bear some Resemblance to a flying Butterfly; for which reason they are also called *Papillionaceous* Flowers.

*Papillionaceous* Flowers, consist of four or five Leaves, whereof the uppermost is called *Vexillum*, or Standard; and the lowest Carina, as resembling the Bottom or Keel of a Boat : Those between the two, are called *Lateral* Leaves or *Alæ*. From the Bottom of the Calix arises a Pistil, which is incompass'd with a Sheath, or Cover, fringed with Stamina. This Pistil always becomes the Fruit, and is usually called the Pod, in Latin, *Siliqua*.

*Umbelliform* Flowers, are those with several Leaves doubled, and dispos'd in manner of a Rose; and whose Calix essentially becomes a fruit of two Seeds, join'd, before they come to Maturity; but afterwards easily separated again.

They have this Denomination, by reason they are generally sustain'd by a Number of Threads, which proceeding from the same Centre are branch'd all around, like the Sticks of an Umbrella. Of this kind are the Flowers of Fennel, Angelica, &c.

*Verticillate* Flowers, are also those ranged, as it were, in Stories, Rings, or Rays along the Stems : Such as those of Horehound, Clary, &c.

**FLOWERS**, in Chymistry, are the finest, and most subtle Parts of dry Bodies, rais'd by Fire, into the Head, and Aludels; and adhering to them , in form of a fine Powder, or Dust. Such are the Flowers of Sulphur, Benjamin, &c.

Flower *of Sulphur*, or *Brimstone*, is prepared by putting the Sulphur grossly powder'd into a Glass Body, placed in a small open Fire, with another earthen Vessel of the same form over, or in it, Neck to Neck. This disposed, the Fire will sublime, or raise the *Flowers*, and gather them in the upper Vessel.

**FLOWERS**, in the Animal Œconomy, are Womens monthly Purgations, or Menses. *Nicod* derives the Word in this sense from *fluere*, q.d. *Fluors* : Others will have the Name occasion'd hence, that Women do not conceive, till they have had their *Flowers*; so that these are a sort of Forerunners of their Fruit.

**FLUIDITY**, in Physicks, that State or Affection of Bodies, which denominates, or renders them fluid. *Fluidity* stands in direct Opposition to Firmness, or Solidity.

It is distinguish'd from *Liquidity*, and *Humidity*, in that the Idea of the first is absolute, and the Property contain'd in the thing it self; whereas that of the latter is relative, and implies wetting, or adhering; *i.e.* somewhat that gives us the Sensation of Wetness, or Moisture, and which would have no Existence, but for our Senses.

Thus, melted Metals, Air, Æther, and even Smoak and Flame itself are fluid Bodies, but not Liquid ones; their Parts being actually dry, and not leaving any Sense of Moisture.

The Nature, or Cause of *Fluidity* has been variously assign'd. The *Gassendists*, and antient Corpuscularians, require only three Conditions as necessary thereto, *viz.* a Smallness and Smoothness of the Particles of the Body; Vacuities interspersed between them; and a Spherical Figure.

The *Cartesians*, and after them Dr. *Hook*[1], Mr. *Boyle*, &c. beside the Circumstances above mentioned, require a various, perpetual, intestine Motion of the Particles of the Bodies, as that which principally contributes to *Fluidity*.

*Fluidity* then, according to these Philosophers, consists in this, that the Parts of the Body being very fine, and small, are so disposed by Motion, or Figure, as that they can easily slide over one another's Surfaces all manner of ways; and that they be in a constant, various, separate Agitation to and fro; and that they only touch one another in some Parts of their Surfaces.

Mr. *Boyle* in his *History of Fluidity* mentions these three as the Conditions principally required to *Fluidity*, viz.

1° The *Minuteness of the Parts* : As, in effect, we find that Fire, by dividing Metals into fine, small Parts, renders them fluid; and that acid Menstruums dissolve and render them fluid after the like manner; and that Fire turns the

[1] This is probably Robert Hooke (1635 – 1703), an English natural philosopher and scientist.

hard Body of common Salt almost wholly into a Liquor, by Distillation : Not but that the Figure of the Particles may have a considerable Share in *Fluidity*.

Thus Mercury, whose Parts are doubtless much grosser than those of Oil and Water, is yet more fluid than either of them : And thus Oil, by the Action of Fire, may be converted into a consistent Substance, like Butter.

2° *Store of Vacuities* interspersed between the Corpuscles, to give room for the several Particles to move among themselves.

3° A *Motion* and *Agitation* of the Corpuscles; either from some Principle of Mobility within themselves, or from some extraneous Agent, penetrating and entering the Pores, moving inwards variously among them, and communicating to them part of its Motion.

That this last is the Qualification chiefly required in *Fluidity*, he argues from divers Observations and Experiments. Thus, a little dry Powder of Alabaster, or Plaister of Paris finely sifted, being put in a Vessel over a Fire; it soon beings to boil like Water; exhibiting all the Motions and Phænomena of a boiling Liquor. It will kindle variously in great Waves like that; will bear stirring with a Stock or Ladle like that, without resisting; Nay, if strongly stirr'd near the Side of the Vessel, its Waves will apparently dash against them : Yet it is all the while a dray, parch'd Powder.

The like is observ'd in Sand : A Dish of which being set on a Drumhead, briskly beaten by the Sticks; or on the upper Stone of a Mill, it in all respects emulates the Properties of a fluid Body. A heavy Body, *e.gr.* will immediately sink in it to the Bottom, and a light one emerge to the Top : Each Grain of Sand has a constant vibratory and dancing Motion; and if a Hole be made in the Side of the Dish, the Sand will spin out like Water.

That the Parts of Fluids are in continual Motion, the *Cartesians* bring divers Considerations to prove; as 1° The Transmutation of Solids into Fluids, *e.gr.* Ice into Water, and *vice versa*; the chief Difference between the Body in those two States consisting in this, that the Parts being fix'd and at rest in one, resists the Touch; whereas in the other, being already in Motion, they give way upon the slightest Impulse.

2° The Effects of Fluids, which commonly proceed from Motion : Such are the Insinuation of Fluids among the Pores of Bodies; the softening and dissolving of hard Bodies; the Actions of corrosive Menstruums, &c. Add, that no Solid can be brought to a State of *Fluidity*, without the Intervention of some moving, or moveable Body, as Fire, Air, or Water.

Air, the same Gentlemen hold the first Spring of these Causes of *Fluidity*; it being this that gives Motion to Fire and Water, though it self receives its Motion and Action from the Æther, or subtile Medium.

The learned *Boerhaave*, in his late Excellent *Institut. Chymiæ*, pleads very strenuously for Fire's being the first Mover, and the Cause of all Fluidity in other Bodies, as Air, Water, &c. without this, he shews, that the Atmosphere it self would fix into one solid Mass.

Sir *I. Newton* sets aside this Theory of the Cause of *Fluidity*, and substitutes a new one, the great Principle of Attraction.

The Corpuscular System, with all the Improvements of *Des Cartes*, and Mr. *Boyle*, did not sufficiently account for the primary Condition, requisite to constitute a Body fluid, *viz.* the various intestine Motion and Agitation of its Particles.

But, this Motion is naturally enough accounted for, by supposing it a primary Law of Nature, that, as all the Particles of Matter attract each other, when within a certain Distance; so at all greater Distances, they fly from, and avoid one another.

For then, tho' there common Gravity together with the Pressure of other Bodies upon them, may keep them together in a Mass; yet their continual Endeavour to avoid one another singly, and the adventitious Impulses of Heat, Light, or other external Causes, may make the Particles of Fluids continually move round about one another, and so produce this Quality.

There is a Difficulty indeed, in accounting, why the Particles of Fluids always keep at such a Distance from one another, as not to come within the Sphere of one another's Attraction.

The Fabrick and Constitution of that fluid Body, Water, is amazing; that a Body so very rare, and which has a vast Over-proportion of Pores, or interspers'd Vacuity, to solid Matter, should yet be perfectly incompressible by the greatest Force : And yet this Fluid is easily reducible into that form, transparent, friable; Body, which we call Ice, by being only exposed to a certain Degree of Cold.

One would think, that tho' the Particles of Water cannot come near enough to attract each other, yet the inventing frigorifick Matter doth, by being mingled *per minima*, strongly attract them, and is it felt likewise strongly attracted by them, and so wedges or fixes all the Mass into a firm solid Body; which solid Body loses its Solidity again, when by Heat the Vinculum is solved, and the frigorifick Particles are disjoined from those of the Water, and are forced to fly out of it : And just thus may the Fumes of Lead perhaps fix Quicksilver.

When a firm solid Body, such as a Metal, is by Heat reduced into a Fluid, the Particles of Fire disjoined separate its constituent Parts, which their mutual Attraction caused before to cohere; and keep them at such a distance from one another, as that they are out of the Sphere of each other's Attraction, as long as that violent Motion lasts; and when by their Lightness and Activity they are flown off, unless they are renewed by a continual Supply, the component Particles of the Metal come near enough again to feel one another's Attractions.

As therefore the Cause of Cohesion of the Parts of solid Bodies appears to be their mutual Attraction; so the chief Cause of *Fluidity* seems to be a contrary Motion, impress'd on the Particles of Fluids, by which they avoid, and fly one another, as soon as they come at, and as long as they keep at such a Distance from each other.

It is observ'd also in all Fluids, that the Direction of their Pressure against the Vessels which contain them, is in Lines perpendicular to the Sides of such Vessels; which Property being the necessary Result of the Particles of any Fluid's being spherical, it shews that the Parts of all Fluids are so, or of a Figure very nearly approaching thereunto.

**FLUOR**, in Physick, &c. a Fluid; or more properly, the State of a Body, which was before hard, or solid, but is now reduc'd by Fusion or Fire into a State of Fluidity. Gold and Silver will remain a long time in a *Fluor*, kept to it by intensest Heat, without losing any thing of their Weight.

*Fluor*, is also us'd by the modern Mineral Writers for such soft, transparent, starry kinds of mineral Concretions, as are frequently found amongst Oars, and Stones, in Mines and Quarries.

**FLUOR** *Albus*, or *Uterinus*, a kind of Flux, incident to Women, popularly called the *Whites*. It consists in an irregular, disorderly Discharge of some corrupt Humour, sometimes white, and pale, like Whey; sometimes yellow, green, or blackish : At first, it is usually soft and harmless, but in time grows hot, sharp, and corrosive, and excoriates all the Parts it touches.

It is attended with a Pain in the *Spina Dorsi*, a Swelling of the Feet and Eyes, Weariness, Lumbago, a Loss of Appetite, Change of Complexion, &c. It is frequently produced from a too heavy and lasting Grief. It must be well distinguish'd from an Ulcer in the Uterus, and a Gonorrhæa.

It happens to all Ages; from Girls of three Years old : And at all times; before, after, or even along with the Menses; and even to Women with Child.

*Etmuller* takes it for a *Gonorrhæa muliebris*, analogous to a non virulent Gonorrhæa in Men, and flowing out of the Glandulæ of the Prostrates.

What the Coryza is in the Nostrils; too much weeping in the Eyes, coughing and hawking in the Fauces; that, according to *Etmuller*, is this *Fluor* in Women.

**FLUX**, *Fluxus*, in Medicine, an extraordinary Issue, or Evacuation of some Humor. *Fluxes* are various, and variously denominated, according to their Seats, or the Humours thus voided; as, *a Flux of the Belly*; *Uterine Flux, Hepatic Flux, Salival Flux*, &c.

The *Flux of the Belly* is of four kinds, which have their respective Denominations, *viz.* the *Lientery*, or *Fluxus Lientericus*; the *Cæliac*, or *Fluxus Chylosus*; *Diarrhæa*; and *Dissentery*, or *Bloody Flux*.

A Wound, or Scarification cross the Crown of he Head is used in *Scotland* to cure *Fluxes* and Dissenteries. *Phil. Transact.* No. 321.

The *Hepatic* Flux of the Antients is a mere Name; being, in reality a hæmorrhoidal *Flux*, out of the hæmorrhoidal Veins; and so reducible to the *Dissentery*.

Women are subject to three kinds of *Fluxes* extraordinary : The first, call'd the *Menses*, or *Menstrual Flux*, as happening every Month; sometimes Courses, as keeping pace with the Moon; and sometimes *Flowers*. The second is after Delivery, call'd *Lochia*. The third is irregular, and præternatural; and for want of a better Name called *Fluor albus*, or *Whites*.

**FLUX** *Powders* are those prepared to facilitate the Fusion of the harder Metals; as also to melt Oars, in order to discover what Proportion of Metal they contain. Powder of Antimony is a very good *Flux* Powder. By this alone may you readily melt Iron or Steel in a Crucible, with an ordinary Charcoal Fire.

**FLUXION**, in Medicine, a sudden Collection of morbid Matter in any Part of the Body. *Fluxions* are occasion'd by Motion, Heat, Pain, Fomentation, &c. A *Fluxion*, or Defluxion on the Lungs, is called a Catarrh. *Fluxions* arise either from the Weakness, Flaccidity, and Inactivity of the Part affected, which does not disperse, protrude, or expel the Humors naturally receiv'd into it : Or from the Derivation of some extraordinary Quantity of peccant Matter from some other Part. This latter is properly called *Defluxion*, and by the Antients, Attraction.

**FOETOR**, in Medicine, stinking, or fœtid Effluvia, proceeding from the Body, or the Parts thereof. *Fœtors* arise from stagnant, extravasated, corrupted, or poison'd Humors; as also from any things capable of attenuating and volatizing the Oil and Salts : As, Abstinence, Heat, too much Motion, Acrimony of Food, &c.

**FOETOR** *Narium*, Stench of the Nostrils, a sort of Disease, arising from a deep Ulcer, within side the Nose, yielding a foetid Smell. Its Cause, according to *Galen*, is a sharp Humor, falling from the Brain upon the Mamillary Processes. This is one of the Causes that annuls Marriage.

**FOLLICULUS**, among Gardeners, the Seed-Vessel, Case, Coat, Husk, or Cover, which some Seeds and Fruits have over them.

**FOMENTATION**, in a liquid Medicine, applied on any diseas'd Part. *Fomentations* are either *Simple*, or *Compound*. *Simple* Fomentations are those made with luke warm Water, Milk, Oil, Oxicrat, or other the like Liquor.

*Compound Fomentations* are Decoctions of Roots, Leaves, Flowers, Seeds, made in common Water, or other proper Liquor; to which are sometimes added Salts, Axungiae, Oil. &c. To use, or apply, them, they dip a hot linen Cloth or Flannel in the Liquor, and spread it on the Part affected.

There are also *Fomentations* made another way; *viz.* by boiling certain Drugs in linen Bags, and then applying 'em, Bags and all, on the Part.

There are also a sort of *dry Fomentations*, being Bags fill'd with Medicines, but not boil'd, only sometimes sprinkled with a little Wine or Brandy.

The Intention of *Fomentations* is to resolve, discuss, soften, assuage, fortify, constringe, &c. the Parts they are applied on.

*Fomentations* are also called Local Baths, or Partial Bathings; because, being applied on a diseased Part, they have much the same Effect as a Bath, or Half-bath has on the whole Body.

**FONTICULUS**, or *Fontinella*, in Chirurgery, a general Name for Issues, Seatons, Cauteries, and other small artificial Discharges. The Word is a Diminutive of *Fons*, Fountain.

**FORCEPS**, Pair of Tongues, a Chirurgeon's Instrument, wherewith dead, and corrupt Parts are seiz'd, and cut, or pulled off, &c. As also foreign Bodies extracted out of Wounds, &c. They are of divers Forms, long, crooked, with Teeth, with Beaks, half-moon'd, &c.

**FORM**, in Philosophy, is the manner of being peculiar to each Body; or that which constitutes it such a particular Body, and distinguishes it from every other.

The Philosophers generally allow two Principles of Bodies : *Matter*, as the common Basis, or Substratum of all; and *Form*, as that which specifies and distinguishes each; and which added to a Quantity of common matter, determines or denominates it this, or that; Wood, or Fire, or Ashes, &c.

*Aristotle* calls Form λογος της ουσιας, the *Reason*, or Manner of the *Essence*, or Being of a thing : But as ουσια denotes *Substance*, as well as *Essence*, a mighty Controversy has arose in the Schools, in which sense the Word is here to be us'd; and whether *Forms* are to be accounted *substantial*, or only *essential* : *i.e.* Whether the *Forms* of Bodies be any real Substances, and have an Existence distinct from that of Matter, or not.

'Tis certain, the most antient Philosophers never dreamt of making *Form* a Substance. *Parmenides* and *Telesins* expressly assert, all natural Things to consist of one and the same kind of Substance, and only to differ in Accidents. And tho' *Empedocles* allow'd of a substantial *Form* in mixt Bodies; yet he deny'd it in the Elements, and only held an essential one.

*Galen* allow'd of nothing in Matter more than the Temperature of the primary Elements, in which he was seconded by *Alex. Aphrodisaeus, Philoponus*, and others.

*Substantial* Forms seem to have been first broch'd by the Followers of *Aristotle*, who thought Matter, under different Modes or Modifications, not sufficient to constitute different Bodies; but that something substantial was necessary to set them at a sufficient Distance : And thus introduc'd substantial *Forms*; on the footing of Souls, which specify and distinguish Animals.

The Consideration which the Peripateticks principally insist on, in confirmation of this Doctrine, are :

1° That without substantial *Forms*, all natural Things would be of the same Species, Nature, and Essence; which is suppos'd an Absurdity.

2° That everything has its peculiar Pow'r, Motion, and Operation; as the Magnet, *e.gr.* has of attracting Iron; but that this Pow'r, does not flow form the Matter of the Body, which is only passive; nor from the Accidents : And therefore must arise from a substantial *Form*.

3° That without substantial *Forms* there would be no Generation; for a Production of Accidents is only an Alternative.

4° That without such Form, the Nature of a Man and of a Lyon would not differ.

What contributed much to their Error, was the Circumstances of Life and Death : For, observing, that as soon as the Soul was departed out of a Man, all Motion, Respiration, Nutrition, &c. immediately ceas'd; they concluded that all those Functions depended on the Soul; and consequently that the Soul was the *Form* of the animal Body, or that which constituted it such : And that the Soul was a Substance, independent of Matter, no body doubted; whence the Forms of other Bodies were concluded equally substantial.

But to this is answer'd, that tho' the Soul be that by which a *Man* is *Man*;

and consequently is the *Form* of the *human* Body, as *human*; yet it does not follow, that it is properly the *Form* of this Body of ours, as it is a Body; nor of the several Parts thereof, consider'd as distinct from each other.

For those several Parts have their proper *Forms* so closely connected with their Matter, that it remains inseparable therefrom, long after the Soul has quitted the Body: Thus, Flesh has the *Form* of Flesh; Bone, of Bone, &c. after the Soul is remov'd, as well as before.

The Truth is, the Body does not become incapable of performing its accustom'd Functions, by reason the Soul has deserted it; but the Soul takes its leave, by reason the Body is not in a Condition to perform its Functions.

The antient and modern corpuscular Philosophers therefore, with the *Cartesians*, exclude the Notion of substantial *Forms*; and shew by many Arguments, that the *Form* is only the Modus, or manner of the Body it is inherent in.

And as there are only three primary Modes of Matter, *viz*. Figure, Rest, and Motion; with two others arising therefrom, *viz*. Magnitude, and Situation : The *Forms* of all Bodies they hold to consist therein; and supposed the Variations these Modes are capable of, sufficient to present all the Variety observable in Bodies.

Many Varieties we actually see result from changes in these Modes; which may very well pass for Differences of *Form* : Thus an Awl only differs from a Needle in Magnitude; a Globe from a Cube in Figure : Transparent Glass being pulveriz'd, will reflect the Light, and appear white; and yet all the Alteration consists in the Order and Arrangement of the Parts : When Wheat is ground into Flower, all the Change consists in a Separation of the contiguous Parts; and when the Flower is bak'd into Bread, what is it but the same Particles associated again, in another manner. By agitating Water, a Froth is form'd; if the Agitation be increas'd, the Particles will exhale, and form Clouds; which being con-gregated again, return in Dew, Snow, Hail, or Rain : And the same Water, by the Accession of Cold, might have been form'd into Ice. So many different Bodies, endued with different Qualities, and which the Peripateticks themselves allow specifically different, arise from one and the same Body, by mere Motion, and Rest.

The Philosophy of substantial Forms, its Rise, Use, and Extent, are set in an excellent light by Fa. *Mallebranch*.

The way of thinking, that first introduc'd it, is this : Every thing I perceive in tasting, seeing, and handling this Honey, and Salt, is in the Honey, and Salt : But it is certain, that the things I perceive in the Honey, *e.gr*. the Colour, Taste, &c. differ essentially from those I perceive in the Salt; consequently, there is an essential Difference between the two.

Hence it follows, that they are grossly deceiv'd, who take all the Differences between those Bodies to consist in the different Configurations of the component Parts; since the different Figure is not at all essential to the different Bodies : For change the Figure of the Parts of Honey how you will; and even give them those of the Parts of Salt; yet it is Honey still.

There must therefore be some Substance added to the common Matter of all Bodies, to make them essentially different. And thus are *substantial Forms* hook'd in; those fertile Substances, which perform every thing that we see in all nature.

Since then in every natural Body there are two Substances; the one common to Honey, Salt, and all other Bodies; and the other, that which makes the Honey, Honey; the Salt, Salt; and all other Bodies what they are : It follows, that the first, *viz. Matter*, having no contrary, but being indifferent to all Forms, must remain without Force, and Action; as having no occasion to defend it self.

But for the others, *viz.* the substantial *Forms*, there is a Necessity of their being accompany'd and invested with Faculties and Qualities for their Defence, and Subsistence. These must be always on their Guard, for fear of being surpriz'd : They are in possession of a thing, which they are to hold against numerous Pretenders; and therefore must be continually at work, to fortify themselves, and extend their Dominion over the neighbouring Matters, and push their Conquests as far as they can: Were they to remain unactive, and unprepar'd, other *Forms* would lay hold of them, and banish and destroy them for ever. To guard against this, they keep constant watch; and entertain mortal Enmities and Antipathies against those other *Forms*, which only wait to destroy them.

If now it happens, that one *Form* seize the Matter, or Receptacle of another; that the *Form* of a Carcass, for instance, seize the Body of a Dog; it is not enough, that this new *Form* annihilate the former; but its Hatred must be further gratify'd with the Destruction of all the Qualities, that took its Enemy's part.

The Hair of the Carcass, then, must be turn'd white; by a Creation of a new Colour: Its Blood must become red, but of such a red, as is not to be suspected in the Interest of the Enemy; and the whole Body to be invested with Qualities, trusty to their new Master, whom they are to defend with all the Power the Qualities of a Carcass can have; till such time as being overpower'd, this Form gives way too, in its turn, to the *Form* of Maggots, Worms, &c.

But, as nothing can be in perpetual War; but every thing has its place of Rest; it follows, that even the Fire must likewise have its Centre, whither its natural Levity always prompts it, that it may remain at rest, cease to burn, and even quit its Heat, which it only maintains here below for its Defence.

These may serve as a Taste of the Consequences, drawn from that important Principle, *Substantial Forms*; which is infinitely fertile, and furnishes every Philosopher with all sorts of Solutions, according to his Ability, Address, Inclination, &c.

Forms are distinguished into *Essential*, and *Accidental*.

*Essential* Forms. Though the five Modes above mention'd, generally taken, be adventitious; yet, to this, or that Body, *e.gr.* to Fire, or Water, they are essential: Thus, it is *accidental* to Iron, to have this, or that Magnitude, Figure, or Situation; since it might exist in different ones; yet, to a Knife, or Hammer, the Figure, Magnitude, and Position of Parts, which constitute it a hammer, or Knife, are *essential*; and they cannot exist or be conceiv'd without them.

Hence it is infer'd, that tho' there be no *Substantial*, there are *Essential Forms*, whereby the several Species of Bodies become each what they are, and are distinguish'd from all others.

*Accidental* Forms are those really inherent in Bodies; but in such manner, as that the Body may exist in all its Perfection, without them. Such is Whiteness in a Wall; Heat in Water; a Figure of a Man in Wax, &c.

*Metaphysical* Form is nothing else but specific Difference; as metaphysical Matter is nothing else but Genus. Thus, *Rational*, is the Metaphysical *Form* of Man.

*Syllogistic* Form is a just Disposition, both of the Terms, in respect of Predicate, and Subject; and of the Propositions, in respect of Quantity, and Quality. But just Disposition we mean such an one, wherein the Conclusion follows duly and legitimately from the two Premisses; there being no Form, where there is no Conclusion.

The Disposition of the several Terms, being, as it were, so many Steps or Degrees of a *Syllogistic Form*; is call'd the *Figure* of the Syllogism. The Disposition of the Premisses alone, being as it were another Degree, is call'd the *Mode of the Syllogism.*

*Forms*, again, are distinguish'd into *Simple*, and *Compound*. *Simple* Forms are those of Simple Bodies, *i.e.* of such as have but few Properties. *Compound* Forms are those of more Compounded Bodies; or such, as have more Properties.

Thus, *e.gr*. If the *Form* of a *hard Body* be compar'd with the *Form* of Wood; the former may be accounted *Simple*, and the latter *Complex*; inasmuch as a hard Body, consider'd only as *hard*, has fewer Properties than Wood. Absolutely speaking, however, *Simple* Forms are those of the Elements; and Compound, of mixt Bodies.

Lastly, some distinguish *Forms* into a *Natural*, and *Artificial*. Natural, are those inherent in Bodies, without any thing contributed thereto on the part of Man. Such is the *Form* of Marble. Artificial, are those arising from human Industry : Such is that of a Statue. But this Difference is useless; and does not imply any intrinsic Difference in the *Forms* themselves.

**FORMICA**, literally signifies an Ant, and is us'd to express little Tumours, which appear like the Bites of those Creatures.

**FORMULA**, is particularly us'd for a little Form, or Prescription; such as Physicians direct in extemporaneous Practice; in Distinction from the greater Forms, which are the Official Medicines.

**FORMULARY**, a Writing, containing the Forms, or Formula of an Oath, Declaration, Attestation, or Abjuration, &c. to be made on certain Occasions. There are also *Formularies* of Devotion, of Prayers, &c. Liturgies are *Formularies* of the publick Service in most Churches,.

**FOSSIL** Kingdom. The Chemists divided all Bodies into three Classes, or Kingdoms; *viz*. Fossil, or Minerals; Vegetable; and Animal.

**FOSSIL**, in Natural History, is us'd, in a general Sense, for any thing dug up, or found under Ground. Such are all Minerals, Metals, Rock Salts, &c. *Fossils* may be distinguish'd into 1° Such as are *Natives* of the Earth; and 2° Such as are *adventitious* and reposited therein by any extraordinary Means, as Earthquakes, Deluges, &c.

*Native Fossils*, or *Fossils* properly so called, are strictly defin'd to be sensible Bodies generated, and growing in, and of the Earth; whose constituent Parts are so simple, and homogeneous, that there is no apparent Distinction of Vessels, and Juices; between the Part, and the Whole.

Native *Fossils* are either *Simple*, or *Compound*. *Simple Fossils* are those, whose Parts, however divided, are all of the same Nature, *i.e.* of the same Gravity, Magnitude, Figure, Hardness, and Mobility, Such is Quicksilver, which, however divided, is always found the same.

*Compound Fossils* are those which may be divided into different, or dissimilar Parts. As Antimony, which may be resolv'd by Fire into Sulphur, and a Metalline Part.

The Simple *Fossils* are all *Metals, Salts, Stones*, both vulgar and pretious, and Earths. The Compound *Fossils* are all Sulphurs, all Semimetals, or what we properly call *Minerals*; and all Bodies combin'd of two, or more or the preceding, either Simple or Compound Fossils.

*Adventitious*, or *Foreign Fossils*, include the subterraneous Exuviæ of Sea and Land Animals, and even vegetables; as Shells, Bones, Teeth, Leaves, Stalks, &c. which are found in great Abundance, in divers Parts of the Earth.

These Extraneous *Fossils* have employ'd the Curiosity of several of out latest and best Naturalists, who have each their several System to account for the surprising Appearances of petrify'd Sea-fishes, in Places far remote from the Sea, and on the Tops of Mountains : Shells in the Middle of Quarries of Stones : Elephants Teeth , and Bones of divers Animals, peculiar to the Southern Climates; and Plants only growing in the East, found in our Northern and Western Parts.

Some will have these Shells, &c to be real Stones, and Stone Plants, form'd after the usual manner of other figur'd Stones, and Stone Plants : Of which Opinion is our learned Dr. *Lister*.

That Author, tho' he allows of petrify'd Shells on the Sea Shores, will by no means agree, that there are any such Petrifactions in the Midland Countries. The Shell-like Stones, found in our Quarries, he contends, are *Lapides sui generis*; and never were any Part of an Animal.

His Reasons are, that their matter, and Texture, is perfectly the same with that of the Rock, or Quarry, where they are taken; as Iron-stone Shells are all iron-stone; Spar, or Crystalline, all Sparr, &c. That Quarries of different Stone yield different Sorts of these Shells : And that there are no Animals in Nature, which yield any thing exactly like them.

But 1° These Shells found under Ground, are perfectly conformable to those in the Sea in Figure, Substance, Magnitude, &c. 2° The Substance of these *Fossils* differs essentially from the common Substance of Stones. 'Tis true, we frequently find them cover'd, or incrusted with a Mineral, or Stony Matter, which has gradually insinuated it self into the Pores; but it is easy distinguishing that Matter from the Substance of the Shell.

The common Opinion is, that these *fossil* Shells, with all other foreign

Bodies, found within the Earth, as Bones, Trees, Plants, &c. were buried therein at the time of the universal Deluge; and that having been penetrated either by the Bituminous Matter, abounding chiefly in watery Places; or by the Salts of the Earth, they have been preserv'd entire, an sometimes petrify'd.

Others think, that those Shells, found at the Tops of the highest Mountains, could never have been carried thither by the Waters, even of the Deluge; inasmuch as most of these aquatic Animals, by reason of the Weight of their Shells, always remain at the Bottom of the Water, and never move but close to the Ground.

They imagine, that a Year's Continuance of the Waters of the Deluge, intermix'd with the salt Waters of the Sea, upon the Surface of the Earth, might well give occasion to the Production of Shells of divers kinds in different Climates; and that the universal Saltness of the Water as the real Cause of their Resemblance with the Sea Shells. The Lakes form'd dayly by the Retention of Rain, or Spring Water, produce different Kinds.

Others think, that the Waters of the Sea, and the Rivers, with those which fell from Heaven, turn'd the whole Surface of the Earth upside down; after the same manner as the Waters of the *Loire*, and other Rivers, which roll in a Sandy Bottom overturn all their Sands, and even the Earth it self, in their Swellings and Inundations : And that in this General Subversion, the Shells come to be interr'd here, Fishes there, Trees there, &c. See the *Journ. Des Scavans, MDCCXV*. p. 19. and the *Mem. de Trev*. 1713.

But no body has set this Sentiment in a better Light, than Dr. *Woodward*, in his *Nat. History of the Earth*. That Ingenious Author maintains the whole Mass of Earth, with every thing belonging thereto, to have been so broke, and dissolv'd, at the Time of the Deluge, that a new Earth was form'd in the Bosom of Water, consisting of different Strata, or Beds of terrestrial Matter, ranged over each other nearly, according to the Order of their specifick Gravities. By this means, Plants, Animals, and specially Fishes, and Shells, not yet dissolv'd among the rest remain'd mix'd and blended among the Minerals and Fossil Matters; which preserv'd them, or at least assum'd and retain'd their Figures and Impressions, either indentedly, or in Relievo.

*Camerarius* attacks this Sentiment of Dr. *Woodward*, and goes yet higher. He supposes 1° That the greatest Part of the Shells now dug from under Ground, had been plac'd there before the Deluge, that is, at the Time of the Creation, when God separated the Earth from Waters.

2° That without having recourse to the Dissolution of the Earth by the Waters, one might suppose most of them to have slipp'd in at the Chinks and Crevices naturally happening after the Waters were retir'd, and the Earth sufficiently drain'd.

3° That particular Inundations might have swept most of these Shells into the Places where we now find them.

4° That the Sea may have wrought, or cast up most of these Shells through subterraneous Spiracles and Canals.

5° That God has created dives Stony and Metalline Bodies, perfectly like the Vegetables and Animals, we see on Earth, and in the Sea.

To all these Suppositions, Dr. *Woodward* answers,

1° That it is no ways probable, God should create such a Number of Shell-fish of the same Species at once; and that purely with a Design to destroy them all again so soon after : That among the *fossil* Shells of the same Species, 'tis easy to distinguish different Ages : That some appear precisely such as we now find them in the Spring, the Season when the Deluge began: That 'tis not only Shells, we find under Ground, but also Bones of Quadrupeds, Plants, and Trees of extraordinary Sizes; and which are not of the Number of Aquaticks : And lastly, that the Waters were separated from the Earth on the third Day; and that none of these Things were crated, till afterwards.

2° That, on the second Supposition, these Shells would be dispos'd perpendicularly, and not horizontally, as they are always found : That we should sometimes find of them in the Clefts of the Earth, of which there is none but where they are broke.

3° That we have no Acquaintance with any of these pretended Inundations: That they could never have brought Shells, Stag Horns, and Elephants from *America*, and the *East Indies*, to *England* and other Parts of *Europe*; None those Pines and Beeches, frequently found far greater than any of our Growth. Add, that these particular Inundations must have risen to the Tops of the highest Mountains, and of consequence must have been general.

4° On the fourth Supposition it must be held, that God did not only create all these several Bodies in the Entrails of the Earth; but their several Parts, and the separate Pieces and Fragments of those Parts; a Piece of a Shell, for Instance; a Side of a Shell, which consists of two; a Shell void of the Fish it should contain; Beards of Corn, without the Grain; Pieces of Cedar Bark, without Wood; Pieces of Bullocks Hides without Flesh and Bones; human Skins without Bodies; a Bone without the rest of the Skeleton; a Tooth without the Jaw, &c.

Add, that the *fossil* Shells have not only external, but essential Resemblages to Sea Shells; both, *e.gr.* Yielding by Analysis, a Quantity of Sea Salt : That among the *fossil* Teeth of Fishes, we meet with some apparently worn : And lastly, that the Shell Fish called *Purple*, has a long sharp Tongue, by means whereof it pierces other Shells, and picks the Fish out of them; and that in digging under Ground we actually meet with dives of these Shells thus pierc'd. Can such minute, tho' paced Resemblances be the accidental Effect of a *Lusu Naturæ*?

**FOTUS**, in Medicine, the same as Fomentation.

**FRANGIPANE**, an exquisite Perfume, frequently given to the Leather whereof Gloves, Purses, Bags, &c are made. It takes its Name from a *Roman* Nobleman, of the antient Family of *Frangipani*; who was the Inventor of thereof.

There is also a kind of perfum'd Liquor of the same Denomination, said to have been invented by a Grandson of *Mutio Frangipani*; and a perfum'd kind of *Ros Solis*, call'd by the same Name.

**FRANKINCENSE**, or Incense, an odoriferous aromatic Gum, or Resin, antiently burnt in Temples, and still us'd in Pharmacy. For all the great Use of this Gum, both in the antient Religion, and the modern Medicine; the Tree that produces it, or even the Place where the Tree grows, is but little known.

The most common Opinion has always been, that it was brought from *Arabia Fælix*, and was found near the City of *Saba*; whence its Epithet *Sabæum* : And yet the Name *Olibanum*, which it sometimes bears, seems to intimate that there are of these thuriferous, or Incense bearing Trees in the *Holy Land* near Mount *Libanon*. And Travellers are positive, that there are others in the *East Indies*.

Nor are we less at a loss as to the Form of Kind of the Tree from which it flows. *Pliny* contents himself to say, that it at first resembles the Pear Tree; then the Mastic Tree; then the Laurel; but that in reality it is the Turpentine Tree.

*Frankincense*, is either Male, or Female. The *Male Incense*, call'd also *Olibanum*, is in fair, white Bits, or Tears, a little yellowish, of a bitter disagreeable taste; and when chew'd, promotes the Flux of Saliva.

That brought from the *Indies*, is not near as good as that from *Arabia*, or Mount *Libanon*. It is usually call'd *Incense of Mocha*, or Female Incense; tho' it be not brought from that City. 'Tis usually in a Mass, but sometimes in Drops or Tears; somewhat reddish, and bitter to the Taste. Some sell it for the true *Bdellium*.

The Manna of *Frankincense* is only little, round, clear, transparent Grains of the Incense it self. *Soot of Incense* is the fine Flower, rubb'd or ground off the Gum in Carriage, and burnt like Rosin, to make Lamp-black. *Bark of Incense*, is the Bark of the Tree that produces it. It has much the same Qualities, and the same Smell as the Incense it self. *Jewish Incense* is only red Storax.

*Male Incense*, or *Olibanum*, is an Ingredient in divers *Galenical*, and *Chymical* Preparations. It is also us'd to assuage the Tooth-ache: But it is apt to spoil the sound teeth. The Female is inferior to it in all respects.

**FRICTION**, the Act of rubbing, or grating the Surface of one Body against that of another; called also *Attrition*. The Phænomenon arising upon the *Friction* of divers Bodies under divers Circumstances, are very numerous and considerable.

Mr. *Hawksbee* gives us a Number of Experiments of this Kind : Particularly that of the Attrition, or *Friction* of Glass, under various Circumstances; the Result of which was, that it yielded Light, became Electrical, &c.

All Bodies by *Friction* are brought to conceive Heat; many of them to emit Light; particularly a Cats-back, Sugar, beaten Sulphur, Mercury, Sea Water, Gold, Copper, &c. But above all, Diamonds, which when briskly rubb'd against Glass, Gold, or the like, yield a Light, equal to that of a live Coal, when blowed by the Bellows.

**FRICTION**, in Medicine, and Chirurgery, the Act of rubbing a diseased Part with Oils, Unguents, or other Matters, in order to ease, relive, and cure it.

*Frictions* are much used, especially abroad, in Venereal Cases; where they prefer the applying of Mercury externally, by way of *Friction*; to that of giving it internally to raise a Salivation. There are also *Frictions with the Flesh-*

*brush*, a *linen Cloth*, or the *Hand* only : For the Effect of which last, see Stroaking,

*Frictions* in the general, and of any kind, are a sort of Exercise that contributes very greatly to Health; as they excite and stir up the natural Warmth, divert Defluxions, promote Perspiration, open the Pores of the Skin, and carry off Humors.

The *Fleshbrush*, Dr. *Cheyne* observes, is an Exercise most useful for promoting a full and free Perspiration and Circulation. Every Body knows the Effect of currying of Horses; that it makes them sleek, gay, lively, and active; so as to be judg'd equivalent to half the Feeding.

This it can no otherwise effect, but by assisting Nature to throw off the Recrements of the Juices which stop the free Circulation; and by constant *Friction*, Irritation and Stimulation, to call the Blood and Spirits to the Parts most distant from the Seat of Heat, and Motion, and so plump up the superficial Muscles. And the same Effects it would have in other Creatures, and Man himself, if managed in the same manner, and with the same Care and Regularity.

Persons, therefore, of weak Nerves and sedentary Lives, would do well to supply the Want of other Exercise with spending half and Hour, Morning and Night, in currying and rubbing their whole Body, especially their Limbs, with a Flesh-brush.

**FRICTION**, or Frixion, in Chemistry, is the same with what in Cookery we call Frying, *viz.* a Preparation of certain Matters in a Pan, with the Addition of some unctuous thing, as Oil, Fat, &c. The *Frixion* of Medicines is perform'd over a slow, moderate Fire; and that of Foods over a quick one.

**FRIGORIFIC**, in Physicks; something that occasions cold. Some Philosophers, particularly, *Gassendus*, and other Corpuscularians, denying Cold to be a mere Privation or Absence of Heat, contend that there are actual frigorific Corpuscles, or Particles as well as fiery ones : Whence proceed Cold and Heat. But the later Philosophers allow of no other frigorific Particles, beside those nitrous Salts, which float in the Air in cold Weather, and occasion Freezing.

**FRONTALE**, or Frontal, in Medicine, an extern Form of Remedy, applied on the forehead, with a Bandage; for the Cure of the Head Ach, Medrim, Vapours, &c.

*Frontals* are composed of Roses, Elder Flowers, Betony, Marjoram, Lavender, &c. wrap'd in a Linen Cloth, and applied over the Forehead and Temples. There are also *Frontals* in manner of Linements, made of *Unguentum populeum*, Extract of Opium,; or of Pastes, Powders, Seeds, &c.

In *Frontals* applied to ease the Violence of the Head ach in the height of Fevers, they frequently mix the Kernels of Cherries.

**FRONTATED**, a Term us'd by the Botanists, to express that the Petalum or Leaf of a Flower grows broader and broader; and at last, perhaps, terminates in a Right Line. In opposition to cuspidated, which expresses that the Leaves terminate in a Point.

**FRUMENTACEOUS**, a Term applied to all Plants which have a Conformity with Wheat, or Frumentum; either in respect of their Fruits, Leaves, Ears, or the like. Thus, Barley, Dogs-grass, &c. are *Frumentaceous* Plants.

**FRUTEX**, Shrub, a Vegetable, of a Genus between a Tree and Herb; but of a woody Substance.

**FUCUS**, in Natural History, a Sea-plant, call'd also *Alpa*. The Flowers of the *Fucus* grow on the whole Extent of its Leaves; in form of little Tufts, composed of a great Number of exceedingly fine Elements, about the length of a Line. The Seed is inclos'd in a viscid Matter, at the Extremity of the Leaves.

**FUCUS** is also us'd for a Paint, or Composition applied on the Face, to beautify it, and heighten the Complexion. Old Women make use of *Fucus's* and Pomatums, to appear young. The *Fucus* made with Ceruss, is corrosive; and pernicious to the Skin.

The Chymists abuse the Ladies in selling them Oil of Bricks, as an excellent *Fucus*. *Pliny* says, that the *Fucus* of the *Roman* Ladies was a kind of white Earth, or Chalk brought from *Chio*, and *Samos*, dissolv'd in Water.

The *Fucus Solimanni* is a Composition of prepared Sublimate, in great Repute among the *Spaniards* of *Peru*.

**FULMINANT**, *Fulminans*, or Fulminating, an Epithet applied to something that thunders, or makes a Noise like that of Thunder; *Jupiter Fulminans, Aurum Fulminans, Pulvis Fulminans*. *Pericles* was call'd the *fulminating* Orator.

*Aurum Fulminans*, is a Preparation of Gold, thus called, because when laid on the Fire, it produces a huge Noice. It consists of Gold dissolv'd in Aqua Regia, and precipitated by means of Oil of Tartar *per Deliquium*; or Volatile Spirit of Sal Ammoniac.

*Pulvis Fulminans*, is a Composition of three Parts of Nitre, two Parts of Salt of Tartar, and one of Sulphur.

Both the *Aurum* and *Pulvis Fulminans* produce their Effect principally downwards: In which they differ form Gunpowder, which acts *in orbem*; but principally upwards. If they be laid in Brass Ladles, and so set a fire; after Fulmination, the Ladles will be found perforated.

**FUMIGATION**, in Medicine, and Chymistry, is understood of Things taken in *Fume*, or Smoak; or that are turn'd into Smoak : And particularly for the Corrosion of a Metal, by the Fumes, or Steam of Lead, Mercury, Vinegar, or other acrimonious Matter.

'Tis dangerous taking Mercury by *Fumigation*. This *Fumigation* is a kind of potential Calcination; the Vapour of Mercury laid on the Fire, corroding and reducing into a Calx, the little Laminæa of Metals suspended over it.

Ceruss is made by the *Fumigation*, or Vapour of Vinegar, gnawing and corroding Plates of Lead.

**FUMIGATION** is also used for the Act of making a suspended Body receive the Fumes, or Steam of one or more other Bodies; in order to calcine them , to correct them, or impart to them some new Quality.

**FUNDAMENT**, the Anus, or Aperture thro' which a Man voids his Excrements.

**FUNGUS**, in Medicine, a fleshy Tumor, or Excrescence, very spongeous, soft, and pale; arising on the Membranes, Tendons, and other nervous Parts, in consequence of Ulcers, Wounds, Contusions, and Strains.

*Fungus's* are frequently form'd on the Meninges, or Membranes of the Brain, in Wounds of the Head when not well cover'd, or defended fro the external Air : They are also frequent about the Joints; which last grow very insensibly. But where the Skin is open, finding more room, they grow to a prodigious degree in a very little time, assuming the Form of a Mushroom or *Fungus*.

There are also *Fungus's* of the *Anus* and *Uterus*. They are all suppos'd to proceed from a Retention and Depravation of the nutritious Juice.

The *Fungus* is a general kind of Excrescence, whereof they are divers particular Species; as the *Ficus, Sarcoma, Condyloma*, &c.

**FUNGOUS** *Flesh*, is a spongeous, excrescent, or (as we popularly call it) *proud* Flesh, frequently growing on the Lips of Wounds, Ulcers, &c. The *Sarcocele* is sometimes the Result of a *fungous* Flesh.

In Ulcers, *Wiseman* observes, there frequently arises a spongious, or *fungous* Flesh, either from the too great Afflux of the Humors; or thro' the Surgeon's Unskilfulness.

It must be suppress'd, or taken off by drying Medicines, or even Causticks : As *Lapis Tutiae*, burnt Alum, Precipitate of Mercury, Roman Vitriol, &c.

**FURFUR**, literally signifies Husk, or Chaff; and there is used for the Scales, Scurf, or Dandruff, which grows upon the Skin with some Likeness thereto.

**FURNACE**, an Utensil, or Vessel, proper to contain Fire; or to raise and maintain a vehement Fire in; whether of Coal or Wood.

There are divers kinds of *Furnaces*, of various Forms, and for various Uses. The Domestick *Furnace*, us'd in making Confections, &c. is usually of Iron, or Earth. Those us'd by the Goldsmiths, Refiners, &c. are much larger, and of a different Structure. Those wherein Line, Brick, &c. are burnt, are called Kilns.

*Furnace* is particularly us'd for a kind of Oven, wherein the Ores of Metals, after beating, washing, &c. are melted down, by a huge Coal or Wood Fire. The Structure and Application of these *Furnaces* is somewhat different in the different Metals.

*Furnace* is more strictly applied to those us'd in the melting of Iron; which Authors frequently confused with iron *Forges*; tho' there is a considerable Difference between them.

The *Furnace* is a Brick Structure, much in the Shape of an Egg set an end, wherein the Iron Ore, after it has been burnt in a Kiln, is put, intermix'd with

Cinders and Charcoal; and the whole melted, till it trickle down into a Receiver underneath; where the Scum and Dross being taken away, the Metal is thrown into Furrows made in a Bed of Sand, and thus cast into Sows or Pigs of Iron.

The Forge is a Place, where the Pigs are heated and fused a second, and even third time, to prepare and fit them further for use.

*Glass-house* **FURNACE**, is the Place wherein the Materials of Glass are fused, and vitrified. There are three kinds of Furnaces us'd in the Glass-works.

The first is called the *Calcar*, serves to prepare or calcine the *Frit* in. It is made in fashion of an Oven, ten Foot long, seven broad, and two deep. The Fuel, which is Sea Coal, is put in a Trench, on one Side of the *Furnace*; and the Flame reverberates from the Roof back upon the Frit. The Coals burn in an iron Grate, and the Ashes fall hence into a Hole underneath.

The second, is the *Working Furnace*, serving to melt the Metal in, or make the Glass. Its Figure is round, three Yards in Diameter, and two high, being arch'd over. Round the Inside are eight, or more Pots plac'd, and piling Pots on these. The Number of Pots is always double that of the *Boccas* or Mouths, or that of the Workmen; that each may have one Pot refined, to work out of; and another for Metal, to refine in, while he works out the former.

The *Furnace* has two Partitions; the lower, separating the Pots from the Fire Place, has a circular Hole in the Centre, cover'd with a Grate, through which the Flame passes from the Fire Place into the *Furnace*; from the arched Sides and Roof whereof it is reverberated into the Melting-pots.

The second Partition divides this from the Leer, or Annealing Furnace. Thro' the Boccas, or Working-holes the Metal is taken out of the Pots, and the Pots put in the Furnace. These Boccas are stopp'd with moveable Covers, made of Lute and Brick, to screen the Workmens Eyes from the Fire. On each Side the Bocca is a Boccarella, out of which colour'd Glass, or the finer Metal is taken from the Piling-pot. The *Furnace* likewise belong Ovens or Holes near the Leer, for calcining of Tartar, Iron, &c.

The *Leer*, which serves to anneal and cool the Vessels; and which *Agricola* makes a particular *Furnace*, consists of a Tower, and the Leer. The Tower lyes directly over the Melting *Furnace*, which a Partition betwixt the Aperture; having an Aperture, call'd *Occhio*, or *Lumella*, thro' which the Flame or Heat ascends out of the Furnace into the Tower : On the Floor or Bottom of this Tower, the Vessels fashion'd by the Masters, are set to anneal. It has also two Boccas or Mouths, by which the Glasses are put in with a Fork, and set on the Floor.

The *Leer* is an Avenue, five or six yards long, continue to the Tower : Thro' this the Glasses, when anneal'd, are drawn in iron Pans, called *Fraches*; by which they come to cool by degrees; being quit cold, by that time they reach the Mouth of the Leer, which enters the *Sarosel*, or Room where the Glasses are to be set.

The third, is the *Green Glass Furnace*, which is a kind of Compound of all the former. It is made square (the two former being circular) having an Arch, at each Angle thereof, for annealing and cooling the Glasses. The Metal is wrought on two opposite Sides; and on the other two, they have their Calcars, into which are made *Linnet Holes* for the Fire to come from the *Furnace* to bake the Frit; as also to discharge the Smoak. Fire are made in the Arches to anneal the Vessels; so that the whole Process is done in one *Furnace*.

The Stones wherewith the Insides of these *Furnaces* are built, are not Brick (which would soon melt down into Glass, as also all the softer Stones); but hard, and sandy, by *Imperat.* call'd *Parychima.*

*Founders* **FURNACE**, is of divers kinds, according to the different kinds of Work to be cast. That us'd by the Founders of Small Work, is much like the Smiths Forge, with this only Difference, that the Fire is made on the Massive, built in a Cavity in the Middle of the *Furnace*, to which the Pipe of the Bellows reaches. This Cavity goes to the Bottom of the Massive : A-cross the Middle of it is plac'd a Grate, which holds the Fire and the Crucible : And below is the Place for the Ashes, &c.

*Glass Painters* **FURNACE**, is made of Brick, nearly square, and about two Foot and a half each way. It is cut horizontally in the Middle by a Grate, which sustains the Pan or Shovel the Glass is baked in. This *Furnace* has two Apertures; one below the Grate, to put the Fuel in at; the other above it, thro' which the Workman spies how the Coction of the Colours goes on.

*Letter Founders* **FURNACE**, is very small, not exceeding a Foot and a half in Height, and one in Diameter; being plac'd on a wooden Stand, or Bench, to raise it to a proper Height for the Artist, who works standing. It is made of the same Earth with Crucibles.

*Plumbers* **FURNACE** is of three Kinds : In the first, they melt the Lead, whereof Sheets are to be cast. This is only a sort of large Copper, or Receptacle like a Copper, made of Free-stone and Potters Earth, well plaister'd round with a little iron Pan at bottom.

In the second, they melt the Lead to be cast in Moulds, for Pipes, &c. which are not to be solder'd.

The third, is the Tinning *Furnace*, which is a square Frame of Wood, or sometimes a Massive of Stone work, with a Brick Hearth, whereon is made a Charcoal Fire, which serves them for the applying of thin Tin Leaves on their Works.

*Hatters* **FURNACES** are of three Kinds : A little one under the Mould, whereon they form their Hats : A larger, in the Fullery under a little Copper full of Water and Lees : And a very large one under the great Copper they dye their hats in.

*Bellows* **FURNACE**, is one of the two kinds of Furnaces us'd in the Mintage, for the fusing of Metals. It consists of a flat Hearth at Bottom, into which the Air may be admitted by a Hole contriv'd therein.

On a Level with the Hearth is a second Aperture, which gives Passage to the Pipe of the *Bellows*, from which the *Furnace* is denominated. About a Foot over this is a moveable Grate, which may be taken off and out on at pleasure.

Lastly, over this is the Place where the Crucible is set; which is square, and made of the same Earth with the Crucible; of Breadth sufficient to bear a Range of Coals around the Crucible.

To melt a Metal in this *Furnace*, they lay a little Plate of forged Iron over the Grate; and on this they se the Crucible, which is likewise cover'd with an iron, or earthen Lid. They fill the *Furnace* with Charcoal; and when it is well lighted, and the Crucible sufficiently hot, they stop the Vent-hole. Lastly, throwing on fresh Coals, they stop the *Furnace* with an iron Lid : Thus, continuing to work the Bellows, and supply fresh Fuel, till the Metal be in Fusion.

*Wind* **FURNACE** is the second *Furnace* us'd in the Fusion of Metals for Coinage. At Bottom it has a Hearth made hollow, in manner of a Coupel, with a Vent-hole in the Fore-part thereof. Over the Vent-hole is a Grate seal'd in the Massive of the *Furnace*. Over the Grate is the Place for the Crucible, which is usually of forged Iron.

The Fire being lighted, the Crucible is set in, with a Cover over it; and a Capital or Cover of Earth or Iron laid likewise over the *Furnace*. A-top of this Capital is a Hole five or six Inches in Diameter.

It is called *Wind Furnace*, by reason the Air entring thro' the Vent-hole at the bottom, which is always open, serves the same purpose as the Bellows in other *Furnaces*.

Gold is usually melted in the *Bellows Furnace*, as requiring an intenser Heat before it fuses. Silver, and Copper, are commonly melted by the Wind Furnace.

**FURNACE**, in Chemistry, is an earthen Vessel, wherein the Fire necessary for the several Operations, is contain'd, determined, and directed. The *Furnace* consists of several Parts; as, a Place for the Vessel, or Body to be wrought on; a *Focus* or Hearth for the Ashes; a *Chimney*; a *Grate*; a *Door*; a *Dome*, and a *Fan*; or else *Registers*, whereby to let in Air, to increase, or abate the Fire.

The Perfection of a *Furnace* consists in its maintaining a constant equable Fire; and this easily temper'd; and at an easy Expence. To have the Expence easy, the whole Action of the Fire or Fuel must be employ'd on the Subject or Matter of the Operation.

It must be *equable*, since different Degrees of Fire have different Effects; so that if any given Degree would answer any given Intention; an Alteration of that Degree will prevent the Intention from taking place. And on these Circumstances does all the Variety of *Furnaces* depend.

*Furnaces* are either fix'd and immoveable, call'd *Athanors*; or portable, call'd *Catholic*, or Universal, being proper for all operations, where the Body to be operated in is not too large.

The first Species of Anthanor, or fix'd *Furnace* is fitted to give a Heat equal to that of a healthy Man. The second is the *Furnace* of the *Balneum Mariæ*, fit for the Distillation of the more subtile Spirits. The third is the *Digesting Furnace*.

The fourth, the Anema, or *Wind Furnace*, call'd also Melting *Furnace*, and

Metallic *Furnace*; us'd in the Fusion of Metals, Minerals and Vitrifications. It is call'd Wind Furnace, by reason the Air drives forcibly in at the same, to blow up the Coals : Its Form is much like that if the Reverberatory Furnace, only less.

**FUSION**, the Solution, or melting of Metals, Minerals, &c. by means of Fire : Or, the Act of changing them from their solid State to a Fluor. To give the Ore its metallic Form, they *fuse* it : When it is in *Fusion*, the metalline Substance, being the heaviest, sinks to the Bottom of the Furnace; the other terrestrial Matters rising in Form of Scoria to the Surface.

'Tis commonly imagin'd, that the *Fusion* and metalline Form of *Minerals* is wholly the Effect of Fire; and we have Theories of Fusibility built on this Principle : But 'tis a mistaken one. Fire, no doubt, is the principal Agent : But Fire alone is not sufficient.

A Mineral, or piece of Metal not purify'd, being put alone in a Crucible, melts with a world of Difficulty, and never becomes a perfect Metal : Copper Ore, for instance, being thus applied, its impure Part forms a Scoria, and vitrifies; the metalline Part residing at Bottom, under the Appearance of a black Regulus.

To promote *Fusion* and Separation, they mix Coals, or Stones, or Cinders, or old Scoria along with the Ore; the inflammable Principle in which, by help of Fire, fuses them perfectly, sets the heterogeneous Part at liberty, and attaches it to the Top.

The general reason of *Fusion* is pretty easily assign'd. The Firmness, or Solidity of the Body arises from the Force wherewith its Particles cohere. And the Cohesion in all Bodies is as the Quantity of Contact in the component Particles.

Now, the Corpuscles of Fire entering with Rapidity into the Pores of the Metal agitates, and by degrees, loosens, divides and diminishes their Contact, till at length there is not enough to hinder their rolling over each other; and giving way to the least Impulse. The Dilatations observable in all *Fusions*, is a Proof that their Particles are separated and set at a distance from each other, and consequently their Contacts and Cohesions diminish'd. In effect, Rarefaction and Dilatation is the necessary Consequence of Fire and Heat.

From the Difference of Cohesion proceeds that Variety we observe in the Fusion of Bodies: for such as have least Contact of Parts, soonest give way to the Fire; and some will melt away by the warmth of a Vapour only, when others, which have a stronger Contact, are not to be separated, but with Difficulty. Upon this account, Vegetables very easily disunite; Minerals slower, and Metals slowest of all : And of the last, those wherein the Contact of Parts is least, as in Lead and Tin, most readily melt; but those which are more compact as Gold, and Silver, are not to be managed, but by a violent Heat.

If now the Force of Cohesion were proportional to the Quantity of Matter, or to the Weight of Bodies, we might from Staticks account for all the Variety that occurs in *Fusion*; for by knowing the specifick Gravity of a Body, we should then know, what Force is required to melt it : But because the same Quantity of Matter may be so variously disposed, that in one Body there shall be a much greater Contact, than in another, tho' the Gravity be equal, or even less at the same time; therefore the Force of Cohesion cannot be estimated by Gravity : For Lead, tho' more ponderous than all other Metals, except Gold; yet in the Fire is more easily melted, than any other : So that it necessarily follows, that in this Metal there must be a less Cohesion, or Contact of Parts, how much soever it may exceed others in the Quantity of its Matters.

Bodies after *Fusion* return again into a solid Mass, upon removing them from the Fire; because their Particles hereupon approach nearer to one another by their attractive Force, and are so compelled to unit.

Such as consist of homogeneous and unalterable Parts, as Wax, Gums, and the purer Metals, recover their antient Form : For when the same Texture of Parts remains in the whole Body, it must of course reassume the same Appearance, when the separating Power ceaseth to act; but other Bodies, whose Parts, with respect to the Density and Surface, are extremely different from one another, while some are carried off by the Force of the Heat, and others are changed as to Figure and Position, must be forced to appear in another Form : For they cannot recover their original Phases, unless every Particle could reinstate it self in that very Situation it had before, which may be hindered infinite ways; as may be experienced easily in heterogeneous Bodies.

The Difference, therefore, observ'd even in homogeneous Bodies after Liquefaction, is no ways to be accounted for but from the changeableness of Surface in its Parts : For those Bodies whose Parts constantly retain the same Surfaces, never lose their Form; but others, by having the Surface of the Parts altered, have a difference Texture, and put on another Appearance.

**GALANGA**, or Galangal, a Medicinal Root, brought from the *East Indies*; the Produce of a Tree of the same Name. There are two kinds of *Galanga's*; the small, and the great : The small is a rough, knotty Root, of a ruddy Colour both within, and without, and of a very pungent aromatic Taste, and Smell. It is brought from *China*, and is used with good Success in all Disorders of the Stomach, Bowels, and Womb, arising from the Weakness of the Nerves. The greater *Galanga*, growing chiefly in Java and Malabar inclines more to an Ash Colour. Its Qualities are of the same kind with those of the other; only less efficacious, and much less used. The Vinegar-makers use both.

**GALBANUM**, in Pharmacy, A Gum issuing out from an Incision in the Root of a ferulaceous Plant, call'd in Latin, *Ferula Galbanifera*; growing in *Arabia, Syria*, &c. The Word is derived, according to *Martinius*[1], from the *Hebrew* Chelbenah, *Fat*.

There are two kinds of *Galbanum*; the one in Tears; the other in Mass : The first is to be chose of a golden Yellow without side, but much paler within; of a bitter Taste, and strong, disagreeable Smell. For the second, take that which is fullest of Tears, very dry, clear, and not stinking. This last is easily sophisticated with broken Beans, Rosin, and Gum Ammoniac.

*Galbanum* is of an emollient, and restorative Nature; good in all Hysteric Case, and in Asthma's and inveterate Coughs ; It provokes the Menses, and brings on Delivery : But it is chiefly used externally, in Plasters for the Belly, which it loosens, what way soever applied.

**GALENIC** *Medicine*, is properly the Manner of considering and treating Diseases, founded on the Principles of *Galen*; or introduced by *Galen*.

*Claud. Galen*, was of *Pergamus* in *Asia*, the Son of a famous Architect, and Pupil of *Satyron* and *Pelops*, two able Physicians. He first distinguish'd himself at *Athens*; then at *Alexandria*, and lastly at Rome; where he wrote a great deal; where he also died, in the Year of Christ 140.

He is said to have composed 200 Treatises, whereof there are 170 still extent. There have been 23 several Editions of this Author : The first is that of *Venice*, in Folio, in the Year 1525: The last is that of *Paris*, in 13 Volumes in Folio, *Greek* and *Latin*, published in 1639.

This Author, collecting and digesting what the Physicians before him had done; and explaining every thing according to the strictest Doctrines of the Peripateticks, set Physic on a new Footing; introduced the Doctrine of the four *Elements*; the Cardinal *Qualities*, and their *Degrees*; and the four *Humours* or Temperaments.

*Galenic* is now more frequently us'd in a wider Signification, *viz.* for that Method of Physick, contradistinguish'd from *Chymical*.

In this Sense, *Galenical Medicine*, *Galenical Pharmacy*, &c. are those which go upon the easier Preparations of Herbs, Roots, &c. by Infusion, Decoction, &c. and attain their Ends, and make their Remedies effectual, by

[1] Martini Martinius (1631 – 1661), an Italian Jesuit missionary.

the combining and multiplying of Ingredients : In opposition to *Chemical Medicine*, or *Pharmacy*, which torture the *Materia Medica* by Fire, and draw their more intimate and remote Virtues by elaborate Preparations; as Calcination, Digestion, Fermentation, &c.

Medicine was wholly *Galenical*, till the Time of *Paracelsus*. *Geber*, indeed, and after him *Raymund Lully*, *Arnoldus de Villa Nova*, and *Basil Valentine*, made some Attempts to apply Chemistry to Medicine; especially the last of them; but no great Advance was made. *Paracelsus*, and after him *Van Helmont*, alter'd the whole of Medicine; exploded *Galenism*, and the Peripatetic Doctrine, and render'd Medicine wholly Chemical.

The late Improvements in Philosophy, have reform'd, and retriev'd the *Galenical* Medicine, which has now very little of *Galen's* in it. 'Tis now all Mechanical and Corpuscular : Instead of Qualities and Degrees, every thing is now reduced to mechanical Affections; to the Figures, Bulks, Gravities, &c. of the component Particles, and to the great Principle of Attraction.

**GALENISTS**, a Denomination given such Physicians, as practice, prescribe, or write on *Galenical* Principles.

The *Galenists* stand opposed to the Chymists ; The *Materia Medica* of the first, is chiefly of the Vegetable Kind; the Virtues of which they procure by the more simple and easy means; and seldom go beyond Decoction. The latter take in Minerals, Salts, Stone, and even Metals, and Semi-metals : These, they hold, afford more efficacious Remedies; and their Virtues, procured by long, artful, labour'd Processes, with the Help of Fire, are had more pure, and in a lesser Compass.

At present, the *Galenists* and Chemists are pretty well accommodated; and most of our Physicians use the Preparations and Remedies of both.

**GALL**, a yellow, bitter Juice, or Humor, call'd also *Bile*, secreted from the Blood, in the Glands of the Liver, and deposited in a peculiar Reservoir, call'd the *Gall-bladder*.

The Bile contain'd in the *Gall* Bladder, properly call'd *Gall*, is somewhat different from the Bile deposited in the *Porus Biliarius*; being of a brighter Yellow, a greater Consistence, and more bitter and acrimonious. For the rest; the manner of Secretion with the Qualities, Use, &c. of the two Juices, are the same; which see under the Article Bile.

The *Gall* of divers Animals, is found of divers Uses : That of a Hog is said to make the hair grow; deterges and heals Ulcers of the Ears : That of a Lamb is recommended for the Epilepsy : That of the Pike, for intermitting Fevers : That of the Carp, clears and strengthens the Sight : That of a Kid, mix'd with the white of an Egg, Bread, and Oil of Laurel, and applied in form of a Poultice on the Navel; is an approved Remedy for a quotidian Fever : That of a Cock, and a Bullock, reputed good in Diseases of the Eyes, and to take away Freckles and other Disfigurements of the Skin.

That of a Roebuck, or Hare, deterges and carries off Clouds, Specks, and Cataracts of the Eyes : That of the Boar, externally applied, is resolutive, and good in scrophulous Tumors : Those of the Sheep and Partridge, serve to deterge and cleanse Ulcers of the Eyes. Fa. *Roger* adds, that the *Mahometans* of *Palestine* use no other Remedy against Poisons, but seven, or eight Drops of the *Gall* of a Bear.

**GALL** *Bladder*, call'd also *Vesicula* and *folliculus fellis*, is a membranous Receptacle, in Figure somewhat like a Pear; situate at the lower Margin of the Liver, on the concave Side, and about the Bigness of a Pullet's Egg.

The *Gall* Bladder adheres to the Liver, both by its Vessels, which it receives from it; and likewise by its Membranes, whereof the external is common with that of the Liver. The lower Part, which hangs out of the Liver, rests on the Pylorus of the Stomach, which it dies yellow with the *Gall* transuding thro; its Membranes.

Its Membranes are reckon'd five : An outer, or common one, from the Peritonæum; an inner one, from the Capsula of the Porta, and Porus Biliarius; and three proper ones : The first *Vasculous*, consisting of white Fibres, interwove with Vessels; the second, *Muscular*, consisting of a double Row of fleshy Fibres, the one longitudinal, the other annular; the third, or inner Coat, *Glandulous*, consisting of a great Number of Glands, like the Crusta Villosa of the Stomach, which separate a Mucus that lines the Inside of the *Gall* Bladder, and defends it from the Acrimony of the Bile.

The Bladder is usually divided into two Parts, the *Fundus*, or Bottom; and the *Collum*, or Neck : At the Orifice of which latter is plac'd a Ring, or Circle of muscular Fibres, which serve as a Sphincter to constringe the Orifice of the *Gall* Bladder, and hinder the too liberal Discharge of the Bile.

There are some Animals without Gall Bladders; as Deer, Horses, Asses, Mules, Camels; and among Fishes, the Sea Calf, and Dolphin. The Gall of these Animals in inclos'd in Ducts, which terminate in the Intestines.

**GALLS**, or *Aleppo* Galls, are a peculiar kind of vegetable Tumors, or Excrescences; used in Dying, making Ink, &c.

These *Galls* are produced on the hardest Species of Oak, called Rouvre, from the Latin *Robur*. Those on other Oaks are less fit for the Purpose. They are hard as Shells; and yet are no other than the Cases of Insects, which are bred in them after the manner above described; and which, when come to Maturity, gnaw their Way out : Which is the Cause of those little Holes observable in them. Of the Insects bred in them, we have a particular Account in *Philos. Transact.* No. 245.

There are three sorts of these *Galls* : The first, Blackish; the second, bordering on Green; the third, Whitish. The Dyers use them all, according to their respective Qualities : The Green and Black, serve to dye in Black; and the White, for Linnens. 'Tis the Black and Green, that are used in the making of Ink.

The *English* and *Dutch* import yearly from *Aleppo*, ten thousand Quintals of *Galls*. The Turks have likewise a kind of ruddy *Gall*, of the Size of a small Nut; which they mix with Cochineel, and Tartar, to dye in Scarlet withal.

**GANGRENE**, *Gangræna*, in Medicine, is a Mortification in its first, or beginning State; while yet the Part retains some Sense of Pain, and a Share of natural Heat : By which this Disease is distinguish'd from a Sphacelus, or thorough Mortification; where there is no Sense or Warmth left at all. The *Gangrene* is a Disease in the Flesh of the Part, which it corrupts, consumes, and turns black; spreading, and seizing itself of the adjoining Parts : And is rarely cured without Amputation.

It arises from a Stoppage, or Interception of the circulatory Motion of the Blood; which by this means, fails to furnish the Part with the nutritious and spirituous Juices, necessary to preserve its Warmth, and Life. This Interception of Circulation, which is the next Cause of the *Gangrene*, is it self occasion'd by divers ways; as, by large Tumors, Erisypela's, great Inflammations, violent Cold, tight Bandages or Compressions, sudden Fluxions of some malignant Humor, Bites of venomous Beasts, Fractures, Wounds, and Ulcers ill managed, &c.

It is distinguish'd by the Colour of the Flesh, which now turns pale, dusky, or sublivid; and by its growing loose, and flabby of vehemently Tense which it was before. In the Progress of the Disease, the Part distils a fetid, discolour'd Water; and emits a cadaverous Smell. Upon the first Seizure, the Skin turns pale, afterwards livid; Vesifications arise, and the Colour at length changes to black; the Flesh becomes fetid, sanious, and moist; then withers, and soon becomes insensible : The Heat and Pulsation of the Parts being likewise diminish'd.

If in a large Wound, the Tumor or the Lips do not suppurate, nor any Flux of Matter, or Inflammation arise; if the Lips do not swell, or after Swelling grow lank and flaccid again on a sudden : 'Tis reckon'd a sure Sign of an approaching *Gangrene*. When a *Gangrene* proceeds from extreme Cold, the Part affected is first benumbed, or seiz'd with a pricking Pain, followed by a Redness, which gradually changes to a Black.

When a tight bandage is the Cause, a Flaccidity of the Part is join'd to the Insensibility thereof : When the Scurvy, it often begins in the great Toe, and appears in form of a blackish Spot, which turns to a dry Crust, succeeded by a Stupor of the Part, &c. When the Bite of any venomous Creature is the Cause, a continual Fever attends, &c. Pain is felt in the Part; which usually brings on a Syncope, or Delirium : Pustules arise about the Bite, &c.

By the Microscope, the *Gangrene* has been discover'd to consist of an infinite Number of little Worms, ingender'd in the morbid Flesh; and which continually producing new Broods, they swarm, and over-run the adjacent Parts.

To stop the Progress of the *Gangrene*, the Physicians prescribe, internally, Sudorifics, and Alexipharmicks; externally, Decoctions of Quick-lime, either simple, or with the Addition of Sulphur, *Mercurius dulcis*, and Spirit of Wine camphorated.

In a severe Stage of the Distemper, they searify deep, to the very Quick; and afterwards apply hot Liquors, Cataplasms, &c. Some recommend Horses Dung, boil'd in Wine, or Urine. The Unguent Ægyptiacum also come into Use.

*Belloste*[1] prescribes the following, as the most efficacious Remedy, known

[1] Auguste Belloste (1654 – 1730), a French military surgeon and author.

for *Gangrene*; *viz.* Quicksilver dissolved in double the Quantity of Spirit of Nitre, or Aqua fortis; a linen Cloth dipt therein, and applied to the *gangrenous* Part. This alone, he assures us, is sufficient. If the *Gangrene* be occasion'd by an intense Frost; Snow Water, or a linen Cloth dipt in cold Water, and applied to the Part affected, *Boerhaave* directs us as the best Cure.

If the *Gangrene* proceeds to an utter Sphacelation, and be sated in any of the Limbs, or extreme Parts, recourse must be had to the operation of *Amputation.*

The Word *Gangræna, Gangrene,* is derived by some Authors from the *Paphlagonean Gangra,* a Goat; it being the Character of a Goat to brooze the Grass all around, without shifting its Place. It is juster, perhaps, to derive it from the *Greek* Verb λραω, λραινω, *manduco, absumo,* I eat, I consume : But 'tis yet safer, to bring it from the Word λαλλραινα, which signifies the same thing.

**GARGARISM**, Gargle, in Medicine, a liquid Form of Remedy, for Disorders of the Mouth, Gums, Throat, &c. The Word is form'd of the *Greek* γαργαειζειν, *colluere,* to wash. Or of the Hebrew Garghera, the Throat. *Gargarisms* are composed of Honey, Salts, Syrups, Spirits, Vinegar, Waters, and Decoctions; and produce their Effect by cleansing, lubricating, &c. An Astringent *Gargarism*, Detergent *Gargarism*, Refrigerent *Gargarism*, &c.

**GAS**, in Chemistry, a Term, us'd by *Van Helmont*, to express the Seeds, or Fermentation, or first Principles of Things : But he applies it so obscurely, and precariously, that 'tis hard reducing it to any one Sense.

Thus, he calls the vital Principle in man, *Gas Vitale*; and the same Denomination *Gas*, he gives to the sulphurous Steams, which occasion Damps : Add, that he calls the Air, *Gas Ventosum*; and Water, the *Gas of Salts.*

Some would fix his Meaning to the Spirit, or subtle and most volatile Part of a Body : And thus, *Gas Cerevisiæ*, is the spirituous Steam, which flies off from Ale, while in working; but this does not take in the whole Idea of Gas.

**GASTRILOQUUS**, or Gastriloquos, a Person who speaks inwardly, or within his Stomach; and whose Voice seems to come a-far off; more usually called *Ventriloquus*. The Word is form'd of the Greek γαςηρ, Belly, and the Latin *loqui*, to speak.

**GASTROTOMY**, the Operation of cutting open the Belly; the same with what is otherwise called the *Cæsarian Section.*

**GAYAC**, Gayacum, or Gayacan, a Medicinal Wood, brought from the *Indies*; much used in Venereal Disorders; called also *Lignum Sanctum*; and by the *Spaniards, Ligno Santo.*

*Gayac* grows equally in the East and West *Indies* : That of the latter is brought in large Pieces, some of them weighting four or five hundred Pounds; by which it is distinguish'd from the former.

The *Gayac* Tree, is the height of our Walnut Tree; and is distinguish'd into two Kinds, male and Female; only differing, as their Leaves are more or less round; being all equally green, the Flowers blue, and of a starry Form; having a little Orange-colour'd Fruit, about the Size of a small Nut, at the Tip thereof.

The Wood *Gayac* is extremely hard and heavy, and on that account used as Ebony, in Mosaic Work, &c. as also for the making of Button Moulds. But its principal Use is in Medicine, being found to warm, rarify, attenuate, attract and promote Sweats and Urine. The usual way of applying it, is in Decoction.

The best is that in large Pieces, of a dusky Colour, fresh, gummy, heavy, of an agreeable Smell, and a brisk pungent Taste; the Bark sticking close to the Wood.

The Bark of the *Gayac* is held of as much Virtue, as the Wood it self : The Rind is of no Efficacy; so that to make a Sudorific Decoction or Ptisan of the Wood, they first pare off all the white Part, which in reality is the Rind; and only chip or rasp the hard, solid Part, which is black, heavy and resinous.

The Chirurgeons frequently substitute Box-wood, instead of *Gayac*, and, 'tis said, with equal Success.

The Resin drawn from *Gayac*, is held much more effectual in Venereal Cases, than either the Wood, or Bark. 'Tis brought us in large Pieces, not unlike common Rozin; but very different in respect of Smell : The former, when cast on the Coals, yielding a very agreeable balsamick Fume.

**GEM**, or Germen, in Botany, a Shoot, or Bud of a Plant.

**GEMMA**, or *Sal Gemmæ*, is peculiarly used for Rock Salt, or Salt dug out of Mines. The name *Gemma* is applied hereto, on occasion of its Lustre, and Brillant; which is not unlike that of Crystal. The principal Mines of this Salt are those of *Wilisca*, in *Poland*; of *Eperie*, in Upper *Hungary*; and of *Cardonna*, in *Catalonia*. The principal Use of this Salt is for the powdering, or pickling of Meats, in Places destitute of Salt-Springs, &c.

**GENEVA**, a popular name for a distill'd Water; procur'd from the Seeds, or Berries of the Juniper Tree; which the *French* call *Genevrier*, and the Berry *Genevre* : Whence the *English* Appellation *Geneva*.

**GENTIAN**, a Medicinal Root, the Product of a Plant of the same Name; which the Antients, to render it the more considerable, denominated from *Gentius*, King of *Illyria*, who is suppos'd to have been the first that discover'd the admirable Virtues thereof.

The Root *Gentian* is of a yellowish Colour, and intolerably bitter; is sometimes as thick as the Arm, but more commonly divided into Branches no bigger than the Thumb : Its Stem is several Feet high, being very smooth and polish'd, tho' divided by Knots from Space to Space, out of which arise the Leaves, which resemble those of *Plantain*. Its Flowers, which likewise accompany the Knots, are yellow; and its Seed, flat, round, smooth, and light.

The Plant affects moist Places, and is found commonly enough in some

Parts of *England*, *Burgundy*, the *Alps*, and *Pyrenæans* : The Root is to be chose dry, new, of a moderate Thickness, free from Earth, and furnish'd with five little Branches or Fibres; and, if possible, that which is dry'd by the Air, which is distinguishable by the Colour, it being blackish within Side, when dry'd in the Oven, and of a golden Yellow, when in the Air.

**GENUS**, *Kind*, in Logicks, and Metaphysicks, is that which has Species under it; Or, it is the Origin, and Radix of divers Species, join'd together by some Affinity or common Relation between them. Or, *Genus*, is a Nature, or Idea, so common and universal, that it extends to other general Ideas, and includes them under it.

Thus, *Animal* is said to be a *Genus*, in respect of *Man*, and *Brute*; in regard Man and Brute agree in the common Nature and Character of Animal : So, a *right lined Figure of four Sides*, is a *Genus*, in respect of a *Parallelogram*, and a *Trapezium*; and so likewise is *Substance*, in respect of *Substance extended*, which is a *Body*; and *thinking Substance*, which is *Mind*.

In the general, *Genus* may be said to be a Class of a greater Extent than *Species*; and which is not convertible therewith. For though we may say, that *all Body is Substance*; yet it cannot be said that *all Substance is Body*. Add, that whatever may be said of the *Genus*, may likewise be said of the Species under it; *e.gr.* whatever is said of *Ens*, Being, will equally hold of the Body.

The Schoolmen define the *Genus Logicum* to be an Universal which is predictable of several Things of different Species; and divide it into two kinds: The one, *summum*, which is the highest or most general; and has nothing above it to respect as a *Genus* : The other *subaltern*, which they likewise call *Medium*. This *Genus summum* is that which holds the uppermost Place in its Class, or Predicament; or it is that which may be divided into several Species, each whereof is a *Genus* in respect to other Species plac'd below it.

Thus in the Predicament of things subsisting of themselves, *Substance* has the Place and Effect of *Genus summum*, and is predicated of all the Things contain'd in that Class; for both *Plato*, and Man, and Animal, and even *Spirit*, are properly call'd Substance. Accordingly there are so many *summa genera*, as there are Classes of Predicaments or Categories.

A *Subaltern Genus* is that which being a Medium between the highest *Genus*, and the lowest Species; is sometimes consider'd as a *Genus*, and sometimes as a Species. Thus Bird, when compar'd with Animal, is a Species; when to a Crow, an Eagle, or the like, a *Genus*.

*Genus* again, is divided into *Remotum*, remote, where, between it and its Species, there is another *Genus*; and *Proximum*, or next, where the Species is immediately under it; as Man, under Animal.

A good Definition, say the Schoolmen, consists of *Genus*, and Difference.

**GENUS**, Gender, in Botany, a System, or Assemblage of several Plants, agreeing in some one common Character, in respect of the Structure of certain Parts; whereby they are distinguish'd from all other Plants.

The Distribution of Plants into *Genera*, and Species, is absolutely necessary to ease the Memory, and prevent its being oppress'd, and overburthen'd with an Infinity of different Names.

The Knowledge of a *Genus*, comprehends, in a kind of Miniature, that of all the Plants belonging thereto; each being denominated from some Circumstance, common to the whole Kind, to save the Embarrass of so many particular Names.

Something like this, even the common People do, especially in the instance of *Ranunculus*; but in most other Plants the Difficulty is infinitely greater, as 'tis hard to find any thing in common among them, whereon to found their *Genus*.

Hence Botanists differ as to the Manner of regulating these Genera, and the Characters whereon they are to be establish'd.

One of the latest and best Writers, Mons. *Tournefort*, after a long and accurate Discussion, has chose in Imitation of *Gesner*[1], and *Columna*[2], to regulate them by the Flowers, and Fruit consider'd together; so that all Plants, which bear a Resemblance in those two respects, are of the same Genus : After which the respective Differences as to Root, Stem, or Leaves, make the different Species, or Sub-divisions.

Mr. *Ray* made some Observations to this Distribution; which grew into a considerable Controversy between the two Authors. The Question was, whether the Flowers and Fruits were sufficient to establish *Genera*, and to determine whether a Plant was of this *Genus*, or that?

The same M. *Tournefort* introduces another higher kind of *Genus*, or Class, which is only regulated by the Flowers : He observes, that he has never hitherto met with above fourteen different Figures of Flowers; which, therefore, are all that are to be retain'd in the Memory; so that a Person who has a Plant in Flower, whose Name he does not know, will immediately see what Class it belongs to in the *Elements of Botany* : The Fruit appearing some Days afterwards, determines its *Genus*, in the same Book; and the other Parts give its Species.

It is a wonderful Ease to the Memory, to have only fourteen Figures of Flowers to retain, and by means hereof to be inabled to descend to 673 *Genera*, which comprehend 8846 Species of Plants; which is the Number of those yet known by Land and Sea.

**GILL**, or *Ground Ivy*, a Medicinal Plant, which gives the Denomination to a sort of medicated Ale, or Drink, called *Gill*, or *Gill Ale*, made by infusing the dried Leaves of the Plant therein. *Gill* is held very abstersive and vulnerary, and is prescribed in all Disorders of the Lungs, and Breast; and is also esteem'd good in Obstructions of the Viscera : Whence it also passes for Hepatic, Diuretic, Splenetic, and Nephritic. It is said to do Wonders in Tubercles and tartarous Indurations of the Lungs. *Willis* commends its Powder in obstinate Coughs; and *Etmuller* gives the History of a Scorbutic Consumption cured by a strong Decoction of this Herb after a Vomit.

[1] Conrad Gesner (1516 – 1565), a Swiss physician and naturalist.

[2] Fabius Columna, born Fabio Colonna (1567 – 1640), an Italian lawyer and botanist.

**GILLA**, in Chymistry and Pharmacy, is an *Arabic* Term for Salt; peculiarly used among us for the Emetic Salt of Vitriol. This Salt is prepared from that Mineral, by three, or four repeated Operations, *viz.* Dissolution, in *May* Dew; Filtration; and Crystallization. In default of *May* Dew, Rain Water may serve. *Gilla* is used in tertian Agues, and all Fevers arising from a Corruption of the Humors of the first Region. It destroys Worms, and prevents Putrefaction. The Dose is from 20 Grains to half a Drachm, taken in Broth, or in Cordial Waters.

**GINGER**, *Gingiber*, an Aromatic Root, of considerable Use both as a Spice, and a Medicine. It is brought chiefly from *Calicut*, in the East Indies; tho' of late it has been cultivated with good Success in the *Antilles* Islands.

The Plant which affords it, resembles our Rush, both in respect of Stem, and Flower. The Root goes no depth under the Ground, but spreads itself near the Surface, in form not unlike a Man's Hand; but very knotty.

When arrived at Maturity, they dig it up, and dry it in Hurdles, either in the Sun, or Oven : The best is that which is new, dry, well fed, hard to break, of a ruddy, brown Colour without, resinous within, and of a hot, pungent Taste.

They use to comfit the Root, when green, with Sugar, and Honey; having first steep'd it some time in Water, to take away part of its Acrimony, and dispose it to part with the Outer-skin. They also make a Marmelade of it, and dry Cakes.

The Northern People make great use of this Confection, as holding it sovereign against the Scurvy. The *Indians* eat the Root, when green, by way of Salade, first chipping it small, mixing it with other Herbs, and seasoning it with Oil and Vinegar.

As to its Medicinal Use, it is held good to strengthen the Stomach, and waken Appetite. It promotes Digestion, prevents Putrefaction, &c.

**GIN-SENG**, or Gin-Sem, in Natural History, a very extraordinary and wonderful Plant, hitherto only found in Tartary. The *Gin-Seng* is one of the principal Curiosities of the Chinese, and Tartars : Their most eminent Physicians have wrote many a Volume of its Virtues.

It is known among them by divers other Names, as the *only Spirituous*; the *pure Spirit of the Earth*; the *Plant that gives Immortality*, &c. It makes, in effect, the whole *Materia Medica*, for the People of Condition; being too pretious for the Populace.

All the Writers of the Chinese Affairs make mention of the *Gin-Seng* : As *Martinius*[1], in his *Atlas*; F. *Kircher*, in his *China Illustrata*; F. *Tachard*[1], in his *Voyages*; and F. *le Comte*[2], in his *Memoirs*.

And yet we know but very little of this Plant, before F. *Jartoux*[3], a Jesuit and Missionary in *China* who being employ'd by Order of the Emperor, in making a Map of *Tartary*, in the Year 1709, had an Opportunity of seeing it

[1] Guy Tachard (1651 – 1712), a French Jesuit missionary.

[2] Louis le Comte (1655 – 1728), a French Jesuit missionary.

[3] Pierre Jartoux (16669 – 1720), a French Jesuit missionary.

growing in a Village about four Leagues from the Kingdom of *Corea*, inhabited by *Tartars*, call'd *Calca-Tatze.*

That Father took the occasion to design the Plant, and give an accurate Description thereof, with its Virtues, and the manner of preparing it; which, being a great Curiosity, we shall here gratify the Reader withal.

The *Gin-seng* has a white Root, somewhat knotty, about thrice the Thickness of the Stem, and which goes tapering to the End : At a few Inches from the Head, it frequently parts into two Branches, which gives it some Resemblance of a Man, whose Thighs the Branches represent : And 'tis hence it takes the Denomination *Gin-seng*.

From the Root rises a perfectly smooth, and tolerable round Stem : Its Colour is a pretty deep Red, except toward the Foot, where, by the Neighbourhood of the Earth, it is turn'd somewhat whiter. At the Top of the Stem is a sort of Joint, or Knot, form'd by the shooting out of four Branches, which spread as from a Centre : The under Side of each Branch is green, mix' with white; and the upper Part, much like the Stalk, of a deep Red : The two Colours gradually decrease, and at length unite on the Sides.

Each Branch has five Leaves, well enough represented in the Figure; and 'tis observable that the Branches divided equally from each other, both in respect of themselves, and of the Horizon; and with the Leaves make a circular Figure, nearly parallel to the Surface of the Ground.

The Fibres of the Leaves are very distinguishable, and on the upper Side are set with small whitish Hairs : The Membrane, or Pellicle between the Fibres, rises a little in the Middle, above the Level of the Fibres. The Colour of the Leaf is a dark Green, above, and a shining, whitish Green underneath; and all the Leaves are finely jagged or indented.

On the Edges, from the Centre of the Branches, arises a second Stalk, very straight, smooth, and whitish, from Bottom to Top, bearing a Bunch of round Fruit of a beautiful red Colour. This Bunch, in the Plant views by our Missionary, was composed of twenty four Berries.

The Red Skin, that covers the Berry, is very thin, and smooth, and contains within it a white Pulp : As these Berries were double (for they are sometimes single) each had two rough Stones of the Size and Figure of out Lentils. The Pedicles, whereon the Berries were supported, all arose from the same Centre; and spreading exactly like the Radii of a Sphere, made the Bunch of Berries of a circular Form. The Fruit is not good to eat; and the Stone includes a Kernel : It has also a small Beard at the Top, diametrically opposite to the Pedicle.

The Plant dies away every Year; the Number of its Years may be known by the Number of Stalks it has shot forth; of which there always remains some mark.

As to the Flower, F. *Jartoux* owns he had never seen it; and therefore could not describe it : Some have assured him, that it is white, and very small; others, that there is no Flower at all, and that no body had ever seen it. He rather inclines to think it so small as to have escap'd Notice; and, what confirms him in the Opinion, is, that those who seek the *Gin-seng*, having nothing in view but its Root, overlook and despise the rest as useless.

As they have sowed the Seed in vain, without any Plant ever arising therefrom; 'tis probable this might give occasion to the Fable which is current among the *Tartars* : They say, that a Bird eats it, as soon as in the Earth; and not being able to digest it, it purifies in its Stomach, and afterwards springs up in the Place where it was cast buy the Bird with its Dung. The Missionary rather believes that the Stone remains a long time in the Ground, before it takes root; which Opinion appears the more probable, as there are some Roots no longer or bigger than ones little Finger, which yet have shot forth at least ten Stalks.

Tho' the Plant, here describe, had four Branches; yet there are some which have but two; others, three; and others, five, six, or seven : But each Branch has always five Leaves.

The Height of the Plant is proportional to its Bigness, and the Number of Branches the Root has : The larger and more uniform it is, and the fewer small Strings or Fibres it has, the better it is accounted.

'Tis hard, to say, why the *Chinese* should call it *Gin-seng*, a Word which signifies Form, or *Representation* : Neither that Father, nor any he inquir'd of, could ever find that it bore more Resemblance to the Figure of a man, than is ordinarily seen among other Roots. The *Tartars*, with more Reason, call it *Ochota*, that is, the *first of Plants*.

Those who gather *Gin-seng*, preserve only the Root; and all they can get of it in ten, or fifteen Days time, they bury together in some Place under Ground. Then they take care to wash it well., and scour it with a Brush : Then dip it in scalding Water, and prepare it in the Fume of a sort of yellow Milet, which it Part of its Colour.

The Milet is put in a Vessel, with a little Water, and boil'd over a gentle Fire; the Roots being laid over the Vessel upon small, transverse Pieces of Wood, being first cover'd with a linen Cloath, or some other Vessel, plac'd over them.

They may also be dried in the Sun, or by the Fire; but then, tho' they retain their Virtue well enough, they have not that yellow Colour, which the Chinese so much admire. When the Roots are dried, they must be kept close in some very dry Place; otherwise they are in danger of corrupting, or being eaten by Worms.

As to the Place where this Root grows, it is between the thirty ninth and forty seventh Degree of North Latitude, and between the tenth and twentieth Degree of East Longitude, reckoning from the Meridian of *Peking*. Here is found a long Tract of Mountains, which the thick Forests that cover and encompass them, render almost unpassable. It is upon the Declivities of these Mountains, and in these thick Forests, upon the banks of Torrents, or about the Roots of Trees, and amidst a thousand other different Sorts of Plants, that the *Gin-seng* is found. It is not to be met with in Plains, Vallies, Marshes, the Bottoms of Rivulets, or in Places too much exposed and open.

If the Forest take fire, and be consum'd, this Plant does not appear till two or three Years after : It also lies hid from the Sun as much as possible, which shews that Heat is an Enemy to it.

The Places where the *Gin-seng* grows, are on every Side separated from the Province of *Quan-tong*, by a Barrier of wooden Stakes, which incompass this whole Province, and about which Guards continually patroll, to hinder the

*Chinese* from going out, and looking after this Root.

Yet, how vigilant soever they are, their Greediness after Gain incites the *Chinese* to lurk about privately in these Deserts, sometimes to the Number of two or three thousand; at the hazard of loosing their Liberty, and all the Fruit of their Labour, if they are taken, either a they go out of, or come into the Province.

The Emperor having a mind that the *Tartars* should reap all the Advantage that is to be made of this Plant, rather than the *Chinese*, gave Orders, in 1709, to the thousand *Tartars*, to go and gather all that they could of the *Gin-seng*, upon Condition that each Person should give him two Ounces of the best, and that the rest should be paid for Weight for Weight, in pure Silver.

It was computed that by this means the Emperor would get this Year about twenty thousand *Chinese* Pounds of it, which would not cost him above one fourth Part of its Value.

We met, by chance, with some of these *Tartars*, in the Midst of those frightful Deserts; and their Mandarins, who were not far out of our Way, came one after another, and offer'd us Oxen for our Subsistence, according to the Commands they had received form the Emperor.

This Army of Herbarists observed the following Order : After they had divided a certain Tract of Land among their several Companies, each to the Number of an hundred Persons, spread itself out in a Right Line, to a certain fix'd Place, every ten of them keeping at a distance from the rest.

Then they search'd carefully for the Plant, going leisurely in the same Order; and in this manner, in a certain Number of Days, they run over the whole space of Ground appointed them.

When the Time is expired, the Mandarins, who are encamp'd with their Tents in such Places as are proper for the Subsistence of their Horses, send to view each Troop, to give them fresh Orders, and to inform themselves if their Number is compleat.

If any one of them is wanting, as it often happens, either by wandring out of the way, or being attack'd by wild Beasts, they look for him a Day or two, and then return again to their Labour as before.

The *Gin-seng*, we have observ'd, is an Ingredient in most of the Medicines which the *Chinese* Physicians prescribe to the better sort of Patients : They affirm that it is a sovereign Remedy for all Weaknesses occasion'd by excessive Fatigues, either of Body, or Mind; that it attenuates and carries off pituitous Humours; cures Weakness of the Lungs, and the Pleurisy; stops Vomitings; strengthens the Stomach, and helps the Appetite; disperses Fumes, or Vapours; fortifies the Breast; is a Remedy for short and weak Breathing; strengthens the vital Spirits, and is good against Dizziness of the Head, and Dimness of Sight, and that it prolongs Life to extreme old Age.

No body can imagine, that the *Chinese* and *Tartars* would set so high a Value upon this Root, if it did not constantly produce a good Effect : Those that are in Health, often make use of it to render themselves more vigorous and string; and I am persuaded it would prove an excellent Medicine in the Hands of any *European* who understands Pharmacy, if had but a sufficient Quantity of it to make such Trials as are necessary to examine the Nature of it chymically, and to apply it in a proper Quantity, according to the Nature of the Disease for which it may be beneficial.

It is certain that it subtilizes, increases the Motion of, and warms, the Blood; that it helps Digestion, and invigorates in a very sensible manner.

After I had designed the Root, I observed the State of my Pulse, and then took half of the Root, raw as it was, and unprepar'd; in an Hour of Time, I found my Pulse much fuller and quicker : I had an Appetite, and found myself much more vigorous, and could bear Labour better and easier than before. Four Days after, finding myself so fatigued and weary, that I could scare sit on Horseback, a Mandarin who was in Company with us, perceiving it, gave me one of these Roots : I took half of it immediately, and an Hour after I was not in the least sensible of any Weariness. I have often made use if it since, and always with the same Success : I have observ'd also, that the green Leaves, and especially the fibrous Part of them ,chewed, would produce nearly the same Effect. The *Tartars* often bring us the Leaves of *Gin-seng*, instead of Tea; and I always find myself so well afterwards, that I should readily prefer them before the best Tea. Their Decoction is of a grateful Colour; and when one has taken it twice, or thrice, its Taste and Smell become very agreeable.

As for the Root, it is necessary to boil it a little more than Tea, to allow time for extracting its Virtue; as is practis'd by the *Chinese*, when they give it to sick Persons; on which occasion they seldom use more than the fifth Part of an Ounce of the dried Root.

To prepare the Root for Exhibition, cut it into thin Slices, and put it into an earthen Pot well glazed, with about half a Pint of Water; the Pot to be well cover'd, and set to boil over a gentle Fire; and when the Water is consumed to the Quantity of a Cup full, a little Sugar to be mix'd with it, and to be drank : Immediately after this as much more Water to be put on the Remainder, and to be boiled as before, to extract all the Juice, and what remains of the spirituous Part of the Root. These two Doses to be taken, the one in the Morning, and the other in the Evening.

**GLAND**, *Glandula*, in Anatomy, a soft, spungy, lax kind of Body; serving to separate some particular Humor from the Mass of Blood.

The Antients took the *Glands* to be nothing more than a kind of *Pillows*, or *Cushions*, for the neighbouring Parts to rest on. Some of them, at length, began to fancy them Sponges; to receive and imbibe the superfluous Moisture of the other Parts.

Later Physicians came to assign them nobler and more important Uses. They consider'd them as *Cisterns*, which contain'd proper Ferments, whereby the Blood, upon its mixing therewith, was put into a Fermentation, in the Progress whereof it work'd or threw off certain of its Parts, and sent them away by the excretory Ducts.

The Moderns, who allow'd them the Organs whereby the vital Fluids are separated for the Uses of the Body, consider'd them as *Filtres*, the pores whereof being all of different Figures, would only admit of similarly figur'd Particles, to pass thro' them. But the latest Authors rather conceive the Glands as *Sieves*, whose Perforations being of different Sizes, tho' of the same Figure, only separate such Particles whose Diameters are less than their own.

The *Glands*, to the Eye, appear a sort of whitish, membranous Masses, composed of an outer Cover, or Integument, within which a vascular plexus Matter is contain'd. They are denominated from their Resemblance in form, to Acorns, which the *Latins* called *Glandes*.

By Dissection, and the Microscope, they are found to be real Plexus's, or Pelotoons of Vessels, variously wound, and implicated among themselves. But the modern Anatomists *Malpighi, Bellini, Wharton*[1], *Nuck, Peyer*[2], &c. have gone further, and discover'd them to be no more than continued Convolutions of the capillary Arteries.

Their Formation appears to be thus – An Artery arriving at a certain Part, is divided into an infinite Number of exceedingly fine Branches or Ramifications : These capillary Branches are laid in various Bends and Circumvolutions; and from the Returns thereof, arise new Branches, or Vesicles, for Veins; which, a little farther, unite, or terminate in some larger Branches.

All these Ramifications, both Veins and Arteries, are rolled up in a Bundle; making numerous Gyres, and Circumvolutions : And from the various Bends and Angles form'd by both Kinds, arise numerous other minute Vessels, which make the principal and most essential Part of the *Gland*.

The Blood brought from the heart-ward, by the Artery, into the *glandular* Plexus, pursues all the Turns, and meanders in the arterial Part thereof, till arriving at the venal Part, it is brought back gain to the Heart. In the mean time, during its Progress thro' the Arterial and Venal Folds, some Part of it is absorbed, or drain'd off, at the Orifices of the Tubules arising from the Flexures thereof.

What is thus received into these, which we may call the *Secretory Ducts*, is commonly taken up by other Tubules, springing out of them : These, joining together, form a single Canal, call'd the *Excretory Duct*; which , passing out of the Body of the Gland, carries off the secreted Matter into some proper Receptacle destined to retain, or receive it. Tho', sometimes, the Secretory Vessels themselves, terminate in a Bason, or Reservoir; and deposite their Contents therein.

A *Gland*, then, is a Composition of divers kinds of Vessels; *viz*. an *Artery*, and a *Vein*; *Secretory* and *Excretory Ducts* : To which may be added a *Nerve*, which is found in every *Gland*, diffused thro' the whole Substance thereof, to furnish Spirits for the promoting the Secretion; and a *Membrane*, which supports the Convolutions of the Vein and Artery, accompanying them thro' all their minutest Divisions; and *Lymphaticks*, which have been discover'd in several Glands.

The Secretory Tubes, however, are what we principally consider as the Organ of the Gland. These alone do sometimes form the greatest Part of what is called the *Gland*, or *glandulous* Body.

M. *Winslow*[3] has discover'd a kind of *Tomentum*, or Down within their Cavity; which he supposes to do the Office of a Philtre, and to be that

[1] Thomas Wharton (1614 – 1673), an English physician and anatomist.

[2] Johann Conrad Peyer (1653 – 1712), a Swiss physician and anatomist.

[3] Jacob Benignus Winslow (1669 – 1760), a Danish physician and anatomist.

whereby such a certain Humor is separated from the common Mass of Blood.

The *Down-Vessel* being the grand Organ of Secretions, its Structure an Application, is diversified according to the different Purposes Nature has in view. Sometimes the Liquor filtrated thro' it, trickles out, Drop by Drop, upon a Membrane, to which one Extremity of the Vessel is fasten'd; as where the Filtration is only intended for moistening and lubricating the Parts, with that Liquor : In which case the Down-Vessel is both Secretory, and Excretory; which is the most simple Case. Such are those innumerable Glands spread thro' the greatest Part of the Viscera.

Sometimes a great Number of these Down-Vessels is spread over the inner Surface of a little, membranous Cell, into which they pour their Liquor, which is discharged hence at a little Aperture in the Cell: Such are the solitary *Glands* of the Intestines, which appear like so many little separate Grains.

Sometimes a Vessel is bent, and has only Down in the first Part thereof, which alone is Secretory, and the rest excretory, pouring the Liquor into some other common Cavity. Such are the *Glands* that compose a Calves Kidney.

The Secretory Vessels are sometimes of a very great Length, notwithstanding that they take up but little room, being wound over themselves again and again; sometimes in a single Pelotoon, or Knot, and sometimes in several, inclosed in a common Membrane. Whence the Distinction of *Glands* into *Conglobate*, and *Conglomerate.*

*Conglobate*, or *Simple Glands*, are those consisting of one continuous Mass, with an uniform Surface. Such are the *Subcutaneous Glands.*

A Conglobate *Gland*, is, more strictly, a little, smooth Body, wrapp'd up in a fine, double Skin, by which it is separated from all the other Parts; only admitting an Artery and Nerve to pass in, and a Vein and excretory Duct to go out. These *Glands* either discharge their secreted Humor into the Chyle, or venous Blood; or else it transpires thro' the Pores of the Skin, or the Coats of the lower Membranes found in most Parts of the Body.

Of the Conglobate Kind are the *Glands* in the cortical Part of the Brain, where the animal Spirits are supposed to be secreted. Such also are the *Labial Glands*, and the *Testes.*

*Conglomerate*, or *Compound Gland*, is an irregular Assemblage of several simple *Glands*, tied together, and wrap'd up under one common Membrane. Such are the *Maxillary Glands*, &c.

The Humors secreted in these Glands, are sometimes discharged at a common excretory Duct, form'd of an Union of the excretory Ducts of all the particular ones; as the *Panchreas* and *Carotides* do. Sometimes, the Ducts uniting form several Tubes, only communicating with each other by cross Canals; as in those of the Breasts. Some again, have several excretory Tubes, without any Communication together; as the *Glandullæ lacrhymales*, and *prostatæ.*

Others, have their several excretory Ducts inserted into a common anal, which opens at last into some of the greater Cavities; as the *Salival Glands*, *Intestinal Glands*, &c. Lastly, in others, each *Gland* has its own excretory Duct, tho' which it transmits its Liquor to a common Bason; such are those of the Kidneys.

The *Glands* are again divided into *Vascular*, and *Vesicular*. Vascular Glands are only Clusters of little Vessels, which uniting together, form the Canal or excretory Duct through which their secreted Juice is discharged. Vesicular Glands are Assemblages of Vesiculæ communicating with each other, and all terminating in two or three larger Vessels; by a Prolongation whereof the excretory Duct is form'd.

The *Glands*, again, are divided into *Adventitious*; and *Perpetual*, or *Natural*. *Adventitious Glands* are those Kernels arising occasionally under the Arm-pits, on the Neck, &c. Such are the Strumæ, and the Tumors sometimes found on the Larynx, and Middle of the Trachea. *Perpetual*, or *Natural Glands* of two Kinds, *Conglobate*, and *Conglomerate*,

**GLANS**, *Acorn*, in Natural History, a Fruit contain'd within a smooth, but hard Bark, including a single Seed; its Hind-part being cover'd with a kind of Cup, and the Fore-part bare.

**GLAUCOMA**, in Medicine, a Disease of the Eye, wherein the crystalline Humour is turn'd of a greenish, or Azure Colour, and its Transparency thus diminish'd. The Word comes from the *Greek* γλαυκος, *glaucus, caesius*, see-green.

Those in whom this Disorder is forming, discover it hence that all Objects appear to them as thro' a Cloud or Mist : When entirely form'd, the visual Rays are all intercepted, and they see nothing at all.

It is reckon'd incurable, when inveterate, and in aged Persons : And even under other Circumstances, is very difficult of Cure; Externals proving of little Service. The Internals best suited to it, are those used in the Gutta Serena.

The *Glaucoma* is usually distinguish'd from the Cataract or Suffusion, in this, that in the Cataract the Whiteness appears in the Pupil, very near the Cornea, but shews deeper in the *Glaucoma*.

Some late *French* Authors, however, maintain the Cataract and *Glaucoma* to be one and the same Disease. According to them, the Cataract is not a Film, or Pellicle form'd before the Pupil, as had always been imagin'd; but an Alteration of the Humor itself, whereby its transparency is prevented; which brings the Cataract to the Glaucoma.

**GLEET**, in Medicine, a Flux of thing Humor from the Urethra. This, or a *Gonorrhæa Simplex*, often succeed the Cure of a *Gonorrhæa Virulenta*, and sometimes remains obstinate, even after the Use of a Salivation.

The *Gleet* may happen either from too great a Relaxation of the Glands in the Urethra, or from a Corrosion or Exulceration of them. It appears most frequently after a Gonorrhæa has been of long standing, or ill managed in the Cure; as by the Use of acrid or corroding Injections, and the like.

The Glands may here also happen to be ulcerated by the Matter of the Running, which is often sharp enough for that purpose.

A *Gleet* is distinguish'd from a *Gonorrhæa Simplex*, not only by the Colour, and Consistence of the Matter evacuated, but also by the manner wherein it comes away : The Matter of a *Gleet* comes away as well at one time as at another; but that of a *Gonorrhæa Simplex* chiefly in Erections, and when the Patient goes to stool. The Matter of a *Gleet* is commonly brownish, but that of a *Gonorrhæa Simplex* white. And the Continuance of a true *Gleet* is unattended with Weakness, or other ill Consequences, and dangerous Symptoms; nor doe sit unfit Men for Procreation, as *Gonorrhæa Simplex* will.

An astringent Regimen is the most proper in both; Coffee and Claret are supposed proper Liquors in these Cases : So are those made acid with Juice of Lemmons, Vinegar, &c.

**GLICYRRHIZZA**, or Glycyrrhiza, call'd also *Radix dulcis, Liquiritia,* and *Liquorice,* a sweet-tasted Root, of considerable Use in Medicine, against Coughs, and other Disorders of the Breast and Lungs.

The Shrub which bears it, is cultivated in divers Parts of *England,* particularly about *Pontefract* in *Yorkshire*; in some Provinces of *France, Spain, Germany,* and *Muscovy*; and especially in *Persia,* where it thrives better than any where else; there being some on the Banks of the *Carusa, Kenki,* and *Kerni-arpa,* whose Roots are thicker than the Arm; and whose Juice, in respect of Strength, Virtue, &c. are preferable to others.

The Root of the *Liquorice* Plant runs, or spreads a great way in the Ground, and emerging into the Air from Place to Place, produces so many new Stems, or Plants, few of which rise above five Foot high. Its Leaves are thick, green, shining, half-round, and glutinous : Its Flower red, like the Hyacinth; and its Seed contain'd in roundish Pods.

In the Culture, care must be taken to have a warm, light, rich Soil, or to amend it with Manure : They plant it in Trenches, three Spits deep, in *February* and *March*; usually in Rows, at a Foot distance from each other. The Parts chose for this purpose, are Sets from the Top of the Plant, or the very Top of the Root; or else the Runners that spread from the Master-root. In moist Weather, the Branches may also be slipp'd and planted.

They are taken about *November*, or *December*, after they have stood three Summers in the Ground; for then the Liquorice weighs most, and will keep with least Loss : Not but that there is a continual Diminution ion this respect from the first taking it.

New, green *Liquorice* should be chose smooth and even, about the Thickness of the middle Finger, ruddy without, yellowish within, easy to cut, and of an agreeable Smell.

This Root being boil'd a long time in Water, till the Fluid has got a deep, yellow Tincture; and the Water, at length evaporated over a moderate Fire; there remains a black, solid Sediment, which is what we call *Liquorice*, or *Liquorice Juice*, or sometimes *Spanish Juice.*

Chuse it black without side, and of a shining Black within, easy to break, and of an agreeable Taste. The whitish, and yellowish Liquorice Juices are good for nought; being usually no other than Compositions of Sugar, Starch, a little Gum Tragacanth, and *Liquorice* Powder.

The native *Liquorice* Juice is very sweet upon the Palate, even more than Sugar, or Honey; and is yet accounted a great Quencher of thirst; on which account *Galen* prescribes it in Dropsies. It is very balsamic, and detergent;

insomuch that there is scarce any medicinal Composition for Diseases of the Breast, but it is an Ingredient in.

**GOLD**, *Aurum*, a yellow Metal; the heaviest, purest, must ductile, and shining, and on those accounts the most valuable of all Metals.

The Chymists call Gold *Sol*, the *Sun*, to denote its Pre-eminence over the other Metals, which are call'd by the Names of the Planets : Its Symbols, or Character is ☉, which in their Hieroglyphical way or writing, denotes Perfection, Simplicity, Solidity, &c.

The Weight of *Gold* is to that of Silver as 19 to 10. A Cubic Inch of pure Gold weights 12 Ounces, 2 Drachms, 52 Grains; and the Cubic Inch of Silver 6 Ounces, 5 Drachms, 28 Gr. The Pound Weight, or twelve Ounces Troy of *Gold* is divided into 24 Caracts.

The Value of *Gold* is to that of Silver as 14 to 1; antiently, it was only as 12 to 1. Indeed, this Proportion varies as *Gold* is more or less plentiful : For *Suetonius*[1] relates, that *Caesar* brought such a Quantity of *Gold* from *Italy*, that the Pound of *Gold* was only worth seven Pounds and half of Silver. Standard *Gold* is worth 44 lib. 10 s. Sterling the Pound-weight : Standard Silver, is worth 3 l. the Pound; or 5 s. the Ounce.

The *first* Characteristic, or Property of *Gold* is that it is the heaviest of all Bodies. So that whoever would make *Gold*, must be able to add to the Weight of other Matters, and make them equiponderate with *Gold*.

In every Mass of Matter, therefore, heavier than Mercury, there must of necessity be a Share of *Gold*; there being no Body in Nature of intermediate Gravity; *i.e.* no Body whose Gravity is to that of *Gold*, more than as 14 to 19.

Its *second* Character is, that of all known Bodies it is the most ductile, and malleable, and of all Bodies its Parts have the greatest Degree of Attraction, *i.e.* cohere with the greatest Force. Our Gold-beaters, and Wire-drawers furnish us with Proof of this Property. They every Day reduce *Gold* into Leaves, or Lamellæ, unconceivably thin; yet without leaving the least Aperture, or Chasm visible to the best Microscope, or even pervious to the Light.

This Tenacity, or cohesive Force of *Gold* depends altogether on its being free from Sulphur: For mix but a single Grain of Sulphur with 1000 times the Weight of *Gold*, and the Mass ceases to be malleable.

The *third* Character of *Gold* is its Fixedness in the Fire; in which it exceeds all other Bodies. This Property seems to result from the Homogeneity, and Equality of its Parts, which equally aid, and support each other, and have equal Pores, or Interstices thro' which the fiery Corpuscles find and easy Passage. The Prince of *Mirandola*, Mr. *Boyle*, and other Chymists furnish divers Experiments to illustrate this wonderful Fixity. After laying a Quantity of *Gold* two Months in the intensest Heat imaginable, it is taken out without any sensible Diminution of Weight.

It must be added, however, that in the Foci of the large Burning Glasses of Mess. *Tschirnhausen*, and *Villette*, even *Gold* itself volatizes and evaporates.

[1] Gaius Suetonius Tranquillus (ca. 71 – 135), a Roman scholar and historian.

After this manner, we are told from the Royal Academy at Paris, a Quantity of pure *Gold* was vitrified; being first fused into a sort of Calx, which emitted Fumes, and lost of its Weight. But the same Calx fused again with a Quantity of Greese was restor'd into *Gold*.

Its *fourth* Character is, not to be dissoluble by any Menstruum in Nature, except *Aqua Regia*, and Mercury. The Basis of *Aqua Regia* is Sea Salt, which is the only Salt in Nature that has any effect on *Gold*. But this Salt has its Effect in what Form or Manner soever applied, whether as a Fluid, or a Solid; in Substance, or in Spirit.

Mr. *Boyle* made a Menstruum of Butter of Antimony, which dissolved *Gold* with great Facility; and hence concluded that *Gold* might be dissolv'd without Sea Salt; But by Mistake, the effective Part even of this Menstruum being still Sea Salt, which is an Ingredient in Sublimate of Mercury wherewith Butter of Antimony is made.

The seventh Character is that it readily and spontaneously, as by some Magnetic Virtue, attracts, and absorbs Mercury; tho' what My Lord *Bacon* writes, *viz*. that *Gold*, in imbibing Mercury, increases its Weight, we doubt, is but ill warranted For 'tis certain it must be increas'd in Bulk, more than in Weight, and consequently must be specifically lighter. It may be added, that as soon as the Mercury enter the *Gold*, the Metal becomes soft, like Paste.

The eight character is, that it withstands the Violence of both Lead, and Antimony, *i.e.* being fused in the Coppel along with either of those Matters, it does not dissipate and fly off with them in Fume, but remains fix'd, and unchanged.

All other Metals, except *Gold*, and Silver melted with Lead, perish with it, and evaporate by Fire; and in Antimony, all other Metals except *Gold*, and even Silver itself, undergo the same Fate. Thus, if a Mass consisting of *Gold*, Silver, Stones Copper, &c. be fused together with Antimony, the several Matters become separated, and all but the *Gold* rises to the Surface inform of a Scoria, and is blow off with Bellows : But the *Gold* remains behind, much purified, as having lost all its heterogeneous Parts along with the other Metals. And hence Antimony is used as the Test of *Gold*.

The ninth Character is that of all Bodies it is the simplest (the primary Elements being here excepted). By simple we here mean that whose minutest Part has all the Physical Properties of the whole Mass. This, if a Grain of *Gold* be dissolv'd in Aqua Regia; and a single Drop of the Solution be taken, a Quantity of Gold may be separated therefrom, which shall only be the Millionth Part of the Grain, and yet have all the Characters of *Gold*. Or, if you fuse a Grain of *Gold* with a large Mass of Silver, and mix the two together, so that the *Gold* becomes equally diffused thro' the whole Mass; you will have in every Particle of the Mass a Particle of perfect *Gold*. Accordingly, dissolve any Part of the Mixture in Aqua fortis, and a Quantity of *Gold* will precipitate to the Bottom, bearing the same Proportion to the Grain that the Part dissolved in did to the whole Mass. On which principle depends the Art of Essaying.

All the known Parts of the Earth afford this precious Metal; tho' with a deal of Difference, in point of Purity, and Abundance : *Europe*, so fertile in other respects, comes short of all the other Quarters, in *Gold*. *America* furnishes the most; and particularly the Mines of *Peru*, and *Chilly*. That of *Asia* is esteem'd the finest, particularly that of *Menaricabo* in the *East Indies* : The *Spaniards* assure us that they get *Gold* out of some of their *Peruvian* Mines, 23 Carats finer before it be purified. Add, that the Gold of *Axima* on the Coast of *Africa* is found from 22 to 23 Carats.

*Glauber*, an eminent Chymist, holds that there is not any Sand, or Stone, but *Gold* may be procured from; Limestone only excepted : Only that in the Expence of separating it, much surmounts the Profits.

*Gold* is chiefly found in Mines : Tho' there is some also found in the Sand and Mud of Rivers, and Torrents; particularly in *Guinea*. This last is in form of a fine Powder, and call'd αμμοχρυσος, *Gold-dust*. *Glauber* holds that there is a third sort of *Gold*, scarce found any where but in the Drains of the Mountains of *Chilly*, which they separate from the Earth by washing; whence the Places where it is found, or separated, are call'd *Lavadero's*.

This Earth is usually reddish, and very fine : At about six Foot deep it is mix'd with Grains of large Dust; and from hence commences the Stratum, or Bed of *Gold*. Between are Banks of bluish Stone, mix'd with yellow Threads which yet are not *Gold*, but only Pyrites, or Marcassites of *Gold*.

When they have discover'd any of this Earth, they endeavour to bring Rivulets to it (which in those Mountains are very frequent) in order, by force thereof, to tear off the upper Earth, and lay the *Golden* Stratum bare. This they forward by digging with Spades, &c. As soon as the Golden Earth is uncover'd, they turn off the Water; and dig up the Soil by Force of Arm; and loading it on Mules, they carry it to the *Lavadero's*, *i.e.* a sort of Basons of Water, where the Earth undergoing divers repeated Lotions, in different Waters the earthy, and impure Part is all separated and carried off by the Stream, and *Gold* left at Bottom.

This Method of getting *Gold* is immensely gainful; the Expences being but trifling, compared with those accruing in the common way by Machines, Fire, and Quicksilver : The richest of these *Lavadero's* is that *de l'Eastancia del Rey*, twelve Leagues from the *Conception*, a Port of the South Sea. *Thuringia*, and some other Places along the Rhine, are the only places in *Europe*, where Gold is got in this manner.

The *Gold* of the Mines is of two kinds; the one in small Pieces, or Grains of various Forms, and Weights. Of this sort, among the Specimens sent by *Columbus* into *Spain*, to let them see the Richness of his Discovery, there were some of 18 Ounces in Weight; and the Relations of those Days assure us, that in 1502 there were others found of thirty two Pounds Weight.

The other kind of Gold is dug up in Stony Glebes, which is what they call the Mineral, or Ore of Gold : These Glebes are of various Colours, and usually 150 or 160 Fathoms deep. Along with the Gold they usually contain some other Mineral Matter, as Antimony, Vitriol, Sulphur, Copper, or Silver; particularly the last; without some Share of which it is scarce ever found.

**GOLD**, in Medicine, and Chymistry. The Chemists make several Preparations of *Gold* for Medicinal Uses; as Salts, Mercuries, and Tinctures of *Gold*; but 'tis a Point not yet well agreed on whether *Gold* have any real Property whereby it may be of Use of Medicine.

The most antient Physicians are all silent in the Matter : The *Arabs* are the first who mention it in this Quality. *Avicenna* attributes extraordinary Virtues to it; but he speaks on Conjecture more than Experiment. And yet it is pretty certain *Gold* must have an Effect : A Quantity of *Gold* Filings being taken by a Person in a Bolus, he was very well purg'd thereby: But this might well be owing to the great Weight of its Particles, which impinging violently against the Glands of the Intestines, promoted their Vibrations, and thus express'd the Humor secreted therein. *Boræus*, in a Letter to *Bartholin* relates, that having heated an Ingot of fine *Gold* several times red hot, and extinguish'd it as often in Water, he found the Weight of the Ingot considerably diminish'd; upon which, proceeding to evaporate the Water, he drew a little Quantity of *Gold* from it. Hence it appears that the subtile Parts of the *Gold* pass into the Liquors it is extinguish'd in; and hence, 'tis argued, it may have considerable Effect.

Notwithstanding the small Number of Experiments whereon the Medicinal Efficacy of *Gold* is founded; the Alchymists will have it contain the Radical Balm of Life, for the retrieving of Health and Youth, and the Removal of all Diseases. *Gold*, according to them, contains a Sulphur friendly to Nature, like that of the Sun, which animates the whole Universe: And on this Principle they have form'd a thousand airy Projects for an Universal Remedy.

In effect, 'tis probable the *Arabs* and Alchemists were only brought to attribute all these Virtues of *Gold*, from their perceiving certain Qualities therein, which they supposed it must communicate to other Bodies. Thus, *e.gr. Gold* being commonly said to be incapable of being destroyed; 'tis hence concluded to be proper to preserve animal Matters,. And defend them from Putrifaction : Which is just as reasonable as some Physicians prescribing the Blood of an Asses Ear as an appealing Remedy, by reason the Ass is a very peaceable Animal.

**GONAGRA**, in Medicine, the Gout in the Knee. The Word is compos'd of γονυ, Knee, and αγρα, *captura*, seizing.

**GONORRHÆA**, or rather Gonorrhea, in Medicine, an involuntary Flux, or Dripping of Seed, or other Humor by the Penis; without Erection, or Titillation. The Word is form'd of the Greek γονος, *genitura*, Seed, and ρεα, *fluo*, I flow. The *Gonorrhæa* is of two kinds : The one *Simple*, the other *Virulent*.

The *Simple Gonorrhæa*, or that without Virus, or Malignity, takes its rise from violent Exercises, and Strainings; the immoderate Use of hot Foods, and particularly, fermented Liquors, as Wine, Beer, Cyder, &c. It is cured by indulging Rest, nourishing Foods, Broths, &c.

This Species is again divided into two; the one *True*, *Gonorrhæa vera*, wherein the Humor discharged is real Seed : The other *Spurious*, *Gonorrhæa Notha*, wherein the dripping Humor is not Seed, but a Matter from the Glands about the Prostates.

This latter Kind bears some Resemblance to the *Fluor Albus*, or Whites in Women; and frequently remains a long time, without much Diminution of the Patient's Strength. Some call it a *Catatarrhal Gonorrhæa*. Its Seat is in the Glands of the Prostates, which are either too much relax'd, or ulcerated.

The *Virulent Gonorrhæa, Gonorrhæa Virulenta*, arises from some impure Commerce, and is the first Stage of the Venereal Disease; being what we popularly call a *Clap*.

The Parts here primarily affected are the *Prostates* in Men, and the *Lacunae* in Women, which being ulcerated by some contagious Matter received in Coition, emit, first, a whitish, watery Liquor, with an acute Pain : This afterwards grows yellowish, then sharper, and at length greenish, or blueish, and frequently fœtid.

It is attended with a Tension and Inflammation of the Yard, and an *Ardor Urinæ*, or Sharpness of Urine, which gives a painful Sensation in the Emission; the urinary Passage being torn and excoriated by the Acrimony of the Humor. Hence arise Tumors of the Prepuce, and Glands, with Ulcers on the same; and sometimes Caruncles in the Urethra.

The Cause of the Virulent *Gonorrhæa*, according to M. *Littre*, is some acid Humor, heated, rarified, and rais'd at the time of Coition, from the internal Parts of the Pudendum of Women infected, and lodg'd in the Urethra of the Man. It has different Seats in the Body : Sometimes it only fixes in *Cowper's*[1] mucous Glands, sometimes on the Prostates; and sometimes on the Vesiculæ Seminales : Sometimes it possesses two; and sometimes all three of the Places at once.

From this Diversity of Seat of the *Gonorrhæa Virulenta*, M. *Littre* makes two Sorts; *Simple*, which only affects one of the three Parts; and *Compound*, or Complicated, where several are affected.

That seated in the mucous Glands, he observes, may remain Simple, thro' the whole Course of the Disease, by reason the Mouths of those Glands open into the Urethra an Inch and a half on this Side the Prostates, and also look down towards the Glans; so that their Liquor is easily discharged. The other two Sorts mutually produce each other; by reason the Ducts of the Vesiculæ Seminales terminates in the Urethra in the Middle of those of the Prostates : So that there is an easy Communication between them.

That seated in the mucous Glands, is much the rarest Case; and the easiest cured. The Cure is effected by emollient Cataplasms, and Fomentations upon the Part, and a Half-bath. *Mem. de Acad. An. 1711.*

For the other Species, more powerful Means are to be used. The principal Remedies are *Mercurial Purges*, an *Emulsion of green Hempseed, Cuttle-fish-bone, Turpentine, Sacch. Saturni*, &c. We have likewise great Commendations of *Green Precipitate of Mercury*, and *Mercur. dulcis. Bals. Saturni Terebinthinatum*, prepared wit a gentle Fire of *Sacch. Saturni*, and *Oil of Turpentine*, is much applauded where the Heat is great about the Reins and Genitals; as also *Camphor*. An *Infusion of Cantharides* in Wine, is the *Nostrum* of a noted Dutch Physician. *Resin* of the Wood *Guaiacum* is also recommended; and *Balsom of Cupaiba* is held a sort of Specifick : To which must be added *Antimonium Diaphoreticum, Bezoardicum Minerale*, Water wherein Mercury has been boiled; *Injections of Line-water, Mercurius dulcis, Saccharum Saturni*, &c.

*Pitcairn's* Method of curing the *Gonorrhæa Virulenta*, is as follows : In the

[1] William Cowper (1666 – 1709), an English physician and anatomist.

Beginning of the Disease, he purges with a laxative Ptisan of Senna, Salt of Tartar, and Melilot Flowers; and gives the Patient Whey for his Drink. After three, or four Days spent in purging, if the Scalding of the Urine, and the Flux, be bated, and the Colour and Consistence of the Matter improved; he administers Bolus's of Turpentine, and Rheum for six or seven Days; and if they keep the Body loose, so much the better. By all means, Astringents to be avoided; the *Gonorrhæa* being scarce ever known to degenerate into a Pox, unless too hastily stopp'd. *Pitcairn in MS.*

*Du Blegny*[1] directs the Cure of the *Gonorrhæa*, to begin with a gentle Cathartic of Cassia , Senna, Crystal Mineral, Tamarinds, Althæa, and Rhubarb, administer'd every other Day : Then, Diuretics, particularly those of Turpentine; and lastly, gentle Astringents; as Mineral Waters, *Crocus Martis astringens*, Tincture of Roses, Tincture of Coral in Cochineel.

A Ptyalism, or Salivation never cures a *Gonorrhæa.*

**GOUT**, Arthritis, in Medicine, a painful Disease, occasion'd by a Flux of sharp Humor, upon the Joints of the Body. Some Physicians define the *Gout*, an Inflammation, Swelling, and Painfulness of the Joints. Its prime Cause is usually attributed to Wine, Venery, Gluttony, and Idleness.

The *Gout* is supposed to arise from two Causes : A Redundancy of Humors, and a Weakness of the Joints. Its proper Seat is in the Limbs; not in the Trunk of the Body : In the latter Case it frequently proves mortal, not in the former.

*Musgrave* makes the Apoplexy a *Gout*, because arising from the Abundance of Pituita, or Phlegm. According as this redundant Pituita throws itself on the lungs, the Liver, or any other Part, it makes, according to him, an *Apoplexy*, a *Gout of the Liver*, *of the Lung*, *of the Spleen*, &c.,

The *Gout* is a Painful, Periodical, and Critical Paroxysm, tending to free the Body of an offensive, or corrosive Matter, by throwing it upon the Extremities; breathing it out insensibly; or comminuting it so as to render it harmless, or capable of circulating freely along with the Juices, till by collecting again, gradually increasing, or separating from the Blood, it cause another Paroxysm.

The *Gout* is either Regular or Intensive. *Regular*, when it appears to be seated in the Extremities of the Body, returns at stated Periods, and with a gradual Increase and Decline of the Symptoms : *Irregular*, when the Paroxysms are frequent, and un-certain; when the Symptoms vary, or happen promiscuously, and the Disease appears to be seated in the internal Parts of the Body; as the Stomach, Brain, &c. leaving the extreme Parts, as the hands, Feet, &c. free from Pain.

According as different Parts are affected by this Distemper, it goes by different Names : When it seizes the Feet, it is called *Podagra*; when the Knees, *Gonagra*; when the Hands, *Chiragra*; and when the Hip Joint, *Sciatica*, &c.

Sometimes it attacks the whole Body at the same time, and then it is called the *General*, or *Universal Gout.*

[1] Nicolas de Blegny (1652 – 1722), a French physician and surgeon.

The *Gout* may be Hereditary, or Natural to the Constitution, proceeding from a too great Constriction of the Capillary Vessels, whence the gouty Humor is more easily lodged,. Or detained in them. It may also proceed from High-living, Crapula's, and eating such things as are hard of Digestion; a sedentary Life, drinking too freely of tartarous Wines; irregular living, Excess in Venery; an obstructed Perspiration, and a Suppression of the natural Evacuations.

The immediate Cause of the *Gout* appears to be an Alkaline, or acrimonious Matter in the Blood; which being separated from it at particular times, falls upon the Joints, but most frequently upon the Feet, and Hands; which, if it be repelled, or of the Blood be overcharged therewith, so that a Crisis cannot be procured in the Extremities (as generally happens in old Age) it falls upon the nobler Parts; and then produces the Irregular *Gout*.

The Regular *Gout*, chiefly and immediately affects the Tendons, Nerves, Membranes, and Ligaments of the Body, about the Joints. Sometimes a cold shivering Fit precedes, and generally a Fever accompanies, its first Appearance, which soon goes off, and returns by Intervals. A slight Pain is felt in the Joints, where the Crisis is perform'd, which increases gradually; and in the Podagra generally fixes first on the great Toe, thence proceeding to the Tarsus and Metatarsus; sometimes, especially in old Age, it attacks the Knees and Hands; and wherever it is, by distending and irritating the Parts, causes a violent Pain, not unlike to that if a dislocated Bone. When the Pain is at its State, there appears an Inflammation, and a Swelling; both which increase as the Pain increases; and upon their Remission the Paroxysm, is ended : Tho' the tenderness and Swelling in sever Fits, will sometimes remain a longer Time, and cause an Uneasiness upon Motion.

It is observed, that Women, Children, and young Men, are seldom troubled with the *Gout*, unless it be hereditary; that it rarely attacks, before the Patient is 35, or 40 Years old, and sometimes not till the Decline of Life; that the Corpulent are more subject to it, than those who are spare, and lean; that the Pain increases towards Night, and decreases towards the Morning; that the longer the Interval between the Paroxysms, the more severe they prove, and the longer they generally continue.

The Disease usually returns twice a Year, *viz.* in the *Spring*, and *Autumn*; and in the latter the Paroxysm is sometimes two, or three Months, before it comes to a Period; tho' its Duration is sometimes not above three, or four Weeks.

These are called *Cardinal Paroxysms*, to distinguish them from others of less Duration, which happen between the *Spring* and *Autumn*. The more high-colour'd the Urine, and the less Sediment it deposites; the further is the Disease from the State of *Concoction*, as 'tis termed. According to the Violence and Continuance of the Fever, the Paroxysm proves more or less severe.

In Constitutions much broke or shatter'd with the *Gout*, there are usually stony, or chalky Concretions form'd in the Joints of the Fingers, or Toes, and thence translated to the Viscera; which case is often attended with irregular, frequent, and short Paroxysms in the Extremities. In the Decline of Life, when the usual Fits do not happen; or if the gouty Matter be suddenly repelled fro the Extremities by an improper Regimen, or Medicines; it usually seizes the internal Parts, and frequently the Stomach, Head, Intestines, &c. Causing Want of Appetite, Reaching to vomit, Indigestion, a Cachexia, the Jaundice, Asthma, Diarrhæa; and at last, so obstructs the fine capillary, nervous Tubes (especially those of the Stomach, and Brain) as possibly to hinder the Flux of the Animal Spirits : Upon which Death suddenly ensues.

*Sydenham* gives us an accurate History of a Fit of the *Gout* in the Feet : It begins towards the close of *January*, or Beginning of *February*, without the least previous Notice; except, perhaps, a Crudity, or Apepsy for some Weeks beforehand; with a sort of windy Intumescence, and a Heaviness of the Body, which continually increases, till at last, a Paroxysm breaks out; being preceded, some Days, with a sort of Torpor, and a sensible Descent of the Flatulences thro' the Flesh of the Thighs, with some spasmodic Symptoms. The Day before the Paroxysm, his Appetite is very greedy; an our or two after Midnight, he is waked by a Pain, commonly in his great Toe, sometimes in the Heel, Ankle, or the Calf of the Leg, not unlike the Pain felt upon a Dislocation of the said Bones; with a Sense as if Water were sprinkled on the Part affected. This is succeeded by a Chilliness, and some Approach to a Fever : The Pain in the mean time, which at first was more remiss, gradually increases; in proportion to which the Chilliness abates. By Night, it is arrived at its Height, and settled about the Ligaments of the Bones of the Tarsus, and Metatarsus; where it sometime resembles a violent Tension; and sometimes a Laceration of thee Ligaments; sometimes the Biting, or Gnawing of a Dog; a Squeezing, or Coarctation. Thus far the Part affected has such an exquisite Sense, that it cannot bear the Weight of the Linnen, nor even the Shaking of the Room occasion'd by a Person's Stepping.

Hence, a thousand vain Endeavours to Ease, by changing the Posture of the Body, the Position of the Foot, &c. till about two o three a-Clock in the Morning (the Space of a Nychthemeron from its Access), when a Remission is first perceived; the morbid Matter being by this time tolerably digested, or even dissipated. The Patient, here-upon, drops a-sleep, and at his Waking finds his Pains much abated, but the Part newly swell'd. A few Days hence, the other Foot undergoes the same Fate : Sometimes, both are attack'd from the first. From the Time it has seiz'd on both Legs, the Symptoms become more irregular, and precarious, both as to the Time of Invasion, and the Duration thereof. But this still holds, that the Pain recruits in the Night, and remits again in the Morning. A Series of these little, alternate Accesses, &c. constitutes a *Fit*, or *Paroxysm of the Gout*, which holds longer, or less, according to the Age, &c. of the Patient. In strong People, and those who have not had it often, Fourteen Days is a moderate Paroxysm ; In old People, and those long used to it, it will hold two Months.

For the first fourteen Days the Patient is usually bound : A loss of Appetite, Chilliness towards Evening, and a Heaviness, and Uneasiness even of the Parts not affected, attend the whole Paroxysm. As it goes off, he is seiz'd with an intolerable Itching, especially between the Fingers; the Furfur falls, and his Toes scale, as if he had drank Poison.

Such is the Course of a Regular *Gout*; but when thro' improper Treatment it is disturbed, or prolonged it seizes the Hands, Wrists, Elbows, Knees, and other Parts : Sometimes distorting the Fingers, and taking away their Use; sometimes generating tophaceous Concretions, or Knots about the Ligaments of the Joints, resembling Chalk, or Crabs Eyes; sometimes raising a whitish, inflammable Tumor, almost as big as an Egg, about the Elbow, &c.

It may be added, that where a Person has labor'd under the *Gout* for many Years; the Pain is sensibly lessen'd each Paroxysm, till at length it becomes rather an Uneasiness than a Pain : Hence that Reflexion of the Great *Sydenham, Dolor in hoc Morbo amarissimum est Naturæ Pharmacum.*

Bleeding and purging are found absolutely prejudicial; and Diaphoreticks of no Service. Emeticks, according to *Pitcairn*, and *Etmuller*, may do good in the Beginning of the Disease. But, upon the whole, nothing, in *Sydenham's* Opinion, proves of more Service than Digestives, or Medicines which strengthen the Stomach, and promote Digestion : As, Angelica Root, *Enul. Campan.* The Theriac Andromach. the Jesuit's Bark : These chiefly to be administer'd in the Intervals between the Paroxysms. *Musgrave*, however, recommends internally Repellants, and principally Cardiacks; externally, Emplasters of *Gum. Caran.* or *Oxycroc*, or Cephalic, with *Burgundy* Pitch; or green Sea-cloth, commonly called *Hat-case*, &c. Yet *Dolæus* affirms, that Repellants do more harm than good; and gives us the following Recipe, as more than equal to all others.

R, *Confect. Hamech. 1 ounce Pulv. Jalap. 1 semi-ounce extract. Trifol. fibrin. two ounces. Litharg. aur. 6 ounces. Sapæ Antimon. 1 semi-ounce. Sacchar. Canth. 6 ounces. Ol. Olivar. q. s. Ceræ & Picis parum f. s. a.* An Emplaster to be laid on the Joint affected, till the Pain, and the morbid Matter be driven away.

**GRAIN** is also a small Weight, us'd in estimating divers Substances. The *Grain* is the smallest of all the Weights know on England. It is taken from the Weight of a *Grain* of Wheat, gather'd out of the Middle of the Ear, and well dried. 24 Grains male a Penny-weight, and 20 Penny-weight an Ounce.

The *Grain* is a Troy Weight, and used in the weighing of Gold, Silver, Jewels, Bread, and Liquors.

Among the Antients, the *Grain* was the fourth Part of the *Siliqua*, or twelfth of the *Obolus*, and the 72d of the *Drachma*. It comprehended a Lens and an half.

*Fernelius L. IV. c. 6. Method. Medend.* Affirms it as a thing known and certain, that the Grain is of the same Weight, every where; but he is mistaken. Mr. *Greaves*[1] in his Treatise of the *Roman Foot* has shewn, that 179 *Dutch Grains*, which *Snellius*[2] had found to be the Weight of a *Philip* of Gold, only amount to 134 ½ *English Grains*. Add, that Mons. *Perrault*[3] has computed the French *Grain* to be less than the *English*; and yet bigger than the *Dutch* : To the *English*, it is as 158 to 134 1/2; and to that of the *Holland*, as 158 to 179.

The *Grain* used by the Apothecaries, is the same with that of the Goldsmiths; tho' they make a Difference in the Weights rais'd therefrom.

[1] John Greaves (1602 – 1652), an English mathematician and astronomer.

[2] Willebrord Snellius, born Willebrord Snel van Royen (1580 – 1626), a Dutch mathematician and astronomer.

[3] This may be Charles Perrault (1628 – 1703), a French lawyer and writer

Thus, 20 *Grains*, with them, make a Scruple, 3 Scruples, a Drachm, 8 Drachms, an Ounce, &c.

The Carat used in weighing Diamonds and precious Stones is also divided into four *Grains*.

**GRANATE**, a Gem, or pretious Stone, of a high, red Colour; thus called from the Resemblance it bears to that of the Kernel of a Pomgranate. *Granates* are either *Oriental*, or *Occidental* : The first are brought from divers Parts of the *East Indies*; the second from *Spain, Bohemia*, and *Silesia*.

These, from the East, are distinguish'd by their Colour into three Kinds : The first, of a deep, brownish Red, like black clotted Blood; of which Kind there are some as big as an Hen's Egg : The second, are nearly the Colour of a Hyacinth, with which it were easy to confound them, but for their superior Redness. The last, having a Mixture of Violet with their Red, are called by the Italians, *Rubini della Rocha*.

The Occidental *Granates* are of divers Reds, according to the Places they are found in. Those of *Spain*, imitate the Colour of the Kernel of a Pomgranate : Those of *Bohemia* have a golden Cast with their Red, glittering like a live Coal : Those of *Silesia* are the darkest of all, and seldom thoroughly transparent.

Of the Occidental *Granates*, those of *Bohemia* are the most valued : Some even give them the Preference over the Oriental Kind. They are found near *Prague*; not in any particular Mines, but are pick'd up by Peasants in their Fields, from among he Sands, and Pebbles.

The *Granate* is of some Use in Medicine : Its Powder is sometimes an Ingredient in the Cordial Electuaries. The Antients held it excellent against Heaviness and Melancholy.

**GRANIT**, Granites, a sort of Marble, extremely hard, rough, and incapable of taking a thoro' Polish : Thus called as being sprinkled over with a great Number of little Stains, resembling Grains of Sand.

There are three sorts of *Granit*; that of *Egypt*; that of *Italy*, and that of *Dauphiny*. The first has brownish, or greenish Spots, on a dirty, white Ground. It is found in very large Places; and is that chiefly used by the *Egyptians*, in their Obelisks, and Pyramids on the Tombs of their great Men. There are Columns of this Stone above 40 Foot high.

The *Granit* of *Italy* is softer than that of *Egypt*; especially in the Quarry, were it cuts with much more Ease. There is also a sort of Green Granit, which is a Species of Serpentine, spotted with green, and white Spots.

**GRATIOLA**, a Medicinal Plant, of considerable Virtues; tho' little known in the ordinary Practice; as being suppos'd dangerous of Application. Its most noted Effects are to evacuate hydropic Waters, both upwards and downwards, taken in Infusion, or Decoction; to cleanse Wounds, and to kill Worms.

Its Bark, taken in Powder, is said to be scarce inferior in Virtue to Ipecacuanha for Dysenteries. It is of a very bitter Taste; whence, probably its vermifugous Power; and its Root astringent, whence its use in the Dysentery.

M. *Boulduc* made an Extract of this Plant, which purged gently and was very Diuretic: Another Extract made of the Fæces or Refuse, proved much more efficacious. *Hist. de l'Acad. An.* 1705.

**GRAVEL**, in Medicine, a Disease of the Bladder, and Kidneys, occasion'd by a sandy or gritty Matter gather'd therein, which cohering into a stony Mass, prevents the due Secretion and Excretion of the Urine. The gravel is generally consider'd as the same Disease with the Calculus, or Stone.

**GRIPES**, *Tormina Ventris*, in Medicine, a sort of Colick, or painful Disorder of the Lower Belly, occasioned by some sharp pungent Matters vellicating the Parts, or by Winds pent up in the Intestines.

The *Gripes* are a very common Symptom in young Children, and may be caused by the Aliment they use, which is considerably different from what they had been accustom'd to in the Uterus.

The Retention of a Part of the Meconium may also give occasion hereto, as being somewhat acrimonious.

This Disorder sometimes proves so violent, as to throw the Child into universal Convulsions, or to cause what is vulgarly called Convulsions of the Bowels.

**GRUBBS**, in Medicine, a white, unctuous kind of Pimples or little Tumors, arising upon the Face, chiefly the Alæ of the Nose. They are usually owing to hard Drinking, and an obstructed Perspiration; though natural in some Constitutions. They begin with a small black Point, which gradually spreads; and sometimes the Matter tends to Suppuration, upon which the Heads of the Eruptions grow white or yellow. They are usually reputed salutary; whence to check their Growth suddenly, has proved of ill Consequence. They are cured by Evacuation, and acrimonious Lotions.

**GRUME**, *Grumus*, in Medicine, &c. A particle of Blood, Milk, or other Fluid, which is coagulated, thicken'd, harden'd, or not sufficiently thin, and diluted. Phthisical People frequently spit up *Grumes, i.e.* Clots of Blood. *Grumes* of Milk, are what we popularly call Curds.

**GRUMOUS** Blood, is that State or Consistence of the Blood, wherein it is too viscid, and thick, for a due brisk Circulation : The Effects whereof are, that it stagnates in the Capillary Vessels, and produces divers Diseases.

**GUADAM**, Guoad, in Natural History, an Herb by the antient *Romans* called *Glastum* and *Vitrum*; by the *Greeks Isatis*; by the *Britains Guadam*; and by us now, *Woad*. The antient *Britains, Caesar* informs us, painted their Faces with this Herb to appear the more terrible to their Enemies. And *Pliny* relates, that the same was practised by the Women in divers Sacrifices.

**GUM**, *Gummi*, a vegetable Juice exsuding thro' the Pores of certain Plants, and there hardening into a tenacious transparent Mass. *Gum* is properly one of the Juices of the Bark : It is drawn thence by the Sun's Warmth, in Form of a glutinous Humour; and by the same Cause is afterwards inspissated, concocted, and render'd tenacious.

The Character of *Gums,* whereby they are distinguished from Resins and other vegetable Juices, is, that they are dissoluble in Water, and at the same Time inflammable by Fire. In the general they are more viscid, and less friable, and generally dissoluble in any aqueous Menstruum; whereas Resins are more sulphurous, and require a spirituous Dissolvent. *Boerhaave* considers a *Gum* as a sort of saponaceous Fat; which beside its oily Principle in common with Resin, has some other Ingredient that renders it miscible with Water.

*Gums* are different, according to the different Trees, Roots, &c. they ouze from : Some Authors distinguish them into *Aqueous,* and *Resinous Gums* : The first, those dissoluble in Water, Wine, and the like Fluids; The second those, only dissoluble in Oil. To these two some add a third *anomalous* Kind, *viz.* those soluble with much Difficulty either in Water or Oil.

Among the Class of *Gums* are usually ranked, *Gum-Anima, Arabic, Gutta, Adraganth, Ammoniac, Assa Fœtida, Bdellium, Balm, Benjoin, Camphor, Copal, Elemy, Frankincense, Euphorbium, Galbanum, Lacca, Manna, Myrrh, Olibanum, Sagapenum, Sanguis Draconis, Sarcolla, Stacte, Storax, Taca-mahacha, Turpentine.*

*Theophrastus* speaks of a way of multiplying Plants, perform'd *per Lachrymas,* by means of the *Gum* or Resin; but *Agricola* takes this to be only possible where there are Seeds in the *Gum.*

**GUM**-*Anima,* or *Animi,* is a resinous Juice ouzing from a Tree by the *Portugueze* called *Courbari,* growing in divers Parts of *America.* This Gum is very hard and transparent, of an agreeable Smell, not unlike Amber ; It neither dissolves in Water nor Oil, and consequently is not properly accounted a Gum. In lieu of this, they frequently substitute Copal.

**GUM**-*Arabic,* call'd also *Thebaic, Sarracenaic, Babylonish,* and *Achantine,* from the Places or the Tree which produce it, is the Juice of a little Tree growing in *Egypt,* of the Cassia Kind, called in Latin *Acacia foliis Scorpoides Leguminosa.*

'Tis very transparent, glutinous upon the Tongue, almost insipid to the Taste, and twisted somewhat in form of a Worm. It is esteem'd good to incrassate, to stop the Pores, blunt the Points of too pungent Medicines, and temper the Acrimony of the Trachea in Coughs, &c.

**GUM**-*Gutta,* or *Gutta-Gamba,* or *Gutta-Gemou,* or *Gamandra,* popularly *Gamboche,* is a resinous *Gum* brought from the Kingdom of *Siam,* &c. in large Pieces fashion not unlike Saucidges, hard, brittle, and very yellow. It ouzes from Incisions made in a kind of prickly Shrub, which climbs up the neighbouring Trees. It purges violently both upwards and downwards; and is particularly used in Dropsies, the Itch, &c. but it is dangerous. It serves also to make a yellow Colour, for painting in Miniature.

**GUM**-*Senegal,* is the *Gum* ordinarily sold by the Druggists for *Gum-Arabic,* which it resembles very nearly both as to Form and Virtue : It is either white bordering on the yellow, or of a deep Amber Colour, transparent, &c. It ouzes out of a prickly Shrub common enough in *Africa*. The *Gum* is brought us from *Senegal*, whence its Name.

**GUMMO**-*Resin*, or *Gum-Rosin*, is a harden'd Juice of a middle Nature between a *Gum* and a *Resin*, being both dissoluble in aqueous Menstruums like a *Gum*; and in oleaginous ones like a *Resin*. Such are *Mastic, Camphor, Storax*, &c. Some Naturalists make a Class of *Irregular* Gummo *Resins*, being such as dissolve, tho' with Difficulty, and not perfectly, both in aqueous and oleaginous Liquors; as *Bdellium, Myrrh*, &c.

**GUN-POWDER**, a Composition of Salt-petre, Sulphur, and Charcoal, mixed together, and usually granulated; which easily takes Fire, and raises of expands with great Vehemence, by means of its Elastic Force. 'Tis to this *Powder* we owe all the Action, and Effect of Guns, Ordnance, &c. so that the modern military Art, Fortification, &c. depend wholly thereon.

The Invention of *Gun-powder* is ascribed by *Polydore Virgil* to a Chymist, who having accidentally put some of this Composition in a Mortar, and cover'd it up with a Stone; it happen'd to take Fire, and blew up the Stone. *Thevet*[1] says, the Person here spoke of was a Monk of *Frybourg* named *Constantine Aneleze* : But *Belleforet*[2] and other Authors, with more Probability, hold it to be *Bartholdus Schwartz*, or the Black : At least it is affirm'd, he first taught the Use of it to the *Venetians*, in the Year 1380, during the War with the *Genoese*; and that it was first imployed in a Place antiently called *Fossa Caudeana*, now *Chioggia*, against *Laurence de Medicis*; and that all *Italy* made Complaints against it, as a manifest Contravention of a fair Warfare.

But what contradicts this Account, and thus shews *Gun-powder* of an older Æra, is, that *Peter Messius*, in his various Readings, mentions, that the *Moors* being besieged in 1343, by *Alphonsus* XI. King of *Castile*, discharged a sort of Iron Mortars upon them, which made a Noise like Thunder ; which is seconded by what Don *Pedro* Bishop of *Leon* relates in his Chronicle of King *Alphonsus* who reduced *Tunis*, and the *Moorish* King of *Sevil*, above 400 Years ago, those of Tunis had certain Iron Tuns, or Barrels, wherewith they threw Thunder bolts of Fire.

*Du Cange*[3] adds, that there is mention made of it in the Registers of the Chambers of Accounts in France as early as the Year 1338.

To say no more, it appears that our *Roger Bacon* knew of Gun-powder 150 Years before *Schwartz* was born : That excellent Friar mentions the Composition in express Terms, in his Treatise *de Nullitate Magiæ*, publish'd at *Oxford* in 1216. "You may raise Thunder and Lightening at pleasure," says he, "by only taking Sulphur, Nitre, and Charcoal, which singly have no Effect, but mix'd together, and confined in a close Place, cause a Noise and Explosion greater than that of a Clap of Thunder."

There are divers Compositions of *Gun-powder*, with respect to the Proportions of the three Ingredients; to be met withal in Pyrotechnical

[1] This might be Andre de Thevet (1502 – 1590), a French Franciscan priest and explorer.

[2] This is probably Francois de Belleforet (1530 -1583), a French historian.

[3] Charles du Fresne (1610 – 1688), sieur du Cange, a French scholar.

Writers : But the Process is much the same in all.

The Sulphur and Salt-peter being purified, and reduced to Powder, are put, with the Charcoal-Dust, in a Mortar, moisten'd with Water or Spirits of Wine, or the like, and pounded 24 Hours together; taking Care to wet the mass from time to time, to prevent its taking Fire : Lastly, squeezing it through a Sieve, it is formed into little Grains, or Globules; which being dried, the Powder is compleat; and the least Spark being struck thereon from a Steel and Flint, the whole will be immediately inflam'd, and burst out with extreme Violence.

The Effect is not hard to account for : The Charcoal of the Grain whereon the Spark falls, catching Fire like Tinder, the Sulphur and Nitre are readily melted, and the former also breaks into Flame; and at the same time the contiguous Grains undergo the same Fate. Now 'tis known that Salt-peter, when ignited, rarifies to a prodigious Degree.

Sir *I. Newton* reasons thus on the Point : The Charcoal and Sulphur in *Gun-powder*, easily take fire, and kindle the Nitre; and the Spirit of Nitre being thereby rarified into Vapour, rushes out with an Explosion much after the manner that the Vapour of Water rushes out of an Æolipile; the Sulphur also being volatile, is converted into Vapour, and augments the Explosion : Add that the acid Vapour of the Sulphur, namely, that which distils under a Bell into Oil of Sulphur, entering violently into the fix'd Body of the Nitre, lets loose the Spirit of Nitre, and excites a greater Fermentation, whereby the Heat is farther augmented, and the fix'd Body of the Nitre is also rarified into Fume, and the Explosion thereby made more vehement and quick.

For if Salt of Tartar be mixed with *Gun-powder*, and that Mixture be warmed till it takes Fire, the Explosion will be more violent and quick than that of *Gun-powder* alone, which cannot proceed from any other use than the Action of the Vapour of *Gun-powder* upon the Salt of Tartar, whereby that Salt is rarified.

The Explosion of *Gun-powder* arises, therefore, from the violent Action whereby all the Mixture being quickly and vehemently heated, is rarified and converted into Fume and Vapour; which Vapour, by the Violence of that Action, becoming so hot as to shine, appears in the Form of Fume.

M. *de la Hire* ascribes all the Force and Effect of *Gun-powder*, to the Spring or Elasticity of the Air, inclosed on the several Grains thereof, and in the Intervals or Spaces between the Grains : The Powder being kindled, sets the Springs of so many little Parcels of air a-playing, and dilates them all at once; whence all the Effect; the *Powder* it self only serving to light a Fire which may put the Air in Action; after which the whole is done by the Air alone.

**GUTTÆ** *Anglicanæ*, the *English Drops*, or the *Volatile English Drops*, or *Goddard's Drops*, is a medicinal Liquor prepared from divers Ingredients; of sovereign Efficacy against Coagulations of the Blood, malignant Fevers, and particularly the Small-Pox, Obstructions, Epilepsies, drousy Diseases, Vapours, &c.

The Inventor of these celebrated Drops, was Dr. *Goddard*, a Physician of

*London*. The Secret of their Composition was purchases by King *Charles* II at the Price of 6000 Pounds Sterling; whence the Denomination *Guttæ Anglicanæ*.

This costly Recipe, we shall here gratify the Reader withal, *a Meilleure Marche* : "Take five Pounds of human Cranium of a person hang'd, or dead of some violent Death, two Pounds of dried Vipers, two Pounds of Hart's-Horn, and two of Ivory; mince the whole small, put it in two or three Retorts, and distill it in a reverberatory Furnace, with the same Precautions as are ordinarily used in distilling Hart's-Horn and Vipers, to extract their volatile Salt. When the Vessels or Receives are cold, unlute 'em, and shake them well, in order to loosen the volatile Salt from the Sides of the Vessels. Pour the whole into a large Glass Cucurbite, and filtrate it through a Brown-Paper, in order to separate the Oil, which is here useless : Put the filtrated Liquor in a Glass Retort, with a Sand-Heat, and fit a Glass Retort thereto, as a Recipient: Take care all Things be well luted, and make a Cohobation of the said Matter at three Times.

But, by the way, add all the Salt before separated from the Receivers; and after the said three Cohobations, unlute the Retorts, and pour the whole into a Matrass with a long Neck, to which fit a suitable Capital, and a Receiver; lute all the Joinings on each Side with a wet Bladder, and set the Vessel in a Sand Heat : By this means, the volatile Salt will be sublimed, and stick to the Capital, and upper Part of the Matrass. Continue the Fire till Spirit enough have rose to fuse and dissolve the Salt which arose first : Then take all the Fire out of the Furnace, that the Distillation may proceed no further; which is a Circumstance of the last importance; without which the Medicine would be weaken'd by too much Phlegm." *Biet*, in the *Mem. de Trev. An.* 1713.

As to the Dose of this Remedy, they begin with 7 or 8 Drops increasing, by Degrees, to 40 or 50, on pressing Occasions, as in Apoplexies, Lethargies, Weaknesses, &c.

The real Composition of the *Guttæ*, however, is somewhat controversial. M. *Tournefort* assures us, that he had the Secret communicated to him by Dr. *Lister*; and that it is no other than the volatile Spirit of Raw-Silk rectified with Oil of Cinnamon, or other essential Oil.

The same Author assures us, he had found by Experience that the *Guttæ Anglicanæ* were not in any respect preferable to the common volatile Spirits of Hart's-Horn and Sal Ammoniac, except that the Smell is more supportable. *Mem. de l'Acad. An.* 1700.

**HABIT**, in Medicine, is what we otherwise call the *Temperament*, or *Constitution* of the Body, whether obtain'd by Birth, or Manner of Living. An ill distemper'd Habit, without any particular apparent Disease, the Physicians usually call a *Cachexia*, or *Cacochymia*. A Thing is said to *enter the Habit*, when it becomes intimately diffused throughout the Body; and is convey'd to the remotest Stages of Circulation.

**HÆMATOSIS**, in Medicine, the Action whereby the Chyle is converted into Blood; call'd also *Sanguification*. The Word is form'd of the *Greek*, αιμα, *Sanguis*, Blood. The chief of the vital Actions, are the *Chylosis*, and *Hæmatosis*.

**HÆMOPTYSIS**, or Hæmoptoe, in Medicine, a spitting of Blood; occasion'd by the Rupture, or Erosion of some Vessel of the Lungs; and accompanied, usually with a Cough, and a Sense of Pressure on the Breast. The *Hæmoptysis* differs from a Vomiting of Blood, in that in the *Hæmoptysis*, the Blood comes from the Lungs, and for that Reason is florid and frothy; where in the Vomiting of Blood, it comes from the Stomach, and is blackish.

The *Hæmoptysis* is occasioned by violent Shouts, or Cries; by Strains, Falls, vehement Coughs; by the Suppression of some ordinary Evacuation, or by the Abundance of some sharp corrosive Humor. The *Hæmoptysis* is either accidental, or habitual. The latter is a Symptom of the *Phthysis*. It is best cured, according to *Morton*, by the *Cortex* : It is stopp'd by Astringents, as *Armen. Bol. Sang. Dracon. Lapis Hæmat.* &c. The Word comes from αιμα, *Blood*; and πτειν, *to spit*.

**HÆMORRHAGE**, in Medicine, a Flux of Blood, at any Part of the Body; arising either from a Rupture of Vessels, as when they are too full, or too much press'd; or from an Erosion of the same, as when the Blood us too sharp and corrosive. The Word is compounded of the *Greek*, αιμα, *Sanguis*, Blood, and ρυαστω, or ρυγνυμαι, *frango, rumpo, erumpo*, I break, burst forth, &c.

The *Hæmorrhage*, properly speaking, as understood by the *Greeks*, was only a Flux of Blood at the Nose; but the Moderns extend the name to any Kind of Flux of Blood, whether by the Nose, Mouth, Lungs, Stomach, Intestines, Fundament, Matrix, or the like. An *Hæmorrhage* at the *Anus*, is more usually call'd *Dysentery*.

Hypochondriac, Scorbutic, and Cachectic Persons, are liable to various and immoderate *Hæmorrhages*. The Cure of *Hæmorrhages* arising from a Plethora, is by Evacuants, and particularly Phlebotomy, to cause a Revulsion. That from an increas'd Velocity of a thin acrimonious Blood, is to be attack'd with Coolers, and Agglutinants.

The principal simple Remedies in *Hæmorrhages*, are *Album Græcum*, Spirit or Oil of Vitriol, *Calcanthum* rubified, Colophony pulverized, Oil of Turpentine, Decoction of *Catechu, Cortex Peruv.*, &c. A Ligature on the Limb has frequently a good Effect : So *Elect. Boylean. Pulvis Galenia; Elect. Styptic. Tinctur. Rosar. Epithem. De Sacchar. Saturn.* &c.

**HÆMORRHOIDAL**, an Epithet given to the Veins and Arteries of the Intestinum Rectum, and the Fundament; as being the Seat of the *Hæmorrhoids*.

The *Hæmorrhoidal* Arteries are two; the one *internal*, the other *external*. The internal is a Branch of the lower Mesenteric, which running along the Rectum, terminates at the Fundament; the external springs from the Hypogastric Artery.

The *Hæmorrhoidal* Veins are also internal and external. The internal carries back the Blood of the *Rectum* and Fundament, which it embraces regularly; and is inserted sometimes into the splenic Branch of the *Porta*, and sometimes into the Mesenteric : The external brings back the Blood from the musculous Parts about the Fundament, and terminates in the Hypogastric Vein.

**HÆMORRHOIDS**, in Medicine, a Disease of the Fundament, popularly call'd the *Piles*. The *Hæmorrhoids* are a painful, periodical Tumor, in the lower Part of the *Intestinum Rectum*; usually appearing externally in the Anus. They may be consider'd as a Sort of varicose Tumors in the *Hæmorrhoidal* Veins; arising from the too great Abundance of morbid Blood therein.

The Disease is either *simple*, as when the Veins alone are tumified; or *compound*, as when the neighbouring Parts become infected, or an Excrescence arise therefrom, as a *Ficus, Crista Galli, Condyloma*, or the like.

*Hæmorrhoids* are either *open, fluentes*, that is, yield Blood; or *blind, cœcæ*, where the Parts are only tumid. In the first, the Vessels of the Rectum are open; in the latter, there is some Obstruction, which occasions them to swell.

The *Hæmorrhoids* sometimes are internal, and cause great Pain in going to Stool; especially if the Faeces be indurated : After which they often appear externally, and Blood is seen upon the Excrements.

*Etmuller* is careful in distinguishing the genuine, *hæmorrhoidal* Flux, from a bloody Diarrhœa, frequent in scorbutic Cases. The *Hæmorrhoids* are usually open'd by the Attrition of the Excrements in a Stool, so that the Blood flows at the same Time with the Excrements; but if it flows promiscuously before, as well as after the Excrements, and without Pain, 'tis a scorbutic Flux.

Where the Flux is excessive, Phlebotomy, and Cupping, are good, by way of Revulsion; and internally, Astringents and Opiates. Upon a Suppression of the usual Flux, without removing the Cause, the open *Hæmorrhoids* degenerate into the blind : In which Case they must be open'd again with Aloeticks, &c. Tamarinds are held excellent to asswage the Flux. Chalybeats strike at the Cause of the Evil. Scrophulary, Onion, and Leek, are much commended.

The Word is form'd of the *Greek*, αιμοροις, *Sanguinis profluvium*, Flux of Blood; which is compounded of αιμα, *Blood*, and ρεω, *I flow*.

**HEAD-ACH**, a painful Sensation in the Muscles, Membranes, Nerves, or other Parts of the Head. It is supposed to arise from an extraordinary

Distention of those Parts, either by the Fluids therein being rarified, or their Quantity and Motion increas'd.

When attended with a Vomiting, Deafness, and Watching it portends Madness; with a Noise in the Ear, Dullness of Feeling in the Hands, &c. an Apoplexy or Epilepsy.

The Cure is by Bleeding in the Jugular; Cupping, or applying Leeches to the Temples, and behind the Ears and Neck. Issues, Emeticks, and Diaphoreticks are also occasionally used; with Anti-epilepticks and Apoplecticks. A Vesicatory applied to the whole Scalp, is the last Remedy.

M. *Homberg* gives us an extraordinary Instance of the Cure of a most vehement and inveterate *Head-Ach*, by an accidental Burn of the Head.

**HEAD** *Mould-Shot*, a Disease in Children, wherein the Sutures of the Skull, generally the Coronal, *ride*; that is, have their Edges shot over one another; and so close lock'd together, *e.gr.* as to compress the internal Parts, the Meninges, or even the Brain it self. The Disease usually occasions Convulsions; and is supposed to admit of no Cure from Medicines; unless Room cou'd be given, by manual Operation, or a Divulsion of the Sutures. The *Head Mould-Shot*, is the Disorder opposite to the Horse-Show Head.

**HEALING**, in its general Sense, includes the whole Process of curing or removing a Disorder, and restoring Health. In this Sense, Medicine is defined the Art of Healing. In its more restrained Sense, as used in Chirurgery, &c. *Healing* denotes the uniting or consolidating the Lips of a Wound or Ulcer. The Medicines, proper for this Intention, are call'd Incarnatives, Agglutinatives, Vulneraries, &c.

**HEALTH**, *Valetudo*, *Sanitas*, a due Temperament, or Constitution, of the several Parts whereof an Animal is composed, both in respect of Quantity and Quality. Or it is the State of the Body, wherein it is fitted to discharge the natural Functions perfectly, easily, and durably. *Health*, is the State or Condition, opposite to Disease.

The Preservation, and Restoration of *Health*, makes the Object of the Art of Medicine.

The Condition, or Continuance of *Health*, depends principally on the six Non-Naturals, *viz. Air*, *Food*, *Exercise*, the *Passions*, *Evacuation* and *Retention*, and *Sleep* and *Waking*.

The Antients personified and even deified *Health*; or rather, erected a Goddess to whom they supposed the Care of *Health* to belong. The *Greeks* worshipp'd her under the Name *Hygeia*, and the *Latins* under that of *Sanitas*. The Place of her Worship at *Rome* was on the Mons *Quirinalis*, where she had a Temple; and a Statue crown'd with Medicinal Herbs.

We frequently find the Goddess *Health* on the Reverse of Medals. She is represented with a Serpent stretch'd on her left Arm, and holding a Patera to it with the left. Sometimes she has an Altar before her, with a Serpent twisted around the same, and raising its Head to take something out of the flame. The Inscription is SAL. AUG.

**HEART-BURN**, a Disease, among Physicians usually call'd Cardialgia. The Testaceous Powders, as Oyster-Shells, Crabs-Eyes, &c. are the usual Remedies.

**HECTIC**, or Hectic *Fever*, in Medicine, a Sort of slow habitual Fever, gradually preying on and consuming the Moisture of the Body, and ending in a *Tabes*, or Consumption. The *Hectic* is also an Attendant of a Consumption; and is reputed one of the Diagnostic Signs thereof.

The Word is *Greek*, εκτικος, form'd of εξις, *Habitus*; a Quality hard to separate from its Subject.

The *Hectic*, Dr. *Quincy* observes, is the Reverse of those Fevers which arise from a *Plethora*, or too great a Fullness from Obstruction. This being attended with too lax a State of the excretory Passages, and particularly of the Skin, whereby so much runs off, as leaves not Resistance enough in the contractile Vessels to keep them sufficiently distended, so that they vibrate oftener, agitate the Fluids more, and keep them thin and hot.

The Remedy consists in giving a firmer Tone to the Solids, and laying more Load upon the Fluids, and thus brining them to a better Consistence; which is effected by Means of Balsamicks, Agglutinants, and Foods of the best Nourishment. All Evacuation herein is bad.

A Milk Diet, is much recommended in *Hecticks*, and particularly Asses-Milk, as being the least viscid and heavy. Dr. *Baynard*[1] proposes Butter-Milk as a Seccedaneum to Asses-Milk. According to him, it answers most of the Indications in this Case, as it cools, moistens, nourishes, &c. He adds, that he has known many Persons cured of obstinate *Hecticks* by a continued Use thereof.

**HELIOTROPE**, *Heliotropium*, in Natural History, a Plant popularly call'd the Sun-flower; as also *Tournsol*, or *Turnsol*. The Word is compounded of the *Greek*, ηλιος, *Sun*, and τρεπος, *verto*, I turn.

**HELLEBORE**, *Helleborus*, *Helleborum*, *Ellebore*, a medicinal Plant, reputed, among the Antients, a specific for the Cure of Folly, Melancholy, and Madness. There are two Sorts of Hellebore, the Black and the White.

The *Black Hellebore*, *Helleborus Niger*, call'd also *Melampodium*, has a dark-coloured Root, furnished with Abundance of little Fibres; its Stem green, its Leaves dented, and its Flowers of a Carnation Hue, not unlike the Rose.

The *White Hellebore*, *Helleborus Albus*, call'd also *Veratrum*, to distinguish it from the former, has a whitish Root, beset with Fibres of the same Colour, shooting out at a Sort of Bulb, not unlike the Head of an Onion. Its Leaves are broad; at first green, afterwards of a yellowish red. From the middle of the Leaves rises a Stem, two or three Foot high, which separate about the middle into Branches, each whereof bears a considerable Number of little Flowers like Stars, disposed in Manner of a *Spica*, or Ear.

'Tis only the Roots are used, in each Kind; which are to be chosen large and

[1] Edward Baynard (1641 – 1717), an English physician.

fair, furnish'd with big Filaments : Those of the White, tan coloured without, and white within; and those of the Black, blackish without, and brownish within; dry, clean, and of a very sharp disagreeable Taste.

The Antients, as already observed, had a great Opinion of their Efficacy in Diseases of the Mind; whence various Phrases and Forms of speaking among Writers: As *Caput Helleboro Dignum.* He needs a double Dose of *Hellebore.* The Island of *Anticyra*, situate against Mount *Oeta*, was famous for the Growth and use of this Plant, it being here in its greatest Perfection, and used with the best Effect. Whence the Proverb, *Naviger Anticyras*, send him on a Voyage to *Anticyra.*

They act as Purgative, but so very violently, both upwards and downwards, as frequently to cause Convulsions; whence the Use of them internally is now out of Doors, unless joyn'd with other Purgatives, and even Alterants to correct them; but are still retain'd with Success, for the Farcy in Horses, and the Scab in Sheep.

The chief Use wherein the present Practice acknowledges white *Hellebore*, is in Form of a sternutatory Powder, to clear and open the Head.

The black *Hellebore* used among us, Dr. *Quincy* suggest to be much inferior in Virtue to that of the Antients; for that it will not operate much by Stool, but is only a powerful Alterative, getting far into the habit, and so promoting Sweat. He adds, that he has known it do Wonders in the Gout and Rheumatism, and that it rarely fails in Obstructions of the Menses.

**HELM**, in Chymistry, is the Head of a Still or Alembic; thus call'd, because in Figure it sometimes resembles a Helm, or Helmet. Hence, to bring a Thing *over the Helm*, is the same as to force it by Fire up to the Top of the Vessel, that it may distil down into the Receiver by the Beak of the Head. And when they say, such a Thing cannot be brought over the Helm, they mean, that it is of too fixed a Nature to be raised into Vapour, by the Force of Fire.

**HEMIPLEGIA**, or Hemiplexia, in Medicine, a Palsy of one whole Side of the Body. The Word is compounded of ημι, *half*, and πληοστω, *I strike*, or *seize.*

**HEMITRITÆUS**, in Medicine, an irregular, intermitting Fever, which returns twice every Day; by which it is distinguish'd from the Quotidian, which only returns once in the Day. The Word is compounded of ημι, *half*, and τριταιος, third.

**HEMLOCK**, *Cicuta*, a Narcotic Plant; of some Use in Physic, in that Intention. The common *Hemlock* is a Poison; tho' not of the violent Sort. We have Instances of considerable Quantities being taken without the least Disorder. *Philosoph. Transact.* No. 231. There is a Plaster denominated from it in the College Dispensatory; consisting of the Juice of the plant boiled up with Gums, &c. The Cicuta so much celebrated among the Antients, was the Juice of a Species of this Plant, call'd *Oenanthe Aquatica.*

**HEPATIC**, in Medicine and Anatomy, something that relates to the *Liver*; which the *Greeks* call ηπας, *Hepar.*

**HEPATIC** *Aloes*, is that otherwise call'd *Aloes Succotrina*.

**HEPATITIS**, in Medicine, an Inflammation of the Liver, with an Abscess or Imposthume thereof. The Hepatitis nears a near Resemblance to the Pleurisy; only that its Symptoms are less intense. It usually either kills the Patient, or discusses, or suppurates gradually, or degenerates into a Schirrus.

**HERB**, a Name common to all Plants whose Stalks or Stems, die away every Year, after their Seed is become ripe. There are some *Herbs* whose Root perishes with the Stem : And others, where the Root survives the Stem by several Years.

Of the former, those which to Maturity the first Year, and after they have cast their Seed, die away; are call'd *Annuals* : Such are *Wheat*, Rye, &c.

Those which only bear Flowers and Fruit the second Year, or even the Third Year, and then perish; are called *Bisannuals* : Such are the Garden *Angelica*, and some others.

*Herbs* whose Root does not perish after they have shed their Seed, are call'd *Perennials*; such are *Mint*, *Fennel*, &c. Of these, some keep their Leaves all the Year round, and are call'd *Ever-greens*; as the *Asarabaca*, *yellow Violet*, &c. The rest lose their Leaves, and continue bare, part of the Year; as *Fern*, *Colts-foot*, &c.

*Herbs* are also distinguished into *Kitchin*, or *Sallet-Herbs*, and *Medicinal Herbs*.

The Word *Herb* is form'd of the Latin *Herba*; which some derive from *Arvum*, Field : Others derive it from the *Greek*, φερβειν, *pascere*, to feed; of φερβη, *Pabulum*. Of the Greek *Ferbe*, the *Latins* form'd *Ferba*; and of *Ferba*, Herba, after the Manner of the *Spaniards* who always change the *f* at the beginning of a Word to *h*.

**HERBAGE**, a collective Name, comprehending all Kinds of Herbs. The antient Hermits liv'd altogether of *Herbage*. What makes the principal Difference in the Goodness of Butters and Cheeses, is the Difference of *Herbage*.

**HERBAL**, a Book which treats of Plants; or describes the Figure, Genus, Species, Properties, Virtues, &c of *Herbs*, Trees, Seeds, &c. Such are *Gerard's Herbal*, *Parkinson's Herbal*, &c. *Herbal* is also used for a Set or Collection of Specimens of the several Kinds of Plants, dried and preserved in the Leaves of a Book.

In the *Philosophical Transactions*, we have a Method described for preserving Specimens for such an *Herbal*. The Flowers, Leaves, &c. gather'd perfectly ripe, and in their true Colours, are to be spread on brown Paper, with all the Parts display'd as distinctly as may be. If the Stem, or the Body of the Flower, &c. be thick, one half to be pared away to make it lye flat. Over them is to be spread another brown Paper; and the whole to be put between two Iron Plates, screwed tight together, and thus baked in an Oven for two Hours. When taken out, wash them with a Mixture of Brandy and *Aqua fortis*, and lay them on fresh Paper to dry. Lastly, lick over the Backsides with a Brush dipped in a Dissolution of *Gum Dragon*, to make them stick; and lay them in the Paper Book, where they will lye fast, and always look fresh.

**HERCULEUS** *Morbus*, in Medicine, the Epilepsy; thus call'd, from the Terror of its Attacks, and the Difficulty of Cure.

**HERMODACTYL**, in Medicine, a Drug used as a gentle Purgative. Naturalists are not agreed as to the Origin of this Drug. Some will have it the Root, and others the Fruit of a Plant. To reconcile them, one might probably allow two Kinds of *Hermodactyls*; the one a Root, the other a Fruit. The Fruit is about the Size of a little Chessnut, in Figure resembling a Heart; ruddy without, very white within; of a light fungous Substance; without Fibres; easily broke, and reducible into a Powder like Flower, of a sweetish Taste, but somewhat viscid. It is brought to us dried from *Egypt* and *Syria*. Authors differ as to the Plant which bears it. In the common Opinion it passes for a Sort of *Colchicum* : Others take it for a tuberous *Iris*.

*Hermodactyls* are chiefly used to purge pituitous Humours of the Brain and Joynts. They are so efficacious in scowering the mucilaginous Glands, and preserving them from the Lodgments of gritty Matters, which occasion the Gout and arthritic Complaint; that they are denominated by some Writers, *Anima Articulorum*. They also promote Sweat.

**HERNIA**, in Medicine, &c. a Descent of the Intestines, or *Omentum*, out of their natural Place; or, rather, the Tumour form'd by that Descent; popularly called a Rupture.

When the *Peritoneum* happens to be broken, or extraordinarily dilated; the *Viscera*, and particularly the Caul and small Guts, are apt to fall out of their Place, and to form these Sorts of Tumours called *Hernia's*. They happen most usually in the *Inguen*, or Groin; the Scrotum, and Navel : Tho, sometimes, in other Places; as above or below the Navel; in the Side, far above the *Inguen*, in the upper Part of the Thigh, near the Spine, &c.

*Hernia's* are occasion'd by Blows, violent Concussions, over-stretching in Vomiting, hard Labour, or Wind; form which last Cause it is, that they are so frequent in Children, and so easily help'd by timely Cure : In Adults they are generally incurable. From *Hernia's* frequently arise the Iliac Passion, and sometimes Inflammations, and even Gangrenes of the Intestines.

*Hernia's* are variously denominated, both according to the Parts displaced, and to those wherein they fall. A Descent of the Intestines into the Scrotum, which is the most usual Kind of Rupture, is call'd *Enterocele*. If, instead of the Intestines, the *Omentum* be fallen; it is called *Epiplocele*. A Descent of both, is called *Entero-Epiplocele*. If the Intestines fall on the Navel, it is call'd *Omphalocele*. If they fall thro' the Perforation of the *Obliquus Descendus* into the Groin; it is called *Bubunocele*, or *Inguinalis*.

There are also a spurious Sort of *Hernia's*, or Tumours of the Testes, &c. occasion'd, not by a Descent of any of the solid Parts, but a Coagmentation of some of the Fluids. When the Testicles are swell'd, and distended with a watery Humour, it is called a *Hydrocele*, or *Hernia Aquosa*. When with the Wind, *Pneumatocele*, or *Hernia Ventosa*.

When the Tumour is owing to a Mole, or Excrescence of Flesh, it is call'd

*Sarcocele*, or *Hernia Carnosa*. When to a Dilatation of the Vessels, of in Manner of a Varix, *Circocele*, or *Hernia Varicosa*. A Kind of prominent Tumour in the Throat, is frequently call'd *Bronchocele*, or *Hernia Gutturalis*.

Some late Authors also speak of *Hernia's*, or Descents of the Bladder into the Scrotum; but these are rare. M. *Mery*[1] concludes, that they never arise from mere Accident; but when they do happen, it must be the Effect of an original ill Conformation. His Reason is, that the Bladder of the Urine is too big to pass thro' the Annuli or Rings, which the Intestines pass thro'; beside that it is fasten'd too strongly on all Sides to admit of a Descent.

M. *Petit*, however, is of a different Sentiment; and maintains that *Hernias* of the Bladder may be produced after the ordinary Manner of others.

*Priscian* observes, that the antient *Marsi* gave the Appellation of *Herna* to Rocks : Whence, some will have *Hernia's* thus called *propter duritiem*, on Account of their Hardness. *Scaliger* chuses rather to derive the Word from the *Greek* ερνος, *Ramus*, Branch.

The Word is Latin, *Hernia*, and originally signifies the same with *Tumor Scroti*; call'd also *Ramex*.

**HERPES**, in Medicine, a cutaneous Heat or Inflammation, occasioning a Roughness of the Skin, by Means of a Number of little Pustules spreading this Way and that. The Word is form'd of the *Greek*, ερπω, *paulatim, gradior, repo*, by Reason of the Eruptions creep from Place to Place.

There are divers Kinds of this Disease : The *simple Herpes*, is a single Pustule or two, rising chiefly on the Face, of a whitish or yellowish Colour, pointed, and with an inflamed Base. These dry away of their own Accord, upon letting out the little Drop of Pus contain'd in them. The second Species of *Herpes*, is what we otherwise call *Serpigo*; and in *English*, a *Tetter*, or *Ring-worm*.

*Milliary Herpes*, is an Assemblage of innumerable little Pustules, under the Cuticle, of the Size of Millet Seeds : Popularly call'd the *Shingles*. The *Herpes Milliaris*, according to *Wiseman*, approaches very nearly to the Nature of the *Psora*; and therefore to be cured with Mercurial Cathartics, &c.

*Herpes Exedens*, is of a more corrosive Kind; the Pustules are ruddy, and attended with an itching; and ulcerate the Parts they rise on.

**HICKUP**, Hiccough, or Hicket, *Singultus*, in Medicine, a sudden irregular Inspiration; wherein the Stomach, and the Parts contain'd in the lower Venter, are driven from below, upwards. The *Hickup* is not a Disorder of the Stomach, as is usually imagined, but a convulsive Motion of the *Diaphragma*; whereby that Muscle retiring impetuously downwards, impels the Parts beneath it.

It is occasion'd by sharp Humours; a too great Plenitude of the Stomach; a Bit of any Thing stopp'd at its upper Orifice; or, in general, by any Thing capable of irritating the nerves of the *Diaphragma*.

[1] Jean Mery (1645 – 1722), a French physician and anatomist.

The Remedy for the *Hiccough*, according to *Hippocrates*, is to fetch the Breath very long, or even to stop the breath for some Time. A Sneezing happening upon a *Hiccough* generally cure its; the Diaphragm, shook by the violent Expiration, being apt to throw off what before irritated it.

The Word is form'd of the Flemish *Hick*, which signifies the same Thing. Others derive it *ab hiscendo*; others *a difficili Anhelitu.*

**HIDROTICKS**, or rather Hydroticks, in Medicine, are the same with Sudorificks. Carduus Benedictus, Zedoary, Gayac, Angelica, &c. are of the Number of *Hidroticks*, or *Hidrotic* Medicines. The Word is composed of the *Greek*, ιδρος, *Sweat.*

**HIERA PICRA**, in Pharmacy, a Kind of Electuary, first described by *Galen*; composed of Aloes, Cinnamon, Mace, Asarabacca, Spicanardi, Saffron, Mastic, Honey. It is used to purge and cleanse the Stomach; remove Obstructions, promote the Menses and Haemorrhoids, and sweeten the Blood. Tho' its chief Use among us, is in making the *Tinctura sacra.*

It is denominated from the *Greek*, ιερος, *sacer*, holy, by Reason of its rare Virtues; and πικρος, *amarus*, bitter; Aloes, which is the Base thereof, rendering it extremely bitter.

There is another *Hiera*, call'd *Hiera Diacolocynthidos Pachii*, by Reason *Colocynthis* is the Base thereof, and that it was first used with good Success by *Pachius* of *Antioch*, in divers obstinate Diseases. It is composed of *Colocynthis, Opoponax, Aristolochia rotunda, Agaric,* and other Ingredients.

It is used in Epilepsies, Apoplexies, Palsies, and Lethargies, to excite the Menses, and promote the Expulsion of the After-birth.

There is also a third Sort of *Hiera*, call'd *Liberanus*; but rarely used. Dr. *Quincy* says, 'tis one of the most ridiculous Medleys ever contrived. It passes for a Cordial, &c.

**HIPPOMANES**, a Sort of Poison, famous among the Antients as an ingredient in amorous Philters, or Charms. The Word is *Greek*, ιπομανες, compounded of ιππος, *Equus*, Horse, and μανια, *Fury, Madness.*

Naturalists are not agreed about the Nature of the *Hippomanes*. *Pliny* describes it as a blackish Caruncle, found on the Head of a new born Colt; which the Dam bites off, and eats, assoon as she is delivered. He adds, that if she be prevented herein by any others cutting it off before, she will not take to, nor bring up, the young.

*Servius*[1] and *Columella*[2] describe it as a poisonous Matter, trickling from the *Pudendum* of a Mare, when proud, or longing for a Horse.

At the End of Mons. *Bayle's*[3] Dictionary, is a very learned Dissertation on the *Hippomanes*; and all its Virtues both real and pretended.

[1] Maurus Servius Honoratus (ca. late 4th cent.), a Roman scholar.

[2] Lucius Junius Moderatus Columella (ca. 4 – 70), a Roman scholar.

[3] Pierre Bayle (1647 – 1706), a Huguenot scholar.

**HIPPUS**, in Medicine, an Affection of the Eyes, wherein they continually shake and tremble; and thus represent Objects as if continually fluctuating. It is this called from the *Greek*, ιππος, *Horse*; in regard the Objects appear to shift as much as when we are riding. *Blanchard.*

**HONEY**, *Mel*, a sweet sort of Juice suck'd from Vegetables by Bees, and reposited in their Combs. *Honey* is properly one of the Juices afforded by the Flowers, and is found to exude from all Sorts thereof; the very bitterest, as Aloes and Colocynth, not excepted.

In all Male flowers that have Utricles at the Bottom of the Petals, is found a viscid, ruddy, sweet Juice in good Plenty; whence it is, that we see the Children gather Cowslips, Fox-gloves, *Honey*-suckles, &c. and suck the *Honey* from them. The Bees too visit these Flowers; and putting in their Proboscides, or Trunks, suck out the *Honey-Juice*, and load their Stomachs therewith; to be afterwards discharg'd and laid up in their Combs : So that Honey is a vegetable Substance.

In the Belly of the Bee is a small transparent Bladder, which is the proper Receptacle of the *Honey* : When the Animal finds this full, it returns, enters one of the Cells, and discharges it there by that Part of the Head situate between the two Jaws, which it extends wide than ordinary, moving its Head at the same time this way and that. If a Drop happen to be ill plac'd, it sucks it up again by its Proboscis, and discharges it a-new. When a Cell is fill'd with *Honey*, they stop it up with Wax for Winter Store.

*Honey* was anciently taken for a Dew that fell or descended on the Flowers; but what proves this a Mistake, is, that the Bees only gather it after the Sun is up, when there is no Dew left : It must therefore be either a Liquor prepar'd in the Flower, and excreted by its roper Vessels, like Manna.

Or rather, it appears to be the fine Dust, or Farina Fecundans of the Apices. For, according to the Observations of M. *du Vernay*, the Bees, when in the Search of *Honey*, fix on no other Parts but the Stamina and Apices, and not on such as yield any other Liquor.

What is very remarkable, is, that Honey, in Virtue of its vegetable Nature, is discover'd by M. *Lemery* to contain Iron; which Discovery may serve as an Answer to M. *Geoffroy's* Chymical Question, *viz.* Whether there is any Part of a Plant without Iron? For if so delicate an Extract from the finest Part of the Flower, and this further elaborated in the little Viscera of the Insect, be not void of Iron, we may despair of seeing any so.

We have two Kinds of *Honey*, *white* and *yellow*. The white, call'd also *Virgin Honey*, trickles out spontaneously from the Comb, by turning it up or breaking it.

The second is squeez'd from the Combs in a Press, after having first soften'd them with a little Water over the Fire. Here is also an intermediate Sort, of a yellowish white Colour, drawn by Expression, without Fire.

The *Honey* left to stand two or three Days, purges itself; throwing up a Scum of Wax and other Dross, which is to be taken off.

Some Naturalists will have the *Honey* to be of a different Quality, according to the Difference of the Flowers, or Plants the Bees suck it from. Accordingly *Strabo* relates, that there is a Kind of Honey in Pontus, which is a string Poison; being procur'd by Bees which feed upon Aconite and Wormwood.

F. *Lamberti*[1], in his Account of the *Mingrelia*, assures us of the contrary; and affirms it the best *Honey* in the World, by reason of the great Quantity of Bawm growing there. He adds, that there is another very white Kind of *Honey*, hard as Sugar, and which does not stick to the Hands.

*Honey* has considerable medicinal Virtues; being reputed a good Detergent and Cleanser; and in that Quality used both internally and externally, for the Viscera, Wounds, Ulcers, &c.

*Honey* is the Base of several Compositions in Pharmacy. Of *Honey*, with the Addition of Roses or Violets, Mercurialis, &c. is made *Mel Rosatum, Mercuriale*, &c.

There is also a *Mel Scilliticum*, or a Preparation of Squillæ : *Mel Passulatum Violatum*, made with Raisins boil'd in hot Water : And *Mel Anthosatum*, made of Rosemary Flowers.

*Honey* is also an Ingredient in several Drinks, as *Mum, Metheglin*, &c. The Ancients rank'd Sugar and Manna among the Species of *Honey*. The Chymists also draw a Water, a Spirit, an Oil, &c. from *Honey*.

*Wild* **HONEY**. *S. Adauman*[2], Abbot of *Hii*, in his Description of the holy Places, observes, that in the Place where St. John Baptist liv'd in the Desart, there are Locusts which the poor People boil with Oil, and a Sort of Herbs with large long Leaves, of a Milk Colour, and a Taste like that of Honey; and that this is what in Scripture is call'd *wild Honey*.

**HONEY-DEW**, is a sweet-tasted Dew, found early in the Morning on the Leaves of divers Sorts of Plants.

*Honey-Dews*, or *Mildews*, are of a very different Nature from Blastings, being caus'd by the condensing of a fat moist Exhalation, rais'd in a hot dry Summer, from Plants and Blossoms; as also from the Earth; which, by the Coolness and Serenity of the Air in the Night, or in the upper clear Region of the Air, is thicken'd into a fat gluey Matter, and falls to the Earth again; Part whereof rests upon Oak Leaves, and some other Trees, whose Leaves are smooth, and do not easily admit the Moisture into them.

*Gassendus* holds, that a viscid Juice transpiring out of the Leaves, helps to compose this *Honey*, or to concert the Dew falling on them into a *Honey* Substance, which before had nothing of it : And hence he accounts for the Reason why we find it on some Trees, and not others.

This *Honey-Dew* falling on the Ears and Stalks of Wheat, besmears them with a different Colour from the natural; and being of a clammy Substance, so binds up the young, tender, and close Ears of the Wheat, by the Heat of the Sun, that it prevents the Growth and Compleating of the perfect Grain therein. A Shower of Rain succeeding presently after the Fall thereof, or the Wind blowing stiffly, are the only natural Remedies against it.

[1] Arcangelo Lamberti (ca. 1610 – 1660), an Italian Christian missionary.

[2] This is probably St. Adamnan (624 – 704), an Irish monk and Abbot of Iona (aka Hii).

**HOP**, or Hops, a Plant of the reptile Kind, whose Flower is a principal Ingredient in Beer, and other Malt Liquors.

The *Hop* creeps like Snake-weed, unless it find Pales or Shrubs to hand to; or unless they who cultivate it, plant Poles for the Purpose. Its Stem is long, flexible, rough, and hairy. Its Leaf indented like that of the Vine and cover'd with a kind of prickly Down like that of the Cucumber. Its Flowers are of a greenish Yellow, resembling, both as to Form and Size, those of the Female Elm; and grow in a kind of Bunch or Cluster. In this Flower is a blackish bitter Grain contain'd, which the Seed of the *Hop*.

In the Spring time, while the Bud is yet tender, the Tops of the Plant being cut off, and boil'd, are eat like Asparagus; and found effectual to loosen the Body : The Heads and Tendrils are good to purity the Blood in the Scorbutus, and most cutaneous Diseases : Decoctions of the Flowers, and Syrops thereof, are of use against pestilential Fevers : Juleps and Apozems are also prepar'd with *Hops*, for Hypochondriacal and Hysterical Affections, and to promote the Menses.

**HORDEATUM**, a liquid Medicine, made of Barley, beat and boil'd with other suitable Ingredients.

**HORDEOLUM**, in Medicine, a small Tubercle arising on the Palpebræ or Eye-lids. It is thus call'd from the *Latin, Hordeum*, Barley, as resembling a Barley Corn. The Cure of the *Hordeolum* and *Grando*, is by Discutients and Suppuratives.

**HART'S-HORN**, *Cornu Corvi*. The Scrapings or Raspings of the Horn of this Animal are medicinal, and used in Astringent Draughts, Ptisans, &c. with that Intention. It yields by Distillation a very penetrative volatile Spirit.

**HUMECTATION**, Moistening, in Pharmacy, the preparing of a Medicine, by steeping it a while in Water, in order to soften and moisten it when too dry, to cleanse it, or to prevent its subtile Parts from being dissipated in grinding it, or the like. The Term is also us'd for the Application of moistening or suppling Remedies. In this Sense we say, Embrocations, Emplasters, Unctions, *Humectations*, Fomentations, &c. The Word is *Latin, Humectatio*, of *Humor*, Moisture.

**HUMID**, Humidum, *moist*. The School of Philosophers make Water the *primum Humidium*, the first of humid Bodies, and the Cause or Principle of Humidity in others, which are more or less moist, as they partake more or less of this Element.

**HUMIDITY**, or Moisture, the Quality or Power of wetting or moistening other Bodies.

*Aristotle* defines *Humidity*, by a passive Quality which indisposes a Body from being retain'd in its own Bounds, but make sit easily retain'd in those of another : which amounts to the same as his Definition of Fluidity.

Others of the *Peripatetick* School, make *Humidity* a Quality whereby a Body is *humid*, *i.e.* moistens other Bodies, and, in moistening, softens and disposes them to receive any Figure or Impression.

The modern Writers consider *Humidity* as a particular Species of Fluidity; and define it a Fluor, which being apply'd in a solid Body, adheres thereto, and communicates the Quality to other Bodies. Others, somewhat more accurately call *Humidity* the Power whereby a Body moistens another : But what that Power is, they do not shew.

But of this we are certain, that *Humidity* is no more than a Sort of relative Mode. So far as the component Particles of a Fluid, compar'd with respect to the Pores and Particles of other Bodies, or the Texture thereof, are apt and dispos'd to enter those Pores, or stick to those Particles; so far is that Fluid *humid* : On the contrary, so far as there is a Repugnance or Incongruity between the Particles, &c. in respect of such Bodies, the Fluid is not *humid*.

Thus Quicksilver is not moist in respect to our Hands or Cloaths, and other Things, which it will not stick to; but it may be call'd *humid* in reference to Gold, Tin, or Lead, to whose Surfaces it will presently adhere, and render them soft and moist.

Even Water itself, which wets almost every thing, and is the great Standard of Moisture and *Humidity*, is not capable of wetting all Things; for it stands, or runs off in globular Drops on the Leaves of Cabbages, and many other Plants; and it will not wet the Feathers of Ducks, Swans, and other Water-Fowl.

Add, that the Texture alone may cause the Fluid to be *humid*, as is plain, in that neither Quicksilver along, Lead, or Bismuth, will stick upon Glass; yet being mix'd together, they will form a Mass that will do so; as appears from such a Composition being frequently us'd in foliating Looking-Glasses.

**HUMIDIUM** *Radicale*, or *Radical Moisture*. This, in reality, seems to amount to no more than the purest and most defecate Part of the nutritious Matter, in a Condition ready to be assimilated. By too much Heat, as in Fevers, Hectics, &c. this *Humidity* is too hastily exhausted and spent.

**HUMOUR**, in Medicine, is apply'd to any Juice, or fluid Part of the Body, as the *Chyle, Blood, Milk, Fat, Serum, Lymph, Spirits, Bile, Seed, Salival*, and *Panchreatic* Juices, &c.

The four Humours so much talk'd of by the ancient Philosophers, are four liquid Substances, which they suppose to moisten the whole Body of all Animals, and to be the Cause of the divers Temperaments thereof. These are Phlegm, *Pituita, Blood, Bile*, and *Melancholy*.

But the Moderns do not allow of these Divisions. The *Humours* they rather chuse to distinguish into *Nutritious*, or *Alimentary*, as *Chyle* and *Blood*; those separate from the Blood, as *Bile, Saliva, Urine*, &c. and those return'd into the Blood.

*Humours*, again, are distinguish'd into *natural* or salutary, and *morbid* or corrupted. To the former Class belong all the Juices ordinarily secreted for the Uses of the Body.

To the latter belong those compound *Humours* which thicken, and grow putrid; causing Tumors, Abscesses, Obstructions, and most Diseases.

These are distinguish'd by various Names, *Malignant, Adust, Acrimonious,*

*Corrosive, Crude, Peccant*, &c.

**HUMOUR** is also us'd for the particular Temperament or Constitution of a Person, consider'd as arising from the Prevalence of this or that *Humour*, or Juice of the Body. Thus we say, a Bilious Coleric *Humour*; a Phlegmatic *Humour*; a Melancholic, Restless, Hypochondriac *Humour*; a Sanguine, Gay, Sprightly *Humour*, &c.

**HUNGARY WATER**, *Aqua Hungarica*, a distill'd Water, denominated from a Queen of Hungary, for whose Use it was first prepar'd. *Hungary Water* is one of the distill'd Waters of the Shops; and is directed in the College Dispensatory, to be made of Rosemary Flowers infus'd some Days in rectify'd Spirit of Wine, and thus distill'd. Its Virtues are much the same as those of the Simple it is drawn from.

**HYACINTH**, or Jacinth, in Natural History, a precious Stone; thus call'd from its Resemblance of the Purple Flower nam'd *Hyacinth*.

There are four Sorts of *Hyacinths* : those intermix'd with a Vermillion Colour; those of a Saffron Colour; those of an Amber Colour; and, lastly, those of a white, intermix'd with a slight red.

*Hyacinths*, again, are distinguished into Oriental and Occidental. The Oriental come from *Calicut* and *Cambaya*, and are equal in Hardness to the Oriental Amethyst. The Occidental are found in *Bohemia* and *Portugal*, which are a Degree softer.

The Stone graves or cuts fine, and would be more us'd for Seals, &c. but that the Graving frequently costs more than the Stone.

The Antients us'd it for Amulets and Talismans; and bore it about their Neck, or set in Rings, &c. supposing it to have the Virtue of securing them from the Plague, &c.

The *Hyacinth* us'd in Medicine, and whereof the Confection of *Hyacinth* is made, is a different Stone, of which there are three several Sorts : The first about the Bigness and Figure of a Grain of Salt, and pretty soft : The 2d ruddy, and shap'd like the Point of a Diamond, found in divers Parts of *Italy, Silesia, Bohemia*, &c. The third is white, intermix'd with yellow, and some other Colours; being found in the same Places as the red.

In Strictness, only the first Kind should be us'd in the Confection of *Hyacinth*; but the Druggists and Apothecaries frequently substitute the other.

*Confection of Hyacinth*, is a thin cordial Electuary, compos'd of divers Kinds of precious Stones, particularly of that whose Denomination it bears, with certain Earths, Seeds, Roots, Coral, Hartshorn, and divers other Ingredients, well mix'd, and ground together.

**HYDATIS**, in Medicine, a Disease of the Eyes, consisting of a fatty Substance or Excrescence, growing under the Skin of the upper Eye-lid; by which the whole Eye-lid, in Children, is sometimes render'd Oedematous. *Hydatis* is also us'd, among the modern Physicians, for a little Bladder of Water, occasionally found in divers Parts of the Body.

**HYDATIDES**, in Medicine, a little transparent Bags or Bladders full of Water, frequently found in divers Parts of the Body. The Word is form'd of the *Greek*, υδωρ, Water, which in the genitive Case, gives υδατος, whence υδατις, *Hydatis*.

*Hydatides* are most common in dropsical Persons, and are suppos'd to arise from a Distention and Rupture of the Lymphæ-ducts; being found chiefly in the Parts abounding in those Vessels, as the Liver, Lungs, &c. They are also sometimes found in Icterical Cases.

We have Instances of *Hydatides* voided both by Stool, by Urine, and by Vomiting. They are of all Sizes, from a Pin's Head to a Pullet's Egg.

**HYDRAGOGUES**, a Species of purgative Medicines; being such as are suppos'd peculiarly fitted to discharge serous, or water Humours. In the general, all sudorific, aperitive, and diuretic Medicines, are *Hydragogues*. The Word is form'd of υδως, Water, and αγειν, to draw, to lead.

The strongest Catharticks, Dr. *Quincy* observes, chiefly answer to the Character of *Hydragogues*; in that by their forcible shaking and vellicating the Bowels and their Appendages, they squeeze out Water enough to make the Stools appear little else.

The principal *Hydragogues*, on the common Opinion, are the Juices of Elder, of the Roots of Iris, of Soldanella, Mechoacan, Jalap, &c.

**HYDRARGYRUM**, a Name the Chymists give to Mercury or Quick silver. The Word is Greek, form'd of υδως, *aqua*, Water, and αργυρος, argentums, Silver, *q.d.* Water of Silver, by reason of its resembling liquid or melted Silver.

**HYDRELÆON**, or Hydrelæum, in Pharmacy, a Mixture of common Oil and Water. *Hydrelæon* taken internally excites Vomiting; externally, it is Anodyne, and promotes Suppuration. The Word is compounded of the *Greek*, υδως, *aqua*, Water, and ελαιον, *Oleum*, Oil.

**HYDRENTEROCELE**, in Medicine, a Hernia, or Tumor occasion'd by a Descent of the Intestines, and Water along with them, into the Scrotum. The Word is compounded of υδως, Water; εντωρον, Intestine; and κηλη, Tumor.

**HYDROCELE**, in Medicine, a Swelling or Bloating of the outer Integument or Skin of the Scrotum, occasion'd by watery Humours cast or detain'd therein. The Word is form'd of the *Greek*, υδως, *aqua*, and κηλη, Tumor.

The *Hydrocele* is distinguish'd from an Hernia or Descent, in that the first is form'd by slow Degrees, and the latter all at once.

Youth is most expos'd to the *Hydrocele*. It is cur'd by drying Medicines; or by letting out the Water with a Lancet, a Seton, or the like. But these only amount to a palliative Cure : To go to the Bottom of the Disease, recourse must be had to Cauteries.

**HYDROCEPHALUS**, or Hydrocephale, in Medicine, a watery Head, or Dropsy in the Head. The *Hydrocephalus* is a Congestion of Water in the

Head, so as to distend and render it soft. The Word is *Greek*, form'd of υδως, Water, and κεραλη, *Caput*, Head.

There are three Kinds of *Hydrocephali*. The first, when the Water is gather'd between the Skull and the Skin : The second, when between the Skull and the Brain : And the third, when the Water is collected in the Ventricles of the Brain.

Children are more liable to *Hydrocephali*, than Adults; by reason their Head is soft, and has been much compress'd in the Womb; or, perhaps, by their having been too roughly handed by the Midwife. Add, that the Bones of Childrens Heads being very soft, and their Sutures not yet exactly clos'd; they easily open, and give Way to an Influx of Water from without; whereas in Adults, the Bones of the Cranium are very hard, and closely bound together.

The *Hydrocephalus* is a Disease very difficult to cure. There is no Remedy but by serve blistering on the Sutures. It sometimes ends in mortal Convulsions, and sometimes in Lethargies or Apoplexies.

The Head, in this Case, is sometimes extended to a prodigious Bulk; so that the Person cannot bear or sustain it. Of this we have an extraordinary Instance given us by Dr. *Freind*, of a Girl two Years old, whose Head was 26 Inches in Circumference. *Philosoph. Transact.* No. 318.

**HYDROMEL**, a Drink made of Water, and Honey; call'd by the *Greeks* μελικροτον. The Word is compos'd of υδωρ, Water, and μελι, *Mel*, Honey.

*Hydromel* is Honey diluted with a sufficient Quantity of Water, and fermented by a long and gentle Heat. Under the Class of *Hydromels* come out Mead, and Metheglin. *Hydromel* is either *Simple*, call'd also aqueous, where Honey and Water are the only Ingredients, which may be prepar'd at any Time; or *Compound*, when other Drugs are added, to improve and exalt the Flavour and Virtues.

'Tis particularly call'd *Vinous Hydromel*, when it equals the Strength of Wine; which it is brought to do, not only by the great Quantity of Honey us'd in it, but also by its long Coction, Insolation, &c. This is only made in the Heat of Summer.

*Vinous Hydromel*, (the same with what we otherwise call Mead, &c.) is made of Rain Water and the best Honey boil'd together, and skum'd from Time to Time till they become of a Consistence to sustain an Egg. This done, the Liquor is expos'd to the Sun for 40 Days, to dispose it to ferment; then, adding some *Spanish* Wine, and keeping it two or three Months, it acquires a Flavour scarce inferior to Malmsey. It fuddles readily; and the drunken Fit holds longer than that produc'd by Wines, by reason of its more viscid Consistence.

*Hydromel* is the common Drink of the *Poles* and *Russians*, *Diodorus Siculus*, lib. V. and *Aristotle*, relate, that the *Celtiberi* and *Taulantii*, ancient People of *Illyria*, drank *Hydromel* instead of Wine.

**HYDROMPHALUS**, in Medicine, a Tumor in the Navel, arising from a Collection of Water. The *Hydromphalus* is discuss'd by emollient and resolutive medicines. It is also cur'd by a Puncture made in the Middle of the Navel. The Word is form'd of the Greek υδωρ, Water, and ομφαλος, *umbilicus*, Navel.

**HYDROPHOBIA**, in Medicine, an Aversion or Dread of Water; a Symptom arising in person bitten by a mad Dog, or other Beast. Tho' the Term *Hydrophobia* do, in Strictness, only denote this one Symptom; yet it is frequently apply'd to the whole Disease consequent on such Bite, with all its Symptoms. The Word is *Greek*, compounded of υδωρ, Water, and φοβος, *Timor*, Fear, of φοβουμαι, *timeo*, I fear.

The History of this horrible Disease, as given by *Coelius Aurelianus*, Dr. *Mead*[1], *Etmuller*, *Lister*, &c. is as follows : The Bite of mad Dog is attended with this surprizing Circumstance, that its Effects frequently do not discover themselves till after the Cause is forgot; the Wound itself closing and healing like any other common Wound. But, some time after, direful Symptoms ensue : Usually they commence in about forty Days; sometimes in sixty, sometimes not till six Months, and sometimes not till a Year, or even two.

The first Thing observ'd, is a wandering Pain throughout the whole Body, but chiefly about the wounded Part : The Patient grows anxious and melancholly, and very prone to Anger; complaining of every Thing, as the ambient Air, the Heaviness of his Bed Cloaths, &c. He vomits; his Pulse intermits, and somewhat of a Tremor is observ'd, with Convulsions of the Nerves and Tendons : Along with these he feels an inward Heat and Thirst : At last the grand Symptom appears, which denominates the Disease, *viz.* the *Aquæ Pavor*, or Dread of Water, so that he cannot bear so much as the Sight of any Liquid, without the utmost Consternation; much less can he swallow the smallest Drop. This is the Pathogenomic Sign of the Disease's being come to its Height; and never happens till two or three Days before the Patient's Death; the Disease being then, by the unanimous Consent of both ancient and modern Physicians, absolutely incurable.

With this there are other concomitant Symptoms. He foams at the Mouth, his Eyes stare, he cannot swallow his Spittle without Pain, and his Penis is constantly erected : Some bark and snarl like Dogs, and actually fancy themselves transform'd into those Creatures, and, in the Height of their Madness, are ready to fly upon and tear to Pieces the By-standers. *Palmarius*[2] observes, that the *Hydrophobous* Patient cannot bear to look in a Glass, or any transparent Body : And that he never recovers, unless he know himself in a Glass; this being a Sign that the Poison has not yet laid hold of the vital Parts.

It may be added, that the *Hydrophobia* is not only occasion'd by the Bite of a mad Dog, but also of other Brutes, as Cats, Foxes, Wolves, Horses, Mules, Bullocks, and even Cocks, &c. or of a Man in the like Condition.

Nor is any Bite or Wound at all necessary; the Saliva of a mad Dog, &c. being apt to convey the Disease be mere Contact, or Application to the Skin. Thus, we have an Instance in the *Philosophical Transactions*, of two Men catching the Disease by putting their fingers in the Mouth of a Puppy that had been bit by its mad Dam, and feeling its Tongue and Throat : And the like

[1] Richard Mead (1630 – 1699), an English physician.

[2] Petrus Palmarius, born Pierre le Paulmier (1568 – 1610), a French physician.

Instance we have in the same Work, of two Children in *Ireland*, who, by touching and handling the head of a Dog that had been bit by a mad Dog, and washing the Wound, cur'd the Dog, but caught the Disease themselves.

*For the Nature and Cause of Hydrophobia*; Dr. *Mead*, from several Histories of particular Cases, concludes that the *Hydrophobia* is the Effect of a particular Kind of Inflammation of the Blood, accompany'd with so great a Tension and Dryness of the nervous Membranes, and such an Elasticity and Force of the Fluid with which they are fill'd, that the most common Representations are made to the Mind with too great Effect; so that the usual Impressions on the Organs cannot be suffer'd. Hence that Timorousness, unaccountable Anxiety, and Disquietude, which are always the Forerunners of the Dread of Liquids; as also, the Pain often felt in making of Water, and the strange Aversions sometimes found in Patients at the Sight of any thing white, the Retina being hurt and griev'd by the lively Impressions of that Colour thereon. Nor it is hard to conceive, that when the Saliva is hot, and the Throat inflam'd and dry, the Swallowing of Drink should cause such an intolerable Agony.

M. *Tauvry*, from a nice Dissection and Examen of the Parts of a Person dead hereof, conjectures, that the Saliva and Bile are the Fluids first infected; and that the Patient vomiting a Mixture hereof, the Throat becomes excoriated thereby; and hence that Horror for all Foods, and particularly Water, in regard this dissolves those grievous Salts constrain'd in the Saliva and Bile. He adds, That the Nature of the Poison is such, as dissolves the balsamic and nutritious Part of the Blood, whence the Veins are dry'd up, so as not to admit any Blood from the Arteries; and the Arterial Blood by this means sustaining the Action and Impression of its Vessels for so long a Time, is still further dissolv'd, attenuated, and spiritualiz'd, and thus sent, in too great Quantity, and with too great Rapidity, to the Brain; whence those Convulsions, Distractions, &c.

Dr. *Lister*, from the remarkable History of *J. Corton*, whom he attended under this Disease, concludes, 1°. That some of the organic Parts of his Body were actually transform'd into, or affected after the Nature of a Dog, especially the Gula, Tongue, &c. so that any Fluid offer'd him in the erect Posture of a Man, was frightful, as well as difficult to take, as much as it would be for us to get a Dog to drink standing on his hind Legs. But this was not all; for when he was turn'd on his Belly, and would have acted the Dog, he could not drink; tho' the Sight of the Liquor in that Posture gave him as much Pleasure as in the other Posture it did Pain; and tho' he frequently put out his Tongue, and lapp'd, yet he could not endure to take any Thing liquid into his Mouth, as tho' something hinder'd him within. 2°. That his Spittle was envenom'd; for as oft as he swallow'd it, his Stomach vehemently abhorring it, it went to his Heart, as he said, and was present Death to him : And so Liquid Things coming nearer to the Consistence of Spittle, might give him the greater Terror, as they tended to promote the Discharge of Saliva into his Mouth; and for the same Reason might be more difficult to swallow than solid Things.

*As to the Cure of the Hydrophobia*, Dr. *Mead*, after *Galen*, recommends it, in this as in other venomous Cases, to enlarge the Wound by a circular Incision, to apply a Cautery to it, and to keep it open for at least forty Days.

But if this Method seem too cruel, it may suffice to extract the Poison by clasping a Cupping glass in the Place, having first made a deep Scarification. The Doctor adds, he has known a Person fresh bitten, happily sav'd by the sole Application of the *Unguentum Ægyptiacum* exceedingly hot.

If these external Precautions have not been us'd, or not in Time, recourse must be had to internal Remedies : Alexipharmicks must be drank; among which, the Ashes of River Lobsters, or Cray Fish, are principally extoll'd by all the ancient Physicians; so that *Galen* affirms, no Body had ever dy'd who used this Remedy. These Ashes to be taken to the Quantity of one or two Spoonfulls every Day for forty Days successively, either alone, or with Gentian Root and Frankincense in Wine.

But the frequent and sudden plunging of the Patient over the Head and Ears in the Salt Sea Water, is the best and surest Preservative against this Disease.

*Etmuller* recommends Cardiacks and Alexipharmachicks, but all in a double Dose, and long continu'd; and Garlic, Rue, and Salt to be eat together, and apply'd in form of a Cataplasm over the Wound. Purging with Hellebore and *Mercurius Dulcis* is also good; and Cantharides are a Sort of Specific. Scarifying is commended; and after the Scarrification, an Onion roasted under the Ashes, to be apply'd. But the readiest Remedy, he adds, is burning the Place affected with a red hot Iron, which effectually removes all the Malignity. If the Physician be not call'd till late, a Cupping-glass is to be apply'd very hot : An Issue near the Place may likewise be of Service.

Sir *Theod. Mayerne* gives the following Prescriptions for the Bite of a mad Dog. Pluck the Feathers from the Breech of an old Cock, and apply it bare to the Bite : If the Dog were mad, the Cock will swell and die, and the Person bitten will do well : If the Cock dies not, the Dog was not mad. *Philosoph. Transact.* No. 191.

'Tis a common Notion, that a Hair of the same Dog apply'd on the Bite, attracts the Venom, and works a Cure ; But a Physician of *Rostoch*, in a formal Dissertation some Years ago, prov'd this a popular Error; and that the Remedy was more like to do harm than good.

The Marks whereby to know that a Dog is mad, are, his neither eating nor drinking, foaming at the Mouth and Nostrils, looking sad and sullen, and running at anything in his Way, whether Man or Beast, known or unknown, without barking. *Baldus*, a famous Lawyer, dy'd of the *Hydrophobia* four Months after his being bit in the Lip by a little Dog. And the same is said of *Diogenes* the Cynic.

The Members of the Royal Academy of Sciences, furnish us with various Instances of Persons cur'd of the Disease by various Means. M. *Poupart* mentions a Woman perfectly recover'd by bleeding her to a Deliquium, binding her in a Chair for a Year, and feeding her all that Time with Bread and Water. M. *Berger*[1] relates, that of several Persons bitten, two were cur'd by bleeding them in the Forehead. M. *du Hamel* adds, that he has known Salt Water apply'd on the Wound effect a Cure. Divers Cases are produc'd of those cur'd of the *Aquæ Pavor*, by being overwhelm'd with a great Quantity of

[1] This may be Johann Gottfried Berger (1659 – 1736), a German physician.

Water; and one, by being only ty'd to a Tree, and 200 Pails of Water thrown on him. But the best Instance is that of M. *Morin*. A Maid of twenty Years of Age having all the Symptoms, was bath'd in a Tub of River Water wherein a Bushel of Salt had been dissolv'd. They plunged her naked again and again, till, harass'd almost to Death, they left her in it quite senseless. When she came to herself, she was supriz'd to find herself looking at the Water without any Concern. *Histoire del Acad. An.* 1709.

**HYDROPIC**, a dropsical Patient; or a Person swell'd and bloated with the Abundance of Water or Wind. The Word is form'd of υδωρ, Water, and οψς, *Facies*, Face.

**HYDROPS**, in medicine. See Dropsy.

**HYDROPS** *ad Matulam*, a Term sometimes used for a Diabetes.

**HYDROPOTES**, in Medicines, are such as drink nothing but Water. It has long been controverted among Physicians, whether or no the *Hydropotes* live longer than other Persons. The Word is *Greek*, υδιροποτες, of υδωρ, Water, and ποτης, *Potor*, Drinker, of πινω, *bibo*, I drink.

**HYGIEINIA**, that Branch of Medicine which considers *Health*; and discovers proper Means and Remedies, with their Use, in the Prevention and Recovery of that State. The Word is *Greek*, Υγεινη, of υγης, sound, healthy. The Objects of this Branch of Medicine are the Non-Naturals.

*Hygieina* may be divided into three Parts; *Prophylactice*, which serves and prevents Diseases; *Synteritice*, employ'd in preserving Health; and *Analeptice*, whose Office is to cure Diseases, and restore Health.

**HYGROCYRSOCELE**, in Medicine, a Branch of a Vein swell'd with ill Blood, or other Humours. The Word is compos'd of υγρος, *humidus*, and κυρσοκηλη, or rather κιρσοκηλη, *ramex varicosus*.

**HYPERCATHARSIS**, in Medicine, Super-purgation; a too violent and excessive Purgation. The Word is compounded of the *Greek*, υπερ, supra, and καθαριζω, I purge.

**HYPERCRISIS**, in Medicine, am immediate critical Excretion. Thus when a Fever terminates in a Looseness, the Humours sometimes flow off faster than the Strength can bear, and are therefore to be check'd. This is a *Hypercrisis*. The Word is compounded of υπερ, *supra*, and κρισις, *Crisis*, Judgement.

**HYPERSARCOSIS**, in Medicine and Chirurgery, an Excess of Flesh; or rather, a fleshy Excrescence, such as those generally arising on the Lips of Wounds, &c.

**HYPNOTICK**, in Medicine, a Remedy which promotes or induces Sleep; call'd also *Soporific*, *Opiate*, &c. The Word comes from the Greek υπνος, *somnus*, Sleep.

**HYPOCHYMA**, or Hypochysis, in Medicine, a Disease of the Eyes, popularly call'd Cataracts. The Word is *Greek*, υποκαυςον, which literally denotes shedding, Effusion, or pouring out; the Disease having formerly been suppos'd to arise from an Effusion of some viscid Humours upon the Pupil.

**HYPOCYSTIS**, in Medicine, a Juice, us'd in the Composition of Treacle, &c. The Word is *Greek*, form'd of υπο, under, κιςος, *Cistus*.

The *Hypocystis* is the Juice, of a Shoot of the same Name, sprouting out from the Foot of a kind of Citrus Tree, call'd *Laudanum*; common enough in the hot Countries.

The Shoot grows about a Foot high; and one, two, or three Inches thick; somewhat bigger at Top than at Bottom; soft, succulent, of a yellowish Colour, and surrounded from Space to Space with a Sort of Rings, or brownish Knots.

When gather'd, they pound it in a Mortar, and express the Juice : That done, they evaporate it on the Fire till it come to the Consistence of a hard blackish Extract, like *Spanish* Liquorice. Then they make it up into little Cakes for Carriage.

It is of a tart astringent Taste, and us'd to stop Fluxes of the Belly, Vomitings, and Hæmorrhages; tho' anciently much more than at present. It is also an Ingredient in Treacle, and some Unguents. It is sometimes us'd as a Substitute to Acacia. Dr. *Quincy* says, it is the more powerful of the two.

**HYPOCONDRIAC** *Disease*, *Affection*, or *Passion*, is the same with what we popularly call the Spleen, Vapours, &c. The *Hypocondriac* is a very comprehensive Disease : It is variously denominated, according to the various Symptoms it is attended with, and the various Parts where it is suppos'd to be seated, or in which it arises.

When conceiv'd as situate in the *Hypocondriac* Regions, or arising from some Disorder of the Parts contain'd therein, *viz.* the Spleen, Liver, &c. it is properly call'd the *Hypocondriacal Disease, Spleen*, &c.

When conceiv'd as owing to some Disorder of the Womb, it is call'd *Hysteric Affection*, &c. And lastly, when the flatulent Rumblings in the Intestines, Belches, &c. are consider'd, it is call'd the *Vapours*.

The *Hypocondriac* is a very common and obstinate Disease : Few Men of a sedentary Life, and fewer Women, are free from it : Its Symptoms are very numerous : The most usual, are a pain in the Stomach, Windiness, Vomitings, a Swelling or Distension of the *Hypocondrium's* or upper Part of the Belly, Noises and Rumblings in the lower Venter, wandering Pains, a Constriction of the Breast, Difficulty of Breathing, Palpitation of the Heart, Fear, Suspicions, Melancholy, Deliriums, &c. Not that all these Accidents befall every Person seiz'd with this Disease; but sometimes some of them, and at other Times others, according to the Constitution, &c. of the Patient.

In effect, the *Hypocondriacal* is a very vague, indeterminate Sort of Disorder. Dr. *Sydenham* observes, that its Symptoms ape or emulate those of most other Diseases; and that whatever Part it is in, it produces somewhat like the common Diseases of that Part. Thus, in the Head, it produces a Sort of Apoplexy; Fits like the Epilepsy, call'd *Hysteric* Fits; intolerable Head-ach, &c. In Persons affected with the Chlorosis, it produces a Palpitation of the Heart; sometimes, tho' rarely, it seizes the Lungs, and causes a continual dry Cough : It also imitates the Cholic, and Iliac passion, and sometimes the Stone, Jaundice, &c. In the Intestines it produces a Diarrhæa; in the Stomach, Nauseas : Sometimes it seizes the external Parts, and particularly the Back, which it renders chilly and painful; and the Legs and Thighs, which it swells so as to resemble the Dropsy : Seizing the Teeth, it resembles the Scurvy (indeed, *Etmuller* makes the Scurvy itself to be only a great Degree of this Disease). Lastly, which is the most unhappy Circumstance of all, the Patient is more affected in Mind than in Body.

The Seat of this Disease is commonly suppos'd to be in the Animal Spirits, and the nervous System. Its Cause is referr'd to an acid Salt abounding in the Mass of Blood; to which the ill Disposition of the Stomach, and the other Parts contain'd in the Epigastrium, may greatly contribute. *Purcell*[1] assigns Crudities and Indigestions as the prime Cause. According to *Sydenham*, vehement Motions of the Body, or more usually violent Perturbations of the Mind, as Grief, Anger, Fear, &c. are its pro-catarctic Causes.

For the Cure, the principal Indication is to purify and strengthen the Blood, which is to be effected, after proper Evacuations, by Chalybeats, Bitters, Strengtheners, and Volatile Spirits. The Cortex has also notable Virtues in this Disease; as also a Milk Diet. Riding is admirable. *Sydenham.*

**HYPOCONDRIACAL** *Medicines*, are Remedies proper in the *Hypocondriacal Disease*. Such are those which tend to purify the Blood, Humours, and Spirits; as Chervil, Balm, Agrimony, and the other Cephalic and Cardiac Herbs : Such also are those which purge Melancholy or Attrabilis, and those which dispel Wind and Vapours; and all Medicines good for Disorders of the Nerves, particularly Vervain both Male and Female; but above all, frequent, gentle, Anodyne purges.

**HYPOCRAS**, or rather Hippocras, *Vinum Hippcraticum*, a kind of medicated Wine. *Hypocras* is a Drink or Beverage compos'd of Wine, with Spices and other Ingredients infus'd therein; much us'd among the *French* by Way of Dram after Meals. It is recommended as a Cordial, good in Paralytic, Apoplectic, and all nervous Cases.

There are various Kinds of *Hypocras*, according to the Kind of Wine, and other additional Ingredients made use of; white *Hypocras*, red *Hypocras*, Claret *Hypocras*, Strawberry *Hypocras*, *Hypocras* without Wine, Cyder *Hypocras*, &c.

That directed in out College Dispensatory, is to be made of Cloves, Ginger, Cinnamon and Nutmegs, beat, infus'd in Canary, with Sugar; to the Infusion, Milk, a Lemon, and some Slips of Rosemary to be put, and the whole strain'd thro' a Flannel.

*Menage* approves the Conjecture of those who derive *Hypocras* from

[1] John Purcell (1674 – 1730), an English physician.

*Hyppocrates*, as supposing him the Inventor hereof. Others derive the Word from the Greek, υπο and κεραννυμι, to mix.

**HYPOPYON**, in Medicine, a Diseases of the Eyes. It consists in a Collection of Pus, under or behind the Cornea; which sometimes covers the whole Pupil, and obstructs the Light. Some will have it the same with Unguis; but the more accurate make a Difference.

The *Hypopyon* arises from a Rupture of the Vessels in the Uvea; occasion'd either by some external Violence, or the Acrimony of the Blood therein. 'Tis very difficult of Cure. The Suppuration is to be prevented by proper Cataplasms; or, if these have not Effect, is to be promoted.

The Word is *Greek*, υποπυον, form'd of υπο, *sub*, under, and πυον, Pus.

**HYSSOP**, *Hyssopus*, a medicinal Herb, of a deterging cleansing Quality, and chiefly used in Diseases of the Breast and Lungs. It is a standing Ingredient in pectoral Apozems. There is also a syrup, and a simple distill'd Water from it, us'd in the Shops. It has also a Faculty to comfort and strengthen; and is prevalent against Melancholy and Phlegm. It is propagated only by Slips. Its Top and Flowers reduc'd to Powder, are by some reserv'd to strew upon the colder Sallad Herbs.

**HYSSOPIC** *Art*, a Name which *Paracelsus* gave to Chymistry, consider'd as that Art purifies Metals, Minerals &c. In Allusion to that Text in the Psalms, *Purge me with Hyssop, and I shall be clean.*

**HYSTERALGY**, in Medicine, a Pain in the Matrix or Womb, occasion'd by an Inflammation, or other Disorder therein. The Word is compounded of the *Greek*, υστερα, *Matrix*, Womb; and αλγος, *dolor*, Pain.

**HYSTERIC** *Affection*, or *Passion*, a Disease in Women, call'd also *Suffocation of the Womb*, and *Fits of the Mother*.

*Hysteric Affection* is generally used by Authors promiscuously with *Hypocondriac Affection*; the two Diseases being suppos'd to be, in reality, the same. They only differ in Point of Relations and Circumstance. The *Hysteric* is properly a Species or Branch of the Hypocondriac, peculiar to Women, and suppos'd to arise from some Disorder of the Womb.

One of the Symptoms or Effects of Hypocondriac Diseases is Convulsions, and Fits not unlike those of the Epilepsy; these we call *Hysteric* Fits; and the Disease that produces them, the *Hysteric Affection*.

The Name *Hysteric* is form'd of the *Greek*, υστερα, *Uterus*, Womb; the Patient frequently fancying a Ball rolling in the Abdomen, and sometimes rising to the Throat, which some weakly enough have attributed to an Elevation of the Womb.

It is particularly denominated *Hysteric Suffocation*, from one of its principal Symptoms, which is a Contraction of the Breast, and a Difficulty of Breathing.

Some Women under this Disorder, fancy a Rope ty'd about their Necks, ready to strangle them; and others, a Piece got into their Throats, which they cannot swallow, but stops their Breast : Some will even remain a good while as if really strangled, without any Sense or Motion.

The more common Symptoms or Accidents if this Disease, are Swimming of the Head, Dazzling of the Eyes, Inquietudes, Pains of the Abdomen, Belches, Nauseas, Vomitings, Deliriums, Convulsions. It is not always attended with all these Symptoms, but sometimes with more, and sometimes with less, and those more less violent.

Dr. *Purcel* describes a Hysteric Paroxysm, as beginning with a Sense of Coldness creeping up the Back, and afterwards spreading over the whole Body; then ensues a Head-ach, and sometimes a Palpitation of the Heart, with a fainting, from which the Patient soon recovers. Sometimes, after the Coldness, succeeds a remarkable Heat, which brings in the fore-mention'd Symptoms. *Baglivi* adds, that *Hysteric* Women feel a Sense of Cold in the Crown of the Head; and this he takes to be the chief Diagnostic of the Disease.

The ordinary causes of this Disorder are violent Passions, Rage, Love, Grief, ill News, sweet Smells, &c. As for the popular Notion of malignant Vapours rising from the Womb, and occasioning all these Symptoms; the Learned all discard it, and hold Men as subject to the Disease as Women. The real Cause is in the Animal Spirits, and the nervous System; and the Affection does not differ from the Hypocondriac.

For the Cure; as many of the Symptoms are convulsive, Antispasmodicks are indicated. During the Paroxysm, fœtid Things, whether internally or externally apply'd are of Advantage; particularly Castoreum, the Smoak of burnt Horn, or burnt Feathers held to the Nose. Volatile Spirits also help to awake the Patient out of the Paroxysm; as also tickling in the Soles of the Feet. Where 'tis severer than ordinary, recourse must be had to Punction, Scarification, Vesicatories, Causticks, &c.

**HYSTERICKS**, or Hysteric Medicines, are Remedies to remove *Hysteric* Affections; particularly Disorders of the Womb. There are divers Species of *Hystericks* : Some evacuate or cleanse the Womb, by expelling any Impurities lodg'd therein : Others tend to stop immoderate Fluxes thereof: And others strengthen the Tone of the Womb.

According to Dr. *Quincy*, *Hysteric* Affections arise either from too titillating, or too uneasy Sensations : The former proceed from that Irritation of the Nerves, which the Make and Secretion of those Parts have naturally subjected them to, and which, in some Sorts of Constitutions, arise to that Degree, as to draw the while System into Disorder, and occasion a surprizing Variety of Symptoms; *e.gr.* several Sorts of Convulsions, and Species of Madness; which therefore are by some termed *Furores Uterini.*

These Disorders seem most effectually allay'd, by such Things as are in a Manner the Reverse of Cordials, and are both in Smell and Taste very offensive and disagreeable : They seem to answer this End by suffocating, as it were, the Spirits, and damping their inordinate Sallies, so that such Stimulation ceases, and the Fibres return to their natural Tone and Motions : For as what is grateful to the Senses, gives an inexpressible Emotion to the fine nervous Filaments; so does what is foetid and is agreeable quite destroy that Emotion, and deaden it : And as the former Kind consist chiefly of fine subtile volatile Parts, by which, as before explain'd under Cephalicks, they are fitter to enter the Nerves; so these are generally of a clammy viscous Contexture, and thereby the fitter to envelope and entangle that subtile Juice; whereby its motion is much retarded, and consequently the Fibres render'd less spungy.

**ICHOR** strictly signifies a thin watery Humour, like Serum, but it is sometimes also used for a thicker kind, flowing from Ulcers. The word is originally *Greek*, and signifies *Sanies, Rottenness.*

**ICTERIC**, a Term, in Physic, apply'd to such Persons as have the Jaundice, which the *Latins* call *Icterus, Aurigo*, or *Morbus Regius. Icteric* Medicines are such as are prescribed in Cases of Jaundice. The Word is derived from the Greek ικτερος, which some derive further from ικτις, a kind of Weasel with yellow Eyes

**IODIOPATHY**, a Disease or Indisposition proper to some particular Member, or Part of the Body, not caused by any other Disease, or preceding Affection, nor having any thing to do with the rest of the Body. It is opposed to Sympathy, which happens when the Indisposition takes its Rise from a Disorder in some other Part of the Body.

Thus a Cataract in the Eye is an *Idiopathy* : an Epilepsy is either *Idiopathic* or Sympathic; *Idiopathic* when it happens purely thro' some Fault in the Brain, Sympathic when it is preceded by some other Disorder. The Word is derived from the *Greek*, ιδιος, *proper*, *particular*, and παθος, *Passion, Affection.*

**IDIOSYNCRASY**, in Physic, is a Temperament peculiar to some Body, in consequence whereof, whether in Sickness or Health, it has a more than ordinary Aversion or Inclination to certain things, or is more affected with them, than others usually are. The word is derived from the Greek, ιδιος, *proper*, συν, with, and κρασις, *Crasis, Mixture, Temperament.*

**ILIAC**, a Term in Physick, applied to a violent and dangerous Disease, called the *Iliac Passion*, or *Miserere*. It consists in a Expulsion of feculent Matter by the Mouth, accompanied with a Swelling of the lower Ventricle, an intense Pain, and a total Constipation. The immediate Cause of the *Iliac* Passion seems owing to an Irregularity in the Peristaltic Motion of the Guts, *viz.* when it begins with the lower, and is continued to the higher. Other Causes are the Hardness of the Excrements, Inflammation of the Intestines, and their Engagement in the Anus or Scrotum, as it frequently happens in Hernia's, their twisting, and their entering within one another.

Persons afflicted with the *Iliac Passion*, have sometimes been found to return Suppositories and Glisters by the Mouth. Some have been cured of it by swallowing a great Quantity of Quick-silver, or a Musket-ball : When the Guts are twisted, or enter one within another, the Weight of these Bodies sometimes setting them to rights again. The *Iliac Passion* takes its name from the Intestine *Ilion*, in regard of its being usually affected in that Distemper, or perhaps from the *Greek* Verb ειλειν, *to turn, twist*; whence also the *Latins* call it *Volvulus.*

**IMBRICATED**, is used by some Botanists to express the Figure of the Leaves of some Plants, which are hollow like an Imbrex, or Gutter Tile.

**IMPERFECT PLANTS**, among the Botanists are such as either really want Flower and Seed, or are supposed to want them; since no Flower or Seed hath yet been discover'd to belong to the greatest part of them. These Mr. *Ray* distinguishes according to the Place of their Growth, into,

1. Aquatics, or such as grow in the Water : And that either, 1. In the Sea, and then they are called *Marine Plants*; and those are either of an hard and stony Consistence, as the Corals, Corallines; or Porous, that is, of a more soft and herbaceous one. Of these some are like Herbs, and are of two kinds; the greater, which are Cauliferous, as the Fucus; the lesser, as the Alga : the others are more of the Muscus, or Fungus Appearance, as the Spongia; 2. Fresh Water *Plants*, and those have either no Leaves, but are Capillaceous, as the Conservæ; or their Leaves divided into three parts, as the *Lens Palustris, Lenticula.*

2. Such *imperfect Plants* as grow in dry Ground, he divides into, First, Such as have Substance, either woody or fleshy; and these have scarce any thing common to the *perfect Plants*, neither the green herbaceous Colour, nor the Texture of Herbs, nor Flower, Seed, nor Leaf, properly speaking, as all the Fungi, which are 1. Such as grow in Trees, and therefore called Arboreous, as the *Fungus Laricis*, called Agarick, and the *Fungus Sambuci*, which we call Jews-Ear. 2. Terrestrial, and these are either Cauliferous, with Heads either lamellated, or porose underneath, or without Stalks, as the *Pezicæ* of *Pliny*, and *Fungus Pulverulentus, Crepitus Lupi*, or common Puff-Balls. 3. Subteraneous, as the *Tuberæ Terræ*, or Trufles. Secondly, Such as have a more soft and dry Consistence, and more kike that of Herbs; of which some are both cauliferous and branched, as the Musci, or Mosses : Others are without Stalks, adhering like a Crust to the Surface of the Earth, Stones, Trees, or Wood; as the *Lichen Terrestris* and *Arboreus*.

**IMPETIGO**, is a Cutaneous Foulness, divided into many kinds by the Antients; but a better Knowledge in Secretion, and the Office of the Cutaneous Glands, has taught us the Cure of all such Disorders, without having any necessary Recourse to such Distinctions : The Itch and Leprosy take in the several kinds, from the most easy to the most obstinate degree of Infection, according to which the Means of Cure are proportioned.

**IMPLANTATION** : One of the six kinds of Transplantation; used by some People for the Cure of certain Diseases. *Implantation* is performed by placing Plants, or at least the Roots of Plants, in a Ground prepared for that purpose, and water'd with what the Patient used to wash himself withal. By which means 'tis pretended the Disease is translated into the Plant. If the Plant happen to die before the Cure be perfected, by reason of the ill Qualities it imbibes, other Plants must be placed instead of it, and the Process be continued as in the first.

**IMPOSITION**, is also a kind of Transplantation practised for the Cure of certain Diseases. It is performed, by taking some of the implanted Spirit or Excrement of the Part affected, or both together, and placing them in a Tree, or a Plant, between the Bark and the Wood, after which it is covered up with Mud. Instead of this, some bore a Hole in the Tree with an Augur; and shutting up the Hole again with a Tampion of the same Wood, cover it over with Mud.

If 'tis desired the Effect should be lasting, a Tree is chosen that will continue long, as an Oak. If 'tis desired the Effect should be speedy, they chuse a Tree that grows fast; in which last case, the Matter serving as the Medium of Transplantation must be taken out of the Tree as soon as the Effect has followed, because too great Alteration of the Spirit, might be some prejudice to the Patient.

**IMPOSTHUME**, is a Collection of Matter or Pus in any Part of the Body, either from an Obstruction of Fluids in that Part, which makes them change into such Matter; or from a Translation of it from some other Part where it is generated.

**INANIMATE**, a Body that has lost its Soul, or that is not of a Nature capable of having any. Thus a dead Man is an *inanimate* Lump, and Metals are *inanimate* Bodies. The word is derived from the *Latin* Preposition *in* taken privitively, and *Anima, Soul.*

**INANITION**, a Term in Physic, signifying Emptiness, or the State of the Stomach, when it is empty, and needs Food. There are Flatuosities which proceed from Repletion, and others from *Inanition*, which last are the more dangerous.

**INCALESCENCE**, denotes the growing hot of any thing by Motion and Friction, or as Quick-lime does, by pouring Water on it, &c. from *in* and *caleo, to grow warm.*

**INCARNATION** signifies the healing and filling up Ulcers and Wounds with new Flesh; and the Medicines which effect this are commonly called *Incarnatives*, from *in* and *caro, Flesh.*

**INCARNATIVE**, *in Chirurgery*, is something that makes Flesh grown, rejoin, or unite, and is applied to Remedies, Bandages, and Sutures.

An *incarnative* Remedy is such a one as makes the Flesh heal and unite; an *incarnative* Bandage, is a Fillet, with an Eye or Noose at one end of it, so as the other end may be put thro' it. To make use of this Bandage, they apply the middle of it to the Side opposite to the Wound, so that the Aperture may be over the Wound itself; and slipping the other end thro' it, draw the lips of the Wound close to each other, that they may grow together.

An *incarnative* Suture, is such a one as, by rejoining the Lips of a Wound, and keeping them together, by means of a Thread drawn thro' them with a Needle, occasions them to grow up and heal.

**INCARTATION**, in Chymistry, is a Purification of Gold, by means of Silver and *Aqua-Fortis.*

**INCENSE**, an aromatic, odoriferous Resin. It distils from a Tree, that, according to *Theophrastus*, has Leaves like those of a Pear-Tree, and grows in the Country of *Saba*, in *Arabia Felix*, called by the Antients *Thurifera*,

Incense-bearing. The Incision for the Resin to ooze out at, is made in the Dog-Days. The Male Incense is the best; it is in round, in white drops, fat within, and inflames immediately, when laid on the Fire. This is also called *Olibanum*. The Female *Incense* is softer, and more resinous, but of less Virtue than the former. *Incense* is of considerable use in Physic, it warms, dries, and binds. It is used in several Diseases of the Head and Breast, in case of Vomiting, a Diarrhæa, or a Dysentery; externally it is used to fortify the Brain, and in healing of Wounds.

*Bark of Incense*, is a Bark of the Tree whence the Incense flows, which has the same Qualities with the *Incense* itself. There is another Bark brought from the *Indies*, called also *Bark of Incense*, and sometimes *Jews Incense*, in regard the *Jews* make frequent Use thereof in their Perfumes.

*Manna of Incense*, is the Flower or Farina of *Incense*, occasioned by the Friction of the Grains against each other in the Sacks wherein they carry it. There is also a Soot of *Incense*, which is a Preparation of it.

Incense was formerly burnt in the Temples of all Religions, to do honour to the Divinities that were there adored. Many of the Primitive Christians were put to death, because they would not offer Incense to Idols. In the *Romish* Church they still retain the Use of Incense in many of their Ceremonies, particularly at solemn Festivals, as on Prelates, &c. and sometimes also on the People. The word comes from the *Latin, incensum*, burnt; taking the Effect, for the Thing itself.

**INCIDE**. Those Medicines are said to *incide*, which consist of pointed and sharp Particles, as Acids, and most Salts; by the Force or Insinuation of which, the Particles of other Bodies are divided from one another, which before cohered. And thus some expectorating Medicines are said to *incide*, or cut the Phlegm, when they break, it so as to occasion its Discharge.

**INCINERATION**, in Chymistry, is the Reduction of Vegetables into Ashes which is done by burning them gently. Thus Fern is reduced into Ashes for the making of Glass. The Word is derived from the *Latin* Preposition *in* and *Cinis*, Ashes.

**INCLINATION**, a term used in Medicine and Chymistry, when a clear Liquid is poured off from some Fæces, or Sediment, by only gently stooping the Vessel; which is also called Decantation.

**INCRASSATING**, is the rendering Fluids, thicker than before by the Mixture of less fluid Particles.

**INCUBUS**, or the Night-Mare, is the Name of a Disease consisting in the Oppression of the Breast, so very violent, that the patient cannot speak, or even breathe. In this Disease the Senses are not quite lost, but drown'd and astonish'd, as is the Understanding and Imagination; so that he Patient seems to think some huge Weight thrown on him ready to strangle him. Children are very liable to this Distemper; so are fat people, and Men of much Study and Application of Mind : By reason the Stomach in all these finds some difficulty in Digestion.

The Incubus seems to be Cousin-German to the Epilepsy and Apoplexy; for it lasts long, it degenerates into one or other of those Distempers. Other reckon it a kind of Asthma and call it *Asthma Nocturnum*, and say it proceeds from the same Causes, and is helped by the same Means as the common Asthma. The word *Incubus* is derived form the *Latin Incubare*, to lie down on any thing and press it. The *Greeks* called it εφιαλγυς, *Saltator*, Leper, or one that rushes on a Person.

**INDIAN WOOD**, call'd also *Jamaica* and *Campeche Wood*, is taken out of the Heart of a large Tree growing plentifully in the Isles of *Jamaica*, *Campeche*, &c. It is used in Dying; its Decoction is very red : land it has been observ'd, that putting some of this Decoction into two Bottles, and mixing a little Powder of Alum with the one, it will become of a very beautiful Red, which will hold; the other in a day's time becoming yellowish, though both Bottles were stopp'd from the Air alike : and if a little of the same Decoction were exposed to the Air, it would become black as Ink in the same Space of Time.

**INDIGESTION**, a want of Digestion. In the System of Trituration, *Indigestion*, which is a Crudity, may be very naturally accounted for, from the Relaxation of the fibres of the Stomach. A bilious *Indigestion*, in the Opinion of *Hecquet*, a great Advocate for Trituration, is owing to too much Force in the Stomach, too much Vivacity in its Oscillations, which spoil the Digestion, by rendering the Trituration imperfect. But this is hardly satisfactory, for it should seem that Digestion would be the more perfect in proportion as the Force of the Stomach increased. See Digestion.

**INDIGO**, a Drug of a deep blue Colour, brought hither from the *West-Indies*. It is drawn from the Leaves of a Plant which the *Spaniards* call *Anil*, and we *Indigo*. The Method of Preparation is this. When the Plant has attained to a certain height, and its Leaves are in a good Condition, they cut them down, and throw them into a kind of Vat, covering them with Water. These they boil together for the space of twenty four hours : at the Top swims a Scum, with all the different Colours of the Rainbow. Then the Water is let off into another Vessel, where they agitate and churn it, as it were, with five or six long Poles, fitted together for that purpose.

This they continue to do till the Water becomes of a deep Green, and till the Grain, as they call it, forms itself, which they discover by taking a little of it out into another Vessel, and spitting in it; for if then they perceive a bluish Dreg subsiding, they cease to beat. The Matter then precipitates of itself to the Bottom of the Vessel, and when it is well settled, they pour off the Water. After this they take out the Indigo, and put it into little Linen Bags, and let it drain; this done, they put it into shallow wooden Boxes, and when it is dry, they cut it into slices, and let them harden in the Sun.

There are several kinds of Indigo; the best is that called *Serquisse*, from the Name of a Village where 'tis prepared. We chuse it in flat Pieces, of a moderate thickness, pretty hard, clean, light enough to swim in the Water, inflammable, of a fine blue Colour, marked a little on the Inside with Silver Streaks, and appearing reddish when rubbed on the Nail.

*Indigo* is used among the Painters, who grind and mix it with white to make a blue Colour; for without that Mixture it would paint blackish. They mix it with Yellow, to make a Green Colour. It is also used in Dying, and by the Laun-dresses, to give a bluish Cast to their Linen.

In the *Hortus Malabaricus* is an Account of the Plant whence *Indigo* is drawn: The Decoction of whose Root is said to be excellent against Nephritic Cholics; its Leaves, applied to the lower Ventricle, good to promote Urine; and the *Indigo* itself of good Use in drying Tumours.

**INDURATING**, a Term applied to such Things as give a harder or firmer Consistence to others, by a greater Solidity of their Particles, or as dissipate the thinner Parts of any matter, so as to leave the Remainder harder. Thus a Tumour is *indurated*, either by the Addition of earthy and solid Particles, as in *Schirri* and knotty Swellings, or by transpiring the thinner Parts thro' the Skin, whereby the Remainder grows more fixed, as in an *Oedema.*

**INESCATION**, a kind of Transplantation, practis'd for the Cure of certain Diseases; it consists on impregnating a proper Medium or Vehicle, with some of the Mumia or vital Spirit of the Patient, and giving it to some Animal to eat.

'Tis pretended the Animal unites and assimilates that Mumia with itself, correcting it, and imbibing its vicious Quality, and by that means restoring Health to the Person whereto the Mumia belonged. If the Animal happens to die before the Cure be effected, a second Animal must be pitched on, and the Experiment repeated. Some tell us, that the Blood of the Patient well putrefied or fermented, does the Business better than any other Part. The word is derived from the privative Preposition *in*, and *esca*, Food.

**INFECTION**, is the catching a Disease by some Effluvia or fine Particles, which fly off from some distempered Bodies, and mixing with the Juices of others, occasion the same Disorders, as in the Bodies they came from . The word comes from the *Latin* verb *inficere*, which properly signifies *to dye of some other Colour*; *inficere*, i.e. *facere ut aliquid intus sit, to occasion something to be imbibed.*

**INFLAMMATION**, in Physic, is understood of a Tumour, occasioned from an Obstruction; by means whereof the Blood flowing into some Part faster than it can run off again, swells up, and causes a Tension, with an unusual Soreness, Redness, and Heat. The immediate Cause, there of all *Inflammations*, is an overflowing of Blood. Other Causes, more remote, may be the Density and Coagulation of the Blood, or the Relaxation and Contusion of the Fibres. Physicians have given particular Names to the *Inflammations* of several Parts. That of the Eyes is call'd *Ophthalmia*, that of the Lungs *Peripneumonia*, and that of the Liver *Hepatites*. The word *Inflammation* comes from the *Latin in*, and *Flamma*, Flame.

**INFLUENT**, a Term used where any Liquor or Juice, by the Contrivance of Nature, and the Laws of Circulation, falls into another Current and Receptacle. Thus with respect to the common Receptacle in the human Body, the Chyle is its *influent* Juice, and so is the Bile to the Gall-Bladder, and

Venal-Blood to the Hearts in its Diastole; and the like.

**INFUSION**, is a Part of Pharmacy, whereby the Virtues of Plants, Roots, and the like, are drawn out, by letting them step in some convenient Menstruum. *Infusion* is used in Bodies of a lax Texture, whose Parts are so light, as not to admit of a greater Motion, without hazard of flying away in Vapour.

Its Use is to communicate the Virtues out of Bodies to Liquors, either in order to augment their Force, or correct their ill Qualities. Some *Infusions* are made in common Water, others in Wine, Vinegar, Milk ,Spirit of Wine, &c.

*Infusion* is also used to signify the Action of conveying a Liquor into the Body by the Veins. Some Physicians have found out a new Method of Purging, by *infusing* a Cathartic into the Veins, which operates pretty much after the manner of a Clyster.

**INGEMINATED FLOWERS**, are when one Flower stands on, or naturally grows out of another.

**INGUEN** is that Part of the Body, reaching from the Head of the Thigh to above the secret Parts, and is commonly called the Groin. *Inguinalis* is given to any Substance made of that Part, or any thing therein contained, or applied thereunto by way of Medicine, or the like. The word is pure *Latin*, and is derived, according to some, from *Unguen*, Ointment, because these Parts are frequently anointed. Others derive it from *ango*, because Pains happen frequently there; others again from *ingenor*, because the genital Parts are here.

**INJECTION**, in Pharmacy, is any liquid Medicine made to be injected by a Syringe, Clyster-Pipe, or any other Instrument into any Part of the Body. It is likewise a common Term for filling the Vessels with coloured Wax, or any other proper Matter, to shew their Figures and Ramifications; a thing frequent among Anatomists.

**INSEMINATION**, one of the four Kinds of Transplantation, in use for the Cure of certain Diseases. It is performed by mixing the Medium impregnated with the *Mumia* taken from the Patient with some fat Earth wherein has been sown the Seed of a Plant appropriate to that Disease; but Care must be taken from time to time to sprinkle it with the Water wherein the Part affected has been wash'd. 'Tis supposed the Diseases will decline in proportion as the Plant grows. By *Mumia*, is here meant a Part of the viral Spirit of the Patient.

**INSESSUS**, is a kind of Half-Bath, usually prepared with a Decoction of several Herbs, proper for the lower Parts, wherein the Patient sits down to the Navel. It has several Uses, as the easing of Pain, softening of Parts, dispelling of flatulent Matter, and frequently, promoting of the *Menses*.

**INSIPID**, that which has nothing in it sharp or pungent enough to affect the Palate, Tongue, &c. and to occasion that Sensation we call Tasting.

**INSITIO**, a Term in Botany, used in the same Sense with engrafting; signifying in general the Insertion and Uniting of any Cyon, Bud, &c. into the Substance of the Stock.

**INSOLATION**, in Pharmacy, is a Preparation of Fruits, Drugs, &c. by exposing them to the Heat of the Sun's Rays; either to dry them, or to bake or sharpen them, as is done in Vinegar, Figs, &c. The Word comes from the *Latin* Verb *insolare*, which is used by *Pliny* and *Columella*, and signifies *to expose to the Sun.*

**INSPISSATE**, a Term used in Pharmacy for that Operation whereby a Liquor is brought to a thicker Consistence, by evaporating the thinner Parts : and thus Juices, as that of Liquorice, are *inspissated.*

**INTERNODII**, in Botany, are those little Spaces contained between any two Knots or Joints of the Stalk of a Plant; and in Anatomy, the *Extensores Pollicis*, which see, are also so called.

**INTESTINE MOTION**, of the Parts of Fluids. Where the attracting Corpuscles of any Fluid are elastick, they must necessarily produce an Intestine Motion; that is, a visible Motion or Change of Place among the minute Parts of fluid Body : and this greater or less according to the Degrees of their Elasticity, and attractive Forces. For two elastic Particles after meeting will fly from one another (abstracting the Resistance of the Medium) with the same degree of Velocity, with which they met : But when in flying back from one another, they approach other Particles, their Velocity will be increased.

**IPECACUANHA**, a little Root, about the Thickness of a moderate Quill, brought hither from several Places in the *West-Indies*. There are three kinds of it, *viz.* a brown, grey, and a white one; the first is most esteemed in Physic; it is firm, twisted, difficult to break, of a sharp bitter Taste, and grows in *Brazil* in the Gold-Mines. The Root of the grey *Ipecacuanha*, in its Virtue and Colour, is inferior to the former; it grows at the feet of Mountains, and in Meadows, and other most Places. The *Spaniards* call it *Bexugillo.*

The white *Ipecacuanha* differs from both the others, not only in Colour, but rather resembling the Root of white Dittany. The *Ipecacuanha* is purgative and astringent, it is also a gentle Vomitive, and is found one of the best and surest Remedies hitherto discovered for a Dysentery.

**IRRADIATION**, signifies an Emanation or shooting out of subtile Effluvia from one Body to another.

**IRRORATION**, a kind of Transplantation used for the Cure of certain Diseases. It consists in the sprinkling every Day either Trees, or other proper Plants, with the Urine of Sweat of the Patient, or with the Water wherein his Body, or at least the Part affected, has been washed, till such time as the Disease is removed. As soon as the Sprinkling has been made, they throw fresh Earth on it, in order to prevent the Virtue of the Mumia, that is, of the vital Spirit of the Liquid, from evaporating into the Air.

**ISCHURIA**, in Physic, is a Disease that consists in an entire Suppression of Urine. It is occasioned by any thing that may obstruct the Passages of the Reins, Ureters, or the Neck of the Bladder, as Sand, Stone, Phlegm, &c. It may also be occasioned by an Obstruction of the Nerves, which pass to the Reins or Bladder, as we see it is, in a Paralysis of the lower Parts from the Diaphragm.

The too great Distention of the Bladder may also produce the same Effect; for the Fibres being much lengthened, and consequently condensed, the Spirits necessary for their Contraction cannot get Admittance; whence it is that Persons, who have retained their Urine a long time, find a great deal of difficulty in discharging it. The Word is derived form the *Greek* ισχω, *I stop*, and ουρον, *Urine*.

**ISSUES**, in Physic, are small artificial Apertures in a fleshy part of the Body, to drain off superfluous Moisture, or give vent to any noxious Humour. They are usually made in the Arms, Legs, or Back, either by Caustics or Incision. Caution is used to place them about the middle of a Muscle, that the necessary Motion of the Part may not incommode them, or pain the Patient.

There is an easy way of making an issue, which succeeds best in Children; 'tis done after this manner : Having applied a small piece of blistering Plaister, about the bigness of a small Pea, to the Part where you would have an *Issue*, and letting it lie on for a few Hours, it will cause a Blister; the Skin being rais'd, apply a Pea as usual, and compress it tight with a Bandage, till by degrees it sinks in, and forms an *Issue*.

*Issues* are very useful in many Distempers, several of which, when obstinate cannot be cured without them; as an *Hydrocephalus, Ophthalmia, Old Ulcers*, &c.

**JADE**, a greenish Stone, bordering on the Colour of Olive, much esteem'd for its Hardness, which exceeds that of Porphyry, Agat, and Jasper, and only to be cut with Powder of Diamond. It is in mighty esteem among the *Turks* and *Poles*, who adorn all their fine Works with it, and especially the Handles of their Sabers.

This Stone applied to the Reins, is said to be a Preservative from the Nephritic Cholic. Mr. *Bernier*[1] tells us, that the Caravans of *Thibet* carry it to *Cachmire*, and that the *Galibus* prize it as highly as Diamond. The Natives of *South-America* value it on a account of the Virtues they attribute to it in the Epilepsy, Diseases of the Reins, the Stone and Gravel. In a Treatise of it printed in Paris, 'tis called the Divine Stone.

**JALAP**, is the Root of a Plant not much unlike our Bryony, and is therefore by some called *Bryonia Peruviana*; for it is brought to us chiefly from *Peru* and *New-Spain*. The *Mechoacan* and this are reckoned a Species, and therefore as this is sometimes called *Mechoacana nigra*, that goes as often by the Name of *Jalapian album*. As this does not appear to have been known to the Antients, it has its place in Medicine only since those parts of *America*, which produce it, have been traded to by *Europeans*. That which breaks blackest, most brittle, sound, and shining within side, is the best; by reason the resinous Parts, which give it those Properties, are supposed to contain its Medicinal Virtues.

Some take great pains to extract its Resin, which is to be done with any spirituous Menstruum, and afterwards want Correctors for it. The most common, is Salt of Tartar or Loaf-Sugar; but if correcting consists in separating its Parts, as it certainly does, the drawing it from the Root, and making it into a Resin, must be very needless. Monsieur *Bolduc*, who hath made several Experiments upon it, says, it is one of the best Cathartics we have, taken as Nature only has prepared it.

**JAPAN-EARTH**, also called *Catechu*, is an Earth of a dark purple Colour. It is very austere upon the Palate, seems to melt, like the Bole, in the Mouth, and leaves somewhat of a sweetish Taste behind it. It is famous for stopping Fluxes of all Kinds.

**JATRALEPTIC**, the Name of that part of Physick which cures by Frictions, by the Application of Fomentations and Plaisters. It was one *Prodicus*, a Disciple of *Hippocrates*, and a Native of *Corinth*, who first instituted it.

**JAUNDICE**, a Disease, which consists in an overflowing of the Bile. Of this there are three kinds; the first, properly called the *Jaundice*, is owing to the yellow Bile, which, in this Case, is too exalted or too abundant in the Mass of Blood; or perhaps to an Obstruction of the Glands of the Liver, which prevents the Gall's being duly separated from the Blood.

The second, called, the Black *Jaundice*, is owing to the same yellow Bile, mingled with Acids. The third, bordering on Green, takes its Rise also from a

[1] Francois Bernier (1625 – 1688), a French physician.

Mixture of Bile with an Acid; this is usually called the Green-sickness, and is a Distemper pretty common in young Women.

In the *Jaundice*, the White of the Eye and the Skin are yellow, and troubled with an Itching; in the Black *Jaundice* the natural Colour is lost, by reason of an atrabilary Humour spread underneath the Skin; it first appears brownish, and afterwards of a Lead-Colour. The *Jaundice* often proves a Forerunner of the Dropsy. A Doctor of the Faculty of *Montpellier*, calls the Yellow *Jaundice*, attended with periodical Pains, a Rheumatism of the Liver; and another of the same place, calls it a Quartan Ague of the Liver. In the Journal of *Leipsic*, 'tis asserted that the *Jaundice* is not occasioned by Obstructions. The Acid Spirit of *Sal Ammoniac* is said to be an excellent Remedy against the *Jaundice*. The Word is derived fro the *French*, *Jaunisse, Yellowness*, of *Jaune, Yellow*.

**JECTIGATION**, in Physic, is a Trembling or Palpitation felt in the Pulse of a sick Person, which shews that the Brain, which is the Origin of the Nerves, is attacked and threatened with Convulsions.

**JECUR UTERINUM** : The Placenta is by some this called, from the supposed Similitude of its Office with that of the Liver.

**JEWS-EAR**, a kind of Fungus, Mushroom, or spungy Substance, that grows about the Root of the Elder-tree. It is chiefly used in Decoction, which is found Detergent and Vulnerary, and a good Gargle in sore Throats.

**JUDAICUS LAPIS**, a grey, soft, brittle Stone, in form of an Acorn, having Lines drawn regularly on its Surface, as if they were turn'd : It is used in Physic to dissolve the Stone in the Bladder.

**JUJUBE**, the Fruit of a Tree of the same Name, growing very commonly in *Provence*, and some other Parts. The *Jujubes* are about the Size of a Plumb, oval, red without, yellow within, of a sweet, very commonly, vinous Taste; they are pectoral and aperitive, soften the Acrimony of the Humours, and promote a Discharge by the Sputum. *Pliny* tells us, that *Sextus Papinius* brought the first *Jujubes* from *Syria*, and Truffles from *Africa*, towards the End of *Augustus's* Reign.

**JULAP**, in Pharmacy, is an easy agreeable Potion prescribed to sick Persons: It usually consist of distilled Waters, or light Decoctions, frequently sweeten'd with Sugar or clarified Juices. It is sometimes used as the ordinary Drink in certain Diseases, but usually as a Vehicle for other Forms of Medicines; serving to correct the peccant Humours, to restore the declining Strength of the Heart, and to promote Sleep. The word, according to *Menage*, is derived from the *Arabic*, *Guilep*, or rather form the *Greek* ζουλαπια. *Olearius*[1] derives from *Gulap*, a *Persian* Word, signifying *Rose-Water*.

**JULUS**, a Name which the Botanists give to those Wormlike Tufts, or Palms, as they are called, in Willows, which, at the beginning of the Year, grow out,

[1] Adam Olearius, born Adam Oelschlager (1603 – 1671), a German philosopher.

and hang pendulous down from Hazels, Walnut-Trees, &c. Mr. *Ray* thinks them to be a kind of Collection of the Stamina of the Flowers of the Tree, because in fertile Trees and Plants they have abundance of seminal Vessels and Seed-Pods.

**JUNIPER-BERRIES**, the Fruit of a Shrub of the same Name; much used in Medicine. *Etmuller* had a vast Opinion of them, and thought they deserved a whole Treatise to be wrote of them. The Rob (a Form of Medicine now out of use) made of the expressed Juice of the Green Berries, has been called the *Theriaca Germanorum*; so much have they been in esteem amongst them for anti-pestilential Qualities. They are certainly carminative, but their most remarkable Properties are in scouring the Viscera, and particularly the Reins and Urinary Passages, as all of the Turpentine-kind do.

The Wood of this Shrub is also of considerable Use in Physic, it strengthens the Stomach, expels Wind, clears the Lungs, provokes the Menses, and removes Obstructions of the Viscera. It is further said to be Sudorific, Cephalic, and Hysteric. From it they draw a Spirit, a Tincture, an Elixir, Extract and a Ratifia. 'Tis said it will last an hundred Years without corrupting; and the Chymists add, that a Coal of *Juniper*, covered with Ashes of the same kind, will keep fire an entire Year.

**KALI**, a Plant, otherwise called *Glasswort*; it grows in the Sands on the Sea-shore, where the People sow it in order to burn it green. Of its Ashes they make Soap, Glass, Alkali-Salt, &c. Thus Plant grows in great abundance in *Egypt* and *Syria*; its Name *Kali* was given it by the *Arabs*. It is found pretty plentifully, too, in *Languedoc*, where the People turn it to a very good account.

Their manner of preparing it is this : When the Tree is grown up to its pitch, they cut it down, and let it dry; afterwards they burn and calcine it in certain Pits like Lime-Kilns dug in the Ground for that purpose, which are close covered up with Earth, so as no Air may come at the Fire. The Matter by this means is not reduced into Ashes only, but made into a very hard Stone, like Rock-Salt, which they are forced to break with Hammers to get it out, and this Matter they call *Salicor*, or *Soude en Pierre*.

They make such Quantities of it here, that they export it into several other Countries, but principally into *Italy*, where the *Venetians* manufacture it into those beautiful Glasses, which they afterwards return into most Countries in *Europe*. However, the *Salicor* made here is inferior to that brought from *Alicant*. The best is in little dry sonorous Stones, of a blueish grey Colour, and full of little Eyes or Holes.

**KERMES**, a kind of Husk or Excrescence, as 'tis generally thought, about the Bigness of a Juniper-Berry, round, smooth, and shining, of a beautiful Red, and full of a mucilaginous Juice of the same Colour. It is found sticking to the Leaves and Bark of a kind of Ilex or Holm-Oak, in *Spain*, *Languedoc*, and other hot Countries. It has a vinous Smell, a bitter, tho agreeable Taste, and its Liquor contains an infinite Number of little round or oval Eggs. The Origin of the *Kermes* is supposed owing to a little Worm, which pricking the Holm-Oak, to draw its Food from it, raises a little Tumour or Vessel, which fills with Juice, and as it ripens becomes red.

When the *Kermes* is dried, there comes out of it an infinite Number of little Insects and Flies, so small that they are scarce sensible; insomuch that the whole inward Substance seems converted into them : For this reason it is that they sometimes call it *Vermillion*, (unless, perhaps, it be so call'd from its beautiful Vermillion Colour.) To prevent that Inconvenience, they usually steep the *Kermes* in Vinegar before they dry it.

They draw the Juice or Pulp from the *Kermes*, and make a Syrup of it, by adding a sufficient Quantity of Sugar. Sometimes they dry the Pulp separate from the Husk, which Pulp, thus dried, they call *Pastel of Kermes*. It is Cardiac, Desiccative, Astringent, fortifies the Stomach, and prevents Abortion; of this, is made that celebrated Confection, call'd *Alkermes*. It is, however, of greater use in dying Scarlet.

**KIDNEY**, or Rein, a Part of an Animal, whose Use is to separate the Urine. The *Kidneys* are situate on each Side, the one between the Liver and *Musculus Lumbaris*, on the right Side; the other between the Spleen and the same Muscles on the left Side. In Man the right is lower than the left, but in Quadrupeds 'tis usually the contrary; they are fastened to the Loins and the Diaphragm by their exterior Membrane, and to the Bladder by the Ureters;

the right is also fastened to the Intestine Cæcum, and the left to the Colon : their Figure resembles a Bean, or rather a Crescent, being curve on the side of the *Vena Cava*, and on the outside gibbous.

There are ordinarily two *Kidneys*, tho' sometimes there are found three, and sometimes four, and sometimes but one. In Men they are commonly about five inches long and three broad, and one and an half thick : Their Substance is composed of Glands, and very small urinary Pipes, or Canals; the Glands form the Circumference, and serve to separate the Urine; the Papillæ, or urinary Tubes, form the inner part, they come out of the Glands, and carry the Urine into a Cavity, in the concave Part of the *Kidney*, called the *Pelvis*, whence it pass tho' the Ureters into the Bladder.

The *Kidneys* are covered with two Membranes, they have each of them Arteries and Veins; the Arteries come from the *Aorta*, and the Veins terminate in the Cava; these are all called Emulgents. They have Nerves also, which take their Origin from the *Plexus Renalis*, formed by the Ramifications of the intercostal Nerve, and the Nerves of the Loins.

The *Kidneys* secrete the Urine from the Blood, which, by the Motion of the Heart, is driven thro' the Arteries into the emulgent Arteries, and these carry it into the little Glands, where its Serosity being separated, is received in at the Orifices of the urinary Pipes, which go from the Glands to the Pelvis, and thence runs by the Ureters into the Bladder : the Blood, which could not enter the Glands, is brought back by the emulgent Veins.

**KNOT**, in Medicine, is a Tuberosity form'd in the Joints of old Gouty People. Consisting of a thick viscous, crude, indigested Pituita, accompanied with a bilious Humour, hot and acrimonious; the grossest and most terrestrial part whereof clogs and converts into a stony Substance like Chalk : whence Knots are ingendred, like Stones.

**KYSTUS**, in Medicine, is the Name of a Bag, or Membrane, in form of a Bladder, full of unnatural Humours. The word comes from the Greek κυστις, Bladder.

**LABIATE FLOWERS**, from the word *Labium*, a Lip, is a Term applied by Herbalists to such Flowers, as have one or two Lips, some of which represent a kind of Helmet or Monk's Hood.

**LADANUM**, or *Labdanum*, in Pharmacy, the Name of a Gummous or Resinous Matter ouzing out of the Leaves of a Shrub call'd *Cistus Ladaniferam* which is very common in the hot Countries. The gather the *Ladanum* by means of Goats, which brouzing the Leaves of this Shrub, return to the Stable with their Beards loaden with a fat Substance, which the Peasants rake off, with a kind of Combs made for that purpose.

This Matter they thus collect into Lumps, and, as 'tis mixed with the Goat's Hair and other Impurities, called it *Ladanum* in the Beard, or natural *Ladanum*, Others draw Cords over the Leaves and other Parts of the Shrub, and scraping off what had stuck to the Cords, make up the *Ladanum* into little Balls.

*Ladanum* is used in Physick to soften, digest, attenuate and resolve. That which is brittle is of an ash-colour, sweet-scented, &c. is the best. *Pietro della Valle*[1] tells us he was inform'd by the Indians, that *Ladanum* is formed like Dew, and falls from Heaven like Manna, that it is gather'd on the Leaves of a Plant, a Palm and an half high; that after gathering they boil it, by which means it becomes soft like Wax.

*Liquid Ladanum* is a Preparation of the natural *Ladanum*, by melting and purifying it from the Hairs, &c. This is sometimes sold for a black Amber.

**LAMBATIVES**, a Form of Medicines to be lick'd off the End of a Liquorice-Stick. The same with *Linctus's, Lobocks*, and *Eclegmas*.

**LANGUOR**, signifies a Faintness, which may arise from a Want or Decay of Spirits thro' Indigestion, or too much Exercise; or from an additional Weight of Fluids, from a Diminution of Secretion by the common Discharges.

**LANIGEROUS**, any thing that bears Wool. Hence *Lanigerous* Trees among Herbalists, are those Trees that bear a woolly downy Substance, as the black, white and trembling Poplars, Osiers, and Willows of all Sorts.

**LANUGO** signifies a Down , or soft woolly Substance, which grows upon some Plants, which therefore are called *lanuginous* Plants.

**LAPIDESCENT**, from *Lapis* a Stone, any thing which has a Property of turning Bodies into a stony Nature, as many Spring-Waters will do to Pieces of Wood, and other like Substances.

**LAPIDIFCATION**, in Chymistry; an Action by which any Substance is converted into Stone: This is done by dissolving a Metal, for instance, in a corrosive Spirit of Menstruum, and afterwards boiling that Dissolution into the Consistence of a Stone. *Lapidification* is practised in Metals, fixed Salts,

[1] Pietro della Valle (1586 – 1682), an Italian scholar and traveller.

and Salts of Plants. The Term is also used in making artificial Stones.

**LAPIS INFERNALIS**, a caustick Stone prepared various Ways; sometimes of strong Soap-Lees evaporated to a Dryness, and the Remainder kept in a Glass well stopp'd from the Air : sometimes it is made of Vitriol and Tartar, calcined Sal Armoniac, and Quick-Lime boil'd in Water to a strong Lixivium, then strain'd and evaporated till it is dry.

**LAPIS LAZULI**, a Mineral Stone of a blue Colour. *Pliny* and *Dioscorides* make it a Sand, *Agricola* a Mineral found in the Veins of the Earth; but the truth is, 'tis a mere Stone, call'd by way of Excellence *Lapis*, or *Lapis Lazuli*. When perfect, 'tis studded with little Specks or Stars of Gold; for which Reason, *Mesue* calls it *Lapis Stellatus* : and to be good, should be able to resist Fire and Smoak, and to come out of 'em with new Lustre.

It is found in Mines of Gold, Silver and Copper, as also in Pits of Marble; which last is that generally in Use. Naturalists distinguish three Kinds of *Lapis*. The first call'd old Rock, which is pure, smooth, a fine blue, with beautiful yellow Streaks like Veins of Gold, which yet are frequently no more than Veins of Pyrites. The second called the new Rock, is stuffed with common Stones; its Colour is weaker, and its Price lower : these two Kinds are brought from *Persia* and *Siam*; the third Kind is brought from the Mountains of *Auvergne*. This is mix'd with the common Rock whence it is dug, it is of a pale blue, and is sprinkled with greenish Spots, with Veins, of Pyrites. This when sufficiently charged with Spots of Green is sold for the *Armenian* Stone.

The Lapis is of some Use in Medicines; they prepare it by calcining and washing it several times; which done, it makes an Ingredient in the famous Confection of *Alkermes*. Sometimes, in spight of all its Lotions, it continues to be a Purgative, by reason of the Vitriolic Matter it contains.

**LAPIS MEDICAMENTOSUS**, the medicinal Stone, a Composition of green and white Vitriol, Alum, Anatron of *Sandiver*, common Salt, and Salt of Tartar, melted over the Fire, and stirr'd till they thicken; then mix'd with Powder of Venice, Ceruss, and *Armenian* Bole, stirring the whole till it grows hard. This is said to fasten the Teeth, preserve the Gums, heal and dry up Ulcers and Wounds, and is used in Injections, and in Compositions for sore Eyes.

**LASSITUDE**, among Physicians, expresses that Weariness or Heaviness of Members that proceeds from a distempered State of Body, and not from Exercise; either from an Increase of Bulk, from a Diminution of proper Fluid which is necessary to maintain the Force and Spring of the Solids, as in Fevers and Convulsions; or from a vitiated Secretion of that Juice, whereby the Fibres are not supplied either in due Quantity or Quality. The Remedy in the first Case is Evacuation, in the latter proper Diet, or such Alterative Medicines as influence such a Secretion.

**LAUDANUM**, a Name given by the Chymists to certain Preparations of Opium, by reason of their excellent Qualities, as who should say *Laudanum* from *laudere, to praise*. To these several add Coral, Pearls, Treacle, &c.

*Laudanum* is esteemed an excellent Medicine, it assuages Pain, stops the spitting of Blood, the Flux of the Menses and Hemorrhoides, &c.

**LAXATIVE**, in Medicine, is used to signify a loose State or Disposition of the Body, so as to go frequently to stool. Hence *laxative* Medicines are such as promote that Disposition, which they do by some smooth softening Quality, taking away the Tensity of the Fibres, and facilitating the Passage of the Contents of the intestinal Tube thro it; for which Reason all oily Substances come under this Class.

**LEAD**, a coarse, heavy, impure Metal, of all others the softest and must fusible, when purified; called by the Chymists *Saturn*. Those who have made an Analysis of it, find it contains a little Mercury, some Sulphur, and a great deal of bituminous Earth. Lead is found in various Countries, but abounds particularly in *England*. 'Tis found, too, in several kinds of Soils and Stones, some whereof, besides, contain Gold, some Silver, others Tin, &c.

'Tis melted on a Furnace provided for the purpose with a string Coal-Fire upon it; as it melts, it runs thro' a Canal on one Side of it, leaving the Earth, Stone, and Scoria, with the Ashes of the Coals. 'Tis purified by skimming it e'er cold, and throwing Suet and other fat Bodies into it.

Some very able Naturalists observe, that the Weight of *Lead* increases, either in the open Air, or under Ground. Mr. *Boyle* observes this particularly of the *Lead* of Churches, which, he says, frequently grows both in Bulk and Weight, so as to become too ponderous for the Timber that before sustained it; which some account for the Impurity, Heterogeneity, and loose Texture of its Parts, by means whereof the Particles of the Ait getting Admission within its Pores, are attracted, and easily assimilated to it. But others, who rely wholly on Experience, absolutely deny the Effect, as also that it is reproduced in Mines before exhausted, by letting them lie long open to the Air, which others assert. Lead is found of a lighter or deeper Colour, according as it is more or less purified, tho' some make a difference in the Colour of the Ore, always esteeming that most which is the whitest.

*Lead* is a Metal of much Use; it easily melts, and mixes with Gold, Silver, and Copper, and communicates, as they talk, its Humidity to them; but not being able to endure the Violence of the Fire which they undergo, it retires, and carries with it all that was heterogeneous in them; so as neither Gold nor Silver are refined without Lead. To which it may be added, that the coarser kind of precious Stones, boiled in *Lead*, are thereby rendered much more brilliant.

*Lead* is much used in Buildings, particularly for Covering, Gutters, Pipes, and Glass. *Lead* is either cast into Sheets in a Mold, or milled; which last is found by much the least serviceable, not only on account t of its Thinness, but also because 'tis so exceedingly stretched in milling; that when it comes to lie in the hot Sun, it shrinks and cracks, and consequently will not keep out the Water. The *Lead* used by Glaziers is first cast into slender Rods, twelve or fourteen Inches long, called *Canes*, which being afterwards drawn thro' their Vice, comes to have a Groove on either Side for the panes of Glass; and this they call *Turned Lead*.

The Method of paling or soldering *Lead* for fitting on of Imboss'd Figures,

&c. is by placing the Part whereon the Figure is to be paled, horizontal, and strewing on it some pulverized Rosin; under this place some Coals, till such time as the Rosin becomes reddish, and rises in Pimples; then apply the Figure, and rub some soft Sodder in to the joining : when this is done, the Figure will be paled on, and as firm as if it had been cast on it.

*Borrichius* asserts, that *Lead* reverberated into Minium, melted into Glass, reduced into Ceruss, and burnt into Litharge, immediately resumes its original Figure, upon the dexterous Application of a lixivial Salt. The Antients, according to *Schindlerus*[1], used to compose Books of Plates of Leaves of *Lead.*

There are various preparations of Lead, serving for various Purposes : *Lead-Dust,* a Preparation used by the Potters, made by throwing Charcoal-Dust in melted Lead, and stirring them a long time together; to separate the Coal again, they only wash it with Water, and dry it afresh. Its Use is to give a Varnish and Gloss to their Works.

*Burnt-Lead* is a Chymical Preparation used in Medicine, made of Plates of *Lead* melted in a Pot with Sulphur, and reduced into a brown Powder. *White Lead,* used by Painters, is only thin Plates of *Lead* dissolved by Fumes of boiling Vinegar.

Massicots of several Colours, and the Sandix, are also Preparations of Lead. Litharge of Gold or Silver, is only the *Lead* used in purifying Copper. *Red Lead,* a Preparation of Mineral *Lead* calcined, used by Painters, Potters, and Physicians.

By help of Chymistry there are also drawn from *Lead,* Salts, Balsams, Oils, Vinegar, a Magistery, &c. disguised under the Name of Saturn, to amuse the Ignorant.

*Salt or Sugar of Lead,* or *Saccharum Saturni,* is an essential Salt of Vinegar, incorporated with the proper Substance of *Lead,* dissolved in the Spirit of Vinegar. *Balm of Lead,* or *Saturn,* is an Oil drawn from the Salt of *Lead* by Distillation, after having dissolved it in Spirit of Turpentine. Magistery of Lead is the Calx of *Lead* purified and subtilized, which is made of *Lead* dissolved in *Aqua fortis,* pouring a filtrated Salt water into it; whence results a Magistery extremely white, which, when softened by several Lotions, is mixed with Pomatums for the Face and Complexion.

*Black Lead,* a kind of Mineral Stone, of a black Colour, but silvered, and shining, found in *Lead* Mines, and appearing to be nothing else but *Lead* not yet arrived at Maturity; much used for Pencils or Crayons for designing. 'Tis melted like the common *Lead.*

Mr. *Glanvil* observes, that the Smoke of the *Lead*-Works in *Somersetshire* is a prodigious Annoyance, and subjects both Work-men , and the Cattel that graze about them, to a mortal Disease. The Trees that grow near them have their Tops burnt, and their Leaves and Outsides discoloured and scorched.

When the *Lead-Ore* is dug out, they beat it small, then wash it clean in a running stream, and sift it in Iron Rudders. Their Hearth or Furnace is made of Clay or Firestone; this they set in the Ground, and on it build their Fire,

[1] This is probably Valentin Schindlerus (d. 1611), a German scholar and orientalist.

which they light with Charcoal, continuing it with young Oaken Gads, blown with Bellows, by Mens treading on them. After the Fire is lighted, and the Fire-Place hot, they throw their *Lead-Ore* on the Wood, which melts down into the Furnace and then with an Iron Ladle they take it out, and upon Sand cast it into what Form they please.

The Mine-Men sometimes find the Vein run up into the Root of Trees, and yet don't observe any Difference between those and other Trees. When the Mine is near the Surface, the Grass is sometimes found yellow. They make no account of the *Virgula Divinatoria*; yet say, that when a Mine is open, they may guess by it how far the Vein will lead. The Ore runs sometimes in a Vein, sometimes dispersed in Banks; it lies many times between Rocks; some of it harder, others milder; sometimes they have branched Ore in the Spar; about the Ore is Spar and Chalk, and another Substance, which they call *Crootes*.

**LEAVEN**, any thing that will make a Body swell by means of the most subtile and penetrating of its Parts; which being agitated and divided, divide and agitate the more gross, as we may observe in Paste, in several Liquors, &c. The word comes from *levanum, a levando*, because *Leaven* makes the Past, &c. rise.

**LEES**, the grossest and thickest Parts of Wine, Oil, and other liquors; or the Sediment found at bottom of the Vessel. A kind of gravelly Sand is made with the Lees of Wine burnt and prepared, used by Dyers, &c. which ought to stand as a Caution to People troubled with the Stone, &c.

The Word comes form the *French Lie*, and that either from *Limus Mud*, or from *Lyeus* one of the Surnames of *Bacchus*; or, according to *Du Cange*, from *Lia*, a corrupt *Latin* Word signifying the same thing.

The Vinegar-Makers make a great Trade of the Lees of Wine dried and make into Cakes, after having squeez'd out the Remains of the Liquor in Presses.

**LEGUMEN**, in Botany, is that Species of Plants called *Pulse*; which are so named as being gathered with the Hand, by which they are distinguished from Wheat, Corn, &c. which are mowed or reaped. Of this kind are all that grow in Pods, as Beans, Pease, &c. In the general. All Plants, which have a Papillionaceous, or Butterfly-like Flower, are reckoned by Mr. *Ray* among the *Legumina*. The word *Legumen*, according to *Varro* and *Servius*, is formed *ex eo quod Manu legatur, & non secatur; in regard it is gathered with the Hand, and not cut.*

**LEMNIAN EARTH**, a Medical Astringent, used in the same Cases as Bole, which see. It hath its Name from the Island of *Lemnos*, whence it is chiefly brought : Many form it into round Cakes, and impress a Seal upon it, whence it is call'd *Terra Sigillata*.

**LENITIVE**, in Physic, is any softening resolutive Remedy, that moistens the Part diseased, and dissipates any sharp Humour collected there. *Lenitive*, in Pharmacy, is a gentle Electuary, composed of Sena, Polypody, &c. so called in regard it purges easily, and by resolving.

**LENTIGO**, a freckly or scurvy Eruption upon the Skin, such especially as is common to Women in the time of Child-bearing. Authors distinguish this Eruption into several kinds.

**LENTISCUS**, the Wood of a Tree of the same Name, of some use in Physic; it is astringent and fortifying, and much used for Tooth-Picks. It contains a kind of Gum, or rather resinous Pitch, much like Mastic, or perhaps the Mastic itself or Incense or *Persia*, so highly commended by *Strabo*. The *Lentiscus* has nearly the same Properties with the *Saunders*, but has more of the Turpentine in it, and sometimes passes by Urine.

**LEPRA**, *Leprosy*, a foul contagious Disease, seated in the Cuticle or Surface of the Skin , arising, as most other cutaneous Diseases do, from thin salt Humours, thrown off from the Blood, and arrested by the Density and Closeness of the Cuticula.

This Distemper has been much more frequent in former Times than at present, and much more frequent in the hot Countries of the East, particularly among the *Jews*, than among us; for the Salts which by appointment of Nature, are to be eliminated thro' the Pores of the Skin, along with the recrementitious Serum, their proper Vehicle, are, in hot Countries, conveyed in greater plenty to the Surface of the Body, than in these *Northern* Regions they ordinarily are; and sticking in their Passage in the thin dry Membrane of the Cuticle, the aqueous Parts, which are their Vehicle, slip away from them by insensible Evaporation, and leave them there to corrode and fret it, till at length, thro' the Quantity so gathered, the Membrane becomes dry, brittle, white, which is the Cause of that Disquamation, or falling away in white Scales : that Whiteness as well as the Brittleness proceeding merely from the Quantity of these Salts, which are themselves white; and when the Moisture is drawn from them, being aculeated, and having insinuated themselves into the Pores of the Cuticle, dissolve the Continuity of it by their Points and Edges, which, so dead and broken, is apt, on the least Friction, to fall off as above-mentioned. This is what they call the *Lepra Græcorum*, from its Frequency among that People.

*Lepra Arabum* was another Species of the Distemper, which tho' different in Appearance, as carrying a dry scabby Crust, yet seems only a different Degree of the same Disease. For as in the former Case the Salts, being left destitute of their Humidity, are not so active, and therefore affect only the Cuticle; in the latter Case these Salts, with their Vehicle, crowding faster than they can be evaporated thro' the Pores of the Skin (being still *in fluore*, and so more caustic) corrode deeper, and eat not only the Cuticle but the excretory Vessels, and Surface of the Skin itself, which thereby spews out a Liquor somewhat thicker than usual; which, when the thinnest and most aqueous Parts are evaporated, are condensed into that Crust or Scab, which is the distinguishing Character of this Disease.

*Galen* defines the *Lepra* to be an Effusion of thick disorderly Blood, that corrupts the whole Habitude of the Body. *Avicenna* calls it *An Universal Cancer*. The *Greeks* give it the Name of εληφανθιασις, in regard the Patient has his Skin rough, wrinkled, and unequal like that of an Elephant. The *Lepra* begins within-side, a long time before it appears without-side. It was frequent in Europe in the Xth and XIth Centuries, but seems at present quite extinct, unless we allow the Venereal Disease to be the same with the *Lepra*; as it was the Opinion, among many others , of the Great *Pitcairn*, and as has been lately endeavoured to be proved by Mr. *Becket*, in a Treatise expressly in the Subject in the Philosophical Transactions.

The Symptoms of the antient *Lepra*. As laid down by *Galen, Aretæus, Pontanus, Ægineta, Cardan, Varanda, Gordon, Paræus*, and others are as follow : The Patient's Voice is hoarse, and comes rather thro' the Nose than the Mouth; the Blood full of little white shining Bodies, like Grains of Millet, that upon filtration separate themselves from it; the Serum is scabious, and destitute of its natural Humidity, inasmuch that Salt applied to it does not dissolve; it is so dry, that Vinegar poured on it boils; and is so strongly bound together by little imperceptible Threads, that calcined Lead thrown into it swims. The Face resembles a Coal half extinct, unctuous, shining, and bloated, with frequent hard Knobs, green at bottom, and white at top. The Hair is short, stiff, and brinded, and not to be torn off without brining away some of the rotten Flesh to which hit adheres; if it grows again, either on the Head or Chin, 'tis always white. Athwart the Forehead run large Wrinkles or Furrows, from one Temple to the other; the Eyes red and inflamed, and shine like those of a Cat; the Ear swollen and red, eaten with Ulcers towards the bottom, and incompassed with little Glands; the Nose sunk, because of the rotting of the Cartilage; the Tongue dry and black, swollen, ulcerated, divided with Furrows and spotted with Grains of white; the Skin covered with Ulcers, that die and revive each other, or with white Spots or Scales like a Fish; it is rough and insensible, and when cut, instead of Blood, yields a sanious Liquor. It arrives in time to such a Degree of Insensibility, that the Wrist, Feet, or even the large Tendon may be pierced with a Needle, without the Patient's feeling any Pain. At last the Nose, Fingers, Toes, and even Privy Members fall off entire, and by a Death peculiar to each of them anticipate that of the Patient. 'Tis added, that the Body is so hot, that a fresh Apple, held in the hand an Hour, will be dried and wrinkled, as if exposed to the Sun for a Week.

*Matthew Paris* says, that in *Christendom* there were fifteen Thousand Hospitals for *Lepers*; but the Disease having been discontinued for two Hundred Years, the Revenues of those Hospitals were abused, and Persons feigned themselves *leprous*, to be entitled to the Provision; which occasioned their Regulation in some Countries, and their entire Suppression in others. In *France* they were united to the Order of the Religious of St. *Lazarus* and Mount *Carmel* in 1664, and the Administration of then given to the Knights of that Order; in *England* they have been converted to other Purposes.

Formerly the Causes of *Lepers* were committed to the Ecclesiastical tribunals, and it was prohibited to prosecute a *Leper* before a Lay-Judge, in regard they were under the Protection of the Church, which separated them from the rest of the People by a Ceremony still to be seen in the Rituals.

The *Lepra* appeared differently in different Nations, according to the Climate and the Manner of Living; whence it was distinguished into several kinds, as the *Lepra Arabum, Lepra Græcorum*, &c. As to the Cure, that which proved effectual in those *Southern* Countries, fails among us, where the strongest Medicaments, and the most powerful Mercurials are necessary.

Bathing is judged to be of good Use in the *Lepra*. Dogs and Hares are said to be subject to this Disease. Among the *Indians* a white Man is despised, this passing with them for the Mark of a *Leper*. The word *Lepra* is derived from the *Greek* λεπις, *Scale*, in regard this Disease forms a kind of Scales on the Skin.

**LETHARGY**, in Medicine, a Disease consisting in a profound Drowsiness or Sleepiness, wherein the Patient can scarce be awaked; or, if awaked, remains stupid, without Sense or Memory, and presently sinks again into his former Sleep. The Word comes from the *Greek*, ληθη, *Oblivion*, and αργια, *Numbness, Laziness.*

The *Lethargy* is usually accompanied with a Fever and Delirium. The *Lethargy, Boerhaave* makes a gentle Apoplexy, arising from the same Causes, and to be known and cured in the same manner. Some Authors distinguish the *Lethargy* from the *Carus*, in that this latter is without a Fever, or at most is preceded with a slow one, *Celsus* ranks the *Lethargy* in the Number of acute Diseases, the Patient usually dying on the 7th Day. A *Lethargy* frequently succeeds a Frenzy.

**LEUCOMA**, in Physic, is a little white Spot on the Cornea of the Eye, call'd by the *Latins, Albugo*. It is occasioned by an Humour gather'd in this Membrane, or by the Scar following a Wound, or by an Ulcer in this Part, as sometimes happens in the Small-Pox. The Word is *Greek*, and is formed from λευκος, *white.*

**LEUCOPHLEGMATIA**, a kind of Dropsy, otherwise call'd *Anasarcha*. It consists in a Tumor of Bloating of the whole outer Surface of the Body, or some of its Parts; white and soft, easily giving way to the Touch, and preserving the Impression made by the Finger for some time. It may either be owing to some Disorder of the Blood, which in this Disease is of a pale Colour, viscid and cold; or to an aqueous Humour extravasated, and gathered together in the Muscles and the Pores of the Skin. The Word is *Greek*, and comes from λευκος, *white*, and φλεγμα, *Pituita, Phlegm.*

**LEVIGATION** signifies the Reduction of any hard ponderous Bodies, as Coral, Tutty, Precious Stones, &c. into a light subtile Powder, by grinding upon Porphyry, a Sea-Shell, Marble, Stone, &c. as Painters do their Colours. This is much used in Pharmacy and Chymistry, but unless the grinding Instruments are extremely hard, they will wear away, so as some times to double the Weight of the Medicine thus managed.

**LICHEN**, a cutaneous Distemper, in many respects the same with a Leprosy; for which, a Moss of the same name is said to be an extraordinary Remedy : but this the present Practice seldom meets with.

**LIENTERY**, in Physic, a kind of Looseness wherein the Food passes so suddenly thro the Stomach and Guts, as to be thrown out by Stool with little or no Alteration. The *Lientery* is owing either to a Defect in the Ferment of the Stomach, or to a Relaxation of the Pylorus, attended with so brisk an Irritation of the Fibres of the Ventricle, that instead of retaining the Aliment it lets it pass.

Excess of Drinking sometimes occasions this Disease, by relaxing the Stomach, and especially the Pylorus, too immoderately. The Antients were of opinion the *Lientery* was owing to the too great Smoothness and Slipperiness of the Inside of the Intestines, by which they let the Food slip off before it was digested : and hence they gave it this Name, which is formed from λειθος, *polished*, and εντερον, *Intestine.*

**LIME**, Calcined Stone, Marble, Free-stone, Chalk, or other Matter burnt by a large Fire in a Kiln or Furnace built express; to be afterwards used in the Composition of Mortar, for building; the Fire taking away all its Humidity, and opening its Pores, so that it becomes easily reducible to Powder. Quick *Lime* or Unslack'd *Lime* is that which come out of the Furnace; Slack'd *Lime* is that wash'd or steep'd in Water, and reserv'd for the making of Mortar.

The best *Lime* is that made of the hardest and firmest Stones, and which is slack'd at its coming out of the Furnace. Sir. *H. Wotton*[1] looks on it as a great Error in the *English* to make *Lime* as they do, of Refuse, and Stuff without any Choice; whereas *Italians*, at this day, and much more the Antients burnt their firmest Stones, and even Fragments of Marble where it was plentiful; which in time became almost Marble again for its hardness, as appears in their standing Theatres, &c.

We have two kinds of *Lime* in common use in *England*; the one made of Stone, and the other of Chalk; whereof the former is much the strongest. That made of soft Stone or Chalk is fittest for plaistering of Ceilings and Walls within doors; and that made of hard Stones, for Buildings and for plaistering without doors. Good *Lime* may also be made of Mill-Stone, not coarse and sandy, but fine and greasy; as also of all kinds of Flints; tho 'tis hard to burn 'em, unless in a Reverberatory Furnace, as being apt to run to Glass.

*Dieussant* recommends *Lime* made of Sea-shells as the best, but *Goldman* finds fault with it, as being impatient of Moisture, and therefore easily peeling off from the Outsides of Walls. It is, however, the common *Lime* used in the *Indies*.

Before the Stone be thrown into the Kiln, they are to be broke in pieces; otherwise the Air contain'd in their Cavities, too much expanded by the Heat, makes 'em fly with so much violence as to damage the Kiln. According to *Alberti*[2] and *Palladio*[3], *Lime* will not be sufficiently burnt in less than sixty Hours intense Heat.

The Marks of a well-burnt *Lime*, according to *Alberti*, are, that its Weight is to that of the Stone in a sesquilaterate Proportion; that it is white, light, and sonorous; that when flaked it sticks to the Sides of the Vessel : To which *Boeckler*[4] adds, that when slaked it sends forth a copious thick Smoak; and *Dieussant*, that it needs a great deal of Water to slake it.

To preserve *Lime* several Years, slake and work it up; dig a Pit under

[1] Henry Wotton (1568 – 1639), an English diplomat and author.

[2] This is probably Leon Battista Alberti (1401 – 1472), an Italian philosopher and architect.

[3] Andrea di Pietro della Gondola (1508 – 1580), an Italian architect.

[4] Georg Andreas Boeckler or Böckler, (1644 – 1698), a German architect and engineer.

ground, into which let it pass thro a hole open at the bottom of the Vessel. As soon as the Pit is full, cover it up with Sand, to prevent its drying; thus keeping it moist till it be used. *Boeckler* gives another Method : Cover a Stratum of *Lime* two or three foot high with another of Sand of the like Height; pour on Water enough to slake the *Lime*, but not to reduce it to dust after slaking. If the Sand cleave into Chinks, as the Smoak ascends, cover 'em up, so as no Vent may be given thereto.

*Lime* is much used by Tanners, Skinners, &c. in the Preparation of their Leather.

*Lime*, or *Calx*, in Chymistry, is a kind of fine Powder, or Ashes remaining of Metals or Minerals, that have been a long time in a violent Fire.

*Lime* is of some medicinal Use, being applied externally in Desiccative and Consumptive Medicines. Its Water is said to be an excellent Medicine, taken internally. M. *Burlet*[1] has written an ample Account of its Effects in the *French Memoirs*, in good measure from his own Experience. But he observes it succeeded much better in *Holland*, &c. than in *France*. It is a powerful Alterant, and like a pure Alkaline Water, fitted to blunt and destroy acid Ferments, which are the Principles of all Obstructions, and the Cause of most Chronic Diseases.

Its principal Use is in a Cachexy, Green-sickness, Dropsy, Scurvy, Obstructions of the Liver, Spleen, &c. It is made by pouring six Pounds of hot Water on one of Quick-Lime, leaving them to soak and macerate for the space of 24 hours.

**LINCTUS**, a Form of Medicine the same as *Lambative*, and probably from the same Derivation; or from *Lingua* the Tongue, as being to be licked up with the tongue.

**LINE-SEED**, a Grain, that has several useful Properties. It enters the Composition of several Medicines, and yields, by Expression, an Oil that has most of the Qualities of Nut-Oil, and is accordingly sometimes used in lieu thereof in Painting, and to burn. That drawn without the Assistance of Fire, is of much Esteem in Medicine, and supposed good in the Cure of several Diseases.

**LINIMENT**, a Topical Remedy, serving to soften the Asperities of the Skin, and to moisten those Parts that are to be softened, for resolving the Humours that afflict the Patients, and give him Pain. There are various kinds of Liniments used according to the various Occasions. The Liniment is of a mean Consistence, between an Oil, and an Unguent. The word comes from the *Latin linire, to anoint gently.*

**LINUM CATHARTICUM**, Mountain-Flax; this is much used by common People. It is a rough harsh Purge, and powerfully deterges, and evacuates viscid and watery Humours from the most remote Lodgements; which makes them fond of it in Rheumatisms : but it is only for robust Constitutions.

[1] This may be Claude Burlet (1664 – 1731), a French physician.

**LINUM INCOMBUSTIBILE**, a Mineral Substance, of a whitish Silver Colour, and a woolly Texture; consisting of small Threads or Longitudinal Fibres, endued with the wonderful Property of resisting Fire, and remaining unconsumed in the intensest Heat.

This lanuginous Mineral is sometimes called *Amianthus* and *Asbestos*; sometimes *Salamandra*, or *Salamander's Wooll*, from the Candle-Wicks said to be made antiently of it. From a pungent Quality, which *Agricola* says it has on the Tongue without Astringency, it is call'd *Alumen*, having the Epithet of *Plumeum* added to it, taken from its downy Filaments, to distinguish it from the other Alums.

From its light grey Colour it is call'd *Polia* and *Corsoides*; and from its Likeness to the hoary Fibres of some sorts of Mat-Weed, *Spartapolia*. From the Capacity it has of being spun into Thread, it is call'd *Linum*, with some distinguishing Epithet, taken either from the Quality, as *Linum Asbestinum Vivum*, or *Incombustibile*; or from the Place where it is found, as *Linum Fossile, Linum Indicum, Creticum, Cypricum*, and *Carpasium*, or *Carystium*.

But besides the Places whence it borrows Names, it is also found in *Tartary*, at *Namur* in the *Low Countries*, in *Thuringia*, among the Mines in the *Old Noricum* in *Egypt*, in the Mountains of *Arcadia*, at *Puteoli* in the Island of *Corsica*, in the Island of *Anglesey* in *Wales*, and in *Aberdeenshire* in *Scotland*.

The Naturalists generally reckon it among the Stones, whence its Appellation of *Lapis Asbestos*, &c. but Dr. *Plot*[1] rather judges it a *Terra Lapidosa*, or middle Substance, between Stone and Earth. As to its Generation, the same Author take sit to be a Mixture of some Salt, and a pure Earth without Sulphur, coagulated in the Winter, and hardened by the Heats in Summer. The Salt *J. Hessus*[2] says is a liquid Alum, of a milky Substance, inclining to yellow, that sweats out of the Earth, and smells like rotten Cheese.

As to the Art of managing this Mineral, and spinning and weaving it, &c. the Accounts we have are various. Signior *Castagnata*, Superintendent of some Mines in *Italy*, gives us the Art of reducing it either into a very white Skin, or a very white Paper, either of which resists the most violent Fire.

Mr. *Lloyd*[3] took some of that found in *Anglesey*, and pounding it in a Stone Mortar till it became a downy Substance, sifted it thro a fine Searce; by which means the earthy Parts were separated from it : the *Linum* remaining. Hen then brought it to a Paper-Mill, and putting it in Water, in a proper Vessel, stirred it pretty much, ordering the Workmen to proceed on it in their usual manner of making Paper, with their Writing-Paper Mold; only to stir it about constantly before putting their Mold in; considering it as a far more ponderous Substance than what they used, and consequently, if not immediately taken up after it was agitated, it would subside. The Paper thus made of it proved coarse, and apt to tear, but endured both Ink and Fire very

[1] Robert Plot (1640 – 1696), an English chemist and naturalist.

[2] This may be Johannes Hessus (ca. 1614 – 1653), a German physician.

[3] Edward Lloyd or Lhuyd (1660 – 1709), a Welsh naturalist and archaeologist.

well; the Ink only turning Red with the Violence of the Fire.

M. *Paulus Venetus* gives us the Manufacture of the Linum found in the Province of *Chinchinthelas* in *Tartary*, from one *Cursicar* a *Turk*, Superintendant of the Mines of that Country, as follows : The lanuginous Mineral, or Amianthus, being first dried in the Sun, is then pounded in a Brass Mortar, and the earthy part separated from the woolly, which is afterwards well washed from Filth; being thus purged, it is spun into Thread like other Wool, and after, wove into Cloth, which, if foul or spotted, they cleanse, he says, by throwing it into the Fire for an hour's time, whence it comes out unhurt, as white as Snow : Which very Method, according to the Account given us by *Strabo*, seems to have been used in ordering the *Cretan* Amianthus; with this Addition, that after it was pounded, and the earthy Part separated from the woolly, he says it was combed; and so does *Agricola*.

Signior *Campani*, after describing four sorts of the *Linum*, whereof he had Specimens in his *Musæum*; the first sent him from *Corfu*, the second from *Sestri di Ponente*, the third coarser and darer than the rest, and the fourth from the *Pyreneans*; and after observing, tho' he kept it three Weeks in a Glass-house Fire, yet found it unaltered, tho it would not preserve a Stick wrapp'd in it from the Fire : he proceeds to shew the manner of spinning it, and making it into Cloth, which he effected thus : He first laid the Stone in Water, if warm the better, for some time to soak; then opened and divided it with his Hands, that the earthy parts might fall out of it, which are whitish like Chalk, and server to bind the thready Part together. This makes the Water thick and milky. That Operation he repeated six or seven times with fresh Water, opening and squeezing it again and again, till all the heterogeneous Parts were washed out, and the Flax-like Parts were collected and laid in a Sieve to dry.

As to the spinning, he first shews a Method discovered to him, which is thus : Lay the Amianthus, cleansed as before, between two Cards, such as they card Wooll withal, where let it be gently carded, and then clapp'd in between the Cards, so that some of it may hang out of the sides; then lay the Cards fast on a Table or Bench; take a small Reel made with a little Hook at the end, and a Part to turn it, so that it may be easily turned round. This Reel must be wound over with find Thread : then having a small Vessel of Oil ready, with which the Forefinger and Thumb are constantly to be kept wet, both to preserve the Skin from the corrosive Quality of the Stone, and to render the Filaments thereof more soft and pliant; by continuing to twist about the Thread on the Reel in the Asbestos hanging out of the Cases, some of the latter will be worked up together with it; and little by little the Thread may, with Care, be woven into a coarse sort of Cloth; and by putting it into the Fire, the Thread and Oil will be burnt away, and the incombustible Cloth remain. But finding this way of uniting the Stone with the Thread very tedious, instead of the Thread he put some Flax in a Distaff, and by taking three or four Filaments of the Asbestos, and mixing them with the Flax, he found they might be easily twisted together, and the Thread thus made much more durable and strong; so that there is no need of Carding, which rather breaks the Filaments than does any good : only open and separate the Filaments after washing on a Table, and take them up with the Flax, which is sufficient.

As to the making of Paper, he says, in the washing of the Stone there will remain several short Pieces in the bottom of the Water, of which Paper may be made in the common Method. He concludes with the best way of preserving the Cloth, or any thing made of the Linnen, which, by reason of its excessive Dryness, is very apt to break and twist; and it consists in keeping it always well oiled, which is the only Preservative. When the Cloth is put into the Fire, the Oil burns off, and the Cloth comes out white and purified.

This kind of Linnen-Cloth was highly esteemed by the Antients; tho' then better known and more common than among us, being held equally precious with the richest Pearls; nor is it now of mean Value even in the Country where 'tis most generally made, a *China* Cover, (*i.e.* a Piece of twenty-three Inches and three quarters long) being worth 8 Tale, *i.e. 36 l. 13 s. 4 d. Pliny* says, he himself had seen Napkins thereof, which being taken foul from the Board, after a Feast, were thrown into the Fire, and by that means were better scowered than if they had been washed with Water, &c. But its principal Use, according to *Pliny*, was for the making of Shrowds for Royal Funerals; to wrap up the Corps, so as the Ashes might be preserved distinct from that of the Wood, &c. which made the Funeral Pile; and the Princes of *Tartary*, according to the Accounts in the *Philosophical Transactions*, still use it at this day in burning their Dead.

Some of the Antients are said to have made themselves Clothes of it, particularly the *Brachmans* among the Indians. The Wicks for their perpetual Lamps, according to Dr. *Lister*, were made of it; and we are told that *Septalla* Canon of *Milan* had Thread, Rope, Nets, and Paper of it. A Handkerchief or Pattern of this Linnen was presented to the Royal Society, a foot long and half a foot broad. This gave two Proofs if its resisting Fire; tho' in both Experiments it lost above three Drams in its Weight. When taken out red-hot, it did not burn a Piece of white Paper, on which it was laid. Mr. *Villette* pretends, that his large burning Concave usually vitrifies the Asbestos.

**LIPOTHYMIA**, or Liposychia, in Medicine, is a sudden Diminution or Failure of animal and vital Actions, otherwise called a Swooning or Deliquium. In the *Lipothymia* the Pulse is very faint, the Senses both internal and external, and the animal Motions, both voluntary and natural, extremely weakened, and the Respiration scare visible.

The ordinary Causes of the *Lipothymia* are great Losses of Blood, excessive Evacuations, immoderate Exercise, gross hot Air, such as that in the midst of Crowds of People. The word *Lipothymia* comes the *Greek* λειπω, *deficio*, and θυμος, *Animus*; and *Lyposychia* from λειπω, and ψυχη, the *Soul*.

**LIPPITUDO** is a Disorder of the Eyes otherwise call'd *Blear-Eyedness*; consisting in the Oozing out of a thick viscous Humour, which hardening, binds the Eye-lids together. Some, after *Celsus*, give the Name *Lippitudo* the *Opthalmia*.

**LITHARGE**; there are two Kinds of *Litharge*, the one natural, the other artificial. The Word is composed of the *Greek* λιθος and αργυρος, *Silver*.

Natural *Litharge* is a Mineral sometimes found in Lead Mines, reddish, scaly, brittle, and somewhat resembling white Lead. This *Litharge* is so exceeding rare, that the Shops sell none but the artificial.

*Artificial Litharge* is of two Kinds, *viz.* that of *Gold*, and that of *Silver*; or rather 'tis the same, with this difference, that the one having undergone a greater Degree of Fire than the other, has occasioned different Colours, and thence different Names.

Indeed Naturalists are not over well agreed what the *Artificial Litharge* is : Some say 'tis a Metallic Scum rais'd on the Surface of Lead, when melted; after having serv'd to purify Gold, Silver, or Copper. Others say 'tis a Metallic Smoak arising from those Metals mix'd with the Lead, used in purifying them; which sticking to the Top of Chimneys of Furnaces, is there form'd in a kind of Scales. Lastly, others say 'tis the Lead itself used in the refining of those Metals, and especially Copper; which last Opinion appears the most credible; and the rather, on account of the great Quantities of these *Litharges* brought from *Poland, Sweden*, and *Denmark*; where Copper-Mines are much more frequent than those of Gold and Silver.

*Litharges* are desiccative, detersive, and cooling; they make the Consistence of several Plaisters. The Potters use them to give a beautiful Gloss to their Ware; and they are also used by Painters, Dyers, Skinners, and Glaziers. When mix'd with Wine, they give it a bright sprightly Colour, but render it extremely unwholesome.

**LITHIASIS**, in Physic, signifies the Formation of the Stone, or the Manner in which it grows in the Body.

**LITHONTHRIPTICS**, are Medicines proper to dissolve the Stone in the Bladder and Kidneys; of which Kind are the Lithospermum, Saxifrage, &c. The Word comes from the *Greek* λιθος, *Stone*, and τριβειν, to break or wear.

**LIXIVIOUS**, in Chymistry, is understood of Salts extracted by a Lixivium or Lotion. *Lixivious Salts* are the fix'd Salts of Plants, &c. extracted by calcining the Plants or reducing them to Ashes; and afterwards making a Lixivium of those Ashes with Water; whence that Name is derived. Mr. *Boyle* observes, that the difference between *Lixivious* and Urinous Salts consists in this, That the former change the Dissolution of Sublimate in common Water into a yellow Colour.

**LIXIVIUM**, a Liquor made by the Infusion of Wood-Ashes, or any burnt Substances; which is more or less pungent and penetrating, as it is more or less impregnated with Salts, and fiery Particles abounding therein. What is left after the Evaporation of such a Liquor, is called a *Lixivial* or *Lixiviate Salt*; such as all those are, which are made by Incineration. Lixiviums are of notable use not only in Medicine, but also in Bleaching, Sugar-Works, &c. which see.

**LOCH**, or *Lohoch*, in Pharmacy, is a Composition of a Consistence between that of a Syrup and that of a soft Electuary, destined for Diseases of the Lungs. The Word is originally *Arabic*; but continues still in among the Apothecaries. The *Latins* call it *Linctus*, and the *Greeks* εκλεγμα, by reason the manner of taking it is by licking. There are various kinds of *Loches*.

**LOCHIA**, or *Loches*, the Evacuation consequent on the Delivery of a Woman in Child-bed. As soon as the *Uterus* is eased of its Load, its Fibres, as also those of the Peritonæum, Muscles of the Abdomen, &c. which had been extremely distended during the last Period of Gestation, begin to contract themselves and their Vessels; particularly the *Uterus*, which by this means expels the Blood amass'd in it. At first, pure Blood is evacuated, and in considerable quantities; afterwards it is diluted, and comes out more sparingly; at length if becomes viscid, pale, &c. These are called the *Loches*.

**LOCULAMENTA**, strictly signifies little Pockets; and thence the Term is made is of in Botany, to express those little distinct Cells, or Partitions, within the common *Capsula Seminalis* of any Plant : as those within the Seeds of Poppies, &c.

**LOCUSTÆ**, the Beards and pendulous Seeds of Oats, and of the *Gramina Paniculata*; to which the Botanists gave this name, from their Figure, which sometimes resembles that of a Locust.

**LOTION**, in Pharmacy, a Preparation of Medicines, by washing them in some Liquid, either made very light, so as to take away only the Dregs; or made to penetrate them, in order to clear them of some salt or corrosive Spirit; as the *Lotion* of Antimony, Precipitates, Magisteries, &c. Or else intended to take away some ill Quality, or to communicate some good one.

*Lotion* is also the Name of a Remedy, holding a Medium between a Fomentation and a Bath. There are refreshing and somniferous *Lotions* for feverish Persons, made of Leaves, Flowers, and Roots boil'd, wherewith the Feet and Hands of the Patient are wash'd, and after washing, wrapp'd up in Linnen steep'd in the same Decoction till dry. There are *Lotions* also for the Head and Hair, made of the Ashes of Vine-Twigs.

*Lotion of the Philosophers*, in Chymistry, is a Cohobation which Nature makes of what is rais'd up, and afterwards falls back to the bottom of the Vessel.

**LOTION**, Wash, a Form of Medicine made up of liquid Matters, used for beautifying the Skin, and cleansing it from those Deformities which a distemper'd Blood sometimes throws on it; or rather, which are occasion'd by a preternatural Secretion; for, generally speaking, those Distempers of the Skin, which are accounted Signs of a foul Blood, proceed from the natural Salts thrown off by the cutaneous Glands, which ought to be wash'd away thro the Kidneys : so that instead of Sweetners, which are usually prescribed on these Occasions, Dr. *Quincy* thinks the Urinary Discharge should be promoted, or that of the Skin rectified by proper *Lotions*, or Ointments and Frictions.

**LOZENGES**, a Form of Medicine, made into small Pieces, to be held or chewed in the Mouth, till they are melted or wasted.

**LUCID INTERVALS**, the Fits or Paroxisms of Maniacs, wherein the Phrenzy leaves them in possession of their Reason. 'Tis said they are capable of making a Will in their *Lucid Intervals*.

**LUES** properly signifies a Plague or Contagion, tho' according to the modern Use of the Word, especially when joined with *Gallica*, or *Venerea*, it is restrained only to the *French* Pox.

**LUMBAGO**, Pains very troublesome about the Loins and the Small of the Back, such as precede Ague-Fits and Fevers. They arise commonly from Fullness and Acrimony; in common with a Disposition to Yawning, Shuddering, and erratick Pains in other Parts; and go off with Evacuation, generally by Sweat, and other critical Discharges of Fevers.

**LUNA**, in the Jargon of the Chymists, signifies Silver; from the supposed Influence of that Planet (the Moon) thereupon. The Medicinal Virtues of this Metal, Dr. *Quincy* says, are none at all, until hath undergone very elaborate Preparations.

**LUTE**, in Chymistry, any sort of Cement or Plaister; us'd either in the Construction of Furnaces, or in fitting to them Vessels of Glass of Earth; that are to resist a very violent Fire. The Word comes from the *Latin Lutum*, Clay.

It is frequently made of Potter's Earth, River Sand, Horses Dung, Powder of broken Pots, *Caput Mortuum* of Vitriol, Dross of Iron, beaten Glass, Flocks of Wool mix'd with salt Water or Bullock's Blood.

The *Lute* us'd by *Lemery*, was only two Parts of Sand and one of Clay, tempered together in Water; which does very well for joining the Noses of Retorts and their Receivers in distilling of volatile Spirits, &c. In distilling by the Alembic, or Vesica, or Copper Body, with its Head or Serpentine, a wet Bladder serves very well to *lute* the Junctures of the Vessels : But for the Distillation of corrosive Spirits, as also to stop the Cracks of Glasses, &c. the following Composition is recommended, *viz.* Starch boiled, or Fish-Glue dissolved in Spirit of Wine, with Flower of Sulphur, Mastic, and Lime slacked in Milk.

*Lutum Sapientiæ* is the Hermetical Seal, which is made by melting the End of a Glass Mattrass by a Lamp, and twisting it up with the Pliers.

**LUXATION**, in Chirurgery, a Relaxation of the Tendons or Ligaments, occasioning the Bones to slip out of their Junctures, or at least to remain very loosely in their natural Situation. The proper *Luxation* is when the Bone is entirely out of the Cavity it should move in; which may be done various ways, and there are as many ways of reducing it; according to the particular Formation and Articulation of the Joint : for which, see the Books of Practical Surgery.

**LUXATION**, in Medicine and Surgery, the slipping the head of a Bone from its proper Receptacle into another Place; whereby the natural Motion of the Joint is destroyed. *Luxation* is the same with what is otherwise call'd *Dislocation* : being the displacing of a Bone, or rather the disjointing of two

Bones articulated together for the Motion of the Part. The Word is *Latin*, formed from *luxare*, to loosen.

*Luxations* are either violent, proceeding from some external Cause; as falls, strains, blows, leaps, extensions, &c. Or gentle, arising from internal Causes; as a natural laxity of the Ligaments, a fluxion of Humours, or gradual collection thereof between the Joints, &c.

*Luxation* properly, has place only amongst Bones whose Structure determines them to a manifest Motion, as are all those united by *Diarthrosis*; those articulated by *Synarthrosis*, where there is no manifest Motion, are indeed subject to Fracture, Caries, Exostosis, &c. but not to *Luxation*.

*Luxations*, again, are either *perfect* or *imperfect*.

*Perfect*, or *compleat* Luxation, ΕΞΑΡΟΡΗΜΑ, is that where the head of a Bone is actually started out of the Cavity of another. It is known by a Tumour, or Protuberance, form'd by the Head of the separated Bone, which raises up the Skin, and muscular Flesh above its natural Level in the Part not destined to receive it; and a hollowness or sinking in the Place from whence it is started, perceivable by the Touch. It is also attended with great Pain, a total abolition of Motion, and a shortening of the Limb.

*Imperfect*, or *partial* Luxation, ΠΑΡΑΘΡΗΜΑ, called also *Subluxation*, is where the Motion is only much impaired, the Joint weak, and a Deformity perceivable in it, when compared with the opposite Part, which is found. This is otherwise call'd a *Strain*, when it proceeds from an external Cause; or, simply, a *relaxation*, when from in internal one.

A *Luxation* is said to be *Simple*, when it has no other accident or injury accompanying it; *Complicated*, when it is attended with a Wound, Inflammation, Fracture, or the like.

The Cure of a *Luxation* is by a speedy reduction of the dislocated Member to its natural Place. To this are necessary,

1°. *Extension*, αντιζασις, which a *luxated* as well as fractured Member requires; as well on account of the contraction of the Tendons, as that the Head of the Bone may more directly be intruded into its Seat. This *extension* is made either by the Hands alone, which is call'd *modus palæstricus*, because, among Wrestlers, dislocated Members use to be reduced after this Manner; or by Ligatures, or Towels; or by Instruments, or great Machines, when the *Luxation* is difficult, and inveterate.

2°. After *extension*, follows the intruding of the Joint into the natural Cavity; which, likewise, may either be effected by the Hands only, or by the Heel, (as when the Head of the *Os Humeri* is fallen into the Arm-pit) or by means of Ladders, Doors, Pestles, or *Hippocrates's* Instrument, called *Ambe*. This way is termed *Methodical*, by way of distinction from the third, which is call'd *Organical*, because perform'd by large Instruments, and Machines, but now altogether out of use.

*Gourmelinus* to these adds, αποθεσι, the very Act of reducing the Member into it own Place, which is to be known by the Sound usually heard, and from the Use and Motion of the reduced Joint.

Lastly, because on account of the laxity of the Tendons, &c. the reduced Bone cannot remain in its natural Position, it is necessary yet further to apply

Compresses and Bandage; by whose means the Articulation is preserved safe, till the Ligaments may acquire their usual strength of Elasticity and Astriction.

**LYCANTHROPY**, a kind of Phrenzy or Disease, that urges People to run thro the Streets and Fields in the Night; arising from the Bite of a mad Wolf. The Symptoms, &c. are in most respects the same with that of the *Hydrophobia*. The Word comes from the *Greek* λυκος, *Lupus*, and ανθροπος, *Homo*; as who should say, *Man-Wolf*.

**LYMPHATICS**, or Lymphæducts; very small fine, hollow Vessels, generally arising from the Glands, and conveying back to the Blood a transparent Liquor, call'd *Lymph* or *Lympha*. These, tho not so visible as the other Vessels, because of their Minuteness and Transparency, are however existent in all Parts of the Body; but the difficulty of finding them, has prevented their being described in many Parts.

The *Lymphatics* are contracted at small and unequal Distances, by two opposite semi-lunar Valves, which permit the Lymph to pass through them towards the Heart, but shut, like Flood-Gates, upon its returning. They arise in all Parts of the Body, but after what manner, needs no great Dispute; for, without doubt, all the Liquors in the body, excepting the Chyle, are separated from the Blood in the fine Capillary Vessels, by a different Pipe from the common Chanel in which the rest of the Blood moves : but whether this pipe be long or short, whether it be visible or invisible, it is still a Gland, whilst it suffers some part of the Blood to pass thro it; denying a Passage to the rest.

Now the Glands which separate the *Lymph* must be of the smallest kinds, for they are invisible to the finest Microscope; but their excretory Ducts, the *Lymphatic* Vessels, unit with one another, and grow larger, as they approach the Heart : yet they do not open into one common Channel, as the Veins do; for sometimes we find two, three or more *Lymphatics*, running by one another; which only communicate by short intermediate Ducts, and which unite, and immediately divide again.

In their Progress, they always touch at one or two conglobate or vesicular Glands, into which they discharge themselves of their *Lympha*. Sometimes the whole *Lymphatic* opens at several Places into the Glands, and sometimes it sends in only two or three Branches, whilst the main Trunk passes over, and joins the *Lymphatics* which arise from the opposite sides of the Glands, exporting again their Lympha to their common Receptacles.

Now the Glands of the Abdomen, which receive the *Lymphatics* from all its Parts, as likewise from the lower Extremities, are the *Glandular Inguinales, Sacræ, Iliacæ, Lumbares, Mesentericæ*, and *Hepaticæ*; all which send out new *Lymphatics*, which pour their Contents into the *Receptaculum Chili*, as those of the Chest, Head, and Arms, do into the *Ductus Thoracicus*, Jugular, and Subclavian Veins.

These Glands are round and smooth Bodies, about the Bigness of a Hazle Nut, bigger or lesser, according to the number of *Lymphatics* they receive. Their Substance is membranous, and their whole Bulk divided into little Cells, which receive the *Lymph* from the *Lymphatics*; and are therefore improperly call'd Glands, because they separate no Liquor from the Blood : It is true, that their exporting *Lymphatics*, communicating with their Arteries, do receive *Lymph* from them; but this is done without the help of conglobate Glands; as the lacteal Veins do with the capillary Arteries of the Guts: the chief use of their vesicular Bodies seems to be, that the slow-moving *Lympha* may receive a greater Velocity from the elastic Contraction of their membranous Cells, as well as from the new *Lymph* immediately derived from the Arteries.

**MACERATION**, in Pharmacy and Chymistry, is understood of a certain Preparation of Medicines, otherwise express'd by the Word *Digestion*. Others however restrain the Word to that particular kind of Digestion, which is performed in a thick Matter; as when, for instance, having mix'd Roses with Fat to make *Unguent Rosatum*, the Mixture is exposed for some Days to the Sun, that the Virtue of the Roses may be the better communicated to the Fat.

**MACROCEPHALUS**, from μαρκη, *magnus, great*, and κεφαλη, *Caput, the Head*, is sometimes used to signify a Head larger than of a natural Size.

**MADDER**, the Root of a Plant, much used by Dyers, to make the most solid and rich red Colour; it has its Uses in Medicine, being found of Service in Obstructions of the Viscera and Cachectic Constitutions; and is generally made up in forms of Decoctions, Diet-Drinks, and medicated Ales.

**MADNESS**, or Mania, in Medicine, a kind of Delirium without a Fever, attended with Rage, and a total Deprivation of Reason. *Madness* consisting much in a Delirium, to explain the Nature of the former, Dr. *Quincy* premises that of the latter thus : As often as the Species of Things, wherewith we have been acquainted are hurried together, we may be said to dream, and thence in Sleep they are added with other things, and variously compounded, from the manifold Repercussions of the Animal Spirits, which arise from the Cause producing Sleep, and pressing the Nerves, so as to revert the Fluctuations of their Juice.

A Delirium is therefore the Dreams of waking Persons, wherein Ideas are excited without Order or Coherence, and the Animal Spirits are driven into irregular Fluctuations. If therefore the Cause inducing a Delirium be of that nature, that it can excite Ideas or Motions of a considerable Impetus, without any manner of Certainty or Order, such a Delirium will be attended with Boldness or Rage, and violent Motions of the Body; that is, a *Madness* will be produced.

Now it is plain, that all the known Causes of this Distemper give a greater Disposition to the Blood for Motion, and render it fluxile, but not consistent, and uniformly thick enough; and therefore that they dispose Persons likewise to continued Fevers, since they occasion the blood to be thrown out of the Heart with an increased Force, unless some other Cause intervenes, whereby the Efficacies of these are interrupted in disposing the Blood into Febrile Motions; and the Blood is so disposed, as often as it can be rarefied, that it can easily, with any Force by the Motion received by the Heart, go into Parts divisible at the Occursions of those Orifices, into which it ought to be distributed : for then the Cohesion of the Parts, which can be but very small, will not be any Obstruction to the Increase and Propagation of the Blood's Velocity.

But if it happens that the efficient Cause, or the Heart, throws the Blood with a greater Force, or that the Blood can the more easily be propelled in any given Time, it will occasion, at the same time, that some Parts of the Blood be more nearly united, so as to form Moleculæ, consisting of cohering Particles;

which Moleculæ will cohere to one another, and not so easily obey the Direction of the Heart's propelling Force. The Blood hereupon cannot be uniformly rarefied, nor enter so easily into the small Orifices of the Vessels, and so soon travel thro' them, and therefore there will no Fever arise; but a Delirium without a Fever, wherein the Heat of the Blood will be greater, and the Pressure in the Brain uncertain : whence uncertain Recursions of the Spirits, inordinate Undulations, confused Vibrations of the Nerves, and a remarkable Energy of Imagination; whence will proceed Audacity and Passion beyond measure.

'Tis a Disease very hard to cure, and is generally found to baffle the Physician.

**MAGISTERY**, a Term in Chymistry signifying a Precipitate of some Dissolution; made by a Salt, or some other Body, which breaks the Force of the Dissolvent. Thus we say, *Magistery of Bismuth*, which is a very fine Powder made by dissolving the Bismuth in Spirit of Nitre, and pouring on it Salt Water, which precipitates the *Magistery* to the bottom. *Magistery of Lead* is a fine Powder, made by dissolving *Saccharum Saturni* in distill'd Vinegar, and then precipitating it with Oil of Tartar *per Deliquium*.

The word *Magistery* is also used in speaking of Resins, Resinous Extracts of Scammony, Jalap, Turpeth, &c. which are made by dissolving the Matter in Spirit of Wine, and precipitating it with Water.

Mr. *Boyle* takes the proper Notion of a *Magistery* to consists in a Preparation of a Body, whereby it is wholly, or at least in great measure, by means of some extraneous Additament converted into a Body of a different kind; as when Iron or Copper is turned into Chrystals of *Mars* and *Venus*;

**MAGMA**, among Chymists, &c. the Dregs or Residuum after Infusion or Distillation.

**MAGNES ARSENICAL**, in Chymistry, a Mixture of equal Parts of Arsenic, Sulphur, and Antimony melted together over the Fire, and condensed in manner of a Stone. It is a very gentle Caustic, and was first invented by *Angelus Sala*. It has its Name *Magnet*, because being wore during Malignant Diseases, it is supposed to preserve the Wearer from Infection by a Magnetical Power.

**MAGNET**, or *Loadstone*, a Mineral Stone, or rather a Metal, or an imperfect Iron; in Weight and Colour resembling Iron, tho somewhat harder and more heavy. It is usually found in Iron Mines, and sometimes in very large pieces, half *Magnet*, half Iron. Its Colour is different, according to the different Countries it is brought from. *Norman* observes, that the best are those brought from *China* and *Bengal*, which are of an Iron or Sanguine Colour; those of *Arabia* are reddish, those of *Macedonia* blackish; and those of *Hungary*, *Germany*, *England*, &c. the Colour of unwrought Iron. Neither its Figure nor Bulk are determined, but it is found of al Forms and Sizes.

The Antients reckon'd five kinds of *Magnets*, different in Colour and Virtue: the *Ethiopic*, *Magnesian*, *Bœotic*, *Alexandrian*, and *Natolian*. They also took it to be Male and Female : but he chief Use they made of it was in

Medicine; especially for the Cure of Burns, and Defluxions on the Eyes : the Moderns, more happy, take it to conduct 'em in their Voyages.

The most distinguishing Properties of this wonderful Body, are, That it attracts Iron, and that it points to the Poles of the World; and in other Circumstances also dips or inclines to a Point beneath the Horizon, directly under the Pole; and that it communicates these Properties by Touch, to Iron. In which Foundation are built the Mariners Needles; both Horizontal, and Inclinatory, or Dipping Needles.

*The Attractive Power of the Magnet* was known to the Antients, and is mention'd even by *Plato* and *Euripides*; who call it the Herculean Stone; because it commands Iron, which subdues everything else : But the knowledge of its Directive Power, whereby it disposes its Poles along the Meridian of every Place, and occasions Needles, Pieces of Iron, &c. touch'd with it, to point nearly North and South, is of a much later date; tho the exact Time of its Discovery, and the Discoverer himself, are yet in the dark.

The first tidings we hear of it, is in 1260, when *Paulus Venetus* is said by some to have first introduced the Mariners Compass; tho not as an Invention of this own, but as derived from the *Chinese*, who are said to have had the Use of it long before : but others, and with good reason, think the *Chinese* rather borrow'd it from the *Europeans*. *John de Goia*, a *Neapolitan*, who lived in the 13th Century, is the Person usually supposed to have the best Title to the Discovery : And yet Sir *G. Wheeler*[1] mentions, that he had seen a Book of Astronomy much older, which supposed the Use of the Needle; tho not as applied to the Uses of Navigation, but of Astronomy. And in *Guyot de Provins*, an old *French* Poet, who wrote about the Year 1180, there is express mention made of the Loadstone and the Compass; and their Use in Navigation obliquely hinted at.

*The Variations of the Needle*, or its Declination from the Pole, was first discovered by *Seb. Cabot*[2], a *Venetian*, in 1500; and the Variation of that Variation by Mr. *Gellibrand*[3], an *Englishman*, about the Year 1625. Lastly, The Dip or Inclination of the Needle, when at liberty to play vertically, to a Point beneath the Horizon, was first discover'd by another of our Countrymen, Mr. *R. Norman*, about the Year 1576.

**MAGNETISM**, a Term used by some Chymists, to signify a certain Virtue, whereby one thing becomes affected at the same time with another, either in the same or a different manner. This is what they otherwise call Sympathy.

**MALACIA**, a Disease consisting in a depraved Appetite, wherein the Patient covets and longs for some particular kind of Food with extraordinary Earnestness, and east it to Excess. As when a Woman with Child is vehemently desirous of Herrings, or any other usual Dish. Many Authors confound this Affection with another call'd Pica, consisting in a Deprivation of Appetite, which leads the Patient to covet things unnatural and absurd, as Lime, Coals, &c. The *Malacia* seems to arise from an ill Disposition of the

[1] George Wheeler, or Wheler (1650 – 1724), an English traveller and author.

[2] Sebastian Cabot (1474 – 1557), an Italian mariner and cartographer.

[3] Henry Gellibrand (1597 – 1637), an English astronomer and geometrician.

Menstruum in the Stomach; or from some Defect in the Imagination, which determines it to some one thing rather than another. The word seems derived from the *Greek* μαλακος, soft : too lax a Tone of the Stomach being generally the Occasion of Indigestion and unusual Cravings.

**MALGINANT**, in Medicine, a Disease greatly aggravated : The word is generally applied to such Fevers as are Epidermal, or Infectious, and are attended with Spots and Eruptions of various kinds.

**MANDRAGORA**, *Mandrake*, a Medicinal Plant, which makes a principal Ingredient in the Unguent, called *Populeum*. There are two kinds of *Mandrake*, Male and Female, each bearing a kind of Apples; those of the Male, as well as the Leaves, Roots, &c. being twice as large as those of the Female; but the Juice of each is a Poison, equally violent.

Naturalists tell strange Stories of this Plant, but setting aside its soporiferous Virtue, the modern Botanists will scarce warrant any of them, not even that human Figure ordinarily ascribed to its Roots, especially since the Discovery of the Artifice of Charletan's in preparing it, to surprize the Credulity of the People.

*Chinese* **MANDRAGORA** is the Plant *Ginseng*, which see.

**MANIA**, in Medicine, a Disease popularly call'd Madness. The work is *Greek*, μανια, *Fury, Rage.*

**MANIPULUS**, in Physic, is used for a Measure of Herbs, *viz.* an Handful; which is a quantity often used in Prescription among Physicians, and is generally marked with *M.*

**MANNA**, in Pharmacy, a medicinal Drug of great use in the modern Practice. *Manna* is a white Juice, or Liquor, very sweet, oozing either of it self, or by Incision, from the Branches and Leaves of the Ashe, both wild and ordinary, during the Time of Dog-days.

Others will have it to be a Honey of the Air; or a kind of Dew proceeding from a Vapour rais'd from the Earth, and prepared in the Air, condens'd by the Cold and gathered in the hot Countries, before Sun-rise, both on Plants and Trees, and even on Rocks, and the Earth itself. But this must be a Mistake; and 'tis much more rational to rank it amongst the Number of Gums, which exuding from the Juice of the Tree, and mixing with it some saline Particles of the Air, is condens'd into those Flakes in which we see it.

The *Italians* gather three kinds of *Manna*. The first *Manna di Corpo*, which oozes spontaneously from the Branches of the Tree in the Month of *July*. The second *Manna Forzata*, or *Forzatella*, which is not gather'd 'till *August*, after an Incision of the Tree, when the Flux of the first has ceas'd. The third, *Manna di Fronda*, which issues by itself, in little Drops, like a kind of Sweat from the nervous part of the Leaves of the Ash, and gathers into Grains about the bigness of those of Wheat, which are harden'd by the Sun in August. The Leaves are frequently found so loaden with these Grains, that they seem cover'd with Snow. *Manna* is a gentle and safe Purge; and us also used in Broths. *Altomarus*, a Physician of *Naples*, has written a Treatise expressly upon it; and *Donzellus* has seconded it.

*Manna*, tho' accounted a kind of Honey, purges the Bile; whereas common Honey increases it. Formerly the *Syrian* was in the most Repute, but now it gives way to the *Calabrian*. *Fuchsius* observes, that the Peasants of Mount *Libanus* eat *Manna* ordinarily as others do Honey. At *Mexico* they are said to have a *Manna* which they eat as we do Cheese.

*Manna* is brought from several Countries, and in several Forms. Thus we have *Manna* of *Calabria*, and of *Sicily*; *Manna* in Grains, in Tares, &c. The most esteem'd, is that in Tares; which many take to be factitious, and the Work of the *Jews* of *Leghorn*, but 'tis certainly natural : And what give sit this Figure, is, that they put Straws and Slips of Wood in the Incisions; along which the Manna gliding, is condensed as it comes out, and assumes this Form.

**MARASMUS**, in Medicine,; an extreme Macies or Consumption of the whole Body. A Hectic Fever usually produces a *Marasmus*. The word is *Greek*, being derived from the Verb μαραινειν, *to waste*.

**MARS**, among Chymists, signifies Iron, because imagin'd under the Influence of that Planet. Physical Writers prove Iron preferable for all Medicinal Purposes to Steel, which is only a more harden'd, compact Iron, made so by Art; whereby it is rendred more unfit to yield those Principles or Parts in Preparation, which the Physician requires to be drawn out. For the Operation of its Medicinal Properties, see Chalybeat. The Alchymists sometimes call their Mercury by the Name of *Mars*.

*Crocus* **MARTIS**, is the Rust of Iron; or Iron in an impalpable Powder.

**MARTIAL**, is sometimes used to express Preparations of Iron, or such as are impregnated therewith; as the *Martial* Regulus of Antimony, &c.

**MAST** *of a Forest*, the Fruit of a Species of Trees, call'd *Glandiferous*, or Mast-bearing; as Beech, Oak, Chestnut, &c.

**MASTIC**, a clear and sweet resinous Gum, issuing from the Trunk and larger Branches of the *Mastic* or *Lentisk* Tree, either without, or with an Incision. It is temperate in Heat, and of a dry, binding Quality; so that it strengthens the Stomach, stays Vomiting, stops Issues of Blood, and tickling Coughs and Catarrhs. It strengthens the Reins, and is a good Cleanser, and is for that reason prescribed in Seminal Weaknesses. The Goldsmiths mix it with Turpentine and black Ivory, and lay it under their Diamonds, to give them a Lustre.

The *Mastic* is the Product of *Scio*. The Trees that produce it are cultivated with as much Care as the Vines. It brings in a Revenue of 8000 Ducats *per Annum* to the Grand Signior. There is also a kind of black *Mastic* brought from *Egypt*, which serves to sophisticate Camphor. The best *Mastic* is brought from the island of *Chio*; it is in larger Tears, and those more balsamic, than that of the *Levant*. The *Mastic* produced in *Chio* belongs to the Grand Signior, who takes it of this People in lieu of the Tribute he exacts of the other *Grecian* islands. It has its Name *Mastic*, from its being continually chew'd by the *Turks*, especially the Women.

**MASTICATION**, in Medicine, the Action of *chewing*, or of agitating the solid parts of our Food between the Teeth, by means of the Motion of the Jaws, the Tongue, and the Lips; whereby it is broke into small Pieces, impregnated with Saliva, and so fitted for Deglutination, and a more easy Digestion in the Stomach.

The mixture of Saliva with the Food, is of absolute necessity; for the Saliva imbibed within the Parts, dissolves the Salts hid in them; and by so doing, prepares the Food for Fermentation in the Stomach : The Food therefore has the Beginning of its Digestion from the Saliva, and its Conclusion from the Ferment in the Stomach.

**MASTICATORIES**, in Medicine, are such Remedies as are taken in at the Mouth, and chew'd, in order to promote the Evacuation of the salival Humour; as Tobacco, Ginger, Pepper, Sage, Rosemary, Thyme, Mastic, &c.

**MATERIA SUBTILIS**, a fine subtle Matter, which the *Cartesians* suppose to pervade and penetrate, freely, the Parts of all Bodies, and to fill up all their Pores, so as not to leave the least Vacuity or Interstice between them. This Machine they have recourse to, to support the Doctrine of an absolute *Plenum*, and to make it consistent with the Phænomena of Motion, &c. and accordingly make it act and move just at pleasure, but in vain; for were there any such Matter, in order for it to be able to fill up the Vacuities of other bodies, it must, itself, be entirely void of any, *i.e.* be perfectly solid : vastly more solid than Gold, and therefore more ponderous and resists vastly more. Which is inconsistent with the Phænomena.

Sir *Is. Newton*, indeed, allows of the Existence of a subtile Matter, or Medium, vastly finer than Air, penetrating the closest Bodies, and contributing to the Production of many of the Phænomena of Nature. The Existence of such a Matter he argues from the Experiment of two Thermometers, which being inclosed in Glass Vessels, "one of them exhausted of its Air, and both carried from a cold to a warm Place, the Thermometer *in vacuo* grows warm, and rises, almost as soon as that in the Air; and if return'd into the cold Place, both cool and fall about the same. Hence," says he, "is not the Heat of the arm Room convey'd thro the Vacuum by the Vibrations of a much subtiler Medium than Air, which remain'd *in vacuo*, after the Exhaustion of the Air? And is not this Medium the same with that whereby Light is refracted and reflected, and by whose Vibration, Light communicates Heat to Bodies, and is put into Fits of easy Reflection, and easy Transmission? And do not the Vibrations of that Medium in hot Bodies, contribute to the Intenseness and Duration of their Heat? And do not hot Bodies communicate their Heat to contiguous cold ones, by the Vibration of this Medium propagated from them into the cold ones? And is not this Medium more subtile, more elastic and active than Air? Does it not readily pervade all Bodies? And is it not, by its elastic Force, expanded thro all the Heavens?"

Again, "Does not the Refraction of Light proceed from the different Density of this Matter in different Places; the light always receding from the denser Parts of the Medium? Is not this Matter much rarer within the dense Bodies of the Sun, Stars, Planets, &c. than in the empty, celestial Spaces between them? And in passing from them to great Distances, does it not grow denser and denser, and thereby occasion the Gravitation of those Bodies towards one another, and of the Parts to the Bodies; every Body endeavouring to recede from the denser Parts towards the rarer?"

"Vision performed chiefly by the Vibrations of his Matter, excited in the bottom of the Eye by the Rays of Light, and propagated thro the solid, pellucid, and uniform Capillaments of the Optic Nerves into the Sensory?"

"Is not animal Motion perform'd by the Vibrations of this Medium, excited in the Brian by the Power of the Will, and propagated thence thro the solid Capillaments of the Nerves into the Muscles, to contract and dilate them?"

**MATRASS**, or Bolt Head, a Vessel of Glass used by the Chymists in Distillation, and other Operations. It is made in form of a Bottle, with a very long narrow Neck. The *Matrass* is luted with Earth, when it is to be placed on a very hot Fire. When 'tis required it should be stopped very close, they seal hermetically. The Word comes originally from the Language of the antient *Gauls*.

**MATRIX**, or Matrice, any thing serving for the place of Generation of a Body: whether Organical, as the Matrix or Womb of Female Animals, for the Production of the Species; or Inorganical, as those of Vegetables, Metals, and Minerals.

**MATURANTIA**, in Medicine, &c. Ripeners, or such Things as promote Maturation.

**MATURATION**, in Pharmacy, a Preparation of Fruits, or other Remedies, gather'd before their Maturity; to fit them to be eaten, or taken.

**MEASLES**, or *Morrilli*, in Medicine, a cutaneous Disease, consisting in a general Appearance of Eruptions, not tending to Suppuration; with a Fever. This Distemper seems to bear a great Affinity to the Small-Pox, the Symptoms being in many respects the same, the Cause nearly the same, and the Regimen and Cure not much different.

The Eruptions usually appear about the fourth Day, like Flea-Bites, over the whole Body; but thicker and redder, and with greater Inflammation, than those of the Small-Pox, and vanish in four or six Days after appearance : being, when at the height, not larger than Pins Heads. The *Measles* is more sickly than dangerous; tho it often inclines to Consumptions, by a Cough which it leaves behind.

**MECHOACAN**, Macadossin, or *White Jalap*; called also *White Rhubarb*, and *American Scammony*; a medicinal Root, taking its Name from a Province of *New Spain*, from whence it is brought. *Mechoacan* was known and used as a Purgative before Jalap, tho the latter is now in more general

Use, as being found more efficacious. Yet *Mechoacan* is the sweeter and more gentle of the two, and on that account preferable.

The Seat of its Action is chiefly in the extreme Parts, for which reason it is accounted goo in arthritic Pain. It has the advantage of needing no Preparation or Corrective; and purging in it sown proper Substance, such as it grows. M. *Boulduc* found by analysing it, that it contains twelve times as much Salt as Resin; but neither the saline nor resinous Extract purge so freely as the Substance, even tho taken in larger Doses; nor do they yet purge so gently.

In the Choice of *Mechoacan*, prefer those Pieces which are the brownest within; and whose Substance is the closest, and most compact.

**MECONIUM**, in Pharmacy, is the Juice of the Poppy, drawn by Expression, and dried; differing from Opium, in that this last ouzes out after an Incision made in the heads of the Poppies. The Word comes from the *Greek* μηκων, *Poppy*.

*Meconium* is also a black thick Excrement, gather'd in the Intestines of a Child during the time of Gestation. In Colour and Consistence, it resembles Pulp of *Cassia*. It is also found to resemble *Meconium* , or Juice of Poppy, whence it takes its Name.

**MEDICINE**, as Art, ordinarily call'd *Physic*; defined, by *Boerhaave*, to consist in the Knowledge of those Things, by whose Application, Life is either preserv'd sound and healthy, or when disorder'd, again restor'd to its pristine Healthiness.

*Galen* defines Medicine, the Art of preserving present health, or of retrieving it when past : *Hippocrates*, the Addition of what is wanting, and the Retrenchment of what is redundant : And lastly, *Hierophilus*, the Knowledge of Things good, indifferent, and ill, with regard to Health.

Physic must have been nearly coeval with the World. The Injuries and Vicissitudes of the Air, the Nature and Qualities of Foods, the Violence of external Bodies, the Actions of Life, and lastly, the Fabric of the Human Compages; must have render'd Diseases almost as old as Mankind : And the Presence of a Disease, as it brings with a painful Sensation, the Loss of the Use of a Limb, &c. we find, does, by a necessary mechanical Impulse, both n Brutes and Men, compel the Diseased to seek for Help, and to apply Remedies, either by mere Experiment, or by Instinct, and spontaneous Appetite. Hence arose the Art of *Medicine*; which, in this sense, has been always, every where, among mankind. Antient Histories and Fables tell us, that in a little time, from the Flood, it was so well Cultivated by the *Assyrians, Babylonians, Chaldeans*, and *Magi*, that they were able to remove present Diseases, and prevent future ones. Hence it pass'd into *Egypt, Lybia Cyrenaica*, and *Crotone*; and thence into *Greece*, where it flourish'd, principally in the Islands of *Cnidus, Rhodes, Cos*, and in *Epidaurus*.

The first Foundations of the Art were laid by Chance, natural Instinct, and Events unforeseen : These were improved by the Memory of Success of former Experiments; by writing down the Diseases, their Remedies, and their Event, on Columns, Paintings, and the Walls of their Temples; by exposing Sick in the Markets and public Ways, that those who pass'd by, might enquire into the Disease, and communicate a Remedy, if they knew any : and lastly, by Analogy, or Reasoning, from a Comparison of Things already observ'd, with Things present and to come. The Art at length receiv'd a much greater degree of Perfection, by the appointing of *Physicians*; some for the Cure of particular Diseases, and others for Diseases in general; by an accurate Observation of the Disease, and its Symptoms; and by an exact Description of the Remedy, and its Use : immediately, upon which, it got among the Priests, an at length was confined to particular Families; descending, by way of Inheritance, from Father to Son : which, again, proved a great Bar to its Progress.

The *Extispicia*, or inspecting the Entrails of Beasts, used by the Priests; the Custom of Embalming dead Carcases, and even Butchery itself, promoted the Knowledge of the Human Fabric, and of the Causes both of Health, Diseases, and Death. Lastly, the dissecting of live Animals for Philosophical Purposes, distinct Narratives of the Cause, Rise, Increase, Crisis, Declension, End, and Effect of Diseases; and the Knowledge of Medicines, their Choice, Preparation, Application, Powers, and Events, seem'd to have almost brought the Art to its Perfection.

*Hippocrates*, who was Contemporary with *Democritus*, and perfectly acquainted with every thing hitherto laid down, and besides, furnish'd with a great number of Observations of his own, collecting into one all that was valuable and useful; compiled a Body of *Greek Medicine*; and was the first who deserv'd the Title of a true Physician : for being a Matter of the εμπειρια, *Experience*, as well as of Analogy and Reason, and withal well versed in a pure Philosophy; he, first, made Physic rational; and laid the Foundation of the dogmatical *Medicine*, which has ever since obtain'd.

What *Hippocrates* had done, continu'd a long time sacred and unalter'd, and was the standing Practice of many Ages; at length *Aretæus* the *Cappadocian* digested it into a more orderly Body : whence, in various Places, at various Times, and by various Hands, particularly the *Alexandrian* School, it was further alter'd and improv'd; till at length it came to the hands of *Claud. Galen*; who collecting all the scatter'd Parts, digesting those that were confus'd, and explaining every thing by the rigid Doctrines of the *Peripatetics*, did both a great deal of service, and a great deal of mischief, to the noble Art; he being the first who introduced the Doctrine of the Elements, the Cardinal Qualities, and their Degrees, the four Humours, &c. into *Medicine* : and on these he made the whole Art to depend.

After the sixth Century, the Arts were not only extinguish'd, but almost all Memory of them lost, till the ninth; from which, to the thirteenth, Medicine was vigorously cultivated by the *Arabs* in *Asia*, *Africa*, and *Spain* : who applying themselves particularly to the Study of the *Materia Medica*, and its Preparations, and to the Operations of Chirurgery, render'd both more just and more copious at the same time. And yet *Galen's* errors became now more predominant than ever.

At length, however, they were purged out and exploded by two different Means; principally indeed by the Restoration of the pure Discipline of Hippocrates in France; and then also by the Experiments and Discoveries of Chymists and Anatomists : till at length the immortal *Harvey* overturning, by his Demonstrations, the whole Theory of the Antients, laid a new and certain

Basis of the Science. Since his Time, *Medicine* is become free from the Tyranny of any Sect, and is improv'd by the sure Discoveries on Anatomy, Chymistry, Physics, Botany, Mechanics, &c.

*Medicine* is divided into five principal Branches. The first considers the Human Body, its Parts and Fabric, its Life and Health, and the Effects following from them; and this is call'd Physiology, the *Animal Œconomy*, or *Doctrine of the use of the Parts* : and its Objects, now enumerated, are call'd *Res Naturales*, or Things according to Nature. See Physiology, Natural Things, &c.

The second Branch considers the Diseases of the Human Body, their Differences, Causes, and Effects; and is call'd *Pathology*, as it considers the Diseases; *Ætiology*, as it enquires into their Causes; *Nosology*, when it examines their Differences; and lastly, *Symptomatology*, when it explains their Effects. The Objects of this Part are call'd *Res prætor Naturales*, or beyond Nature.

The third Branch considers the Signs or Symptoms, and how to apply them to use; so as to judge both in a sound, and a diseased Body, what, which, is, will be, the Degree, Order, Effect, of the Health, or the Disease : This is called *Semeiotica*. Its Objects are the Things both *Natural*, *Non-natural*, and *Præter-natural*. The fourth Branch considers the Remedies, and their Use, whereby Life may be preserv'd; whence 'tis call'd *Hygeine*. Its Objects are what we strictly call *Non-naturals*.

Lastly, the fifth furnishes the *Materia Medica*, its Preparations, and Manner of Exhibition, so as to restore Health, and remove Diseases; and is call'd *Therapeutica*, comprehending the *Diaetetica*, *Pharmaceutica*, *Chirurgica*, and *Jetrica*.

**MEDICINES**, or *Medicaments*, Preparations of any natural Substances, apply'd to a human Body, in order to answer some Intention of Cure. *Medicines* are distinguish'd, with regard to the Manner of Application, into Internal and External. *Internal*, are those taken in at the Mouth : *External*, or *Topical*, are those apply'd to any particular Part. With regard to the different Manner of their Operation, they are distinguish'd into *Evacuants*, *Astringents*, and *Alterants*, or *Specifics*.

A general Idea of the Manner wherein *Medicines* operate on a human Body, may be conceiv'd from what follows. A few different sorts of Particles, variously combined, will produce great variety of Fluids; some may have one sort, some two, some three or more. If we suppose only five different sorts of Particles in the Blood, and call them a, b, c, d, e; their several Combinations, without varying the Proportions in which they are mix'd, will be these following : but whether more or less, need not be determin'd.

*a b : a c : a d : a e :*
*b c : b d : b e : c d :*
*c e : d e : a b c : a d c :*
*a b d : a b e : a c e : a d e :*
*b d c : b d e : b e c : d e c :*
*a b c d : a b c e : a c d e : a b d e : b c d e : a b c d e :*

No Theory of Secretion has hitherto been able to give any tolerable Account of the Operation of such *Medicines*, as promote Evacuation. For if the Humours are equally mix'd with the Blood, that is, if the Blood is in every part of the Body the same, and its Particles are not more apt to form certain Humours, in some certain Parts of the Body, than in others; or if they are not forced, by the Power of some *Medicine*, to form such Humours : then the Quantities of Humour, separated in equal Times, will always be as the Velocity of the Blood; but the Velocity of the Blood is seldom doubled by any *Medicine*, and never tripled by the most acute Fever. The Quantity of Humour, however, drawn off by evacuating *Medicines*, is often twenty times greater than the natural Quantity; and therefore, upon supposition that the Humours are very where equally mix'd with the Blood, the Operation of evacuating *Medicines* can never be accounted for.

Tho this Argument hath the Strength of a Demonstration, yet there are some who explain the Operation of purgative, and other evacuating *Medicines*, by a stimulating Faculty; whereby the sluggish Juices are not only forc'd out, but the obstructed Canals open'd, and the Motion of the Blood quicken'd. But tho such a Power be allow'd it would remain to be explain'd why certain *Medicines* do only stimulate certain Glands? For it is evident, that evacuating Medicines have some other Power, besides the squeezing out stagnant Juices; because when they are all squeez'd out, they still evacuate as much, if they are repeated, as they did before : as is plain, by continuing a Salivation for many days. Secondly, we cannot suppose, that all Bodies have every where, and at all times, Juices stagnating; but these *Medicines* constantly produce their Effects, more or less, at all times. Thirdly, if the Vessels be supposed to be obstructed, an evacuating *Medicine* could but double the Quantity that was evacuated, before it was taken. Fourthly, if these *Medicines* operate only these ways, then in a healthful Body, where there were no Obstructions, they would have no effect at all. Fifthly, if the removing Obstructions were the Cause of a greater Quantity evacuated, then the Evacuation should still continue in a greater degree than before the Obstruction was removed; whereas, in fact, we constantly find it less, as the *Medicine* works off. Sixthly, tho a *Medicine*, by stimulating a Vessel, may quicken the Motion of the Fluid in that Vessel; yet it can never increase the Quantity of Fluid running thro it, in equal Space of Time; because it quickens the Motion of the Fluid, only by contracting the Vessel : and therefore the faster the Fluid is made to run thro' the Vessel, the less Fluid the Orifice of the Vessel admits; and consequently after the Vessel is contracted by the stimulating *Medicine*, the Secretion will be less, instead of being greater.

That a Stimulus causes the part, on which it acts, to contract, is matter of fact; and that purgative *Medicines* do stimulate the Bowels; but it may perhaps be likewise said, they stimulate the Heart and Arteries, and increase their Force, being they not only quicken, but raise the Pulse : so that a greater Quantity of Blood is sent to the Glands of the Guts. This may be granted; but not that it is the principal Action of purgative *Medicines*; because that, by the same Force, a greater Quantity of Blood is sent to all the other Glands of the Body, whose Fluids are not, however, sensibly increased; and the Glands of the Intestines receive a less Quantity, in proportion, than any others, because they cannot be so much dilated by the greater Force of the Blood, as others, which are not so much stimulated by the *Medicine*. There are others, who will have evacuating *Medicines* endued with an attenuating Quality, by which they dissolve all the Cohesions of the Particles of the Blood, and so set the several Humours at liberty, to pass thro' their proper Glands : but if these *Medicines* have a power universally to dissolve all the Cohesions of the Blood, then every evacuating *Medicine* would equally and indifferently increase the Quantity of every Secretion.

Mercury would as constantly purge as salivate, and Nitre promote Perspiration, as well as Urine; but this is repugnant to Experience. If they have a power to dissolve certain Cohesions, and not others; this is but setting certain Particles at liberty to pass thro' their proper Glands, which were not so before; and is a preparing the Humours, in order to increase the Quantity of Secretion. Evacuating *Medicines* must therefore have a power to affect some Particles, and not others; that is, to repel some, and attract, retain, and alter others; and this is what may be affirm'd to be in all *Medicines*, and is what a thousand Chymical Experiments demonstrate. The several Humours then being form'd, by the different Cohesion of the Particles of Blood, the Quantity of Humour secerned by any Gland, must be in a Proportion compounded of the Proportion, that the Number of the Particles, cohering in such a manner as is proper to constitute the Humour which passes thro' the Gland, bears to the Mass of Blood; and of the Proportion of the Quantity of Blood, that arrives at the Gland.

And hence it follows, that where there is a determinate Quantity of certain Humour to be separated, the Number of Particles, that are proper to compose the secerned Liquor, must be reciprocally proportional to the Quantity of the Blood that arrives at the Gland : and therefore, if the Quantity of the Secretion is to be increas'd, the Number of Particles is to be increas'd; if the Secretion is to be lessen'd, the Number of Particles, proper for such a Secretion, is to be lessen'd in the same Proportion. *Medicines*, therefore, which can alter he Cohesions, and Combinations of the Particles, can either increase or diminish the Quantity of any Secretion. Thus, suppose the Humour, which passes thro; the Glands of the Intestines, to be composed of three or four several sorts of Particles, and cohering, increase their mutual Attractions, so as they unite in greater Numbers at, or before they arrive at the Intestines, than they would have done, if the *Medicine* had not being given, must necessarily increase the Quantity of Humour, which passes thro' the Glands of the Intestines, if the Quantity of Blood which arrives at the Glands, is not diminish'd in the same Proportion, as the Number of Particles is increas'd. After the same manner do Diuretics, Sudorifics, and Medicines which promote all other Secretions, operate.

Why increasing the Quantity of some Secretions, should diminish that of others, is not easy to explain on any other foot : for if the Blood be equally mix'd in every part of the Body, with all the Humours which are separated from it; that is, if the Mixture of the Blood is every where alike, so that every Humour bears the same Proportion to the rest of the Arterial Blood, in one part of the Body, that it does in another; and if every Humour has its own proper Gland, thro' which it is separated : then what is separated by one Gland, is not subtracted from another; and consequently doth not diminish the Quantity of Humour, which flows to this other, but doth indeed rather increase the Quantity of this other Secretion : for the more any one Humour is carry'd off, the greater Proportion any other remaining in the Blood, bears to the remaining Blood : And therefore the more any one Secretion is increased, the more all the rest should be increased likewise. But if all the Humours are composed by a Combination of a few different sorts of Particles, then the more apt these Particles are to run into any one sort of Combination, the less all other Combinations must be : and consequently the increasing any one Secretion, must necessarily diminish the Quantity of all others; but most especially of that, which has the most of the same sort of Particles.

**MEDICINAL HOURS**, are those proper to take Medicines in : Of which there are four in the Day, *viz.* in the Morning fasting, about an Hour before Dinner, about four Hours after Dinner, and going to Bed; but in acute Cases, the Times are to be govern'd by the Symptoms and Aggravation of the Disease.

**MELANOGOGUES**, are such Medicines as are suppos'd particularly to purge off black Choler; from μελας, *niger*, black; and αγω, *duco*, to lead : but there is no such Distinction of Choler now regarded, and consequently this Distinction is but little used.

**MELANCHOLY**, in Medicine, the Name of a Disease, which consists in a Delirium, without a Fever, and is usually attended with Fear, Heaviness and Sorrow, without any apparent Occasion. The Word comes from the *Greek* μελας, *niger*; and χολη, *Bile*.

The Antients attributed this Disease to black and cloudy Spirits, arising as Vapours from a redundant black Bile. Some of the Moderns ascribe it to the irregular Motion of the Spirits, and their acid Constitution; and others, who know it better, to too heavy and viscid a Blood, which permits not a Sufficiency of Spirits to be separated in the Brain, to animate and invigorate the Nerves and muscles : And others to a Dryness of the *Meninges* of the Brain.

This Disease is vary'd an infinite number of Ways, according to the Temperament and Ideas of the Person affected with it. It is a Species of Madness, and only differs from a downright *Mania* in degree.

**MELICERIS**, is a Tumour inclosed in a *Cystis*, consisting of Matter like Honey: it gathers without pain, and gives way upon Pressure, but returns again : It is to be cured by warm Discutients.

**MELITITES**, a greyish Stone, which, when pulveriz'd, yields a milky Liquor, of a Taste somewhat like Honey; whence it takes its Name. It is found in Mines of Metals, and seems to partake pretty much of the Nature of Lead; having a Sweetness somewhat like the *Sal Saturni*, but much fainter. It only differs from the *Galactites*, in that it is milder to the taste. The Antients used it in Inflammations of the Eyes, and to dry Ulcers.

**MEMPHITES**, or *Lapis Memphiticus*, a sort of Stone mentioned by *Dioscorides, Pliny*, and other Natural Historians. 'Tis suppos'd to be found in Egypt not far from the City *Cairo*, the antient *Memphis*; whence its Name. The Property it is famed for, is, that being pulverized, and smear'd on any part of the Body to be cut off, it deadens it so, as that the Patient shall perceive no pain from the Operation.

**MENSES**, *Catamenia*, in Medicine, &c. The Monthly Evacuations of Women not with Child, nor giving suck; so call'd from *Mensis*, Month, the Period wherein they return. They are also called Flowers, Courses, &c.

The *Menses* make one of the most curious and difficult Phænomena in the whole human Body; for the Explanation whereof, many Hypotheses have been framed : tho' the Matter is hey scarcely ascertained.

'Tis generally agreed by all, that the Necessity Women are under for some extraordinary Supply to compensate the Expence, and support them during the time of Gestation, was the final Reason why this Redundance at other times was given them. But this is all they agree in. Some not content with this Occasion alone, will have the *Menstruous* Blood offend in Quality more than in Quantity; which they argue from the Pain it gives many Women in the Evacuation. They add, that its Malignity is so great, that it excoriates the Parts of Men by mere contact; that the Breath of a *menstruous* Woman will give a permanent Stain to Ivory, or a Looking Glass; that a little of the Blood dropp'd on any Vegetable, blasts, or renders it sterile; that if a pregnant Woman be defiled with the Menses of another Woman, she miscarries; that of a Dog taste them, he runs Mad, and grows Epileptic : All which, with many more Fables of the same kind, tho' related by great Authors, Dr. *Drake* rejects, as too ridiculous to need a Refutation.

Others ascribe this Effect to an imaginary Dominion of the Moon over the Bodies of Women. This was formerly the prevailing Opinion; tho' the smallest Reflection would have shewn them the weakness of it : For had this Purgation been owing to the Influence of the Moon, all Women of the same Age and Temperament, would have found it at the same Periods and Revolutions of the Moon, *i.e.* at the same time; which all Experience shews to be false.

There are two other Opinions which carry with them a great deal of Probability, and are argued with a great deal of Strength and Reason. In both which, the Quality of the Blood is allow'd to be Innocent; but they still differ about the Reason of its Issue. The former is that of Dr. *Bohn* and Dr. *Friend*, who maintain this Flux to be the result of a Plethora, or Plenitude; and to be evacuated only for Relief against the Quantity.

Dr. *Friend*, who has maintain'd the Cause of a *Plethora* with the greatest Strength and Clearness, supposes that this *Plethora* arises from a Coacervation in the Blood-Vessels of a superfluity of Aliment, which he thinks remains over and above what is expended by the ordinary ways; and that Women have this Plethora, and not Men, because their Bodies are more humid, and their Vessels, especially the Extremities of them, more tender, and their manner of living generally more unactive than that of Man; and that these things concurring, are the occasion that Women do not perspire sufficiently to carry off the superfluous alimentary Parts, till it be accumulated in such quantity as to distend the Vessels, and force its way thro' the Capillary Arteries of the *Uterus*. It is supposed to happen to Women more than the Females of other Species, which have the same Parts, because of the erect Posture of the former; and the *Vagina*, and other Canals, being perpendicular to the Horizon; so that the Pressure of the Blood is directed towards their Orifices : Whereas in Brutes, they are parallel to the Horizon, and the Pressure wholly on the Sides of those Vessels. The Discharge, he thinks, happen in this Part rather than in any other, as being more favoured by the Structure of the Vessels; the Arteries being very numerous, and the Veins sinuous and winding, and therefore more apt to retard the Impetus of the Blood, and consequently, in a *Plethoric* Case, to occasion the Rupture of the Extremities of the Vessels, which may last, till by a sufficient discharge the Vessels are eased of their Over-load.

This is the Substance of that great man's Theory, from whence he very Mechanically, and very Philosophically accounts for the Symptoms.

To his Argument, why Women have *Menses* rather than Men, we may add from *Boerhaave*, that in the former, the *Os Sacrum* is wider, and stands farther out, and the *Os Coccygis* farther in; the *Ossa Innominata* wider, and farther apart, and the lowest of them, as well as the lower Eminences of the *Os Pubis* farther outwards than in the latter. Hence in Women, the Latitude or Expansion about these Bones, and the Capacity of the *Pelvis*, is vastly great in proportion to those of Men; and yet in a Women not pregnant, there is not much to fill this Expanse. Again, the fore-side of the *Thorax* is smoother in Women than in Men, and the Blood-Vessels, Lymphatics, adipose and nervous Vessels, Membranes and Fibres, are much laxer in Women than in Men : whence all their Cavities, Cells, Vessels, &c. are more easily repleted, and the Humours aggregated in them; besides that, they are found to perspire less than Men, and to arrive much sooner at their Maturity, or ακμην of Increase. To which he adds the Consideration of the soft pulpous Texture of the *Uterus*, and the vast number of veins and Arteries it is fill'd withal.

Hence, a healthy Maid, being arrived at her Growth, begins to prepare more Nutriment than is required for the support of the Body; which, as there is not to be any farther accretion, must of necessity fill the Vessels, and especially those of the *Uterus*, and Breasts, as being the least compressed. These will be dilated more than the others; whence the lateral *Vascules* evacuating their Humours into the Cavity of the *Uterus*, it will be fill'd, and extended : Hence, a Pain, Heat, Heaviness, will be felt about the Loins, *Pubes*, &c. the Vessels of the Uterus at the same time will be so dilated, as to emit Blood into the Cavity of the *Uterus*, its Mouth will be lubricated and loosened, and the Blood issue out. As the Quantity of Blood is diminished, the Vessels will be less press'd, and will contract themselves closer, so as again to retain the Blood, and let pass the grosser part of the *Serum*; till at length, only the usual *Serum* passes. Again, there are more Humours prepar'd, which are ore easily lodged in Vessels once dilated; hence the *Menses* go, and return at various Periods in various Persons.

This Hypothesis, however plausible, is opposed by Dr. *Drake*, who maintains that there is not such Repletion, or at least that it is not necessary to *Menstruation*. Arguing, That if the Menses were owing to a *Plethora* so accumulated, the Symptoms would arise gradually, and the Heaviness, Stiffness, and Inactivity, necessary Symptoms of a *Plethora*, would be felt long before the Period were compleated, and Women would begin to be heavy, and indisposed soon after Evacuation, and the Symptoms increase daily : Which is contrary to all Experience; many Women, who have them regularly and easily, having no warning, nor other Rule to prevent an indecent Surprize, than the measure of the Time; in which, some that have slipp'd, have been put to Confusion and Shifts, no ways consistent with the notice a *Plethoric* Body would give. He adds, that even in those who are difficultly purged this way, the Symptoms, tho' very vexatious and tedious, do not make such regular Approaches, as a gradual Accumulation necessarily requires. If we consider what violent Symptoms come on in an Hour, we shall be extremely puzzled to find the mighty Accession of Matter which should in an Hour or a Day's time make such great Alterations. According to the Hypothesis, the last contributes no more than the first, and of Consequence, the Alteration should not be greater in the one than the other; setting aside the bare Eruption.

This is the substance of what is argued against Dr. *Friend's* Theory; which, it must be own'd, notwithstanding these Objections, is till the most rational and consistent that has yet been advanced.

Those who oppose it, give into the Doctrine of Fermentation, and maintain the Evacuation of Blood, on those parts, to be the Effect of an Effervescence, or Ebullition of the Blood. This Opinion has been maintained by many, particularly Dr. *Charleton*, *Bale*, *De Graaf*[1], and *Drake*. The two first of which supposed a Ferment peculiar to Women which produces this Flux, and affects that part only, or at least principally. Dr. *Graaf*, less particular in his Notion, only supposes an Effervescence of the Blood raised by some ferment, without assigning how it acts, or what it is. The sudden Turgescence of the Blood, occasion'd them all to think that it arose from something till then extraneous to the Blood, and left them to the Parts principally affected, to seek for an imaginary Ferment, which no Anatomical Enquiry could ever shew, or find any receptacle for, nor any Reasoning necessarily infer. Again, that Heat which frequently accompanies this Turgescence, led them to think the Case more than a *Plethora*, and that there was some extraordinary intestine Motion at that time.

Dr. *Drake* improves on the Doctrine of a Ferment; and contends not only that it is necessary there should be a Ferment, but a Receptacle also for this Ferment: Concluding from the Suddenness and Violence of the Symptoms, that a great quantity must be convey'd into the Blood in a short time, and consequently, that it must have been ready gather'd in some Receptacle, where, while it was lodg'd, its Actions were restrained. But he goes farther still, and pretends to ascertain the Place, &c. both of the one and the other, making the Gall-Bladder to be the Receptacle, and the Bile the Ferment. This Liquor he thinks well adapted to raise a Fermentation in the Blood, when discharged into it in a Quantity : And as it is contain'd in a Receptacle that does not admit of a continual Issue, may be there reserved, till in a certain Period of Time, the Bladder becoming turgid and full through the Compression of the incumbent *Viscera*, it emits the Gall : which, by the way of the *Lacteals*, insinuating itself into the Blood, may raise that Effervescence which occasions the Aperture of the Uterine Arteries.

To confirm this, he alledges, that Persons of a bilious Constitution, have the *Menses* either more plentifully, or more frequently than others; and that

[1] Regnier de Graaf (1641 – 1673), a Dutch physician and anatomist.

Distempers manifestly bilious, are attended with Symptoms resembling those of Women labouring under difficult *Menstruation*. If it be objected, that on this foot, Men should have *Menses*, as well as Women; he answers, that men don't abound in Bile so much as Women; the Pores of the former being more open, and carrying off more of the serous part of the Blood, which is the Vehicle of all the other Humours; and, consequently, a greater part of each is discharged thro' them than in Women; wherein the Superfluity must either continue to circulate with the Blood, or be gathered in proper Receptacles, which is the Case in the Bile. The same Reason he gives why *Menstruation* should not be in Brutes; the Pores of these being manifestly more open than those of Women, as appears from the Crop of Hair which they bear; for the Vegetation whereof, a large Cavity, and a wider Aperture of the Glands is necessary, than where no such thing is produced. Yet there is some difference between the Males and Females even among these, the latter having their *Menses*, tho' not so often, nor in the same Form and Quantity, as Women.

He adds, that the several Phenomena of the Menses, whether in a natural, a regular, or diseases Case, flow naturally and readily from this Hypothesis; and that whatever may be accounted for from a Plethora, or from any particular Ferment, may, without any straining, be apply'd to this.

The Root of black *Hellebore* and Steel, are the principal Remedies for Obstructions of the *Menses*; the former, is almost infallible, and in many Cases where the latter is not only ineffectual, but improper; as in *Plethoric* Habits, for with such, Steel will sometimes raise *Hysteric* Commotions, Convulsions, and a kind of Uterine *Furor*; whereas Hellebore thins the Blood, and disposes it for a Discharge without making it more impetuous. So that tho' each provoke the *Menses*, they do it by different ways; Steel by increasing the Blood's Velocity, and giving it a greater Moment against the Uterine Arteries; and Hellebore by dividing it, and rendering it more fluid.

**MENSTRUAL**, or Menstruous, a term in Medicine, applied to the Blood which flows from Women in their ordinary monthly Purgations.

The *Menstrual* Blood is the excess, or redundance of the Blood in the Body. It may be defined an Excrement serving for the Generation, as well as Nutriture of the Foetus in the Womb, and which at other times is evacuated Monthly.

Of all Animals, there is none besides Women, and perhaps Apes, which have their *Menstrual* Purgations. *Hippocrates* says, that the Menstrual Blood gnaws and tears the Earth like Vinegar. *Pliny* and *Columella* add, that it burns Herbs, kills Plants, tarnishes Looking-Glasses, and that Dogs which taste it, run mad. But this is all fabulous; it being certain that this Blood is the same with that in the Veins and Arteries. By the *Jewish* Law, a Woman was unclean while the *Menstrual* Blood flow'd : and the Man who touched here, or the Moveables she had touched, were declare unclean. *Levit*. Chap. XV.

**MENSTRUUM**, or Dissolvent, in Chymistry, any Liquor that will dissolve, *i.e.* separate the Parts of hard Bodies. Thus *Aqua Regalis* is a *Menstruum* for Gold; *Aqua Fortis*, and Spirit of Nitre, for most other metals; Common Water for Salts, &c.

In Pharmacy, it is chiefly defined a Body that will extract the Virtues of

Ingredients by Infusions, Decoction or the like.

The Term *Menstruum* takes its rise from this, that some Chymists pretend the compleat Dissolution of a mix'd Body can't be effected in less than 40 Days, which Period they call a *Philosophical Month*.

*Menstruum* is properly defined a Body, which being applied to, or intermixed with another, does so dissolve it, as that all the dissolving Parts float among the Parts dissolved; and so divides it into its minutest Parts, as that the Parts of the Dissolvent are intermixed with those of the Body dissolved. Whence it appears, that every *Menstruum* in dissolving a Body is likewise dissolved itself; so as with the Body it dissolves, to make up one Body. A Knife therefore divides Bread, but is not on that account a *Menstruum*; as it does not constitute one Body with the Bread; but Water boil'd with Bread is a *Menstruum*, with regard to the Bread, as it only make sup one Body therewith.

The Antient Chymists were very careful in all their Processes, that neither the Degree of Fire, nor the *Menstruum*, might deceive 'em.

All *Menstruums*, at the time they act as such, that is, at the time they are dissolving, act as Liquids; whether such *Menstruum* be a Liquid or Solid. Thus, *e.gr.* Silver is a *Menstruum* with regard to Gold; for if you take an Ounce of Silver, melt it at the Fire, and add a Grain of Gold; all the Parts of the Silver will intermix themselves with the Parts of the Gold : so, as that the Gold and Silver, which before were separate, now make one Mass. But Gold and Silver are only *Menstruums* as they are dissolved by the Fire; *i.e.* as they are fluid.

All *Menstruums* may be divided into two Classes; the first consists of such as are *fluid*; the second of such as are *solid* : that is, they are either actually divided, or they must be so e'er they act.

*Fluid Menstruums* are *Water*, Dew, Oils, Saline and Acid Spirits, *Alkali, Salts*, &c. and *Solid Menstruums* are such as must be made fluid e'er they will dissolve; such are most *Salts, Nitre, Vitriol*, &c.

*As to the Action of Menstruums*; Sir *Isaac Newton* accounts for it from the Acids wherein they are impregnated. The Particles of Acids are found to be endued with a strong attractive Force, wherein their Activity consists, and by virtue whereof they dissolve Bodies. These Acids he supposes of a middle Nature between Water and hard Bodies, and to attract both. By this Attraction they gather together about the Particles of Bodies, and adhere to them very close, so as scarce to be separated from 'em by Distillation, or Sublimation. Thus strongly attracted, and gather'd together on all sides, they raise, disjoin, and shake asunder the Particles of Bodies, *i.e.* they dissolve them; and by the attractive Power whereby they rush against the Particles of the Bodies, they move the Fluid, and so excite Heat, shaking some of the Particles to that degree, as to convert 'em into Air, and so generating Bubbles.

Dr. *Keil* gives us the Theory or Foundation of the Action of Menstruums, in the following Propositions.

1°. Two Corpuscles may be placed so near each other, without touching, as that the Force wherewith they attract each other, shall easily exceed that of their Gravity.

2°. If a Corpuscle placed in a Fluid be every way equally attracted by the ambient Particles, the Corpuscle will not be put in any Motion; but if it be attracted more by some of the Particles than by others, it will then tend towards that Quarter where the Attraction is the strongest : and the Motion thus produced will be correspondent to the Inequality of the Attraction : That is, if the Inequality be great, the Motion will be so; and if little, little.

3°. Corpuscles swimming in a Fluid, and attracting each other more than the interposed Particles of the Fluid; those Particles of Fluid will be driven aside, and the Corpuscles approach each other with a Force equal to the Excess of their mutual Attraction, beyond the Attraction of the Particles of the Fluid.

4°. If a Body be placed in a Fluid whose Parts attract the Particles of the Fluid more strongly than those Particles of the Fluid more strongly than those Particles are attracted by one another; and if in the Body there by several Pores pervious to the Particles of those Fluid, the Fluid will presently diffuse itself through the Pores; and if the Connection of the Parts in that Body be not so strong but that it may be exceeded by the Impetus of the Particles rushing together; the immers'd Body will undergo a Dissolution.

Hence, for a *Menstruum* to be fit to dissolve a given Body, there are three things required. 1*st*, That the Parts of the Body attract the particles of the *Menstruum* more strongly than those are attracted by each other. 2*dly*, That the Body have Pores adequate and pervious to the Particles of the *Menstruum*. 3*dly*, That the Cohesion of the Parts of the Body be not so strong but that it may be torn asunder by the Impetus of the Particles rushing together. Hence also it follows, that the Particles, which constitute Spirit of Wine, are more strongly attracted by each other, than by those of a saline Body immersed in it.

Hence we see the Reasons of the different Effects of different *Menstruums*; why some Bodies, for instance Metals, dissolve in a saline *Menstruum* : Others again, as Resin, in a sulphureous one, &c. particularly why Silver dissolves in *Aqua fortis*, and Gold only in *Aqua Regalis*; all the Varieties whereof are accountable for, from the different Degrees of Cohesion, *i.e.* of Attraction in the Parts of the Body to be dissolved, the different Diameters and Figures of its Pores, the different Degrees of Attraction in the *Menstruum*, and the different Diameters ad Figures of its Parts.

Suppose, *e.g.* the Attraction of Gold to that of Silver, to be as A to B; and of Silver to *Aqua fortis* as *b* to *d*; but that of *Aqua fortis* to *Aqua Regalis*, as *d* to *e*; let *f* signify the Magnitude of Particles in *Aqua fortis*, and *r* those in *Aqua Regalis*; *e* the Cohesion of Gold, and *e* the Cohesion of Silver : If the Diameters of the Particles *f*, are greater than the Diameters of the Pores of Gold, they can never dissolve the Gold, let their attractive Force by ever so strong. But if *b-exr* be greater than *g*, then the Silver will yield to the *Menstruum* whose Particles are *f*, and less than the Pores of the Silver; and if *b-exr* be less than *g*, the Silver will never dissolve in the *Menstruum*, the Particles whereof are *r*, and the attractive Force *e*. But if *a-exr* be greater than *c*, the *Menstruum* made up of the Particles *r*, and whose attractive Force *e*, will be able to penetrate and dissolve the Gold.

How a *Menstruum* may suspend Bodies much heavier than itself, which very often happens, may be conceiv'd by considering, that the Parts of no Fluid can be so easily separated, but they will a little resist, or retard the

Descent of any heavy Bodies through them; and that this Resistance is, *cæteris paribus*, still proportionable to the Bodies do by no means increase, or decrease, in the same Proportion as their Solidities do; for the Solidity increaseth as the Cube, but the Surface only as the Square of the Diameter. Small Bodies, therefore, will have much larger Surfaces, in proportion to their solid Components, than larger Bodies will; and consequently when exceedingly diminished, may easily by buoyed up in the Liquor.

**MERCURY**, in Natural History, a fluid, mineral Matter, perfectly resembling Silver in fusion. *Mercury* is known under a great number of Names : The common Name among the antients was *Hydrargyrum*, *q.d.* Water of Silver. The Moderns commonly call it *Mercury*, from some supposed Relation it bears to the Planet of that Name. In *English* it is popularly call'd *Quicksilver*, from its Appearance. Many of the Chymists call it *Proteus*, from the variety of Forms, Colours, &c,. it passes thro' in their Preparations.

Naturalists are divided what Class of Fossils to range *Mercury* under : Some make it a *Metal*; others a *Semi-metal*; and others an imperfect *Metal.*

*Boerhaave* observes, that it is very improperly call'd a *Metal*, insamuch as it has not all the Characters of such a Body; nor scarce any thing in common with the Other Metals, except Weight and Similarity of Parts : Thus, for Example, it is neither dissolvable by Fire, malleable, nor fix'd : In effect, it seems to constitute a peculiar Class of Fossils : and is rather the Mother, or Basis of all Metals, than a Metal itself.

Perfect Metals, according to M. *Homberg*, &c. are nothing but pure *Mercury*, whose little Particles are penetrated on all sides, and fill'd with the Matter of Light, which unites and binds them together into a Mass, so that the Parts of fluid Mercury, which are supposed to be little solid Globes, in their Metallification are render'd rough and uneven, being pierced on all sides, and having their Pores or Perforations fill'd with the Matter of Light. By such means they lose their first Confirmation, and the Politure or Smoothness of their Surfaces, which is one of the principal Causes of the fluidity of *Mercury*.

The Chymists make *Mercury* one of their Hypostatical Principles : Not, as M. *Homberg* observes, that it answers the Character of a Principle, which is that whose Substance cannot be Analyzed, or reduced into Matters more simple; but because the Analysis has not yet been discovered : Tho' it is possible it may hereafter, there being little doubt but that Mercury is a Compound. This is the more probable, in regard Mercury may be destroy'd, which never happens to simple Bodies. The manner of destroying Mercury, is, first, by changing it into a perfect Metal, by introducing a sufficient quantity of Light within its Substance; and exposing this Metal to a Burning-Glass, where, in a little time, it evaporates almost wholly into Smoke, leaving nothing behind but a light earthy Dust.

*Sweet Precipitate* of **MERCURY**, or *Mercurius Dulcis*, is compounded of crude *Mercury* drove over from Sea-Salt in a Retort, or revived from common Cinnabar, and dissolved in *Aqua fortis*; then a Brine prepared of Spring-Water and Sea-Salt is filter'd thro' a Cap-Paper, and the Solution of

*Mercury* dropp'd gradually into this Brine, whence there is a white Powder precipitated, which is to be wash'd from all its Acrimony with some simple distill'd Water, or warm Spring-Water, and the whole dried.

This is the common Precipitate of the Shops, usually call'd *White Precipitate*. Its Operation is mostly by Stool, sometimes by Vomit, and will salivate, if ordered accordingly. It is frequently mix'd with Pomatums for the Itch, and other Foulnesses of the Skin; for which purpose, 'tis necessary to keep the Body laxative, and to take something inwardly to take hold of the Mercurial Principles, and prevent their raising a Salivation, which they may otherwise do.

*Corrosive Sublimate of* **MERCURY**, is a Composition of Vitriol calcined to a redness, common Salt, and purify'd Nitre, with crude *Mercury*, cleans'd by straining thro' a Leather, all rubbed together in a Mortar, till the Salts are reduced into Powder, and not the least Globule of *Mercury* appears. The Mixture is then put into a Matrass, and that set in a Furnace with a Sand-heat, under which a Fire being kept to its greatest height for 12 or 15 Hours, the Mercury will be sublimed, and stick to the Top of the Vessel.

This Sublimate is a violent Escharotic, and eats away proud Flesh; half a Dram of it dissolved in a Pound of Lime-Water, turns it yellow, which is then call'd *Phagadenic* Water; it is used to wash Ulcers, and tetterous Eruptions.

*Sweet Sublimate of* **MERCURY**, is a Composition of the preceding corrosive Sublimate with crude Mercury, ground together till no Mercury appear, and then put into a Bolt-head, well stopp'd, and set in a Sand-heat, with a gentle Fire, for the Space of two Hours; which Heat is to be then increas'd for three Hours longer, and lastly, made very strong, for as much more. When this is cold, the Glass is broke, and the Sublimate separated from the light Flowers at top, and the Dust at bottom. This is then powder'd a-fresh, and the Operation repeated in the same manner three times. If it be further repeated a sixth time, it is call'd *Calomel*.

**MERCURIALS**, Medicines composed, or prepared of Mercury or Quick-Silver. The principal Class of *Mercurials*, are Mercurius dulcis, or white Precipitate of Mercury; sweet and corrosive Sublimate of Mercury; Calomel; Artificial Cinnabar; Turbith Mineral; Prince's Powder; Æthiops Mineral, &c.

The Medicinal Efficacy of *Mercury* depends on its extreme Divisibility, and Fineness of its Particles, and on their Gravity or Weight : by means of the first, it finds a Passage into the inmost Recesses of the Animal Structure, and, when properly guarded, does not exter itself till it comes in the remotest Scenes of Action; where most other Medicines either don't arrive, or at least not till their Force is rebated. This Property it has in common with Camphor. By the latter, it is enabled to make still more considerable Alterations in the Animal Œconomy, by rendering the Fluids thinner, and breaking open the secretory Passages : But this Effect it has in common with *Chalybeats*.

It may be here added, that the same Property whereby it becomes so powerful a Deobstruent, indicates, that 'tis to be avoided in Hectics, and all Cases where the Constitution is drawn low by too profuse Evacuations; in regard Mercurials tend to keep up or increase the Excess of Impetus in the

Fluids, and that Over-Capacity in the secretory Orifices, wherein the Defect of such a Constitution seems to consist.

**MESENTERY**, or *Mesaræum*, in Anatomy, a fat membranous Body; thus call'd, because placed in the middle of the Intestines, which it connects to one another. The Word comes the *Greek* μεσον, middle, and εντερον, Intestine, Gut; as being in the middle of the Intestines.

The *Mesentery* is almost of a circular Figure, with a narrow Production, to which the end of the *Colon*, and beginning of the *Rectum*, are tied. 'Tis about four fingers and a half in Diameter : Its Circumference, being full of Plaits and Foldings, is about three Ells in length. The Intestines are tied like a Border on this Circumference of the *Mesentery* : There are three Inches of the Intestines fastened.

The *Mesentery* itself is strongly tied to the three first *Vertebræ* of the Loins. It is composed of three *Laminæ*; the inner, upon which the Glands and Fat lie, and the other two which cover each side of the proper Membrane come from the *Peritonæum*. Between the two external *Laminæ* of the *Mesentery*, run the Branches of *Arteria Mesenteriaca*, superior and inferior, which bring the Blood to the Intestines; and the *Venæ Meseraicæ*, which being Branches of the Portæ, carry the Blood back to the Liver. Here the large Branches of the both Arteries and Veins communicating with one another, march directly to the Guts; where, with the Nerves from the *Plexus Mesentericus*, they divide into an infinite Number of small Branches, which spread themselves extremely finely upon the Coats of the Intestines. The *Venæ Lacteæ*, and Lymphatic Vessels, run likewise upon the *Mesentery*, in which there are also several Vesicular Glands; the biggest of which in the middle of the *Mesentery*, is call'd *Pancreas Asellii*; these Glands receive the Lymphs and Chyle from the Lacteal Veins.

The *Mesentery* has been ordinarily divided into two Parts, the *Mesaræum* and the *Mesocolon*. The first appended to the *Intestina Tenuia*; and the latter to the *Crassa* : But this is a Division of no great moment.

The Use of the *Mesentery*, is, first, to gather the Intestines into a narrow Compass, that the Course of the Chiliferous Vessels towards their common Receptacle may be but short; to cover and protect them and the Blood-Vessels; and to connect and dispose the Intestines so as to secure them from any Entanglement that might hinder their peristaltic Motion.

**METAL**, in Natural History, a simple, fossil Body, that fuses, and becomes fluid by Fire, and by Cold coagulates and hardens into a solid Mass, capable of distending under the Hammer.

*Metal* is said to be *Simple*, as it may be affirm'd of every the minutest Particle of Metal, *e.gr.* a Grain of Gold, that it is Gold, or has all the Properties of Gold. *Fusible* by Fire, that is, when exposed to a great Fire, it dissolves into parts which are easily moveable among themselves, or are in actual motion. *Fixed, i.e.* bearing the Fire without flying off in Vapours. Tho' it is only to a certain degree that *Metals* are fixed; for by the large Burning-Glasses of Mess. *Tschirnhausen* and *Villette*, all *Metals* readily evaporate.

Such is the proper Idea of *Metals*, which is no ways applicable to any other Body in Nature: For a Diamond, or other Stone, tho' a simple Body, is not fusible in the Fire, nor capable of being stretched under the Hammer. And Salt, tho' dissolvable by Fire, is not malleable, but breaks under the Hammer.

There are indeed certain Woods which yield in some measure to the hammer; but then they fall to Dust in the Fire : and so of the rest.

We find but six *Metals* in all Nature, *viz. Gold*, *Lead*, *Silver*, *Copper*, *Iron* and *Tin*. To these, a seventh *Metal* is usually added, *viz. Mercury*, or *Quicksilver*; but improperly, as it has not all the Characters of *Metal*, nor scarce any thing in common with the other *Metals*, except Weight and Similarity of parts.

Thus, for Example, it is neither dissolvable by Fire, malleable, not fix'd : In effect, it seems to constitute a peculiar Class of Fossils, and is rather the Mother, or Basis of all *Metals*, than a *Metal* itself. However, as it is usually reckoned among them, and as it wants nothing to render it a *Metal*, but an additional Sulphur to fix and connect its parts together, it may without any great harm be consider'd under that Class.

The common radical Character of *Metals* is, that of all the known Bodies, they are the heaviest. By Dr. *Halley's* Experiments, the Weight of Gold to that of Glass is determined to be as 7 to 1; and the Weight of Tin, the lightest of all *Metals*, to that of Gold, as 7 to 19; which considerably surpasses the Weight of all Stones, Marbles, Gems, and other the most solid Bodies, as appears from the tables of specific Gravities. Nor is there any Body in Nature but a *Metal*, that is one third the Weight of Gold.

*Plato* will have the Cause of *Metals* to be a humid Vapour, inclosed in the Bowels of the Earth, which being intermix'd with Parts of the Earth, produce various *Metals*. *Plotin* will have Sulphur to be the Father of *Metals*; and an oleaginous viscous Humour the Mother. *Lidyat* endeavours to prove all *Metals* generated by a subterranean Fire; urging, among other Reasons, that many *Metals*, when taken out of the Earth, are exceedingly hot. *Du Hamel* shews, that *Metals* don't take their Rise either from any vaporous Exhalation, or from Water, or from Earth; but are generated of Mercury, Sulphur, and Salt. He adds, that *Metals* take their Matter and Weight from the Mercury, and their Tincture and Form from Sulphur.

The same Author owns the first Rudiment of a *Metal* to be a saline Substance swimming in Water, which is by little and little carry'd off. By how much the Terrestrial Parts are more exquisitely mix'd with the aqueous or humid, by so much is the *Metal* more heavy and firm, as having fewer and smaller Parts. Hence its Ductility; for its Parts being extremely small, dense, and complicated, may be drawn out into a very spacious Surface. On which account it is, that Gold exceeds all other *Metals* in both Weight and Ductility; hence also its Fixity, its Parts being too close and dense to be exhaled. The Water defends the Earth from being burnt, and the Earth the Water from flying off; neither forsakes the other, but each is bound in an undissolvable Knot. The Moisture gives Ductility, the Earth Solidity. Where the Mixture is less perfect, whether the Earth of the Water prevail, the *Metal* will neither have so much Weight, as having larger Pores; nor will it bear the Fire so well. For if the Earth prevails, as in Iron, or the Water, as in Lead; Heat will set the one at liberty from the other; the Moisture evaporates, and the Earth is reduc'd into Scoria, &c.

Dr. *Woodward* accounts for the Production of *Metals* found in the Earth, in the following manner. All Metals now found in the Strata owe their present Conditions to the Deluge; when, also he imagines the Strata of Stone, Earth, Marble, &c. were form'd.

The *Metallic* and Mineral Matter now found in the perpendicular Intervals or Fissures of the several *Strata*, whereof the Body of the Earth is compos'd, was, according to him, at the time of the Deluge lodg'd in the Bodies of those *Strata*, and brought thence, and transmitted into these Intervals since that time; the Intervals themselves not existing, till the Strata were form'd and broke again, to let the Water form the Earth.

Now the Water which, he imagines, is constantly ascending from the Abyss towards the Surface of the Earth, continually pervading the *Strata*, detaches out of their Pores and Interstices such *Metallic* and Mineral Corpuscles as it finds loose in its way, carrying them along with it to the perpendicular Intervals, where having a freer Passage than before, it deserts them, and leaves them in those Intervals. And this he takes to be the way in which all *Metals*, bow found in those Places, were brought thither, and still grow.

Those in the *Strata*, however, he observes do not, nor cannot grow; but, on the contrary, are continually lessen'd and diminish'd, by so much as has been convey'd into the perpendicular Intervals, and brought forth of the Surface of the Earth by Springs and Exhalations from the Abyss, &c.

M. *Tournefort* is of opinion, that all *Metals* have their Origin from Seeds, like Plants; that they have Vessels, with Juices circulating in them, &c.

As to the Species of *Metals*, there are four which the Chymists call *Imperfect*, because their Principles are not bound so fast together, but that the Force of a common Fire destroys them; these are, Iron, Copper, Lead and Tin : the others, which are Proof against common Fire, and Gold and Silver. In the four first 'tis easy to see the Principle of Inflammability. They become all fusible by the Addiction of Salt-Petre, either in a greater or less degree. Iron is that wherein this is the most visible; next, Tin; then Copper and Lead. But the Principle is more conspicuous still, in the Dust or small Filings of the *Metals*, let fall in the Flame of a Candle, than in the Lumps. For Gold and Silver, the sulphurous Principle is not so obvious. No Heat but that of the Sun collected into a Focus, is capable to decompound them. But no doubt they have the same Principles with the other *Metals*, tho' not so easily seen. In Gold, as well as in the imperfect *Metals*, the Ground is an Earth capable of Vitrification, as appears by the Glass remaining after the Calcination of Gold in a Burning-Glass; and there is reason to believe, that the greatest Part of what is exhaled in Smoak during the Operation, is the sulphurous Principle mix'd with Salts. As to Silver, there is sometimes in it extremely various. When purify'd with Antimony, it vitrifies in the Sun; but if purify'd with Lead, it leaves nothing behind it but grey Ashes. The Ground of this *Metal* is doubtless an Earth capable of Vitrification; and what exhales in Smoak, is apparently a Mixture of Sulphur, Salts, and a little Earth, volatilized by the Fire.

The excellent *Boerhaave*, after an accurate Survey of the several *Metals*, their Characters, Properties, Preparations, Uses, &c. draws the following Corollaries concerning the Nature of *Metals*.

1. That which distinguishes *Metals* from all other Bodies, as well as from each other, is their Heaviness : Tho, every *Metal* has its peculiar Weight; which no Art is able to imitate, and which depends, as *Helmont* and the Chymists express it, on the Anatic Homogeneity of the Parts. Now, the later Philosophers have proved, that all corporeal Magnitude has just so much reality in it, as Weight; and therefore if you have found the Heaviness of any *Metal*, you have at the same time found un Corporeity. Sir *Is. Newton* treating of Gravity, and *Huygens*[1] of the Pendulum, shew Weight and Reality are correspondent.

2. The *Metals* appear to be Simple, yet are really Compounds. Their component Principles, according to the Antients, are Sulphur and Mercury; to which some of the Moderns have added Salt : but 'tis certain Salt is no constituent Part, or Ingredient of *Metals*, but rather something external adhering to them. All *Metals* consist of two Parts, or Principles; Mercury as the Basis or Matter; and Sulphur as the Binder or Cement : the first, the Substratum, or metallic Matter; and the second, that which renders it fix'd and malleable. The Mercury, it is to be noted, is the same with our Quicksilver, only defæcate, and clear of any heterogeneous Matter; where the common Quicksilver is always mix'd.

As to the Sulphur, it is not the vulgar fossil Sulphur, but a peculiar sort of Matter specifically denominated *Sulphur of Metals*, concluded by some of our latest, and best Chymists, particularly Mons. *Homberg*, to be Fire; which being mix'd with the Mercury, fixes it, and according to the different degrees of its Union and Cohesion therewith, produces different *Metals*.

3. All *Metals* must first be Mercury, e'er they be Gold; and the thing superadded to common Mercury, whereby it is prevented from becoming Gold, is a sharp volatile Body, which, when heated, becomes corrosive, and emits Fumes; which are the Properties of the fossil Sulphur.

4. If any *Metal*, or other Body, could be found that only differ'd from Gold in its wanting Weight, it were impossible ever to make Gold of it; and, on the contrary, if a Body could be had that is as heavy as Gold, all the other Properties, as Colour, Fixity, Ductility, &c. might easily be added. And hence the more knowing among the Alchymists hold the primary Matter of Gold to be Quicksilver; which, say they, is Gold, at heart, as coming nearest to Gold in the point of specific Gravity, Only there is a corrosive Body, *i.e.* Sulphur, adhering to it, which, if it were separated, you would have Gold; or if it were inverted, Silver.

And accordingly on such Principles whoever would make Gold out of any other foreign Matter, must remember, that the more his Matter differs from Mercury in Weight, &c. the less Gold it will make.

5. Therefore *Metals* are transmutable into one another : for if Mercury be the common matter of all *Metals*, and if all the difference lie in the fixing Spirit or Sulphur, which, as it is less or more subtile and pure, constitutes this or that *Metal*; it is in no way improbable they should be transmuted by a purer fixing Sulphur, taking place of a corrosive one, and fixing the Matter into a more perfect *Metal*.

[1] Christiaan Huygens (1629 – 1695), a Dutch mathematician and astronomer.

6. The purest *Metals* result of the purest and most defæcate Mercury, and the smallest quantity of the subtilest Sulphur. Hence, Mercury of Gold is heavier than common Mercury, and has always some impure part that is lighter than Gold; and could that be taken away, and the fixing Spirit be added, it would become heavier than Gold.

7. The imperfect *Metals* consist of impure Mercury and imperfect Sulphur, with some other variable heterogeneous Matter in it : Thus, fused by the Fire, it emits a Fume which whitens Copper, after which the Sulphur exhales yet further. The reality of such a third Matter is evinced hence, that all these baser *Metals* are resolvable not only into Mercury and Sulphur, but also into *Scoria* or *Sordes*, which are lighter and more earthy than either of the other, and accordingly swim therein.

8. Upon the whole it appears, that in the three nobler *Metals*, Gold, Mercury, and Silver, it is principally the greater or less proportion of the Sulphur to the Mercury, that determines them to be Gold, Mercury, or Silver : That it is by this Proportion those several *Metals* are defined and denominated; and that from this difference of Proportion, flow all the specific differences of Colour, Weight, Fixity, Ductility, Volatility, Fusibility, Solubility, Salubrity, &c.

9. That in the other baser *Metals*, besides this different Proportion of the two Principles, there intervenes another Cause of Diversity, *viz.* a third Principle, or Matter of an earthy kind, and very distant from either of the rest; which adhering to the pure elemental Sulphur, corrupts and adulterates, and variously modifies it : And from the different Circumstances of this third Principle, consider'd along with those of the Sulphur itself, result the specific differences of the more imperfect *Metals* as to Weight, Colour, &c.

**METASTASIS**, in Medicine, from μεταστωαι, *transfero*, I change, or remove; signifies the Removal of a Humour from one part, to another, which is most commonly known in nervous Cases : sometimes also in the grosser Humours; the refluent Blood taking up digested Matter from one part, and disposing it upon another.

**METHODISTS**, *Methodici*, an Appellation given to those Physicians who adhere to the Doctrine of *Galen*, and the Schools; and who cure with Bleedings, Purges, &c. duly apply'd according to Symptoms, Circumstances, &c. in opposition to *Emperics* and *Chymists*, who use violent Medicines, and pretended Secrets or Nostrums.

**METOPOSCOPY**, the Art of discovering the Temperament, Inclinations, and Manners of Persons by Inspecting the Lines in their Faces. *Metoposcopy* is no more than a Branch of Physiognomy; the latter taking its Conjecture from all parts of the Body : But both the Body, and the Branch are extremely precarious, not to say vain. See Physiognomy.

*Ciro Spontoni*[1], who has wrote on the Subject of *Metoposcopy*, observes, that there are seven principal Laws consider'd in the Forehead; each of which has its peculiar Planet. The first is the Law of *Saturn*. The second of *Jupiter*,

[1] Ciro Spontoni (ca. 1552 – 1610), an Italian scholar and author.

&c.

The Word comes from the Greek μετωπον, *Vultus*, Face, and σκεπτομαι, *inspicio*, I view.

**MIASMA**, from μιαινω, *inquino*, I infect; is made use of to signify such Particles, or Atoms, as are supposed to arise from distemper'd, putrifying, or poisonous Bodies, and to affect People at a distance.

**MILK**, *Lac*, a white Juice, or Humour, which Nature prepares in the Breasts of Women, and the Udders of other Animals; for the Nourishment of their Young.

*Milk* is thicker, sweeter, and whiter, than the Chyle itself, from which it is derived, and that probably, without much more Artifice or Alteration than the leaving behind of some of its aqueous Parts. The Antients held it form'd from the Blood; but the Moderns are of Opinion, it comes from the pure Chyle convey'd by the Arteries to the Breasts, and without any other Coction filtrated through the Glands whereof they are compos'd, like Urine through the Reins; without undergoing any considerable change.

According to M. *Leewenhoeck's* Observations, *Milk* consists of little Globules swimming in a clear transparent Liquor, call'd *Serum* or *Whey*.

*Milk* is a composition of three different Kinds of Parts, *Butirous*, *Caseous*, and *Serous*. The *Butirous* Parts are the Cream and Oil that swim a-top. The *Careous* are the grosser Parts, and those that coagulate, and are made into Cheese. The *Serous* are properly a Lympha, and make what we call *Whey*.

Dr. *Drake* says, that *Milk* is nothing but Oil and Water united by the Artifice of Nature, perhaps by the Intervention of some peculiar Salts, which, *Milk* itself, however sweet at first, does, after a little standing, discover to be pretty plentifully therein.

*Milk* is first found in the Breasts of Women after they have been pregnant about four Months. The Fermentation of the *Milk* in the Breasts, the first days after a Woman is delivered, occasions a Fever, which take sits Name therefrom.

*Aristotle* says, there are some Men who have Milk in their Breasts. *Cardan* tells us he saw one that had enough to suckle a Child.

In the *Philosophical Transactions* , we have an Account of a Wether brought to Milk by the sucking of a Lamb; which Lamb was maintain'd by it all the Summer, till it was weaned.

*Milk* corrupted in the Stomachs of Children, occasions the several Diseases incident to that Age. *Dobel*, a *Danish* Physician, who has wrote expressly on this Subject, tells us, an excellent Remedy in such Cases, is a Glass of Water with a little Salt dissolved in it ; This acts as an Emetic, and throws up the Corruption that occasion'd the Disorder. *Celsus* mentions this Remedy, L. 1. c. 3.

*Galen* observes, that in Animals fed with *Milk*, the greatest part of the Food of the Mother is converted into that Humour.

There are several kinds of *Milk*, used not only as Food, but as Physic : As Cows *Milk*, Asses *Milk*, Sheeps *Milk*, and Goats *Milk*. These are prescribed as proper to alter a sharp thin Blood into a Crasis more soft, balsamic, and nutritive; and in Constitutions where they fit the first Passages, must be very good for that End, as being already prepared into Nutriment, so far as is required for their admission into the Blood. But where the Juices of the Stomach are sharp, these Liquors are apt to be turn'd into Curd. Whenever the *Milk*, therefore, of what kind soever, is order'd in Consumptions, and as a Restorative, it is with good reason join'd with the testaceous Powders, and such things as are proper to destroy those Acidities.

Asses *Milk* is said to be a great Beautifier and Preserver of the Skin. *Poppea*, Wife of the Emperor *Nero*, used it for that purpose; having four to five hundred Asses constantly in her Retinue, to furnish her every Morning with a fresh Bath.

We have several artificial Milks, so call'd from their resemblance of natural ones. As, *Milk of Sulphur*, a Preparation of Flowers of Sulphur, and Salt of Tartar; prescribed by the Physicians, as a Sudorific. *Virgin's Milk*, *Lac Virginale*, composed of Rock Alum, Spring Water, Litharge, and Vinegar; used as a Cosmetic to drive in Pimples, and check any cutaneous Eruptions, by its cooling, restringent Quality.

**MILK** *of the Moon*, or *of Silver*, is also the Name of a white, porous, friable, insipid Earth, extracted by sublimation from a Matter frequently found in Silver-Mines : Whence also it has the Name of Flowers of Silver. *Milk of the Moon, Lac Lunae,* is also a Name given by the Naturalists to a kind of fossil Agaric.

**MILLEPEDES**, *Wood-Lice*, little Animals of considerable Use in Medicine. Thus call'd from the great number of their Feet.

*Millepedes* are so much in the Acquaintance of the People, that they seem to be Masters of their medicinal uses, and take them in many Cases without any other Direction. They are, by all Experience, found to be very Diuretic and Abstersive; which makes them not only frequent in Prescriptions for Disorders in the Reins, but also in Obstructions of the Viscera, and particularly in the Jaundice.

They abound with a nitrous Salt, which they seem to derive from the earthy Diet they live on. It is somewhat volatilized by its Digestion and Circulation in the Insect; as such Salt is more or less, in proportion to the digestive Powers of the Animal, into whose Blood it enters; yet no so much, but that it is brackish and pungent upon the Palate. This makes their detersive Qualities extend further, than the larger Glands, and enables them to scour even the minutest Passages, and keep the Nerves clear from Viscidities, and such things as would clog their Springs; whereby they are good in Palsies, Epilepsies, and all nervous Distempers.

As they open and cleanse away Viscosities, and by their Minuteness and Asperities cut their way through any Obstructions, they are good in Struma's, and all inveterate Tumours or Ulcers.

Remarkable Cures have been preformed in each way by a long use of them. They are best taken in Substance; or bruised in white Wine, the Liquor being taken without settling.

There are several Chymical Preparations of *Millepedes*, as Spirit, volatile Salt, Oil, and Wine of *Millepedes*.

**MINERA**, in Medicine and Anatomy, a Term apply'd to those Parts of the Body wherein there are collections and coacervations of Humours made; which hardening, form Obstructions, and produce Disease. In this sense, we say, the *Minera morbi*, &c.

**MINIMA** *Naturæ*, or Minima *Naturalia*, among Philosophers, are the primary Particles, whereof Bodies consist; call'd also *Corpuscles* and *Atoms*.

**MISERERE** *mei*, is a kind of Colic, or Disorder of the Intestines, wherein the Excrements, instead of passing off the common way, are thrown up by the Mouth. The *Miserere mei* is the same with what we otherwise call *Volvulus* and *Iliac Passion*. It takes its Name from the intolerable Pain and Anguish it occasions the Patient; which is such, as claims Pity from the Beholders : *Miserere mei* being a *Latin* phrase, which literally signifies, *Have pity on me*.

**MISSELTOE**, Missletoe, or Misletoe, in Natural History, a Plant of the Parasite Kind; growing, not on the ground, but on other Trees, as the Oak, Apple-Tree, Pear-Tree, Plumb-Tree, *Acacia Americana*, Beech, Chestnut, &c.

*Misseltoe*, by Physicians, &c. call'd *Viscum*, grows to the height of about two Feet. It consists of several Stems, which are usually cover'd with a greenish, sometimes a yellowish Bark, about the Thickness of the Finger, hard, woody, and divided by Knots; from which spring the Leaves, which grow by two and two opposite to each other, oblong, thick, of a greenish, or yellowish Colour, vein'd their whole Length, and rounded at the End. Its Flowers grow by three and three, Trefoil-wise, at the Extremes of the Branches : each Flower is a yellow Calyx, one third of an Inch in Diameter, divided into four Parts. The Fruit likewise grows by the three and three, at the Extremes of the Branches. They are a kind of oval Berries, not unlike little Pearls, fill'd with a flattish Seed in form of a Heart; cover'd with a fine silver'd Membrane, and enclos'd with a viscid, glutinous Humour, of a whitish Colour, wherein the Seed naturally buds or germinates, and puts forth two Eyes. From this Juice it is, that the *Latins* denominated the Plant *Viscum*. The Fruit grows on different Branches from the Flowers.

That uncommon Soil, whereon the *Misseltoe* grows, has occasion'd abundance of fabulous Notions both as to its Production and Virtues.

*Pliny* and most Naturalists relate that Thrushes being exceedingly fond of the Berries of the *Misseltoe*; they swallow 'em, and cast 'em out again on the Branches of Trees where they use to perch; and by this means give Occasion to a new Production of *Misseltoe*. By cracking the Berries with their Bills, or Claws, they are supposed to let out the Viscous Juice, which facilitates their Sticking : And hence that Proverb, *Turdus sibi cacat Malum*; the Viscum being sometimes used as Bird-Lime.

Mr. *Bradley* endeavours to refute the popular Opinion of the Antients, that the Seeds of the *Misseltoe* could not vegetate. Their endeavouring to propagate it in the Earth without success, he takes to have led them into the Error : And asserts, that it may be propagated by Seed on any Tree whatever.

The Method too is very easy. About *Christmas*, when the Berries are full ripe, you need only apply them on the smooth Bark of any Tree; the viscid Juices they are encompass'd withal, will make them stick; and, provided the Birds do not devour the Seed, you may, without any further Trouble, expect a young Plant the following Year.

Others rather chuse to account for the Propagation of *Misseltoe* from the System hereafter advanced for that of *Mushrooms*.

For the Virtues of *Misseltoe*, it seems of the most Efficacy in the Epilepsy; against which some will have it a Specific. Dr. *Colbatch* has wrote expressly to prove it such. It is also prescribed in Apoplexies, Lethargies, and Vertigos; and wore about the Necks of Children to prevent Convulsions, and ease the cutting of their Teeth.

The best is the *Misseltoe of the Oak*; tho' it is not this which is commonly used, but that of the Apple or Pear-Tree. Mr. *Bradley* observes, that there is no variety in this Plant, but that the Leaves, Flowers, Fruit, &c. are all alike on whatever kind of Tree it grows : But others pretend to distinguish that of the Oak by several particulars.

The Virtues ascribed to the *Misseltoe*, may perhaps be the remains of the Religious Honours paid it by the antient *Gauls*; among whom the Druids, assembled constantly on the first Day of the Year, went in quest thereof with Hymns, and other Ceremonies and Rejoycings, distributing it again among the People, as a Thing sacred, after having first consecrated it, crying *Au guy l'An neuf*, to proclaim the new Year. The Cry is still kept up at *Picardy*, where they add *Plantez*, to wish a plentiful new Year.

M. *Perrault* observes, that the *Misseltoe* is full of a poisonous Juice, which weakens the Tree whereon it grows; and that the Fruit has always a disagreeable Taste while it sticks on it.

**MITHRIDATE**, in Pharmacy, an Antidote, or Composition serving either a Remedy or a Preservative against Poisons. It is accounted a Cordial, Opiate, Sudorific and Alexipharmic. *Matthiolus* says it is more effectual against Poisons than *Venice-Treacle*; tho' easier to be made.

*Mithridate* is on of the capital Medicines in the Apothecaries Shops; being composed of a vast Number of Drugs, as *Opium, Myrrh, Agaric, Saffron, Ginger, Cinnamon, Spikenard, Frankincense, Castor, Pepper, Gentian*, &c.

It takes its Name from its Inventor, *Mithridates* King of *Pontus*, who is said to have so fortify'd his Body against Poisons with Antidotes and Preservatives, that when he had a mind to dispatch himself, he could not have any Poison that would have effect.

The Receipt of it was found in his Cabinet, written with his own Hand, and was carried to *Rome* by *Pompey*. It was translated into Verse by *Damocrates*, a famous Physician, and was afterwards translated by *Galen*, from whom we have it : Tho there is room to imagine it has undergone considerable Alterations since the time of its Royal Prescriber.

**MIXT**, or Mixt *Body*, in Philosophy, is that which is compounded of divers Elements, or Principles; in contradistinction to those of which the Chymists suppose to be Elementary, or consisting of one Principle only; as they take

Sulphur, Salt, &c. to be.

The Schoolmen define a *Mixt Body* to be a Whole, resulting from several Ingredients, alter'd, or new modified by the Mixture. On which Principle, the several Ingredients don't actually exist in the *Mixt*, but are all changed, so as to conspire to a new Body of a different Form, from the Forms from the Ingredients. Bur the modern Philosophers rarely conceive the Term in so much strictness.

The Business of Chymistry, we say, is to resolve *Mixt Bodies* into their Principles, or component Parts.

The School-Philosophers distinguish *Mixt Bodies* into *Perfect* and *Imperfect*. *Perfect Mixts* are the Class of Vital or Animated Bodies, where the Elements or Ingredients they are composed of, are changed or transformed by a perfect Mixture. Such are Plants, Beasts, and Men. *Imperfect Mixts* are inanimate Bodies, the Forms whereof remain still the same as of the Ingredients that constitute them : Such are Meteors, Minerals, Metals, &c.

**MIXTION**, the Act of Mixing; or the Union and Coalition of divers Corpuscles into one Body. The *Peripatetics*, who hold an Alteration essential to *Mixtion*, define it the Union of several alter'd Ingredients or Miscibles. *Mixtion* makes a considerable Operation in the Chymical and *Galenical* Pharmacy.

**MOLE**, *Mola*, or *Mola Carnea*, in Medicine, a misshapen Mass of hard Flesh, sometimes generated in the Wombs of Women, instead of a Fœtus; call'd also a *false Conception*.

The *Mole* is the Chaos of an Embryo; and would have grown to an Infant, had not the Process of Conception been disturbed. Tho' it be without regular Bone, Viscera, &c. yet the Lineaments frequently are not so far effaced, but that there are some Remains of a Child; sometimes a Hand, and sometimes a Foot, have been spied; but commonly the Secundines.

It is rare that more than one *Mole* is excluded; though *Sennertus*[1] observes that there are Instances of two, three, or even more. He adds, that tho' they usually come alone, yet they have been known to come with a Fœtus, sometimes before it, and sometimes after it.

The *Mole* is distinguished from an Embryo, in that it has no Placenta whereby to receive its Nourishment from the Mother. Instead of that, it grows immediately to the Womb; and is nourished thence. It has a kind of Vegetative Life, and continues growing in bulk till the time of exclusion. Sometimes it has been born in the Womb for two or three Years.

This Production is supposed to arise from some Defect or Indisposition of the *Ovum* or Egg; or, perhaps, from the Male Seed's wanting force to penetrate it sufficiently in order to open, and expand the Parts. Or the Effect may be accounted for, by supposing an *Ovum* to drop into the Womb, without being impregnated by the Seed of the Male : In all which cases, the Egg continuing to grow, and yet wanting something necessary to organize and form it into an Embryo, becomes a shapeless Lump.

[1] Daniel Sennert (1572 – 1637), a German physician.

Authors divided whether or no the Women ever bring forth *Moles* without any intercourse with men. Same say there are *Moles* which derive their Origin from the Menstruous Blood detain'd, coagulated, and harden'd; through which the Blood and Spirits have made themselves Passages, &c.

The *Mole* is distinguished from a true Conception, by its tremulous palpitating Motion; by its rolling from side to side; and by the Belly's swelling equally every way. The Breasts swell as in the case of a just Embryo; but the Humour generated therein is not true Milk, but a crude Matter, form'd of the suppressed Menses.

To bring the *Mola* out of the Womb, Bleeding and violent Purging are used, and at last strong Emmenagogues. If these fail, recourse is to be held to manual Operation.

The *Latins* give it the Name *Mola*, which literally signifies *Mill-Stone*, from its resemblance thereto in Form and Hardness.

**MOLECULE**, *Molecula*, in Physics, a little Mass or part of any thing. Thus we say the Air, by Respiration, insinuating itself into the veins and Arteries, endeavours by its elastic Power to divide and break the Molecules of the Blood, which on their side resist such division.

**MONOPETALOUS**, in Botany, a Term apply'd to Flowers which have only one undivided *Petalum*, or Leaf.

**MONOPYRENEOUS** Fruits, are such as only contain one Kernal or Seed.

**MOORS-HEAD**, in Chymistry, a Copper-Cap made in form of a Head, to be set over the Chimney of a Reverberating Furnace. *Moors-Head* is also the Head of a Copper or Glass-Still or Alembic, which is luted on to the Body or Cucurbit, and hath a Beak or Pipe to let the Spirit run down into the Receiver.

**MORBID**, *Morridus*, in Medicine, is apply'd to signify those Parts, Humours, &c. whereon a Disease lies.

**MORBILLI**, in Medicine, a Disease popularly call'd the Measles.

**MORBUS**, a term purely Latin, signifying Disease.

**MORBUS** *Comitialis*, is the Epilepsy; thus call'd by the *Romans*, because when in any of their public Assemblies Persons fell down with this Distemper, they immediately broke up, and dissolved the Comitia, which was the common Appellation for such Courts.

**MORBUS** *Regius*. See Jaundice.
**MORBUS** *Virgineus*. See Chlorosis.
**MORBUS** *Gallicus*. See Venereal Disease.

**MORPHEW**, is that Freckle or Scurf which breaks out sometimes upon the Skin, particularly about the Forehead.

**MORSELLI**, and Morsuli, antient Names for those Forms of Medicines which were to be chew'd in the Mouth, as a *Lozenge*; the Word signifying a little Mouthful.

**MORTIFICATION**, in Medicine, &c. a Disease, wherein, the natural Juices of any part quite lose their proper Motions; and by that means fall into a fermentative one, and corrupt and destroy the Texture of the Part. There are two Species, or rather Degrees of *Mortification*: The one call'd a *Gangrene*, which is a *Mortification* in its first, or beginning State : The other a *Sphacelus*, which is a perfect, or finish'd *Mortification*.

**MOSSE**, *Usnea*, in Natural History, a little Plant of the Parasite kind, growing on the Barks, &c. of several Trees, as Oak, Poplar, Ash, Cedar, &c. The most esteemed, and odoriferous is that of the Cedar; it is of some medicinal Use, being Astringent, and proper to stop Hemorrhagies and Dysenteries.

The Antients took the *Moss* of Trees to be the Effect of a Disorder or Discomposure of the Texture of the Bark; or at most a kind of little Filaments arising from the Bark. But the Moderns find by several Observations, that Mosses are all real, distinct Plants, whose Seed, being extremely small, is inclosed in little Capsulæ, which bursting of themselves, the Seed is carried off by the Winds, till falling on the Inequalities of the Bark of Trees, it is there stopp'd, takes Root, and feeds at the expence of the Tree, as Mouldiness does on Bread, &c.

The different kinds of *Mosses* are very numerous; Mons. *Vaillant* reckons 137 Species in the single Neighbourhood of *Paris*. There is also a kind of greenish *Moss* growing in human Skulls that have been long exposed to the Air, call'd *Usnea*, or *Muscus calvarius*. The Antients made a deal of Use of it as an Astringent, &c.

*Mosses* make an Article of Commerce; there being several kinds used in Medicine, in Perfuming, &c. Among others, the *Sea-Moss*, call'd *Coralline*, and the *Moss* of Cedar and Firr, which enter the Composition of Cypress Powder.

The *Moss* of common Trees, as Oak, Ash, Poplar, &c. is used for Caulking of Vessels. 'Tis also used by Bird-Merchants, to prepare Cages for certain kinds of Birds to hatch in. The Gardeners, &c. reckon Moss among the Diseases, or Infir-mities of Plants.

Mr. *Mortimer*[1], &c. directs it to be rubb'd, and scraped off with some proper Instrument that will not hurt the Bark of the Tree, or with a piece of Hair-Cloth after a soaking Rain; tho' the surest Cure is by removing the Cause; which is effected by draining the Land well of all superfluous Moisture. Or, it may be prevented, in the first planting of Trees, by not setting them too deep.

**MOTOS**, a Piece of Line, or Linnen Cloth, teaz'd like Wool, to be put into Ulcers, to stop the Flux of Blood, &c.

[1] John Mortimer (ca. 1656 – 1736), an English agricultural writer.

**MUCILAGE**, in Pharmacy, &c. a thick, viscous Juice; so call'd, as resembling Snot, or the Mucus of the Nose. It is prepar'd from Roots, and Seeds pounded in a Mortar, and infused in Hot Water, and strained thro' a Cloth. The Seeds used for this purpose, are those of Althaea, Mallows, Symphytum, &c. *Mucilages* enter the Composition of several Plaisters; they sometimes are also made of Gums and Fruits, as Figs, Quinces, Izing-Glass, &c.

**MUCILAGE** is also a thick, pituitous Matter, evacuated with the Urine in the Gravel, and Dysuria.

**MULTISILIQUOUS** *Plants*, are the same with *Corniculate* Plants, *viz.* those which, after each Flower, have divers distinct, slender, and frequently crooked *Siliquæ*, or Pods, wherein their Seed is contain'd; and which when they ripen, open of them-selves, and let the Seeds drop. To this Class belongs the Bears-Foot, Columbines, House-Leek, Marigolds, &c.

**MUMMY**, *Mumia*, a Carcass, or Body embalmed or dried in the manner of the antient *Egyptians*. The Preparation of the *Mummy* is so old a standing, that it was in use in *Egypt* before the time of *Moses*. The Coffin in which the *Mummy* is contain'd is of Sycamore-Wood, which is found to keep sound for the Space of 3000 Years; but it is very different from our Sycamore.

*Mummy* is said to have been first brought into use in Medicine by the Malice of a *Jewish* Physician, who wrote that Flesh thus Embalmed was good for the Cure of divers Diseases, and particularly Bruises, to prevent the Blood's gathering and coagulating. The *Turks* prevent the Export of *Mummies* into *Europe* as much as possible.

Properly speaking, *Mummy* is not the Flesh of the Deceased, but the Composition wherewith it is embalmed; but in common use *Mummy* is also used for the Body. There are two kinds of Bodies call'd by the Term *Mummy*.

The first are only Carcasses, dried by the Heat of the Sun, and by that means kept from Putrefaction; frequently found in the dry sands of *Lybia*. Some say, they are the Bodies of deceased People buried there on purpose to keep 'em entire without Embalming; others that they are the Carcasses of Travellers, &c. overwhelm'd with Clouds of Sands rais'd by the Hurricanes frequent in those Deserts. Be that as it will, these *Mummies* are of no use in Medicine, and are only preserv'd as Curiosities.

The second kind of *Mummies* are Bodies taken out of the Pits, or Catacombs near *Cairo*, wherein the *Egyptians* deposited their Dead after Embalming. 'Tis this makes the *Mummy* so much valued, and to which such extraordinary Virtues are ascribed.

'Tis said, that all the *Mummy* sold in the Shops, whether brought from *Venice* or *Lyons*, or even directly from the *Levant* by *Alexandria*, is factitious, and the Work of certain *Jews*, who knowing the Value the *Europeans* set on the *Egyptian Mummy*, counterfeit it by drying Carcasses in Ovens, after having prepared 'em with Dust of Myrrh, Caballin Aloes, *Jewish* Pitch, black Pitch, and other coarse or unwholesome Drugs.

The *French Charletans*, it seems, have likewise got the Art of preparing *Mummies*. Their Method is simple enough : Out of the Carcass of a Person hang'd, they take the Brain and Entrails, dry the rest in an Oven, steeping it in Pitch, and other Drugs. And this they sell for right *Egyptian Mummy.*

*Pareus*[1] has a very curious Treatise of *Mummies*, wherein he shews the Abuses thereof; and makes it appear that they can never be of any real medicinal use. *Matthiolus* is of the same Opinion, after *Serapion*. Both these Authors take even the *Egyptian Mummies* to be no more than Bodies embalmed with Pissasphaltum.

*Mummy*, *Mumia*, is particularly used for the Liquor, or Juice oozing from human Bodies Aromatized and Embalmed; gather'd in the Sepulchres. This is the *Mummy* chiefly spoken of among the antient Writers. *Mummy* is also a Medicinal Drug, or a viscous Composition partaking of Bitumen and Pitch found in the Mountains and Forests of *Arabia*, and other hot Countreys of the *East*.

*Dioscorides* speaks of a *Mummy* found on the Sea-Coasts near *Epidaurus*, brought thither by the Torrents from the *Ceraunian* Mountains, and there dried by the Sun into huge heaps. It smells like Bitumen mixt with Pitch. The People thereabouts call it *mineral Wax*. In *Latin*, or rather *Greek*, it is call'd *Pissasphaltus*.

*Menage*, after *Bochart*, derives the Word *Mummy* from the *Arabic Mumia*; of *Mum*, Wax. *Salmasius* from *Amomo*, a kind of Perfume. Tho others hold, that in the *Arabic* Tongue, the Word *Mumia* signifies a Body Embalmed, or Aromatized.

*Mummy* is also used by some Physicians for I know not what implanted Spirit, found chiefly in Carcasses, when the infused Spirit is fled. The infused Spirit is sometimes also call'd *Mummy* in living Subjects; and both the one and the other are supposed to serve in Transplantation.

A Plant, for instance, bringing this *Mumia* from one Subject to another, the *Mumia* joins and unites itself immediately, and closes with the *Mumia* or Spirit of the new Subject; and from this Union arises a natural and common Inclination between the two Spirits. And on this principle they account for Sympathetic or Magnetic Cures. And on this Principle they account for Sympathetic or Magnetic Cures.

**MUNDIFICATIVES**, in Medicine, Cleansers; Medicines, or Unguents that deterge, and dry, and thus cleanse Ulcers of two kinds of Matter, *viz.* Pus and Sanies. The chief Ingredient in these Unguents, are Gentian, Aristolochia, Enula Campana, and Vulnerary herbs.

**MUSK**, a kind of Perfume, of a very strong Scent; only agreeable when moderated by the Mixture of some other Perfume. The Word comes from the *Arabic Moscha*, Musk : whence was form'd the common *Greek* μοσχος.

It is found in a kind of Bag, or Tumour growing about the bigness of a Hen's Egg under the Belly towards the genital Parts of a wild Beast of the same Name; and appears to be nothing else but a kind of bilious Blood there congealed, and almost corrupted.

The Animal is pretty common in the Kingdom of *Boutan, Tonquin*, and

[1] Ambrose Paré (1509 – 1590), a French physician and surgeon.

some other, as *Cochin China*, &c. But the most esteemed are those in the Kingdom of *Tibet*.

They inhabit the Woods and Forests, where the Natives hunt 'em down : when the Beast is kill'd, they cut out the Bladder under the Belly, separate the coagulated Blood, and dry it in the Sun, where it is reduced into a light friable Substance almost of the nature of a Powder, of a dusky reddish Colour; and acquires a very strong and disagreeable Smell. It is then tied up again in Vessels, and exported to other Countreys; and this is the *Musk* which we use.

What the Antients have wrote of it, is fabulous, *viz.* that it comes from the Testicles of a Castor, which, to stop the pursuit of the Hunter, castrates itself. The occasion of their Error may be owing to this, that among the *Indians* the *Musk* Animal goes by the name of *Castor*.

*Musk* is in considerable use among the Perfumers and Confectioners; tho much less now than formerly. It is supposed to fortify the Heart and Brain; and is good against Deafness; but is little used in Medicine, as being apt to occasion the Vapours.

**MUST**, sweet Wine, newly pressed from the Grape; or the new Liquor press'd from the Fruits before it has work'd or fermented.

**MUSTARD-SEED**, in *Latin Sinapi*, gives the Denomination to a Species of Topical Medicines call'd *Sinapisms*.

**MYRMECIA**, in Medicine, a kind of Wart growing on the Palm of the Hand, and Soal of the Foot; hard, and less than those call'd *Thymi* : they have also deeper Roots, and are more painful. They are usually broad at bottom, and narrow at top.

**MYRABOLANS**, a kind of Medicinal Fruit, brought from the Indies; much more used in the *Arabic* than the *Greek* Pharmacy; and more among the Antients than the Moderns; and still more abroad than in *England*.

There are five kinds of *Myrabolans* : The first call'd *Citrine*, of a yellowish red, hard, oblong, and the size of an Olive. The second call'd *black* or *Indian Myrabolans*, the bigness of an Acorn wrinkled, without Stone. The third, *Chebule Myrobalans*, the size of a Date, of a yellowish brown, pointed at the end. The fourth *Emblics*, round, rough, the size of a Gall, of a dark brown. The last call'd *Bellerics*, hard, yellow, round, the size of an ordinary Prune, less angular than the rest.

*Myrabolans* of each kind are slightly Purgative, and Astringent.

The Word comes from the *Greek* μυρον, *Unguent*, and βαλανος, Acorn; as being in form of Acorns, and used in Medicine.

**MYRRH**, a kind of Gum, or Resin issuing, by Incision, and sometimes spont-aneously, from the Trunk, and larger Branches of a Tree growing in *Arabia, Egypt*, and especially *Abyssinia*. The Word comes from μυρα, I run, or trickle.

Authors are not agreed about the Tree which produces this Gum : 'Tis true, they all make it small, and thorny; but disagree about the Form if its Leaves.

The Incisions are made twice a Year, and the *Myrrh* oozing out is received on Rush-Mats, disposed underneath.

The Druggists sell two kinds of Myrrh, *viz.* Myrrh in Tears, which they call *Stracte*; the other *Ungulata*, or *Nail'd.*

Of the first kind, the best is in bright yellow, transparent Drops, friable, light, of a strong disagreeable smell : But this is very rare; and most of that in use is the *Nail'd Myrrh*, so call'd from little white Spots observed thereon, much like those on the Nails of the Fingers. The best is in little Masses, or Tears, red, and transparent; which, when broke, contain a kind of unctuous Liquor, the most precious part of the *Myrrh*, and the real *Stacte* of the Antients.

This Gum enters a great number of Medicinal Compositions. Its Bitterness renders it good for the Stomach, and against Worms; 'tis chewed to prevent Infection from contagious Diseases. Dr. *Quincy* says it is excellent to cleanse and strengthen the Womb, and against tickling Rheums; a good Detergent; and as such much added externally in Unguents for the Healing of Wounds; and makes the principal Ingredient used in Embalming. The Chymists draw from it Oils, Spirits, Tinctures, &c. to which they attribute extraordinary Virtues.

The Antients had Vessels of a kind of Myrrh, call'd *Vasa Murrhina, Myrrhina Pocula*, &c. Some say they were made of what we now call *Agat*, others of *Onyx*, others of *Coralline*, and others of a Gum congealed and condensed.

**MYTRLE**, Myrtles, the Berries, or Fruits of a Shrub well known under the Name of *Myrtle*, growing common in Spain, especially in the Mountains of *Lasierra Morena*, &c. There are two kinds of *Myrtle*, Male and Female; the latter whereof produces the best Berries, and in the greatest Quantity.

The Fruit is at first green, but becomes black insensibly within; it is a white Seed in form of a Crescent, solid, hard, and of an astringent Taste; while the Fruit continues on the Trees, 'tis succulent and smooth, and only becomes acid and wrinkled, because dried in the Sun for the convenience of Carriage.

They are much used in Medicine, especially in *France*, where they prepare Oils, Syrups, &c. from 'em. The Perfumers likewise use 'em in their Perfumes, an draw an Essence from 'em. The *German* Dyers make a blue Colour from 'em. In *England* the Leaves and Branches are used for tanning Leather.

**MYURUS**, in Medicine, a Pulse which is continually weakening by insensible Degrees; so that the second Beat is fainter that than the first; the third than the second, &c. The Word is formed of the Greek μυουρος, like a *Mouse's Tail*; which is compounded of μυς, Mouse, and ουρα, Tail; the Diminution of the Pulse being supposed like that of the thickness of the Tail of that Animal, which grows less from the Root to the Tip.

**NAPTHA**, or Naphta, a kind of liquid Sulphur or Bitumen, very soft, and inflammable, exuding out of the Earth in several Places in *Chaldea*; particularly the place where stood the antient *Babylon*; and still founding several Provinces of *Italy* and *France*, particularly in *Auvergne*, and near *Ragusa*.

That of *France* is soft and black, like liquid Pitch, and of a fœtid Smell; that of *Italy* is a kind of Petrol, or a clear Oil, of various Colours, oozing out of a Rock, situate on a Mountain in the Dutchy of *Modena*.

*Naptha* is esteemed penetrating, resolutive, and vulnerary; but its Virtues are little known in Medicine : its chief Use is in Lamps, &c. on account of its Inflammability.

The *Turks* call the *Naptha, Carab Sakiz*, black Mastic, to distinguish it form Pitch. *Vossius* has an express Treatise on *Naptha, Antient, and Modern*: He says, 'tis a Flower of Bitumen, of more force than any other Bitumen.

The Word, in the original *Chaldee*, signifies *stillare*, to ooze, or drop; *Naptha*, according to *Pliny*, running like a kind of Bitumen.

**NARCOTICS**, in Medicine, Opiates, or Medicines, that excite Drowsiness and Sleep. The Word comes form the Greek ναρκοτικος, of ναρκοσις, *Drowsiness. Narcotics* act, by calming an diminishing the Motion of the Blood and Spirits.

Authors are of various Opinions, as to the Manner wherein *Narcotics* operate. The Antients tell us, 'tis by their being cold in nature. *Etmuller*, after *Willis*, takes the Animal Spirits to be composed of a fluid volatile Salt; and thinks they are dissolved by the Mixtures of Sulphurs and Oils, wherewith *Narcotics* abound. M. *Andry's*[1] Opinion is, that the Salt of *Narcotics*, dissolves in any Liquor whatever, and that their ramous Branches becoming thus disengaged from the Salts, are embarrassed among one another, and thus stop the Course of the Blood and Spirits. Lastly, others think, that *Narcotics* close the Orifices of the Nerves and thus block up the Passage of the Spirits.

*Linder*[2], in his Treatise *de Venenis*, thinks, that the Operation of *Narcotics* is not the same in all; Drowsiness being producible from a great Variety of different Causes.

**NASALIA**, in Medicine, a sort of Remedies to be taken by the Nose; call'd also *Errhines*.

**NATRON**, or Anatron, in Natural History, a kind of black, greyish Salt, taken out of a Lake of stagnant Water in the Territory of *Terrana* in *Egypt*. 'Tis much of the nature of Nitre, whence it is called *Egyptian Nitre*, and is even supposed to be the proper Nitre of the Antients.

'Tis a popular Error, that all Bones or Stones thrown into this Lake, are by

[1] Nicolas Andry (1658 – 1742), a French physician.

[2] Johan Linder (1676 – 1724), a Swiss physician and botanist.

degrees converted into *Natron*. It makes a great Ebullition, when mixed with Acids; whence it is ranked as of the Alkali Kind. 'Tis used in the Whitening of Linnen; but burns them, if not corrected by a Mixture of Ashes.

The *Natron* of *Egypt*, as described by *Pliny, Matthiolus*, and *Agricola*, is an Alkali Salt perforated in manner of a Sponge, and of a Lixivial Taste. Its Principles, Dr. *Leigh* takes to be chiefly two; *viz.* a Sea-Salt, and an Urinous Salt. The first, he take it for granted, it receives from the Earth; the second, from the Air.

Dr. *Huntington*[1], who was in the spot, says the *Natron* is thought to rise from the bottom of the Lake; where, by the Heat of the Sun, it is condensed, and hardened into the Form we see it in : But his Opinion is, that 'tis rather separated by the Sun from the Water.

M. *de le Chambre*[2] adds, that three of four Days before the *Nile* begins to overflow, there falls a certain Dew, of a fermentative Vertue, insomuch as to leaven a Paste exposed to it, and that at the same time the *Natron* rises.

*Hippocrates, Galen, Matthiolus, Dioscorides*, &c. mention it as of use in Physic; and M. *de Clos* is even of the opinion, that all the Mineral Waters of *France* are impregnated with this kind of *Nitre*; and that 'tis hence they derive their Medicinal Vertues.

It is of singular Efficacy in fertilizing of Ground; which Dr. *Leigh* accounts for, by supposing its volatile Particles heated by some subterranean Fire, or by the Warmth of the Sun; and thus readily made to ascend up the minute Tubes of Plants, and carry with them the Juices of the Earth.

*Pliny* derives the Invention of Glass from some of this *Natron* accidentally melted down into the Sand, where it run into Streams of Glass.

This *Nitre* is distinguished from Salt Petre, by its fermenting with Acids, which Salt Petre will not do; by its volatile Spirit, its lixivial Smell, by the clammy insipid Substance it yields, &c. It agrees with Salt Petre, in that, by dropping Spirit of Sulphur upon it, it shoots into pyramidal Crystals. Dr. *Leigh* thinks it comes nearer a Sal Armoniac than Salt Petre.

Dr. *Lister* conjectures, that most of the Salt Water of the Lakes of *Egypt*, having pass'd thro' the Bodies of those vast Animals wherewith they are stocked, as *Crocodiles, Hippopotami*, &c. must of consequence be rendered Urinous, or Salino-Urinous; which is a Composition of Sal Armoniac.

**NATTA**, or Nata, or Nasa, or Napta, in Medicine, a Tumor arising in several Parts of the Body. *Blanchard* defines it, a large, soft, reddish, painful Tumor, arising usually on the Back, sometimes on the Shoulders : Its Root is very small, yet it grows so prodigiously, that it sometimes equals a Melon, or Gourd.

*Nattæ*, or, as some call them, *Nates*, oftenest appear on the Neck, much after the manner of Talpe. They are of the Oedematous Kind, and are to be extirpated by Incision, and their Return prevented by red Precipitate, Vitriol, or burnt Allom strew'd on the Place.

[1] This is probably Robert Huntington (1635 – 1701), an English clergyman, traveller and writer.

[2] Marin Cureau de la Chambre (1594 – 1669), a French physician and physiognomist.

**NATURALS**, *Res Naturales*, in Medicine : In every Animal, howsoever sick and diseased, there is still remaining some degree of Life, an Strength; and the Causes and Effects of each : These are call'd *Naturals, Natural things, things according to Nature*; and sometimes barely *Nature*; in contraindication to *Non-Naturals*.

**NAUSEA**, in Medicine, a Retching, or Propensity and Endeavours to Vomit; arising from a Loathing of Food, excited by some viscous Humour that irritates the Stomach, and urges it thus to discharge itself; or a Nausea is when the thoughts or sight of Food create a Sickness in the Stomach, or a Tendency to Vomit.

The usual Causes of a *Nausea*, and *Anorexia*, are hard Drinking, great Heat, a Fever, Consumptions, Laxness of the Stomach occasion'd by Tea, &c. Narcotics, as Tobacco, Passions of the Mind, Suppression of Evacuations inducing a Plethora, foul Stomach, tenacious Humours lodg'd therein, &c.

*Boerhaave* defines a *Nausea* Anatomically, to be a retrograde Spasmodic Motion of the Musculous Fibres of the *Oesophagus*, Stomach, and Intestines; attended with Convulsions of the Abdominal Muscles, and the *Septum transversum*.

*Nausea* and Vomiting only differ from one another, as more or less Violent. The *Nausea* is properly the Effort the Stomach makes to Vomit, which has not always the Effect.

The Word is *Latin*, form'd from the *Greek* ναυσια, of ναυς, *Navis*, Ship : In regard, People, at the beginning of their Voyages, are usually inclined to Vomiting.

**NECROSIS**, in Medicine, a compleat Mortification of any part; call'd also *Sideratio* and *Sphacelus*. The Word is Greek, νεκροσις, where it has the same Signification.

**NEPENTHE**, in Pharmacy, a name given to an Opiate, or Laudanum, by *Theo. Swingerus*[1], from the great Opinion he had of its giving Ease in all manner of Pain; the Word importing as much, from the Privative, νη, *non*, or *absque*, without; and πενθος, *Luctus*, Sorrow.

The *Nepenthe* mention'd in antient Authors, was a Plant now unknown. *Homer* says it was a Plant of *Egypt*; and adds, that *Helena* made use of it to charm her Hosts, and make 'em forget their Pains.

Some Authors say, it was the Plant we call *Helenium*, and others *Ænopia*. M. *Petit* has a Dissertation on the antient *Nepenthe*.

**NEPHRITES**, or *Nephriticus Dolor*, in Medicine, a Name given to a painful Disease occasion'd by the Stone or Gravel in the Kidneys. The Word is borrow'd from the *Greek* νεφριτες, *Disease of the Reins*; from νεφρος, *Rein*. The *Greeks* give the Name νεφριτις, to the first *Vertebra* of the Loins, from its neighbourhood to the Kidneys.

[1] Theodorus Swingerus, born Theodore Zwinger or Swinger (1658 – 1724), a Swiss anatomist and botanist.

**NEPHRITIC**, something that relates to the Kidneys. The Word is form'd of the *Greek* νεφρος, *Rein*, Kidney.

**NEPHRITIC** *Colic*, is a Colic or Pain arising from a Stone or Gravel in the Reins, &c. This is the most cruel of all Colics.

**NEPHRITICS**, Medicines proper for Diseases if the Kidneys, particularly the Stone. Such particularly are the Roots of Althaea, Dog's Grass, Sparagrass, Sago, Pellitory of the Wall, Mallows, Pimpernella, red Chich-Peas, Peach-Kernels, Turpentine, &c.

**NEPHRITICUM** *Lignum*, a kind of Medicinal Wood growing in *New Spain*, chiefly in the Kingdom of *Mexico*; call'd by the *Indians, Coalt Tiapalcypathy*, as being sovereign against *Nephritic* Pain.

It must be chosen well clear'd of its Bark and Rind; it is of a bitter Taste, and a reddish yellow Colour; but when infused in cold Water, gives it a sky-blue Tincture, when view'd by a false Light, and a gold Colour, by a true one : A little of any Acid being mixed with the Tincture, both Colours disappear, but a little Oil of Tartar restore sits sky-blue.

Some substitute Ebony, and others red *Brasil* Wood for *Lignum Nephriticum*, but the Deceit becomes apparent by infusing it in Water.

**NEPHRITICUS** *Lapis*, a precious Stone, so call'd from its extraordinary Virtues against the Stone and Gravel in the Kidneys.

'Tis a kind of Jasper, of a greyish Colour, mix'd with a little blue, sometimes white and black; and only differs from Jasper, in its being harder, and always without any thing of red. The best for Medicinal Use is of a bluish grey, fat and unctuous, as *Talc of Venice*.

'Tis brought chiefly from *New Spain*, where it is sometimes found in Pieces large enough to make moderate Cups. There is some likewise found in *Old Spain* and *Bohemia*.

This Stone is very dear, by reason of the wonderful Virtues ascribed to it. A Cup made of it was sold for 1600 Crowns in the time if the Emperor *Rudolphus* II.

The *Indians* of *New Spain*, who first discover'd its use, and taught it the *Europeans*, wear it hung about their Neck, after having cut it in various Figures, chiefly Beaks of Birds : Whence some *Charletans* take occasion to counterfeit it, by cutting *Jada*, and other Stones, into like Figures; and sell it at great Prices to those who have an Opinion of its *Nephritic* Faculty.

**NERVOUS** Spirit, or Juice, is a pure, subtile, volatile Humour, better known by the Name of *Animal Spirits*; secreted from the Arterious Blood in the Cortical Part of the Brain, collected in the *Medulla Oblongata*, and thence driven, by the force of the Heart, into the Cavities of the Nerves; to be convey'd by them throughout the Body, for the Purposes of Sensation and Animal Motion.

**NEURITICS**, or Nervines, in Medicine, Remedies proper for Diseases of the Nerves, and Joints. Such are Betony, Lavender, Rosemary, Sage, Laurel,

Marjoram, and other among the Cephalics. The Word is form'd from the *Greek* νευρος, *Nervus*.

**NEUTRAL SALTS**, among Chymists, are a sort of intermediate Salts between Acids and Alcalies; partaking of the nature of both. See Salt, Acid, and Alcaly. Mr. *Boyle* also gives the Appellation *Neutral* to a sort of Spirits, differing in divers Qualities both from Vinous, Acid, and Urinous Spirits. These he also calls Anonymous and *Adiaphorous* Spirits.

**NICOTANIA**, or *Herba Nicotiana*, a Term given to *Tobacco*; from *Nicot*[1] the *French* Ambassador at the Court of *Portugal*, who first sent it into *France* in 1560, and gave it his own Name; as he himself tells us in his Dictionary.

**NIGHT-MARE**, a popular Name for a Disease by the *Greek* Physicians call'd *Ephialtes*, and the *Latins, Incubus*; to which People lying a-sleep on their Backs, and having their Stomach charg'd with heavy Food difficult of digestion, are very liable.

The Disease makes the sleeping Patient appear as if oppress'd with a huge Weight on the Breast; whence he ordinarily imagines some Spectre or Fantom stopping his Breath.

The Disease does not arise, as was antiently imagined, from gross Vapours filling the Ventricles of the Brain; but rather from a too great repletion of the Stomach which prevents the Motion of the Diaphragm, and, of consequence, the Dilatation of the Breast necessary to Respiration. Others take it to be produced by a Convulsion of the Muscles of Respiration.

*Etmuller* observes, That the *Arabs* call this Disease a *Nocturnal Epilepsy*; since upon its prevailing much, it degenerates into an Epilepsy; and is in effect the *Prodromus* hereof in young People, as in old ones of an Apoplexy.

**NITRE**, in Natural History, a sort of Salt, thus call'd by the Antients; by the Moderns, more usually *Saltpetre*. Naturalists differ as to the Point whether out Saltpetre be the Nitre of the Antients. *G. C. Schelhamer*[2] has a particular Treatise on the Subject, *de Nitro tum veterum tum nostro Comentarius*.

Most other Authors hold the antient *Nitre* to be Mineral or Fossil; whereas our Saltpetre is Artificial. *Serapion* says, their Mines of *Nitre* were like those of common Salt, and that it was form'd out of running Water congeal'd in its Progress into a sort of Stone. He adds, That their *Nitre* was of four kinds, distinguish'd by the Countries whence it came; *viz.* the *Armenian*; *Roman*; *African*; call'd *Aphronitre*, and by *Avicenna, Baurach*; and the *Egyptian*, which was the most famous, giving *Name* to all the rest; itself denominated from *Nitria*, a Province in *Egypt*, where it was found in great abundance. He assures us, too, that their *Nitre* was of divers Colours, *viz.* white, red, and livid; that some was cavernous, like a Spunge; others close and compact; others transparent like Glass; and others scaly.

*Schelhamer* gives a different Account : The Antients, he observes,

[1] Jean Nicot (1530 – 1600), a French diplomat and scholar.

[2] Guenther Christoph Schelhammer (1649 – 1712), a German physician.

distinguish'd between Νιτρον, *Nitre*, Αφρονιτρον, *Aphronitre*, and Αφρος νιτρος, *Spuma Nitri*, or *Scum of Nitre*. He adds, That *Agricola*, &c. is mistaken in asserting that there were antiently Mines in *Lydia*, *Magnesia*, *Caria*, &c. out of which *Nitre* was dug like Stones out of a Quarry : And that the *Nitre* used by the Antients was brought out of the several Countries mentioned by *Pliny*, L. xxxi. c. 10.

A Lake in *Macedonia*, whose Waters were *Nitrous*, and in the middle whereof, however, was a Spring of fresh Water, furnish'd the greatest Quantity, and the best : It was call'd *Callustricum* from a neighbouring Cape in the Gulf of *Thessalonica*, and was form'd like a Crust on the Surface of the Water during Dog-days. The Waters of the Lake *Ascanius* in *Bithynia*, and those of certain Springs near *Chalcis*, were sweet and potable towards the Surface, yet *nitrous* at bottom.

There was also *Nitre* gather'd on the Ground near *Philippi*, in *Thrace*; but it was little, and of no great value. The Valleys of *Media* also furnish'd some. And there were *Nitre*-Pits in *Egypt*, as there are Salt-Pits among us.

The chief Virtue the Antients ascribe to their *Nitre*, is, that of drying, deterging, and attenuating; and, as such, it was used in Ulcers, Disorders of the Eyes, the Itch, the Bite of Serpents, Gout, &c. They also took it inwardly to resolve and attenuate viscid Humours : But its cooling Quality, whereof the modern Physicians make so much use, they were unacquainted with. 'Tis excellent in diseases of the Heart, accompanied with a propensity to vomit.

Abundance of our Physicians are full of the notion of a *volatile Nitre* abounding in the Air; and a world of Phænomena they account for from the Operation of the Particles thereof.

That the Atmosphere abounds with Saline Particles, is most certain; for being filled continually with Effluvia from the Earth and Sea, it must needs have from both a great Quantity of Saline Corpuscles; and these will be of different Kinds, according to the Variety of those Salts from whence they are derived.

But why these should be mostly supposed of a *Nitrous* nature, is not so easy to prove; for Saltpetre is by no means found in grater Quantity than the other Salts, especially common Salt; not is it of a much more volatile Nature that they, nor capable of being raised more easily, or by a lesser heat. But since Soot, and that which produces it, Smoak, is found to abound very much with a truly volatile Salt; and since such a kind of Salt is produced frequently by the Putrefaction of Animal and Vegetable Bodies, 'tis probable the Air may abound with Salts of this kind, among many other decompounded ones of different Natures and Names.

**NOCTAMBULI**, a Term of equal import with Somnambuli, applied to Persons who have a Habit of rising, and walking about in their Sleep. *Skenkins*, *Horstius*[1], *Clauderus*[2], and *Hildanus*[3], who have wrote of Sleep, give us divers unhappy Histories of such Noctambuli. The Word is a

[1] Gregor Horstius (1578 – 1636), a German physician and anatomist.

[2] Gabriel Clauder (1633 – 1691), a German physician

[3] Guilhelmus Fabricius Hildanus, born Wilhelm Fabry (1560 – 1634) in Hilden, Germany, was a physician and surgeon.

compound of the *Latin Nox*, Night, and *ambulo*, I walk.

The Disorder consists in this, that the proper Organs of Muscular Motion are at liberty, while the Organs destined for Sensation are bound up, or in a State of Inaction.

To conceive the Cause, it is to be observ'd, that the Laws of the Union of the Soul and Body, are such, as that certain Ideas follow upon certain Motions of the Fibres of the Bràin; and certain Motions of those Fibres upon certain Ideas. Now, by much thinking on any one thing, the Fibres acquire some permanent Situation, which gives a freer Passage to the Spirits towards a certain part of the Body than ordinary. If then the Animal Spirits become too copious, or too much agitated, or consist of parts too solid; they throw themselves into the Passages they find the most open, glide into the Nerves and Muscles corresponding to those Passages, and there produce the Motions proper to those Muscles.

Accordingly, the Body rises and walks; tho the Soul be excluded from thinking on the Objects that use to employ it on such occasions.

The Bilious, according to *Horstius*; the Melancholic, according to *Salius*; and the Sanguine, according to *Libavius*[1], are the most subject to those *nocturnal* Vagaries.

The Remedies are all such things as temper the Agitation of the Spirits, and relax the Fibres; as Bleeding, and all Coolers, either internally or externally : Aperitives too, have a good effect; but the best Remedy is Cold-Bathing.

**NODE**, *Nodus*, in Chirurgery, a Tumour arising on the Bones, usually proceeding from some Venereal Cause. It seems generated of a thick, cold, viscid Humour, which is often found very difficult to resolve. Some Physicians call it *Exostosis*; others give the Name *Nodus* to all tumors arising on the Joints, and Nerves.

They frequently apply to it a leaden Plate cover'd with Mercury. The Cure is first attempted by *Emplast. de Ranis cum Mercurio*; which failing, some Mercurial Unguent is now and then rubb'd on them; and afterwards Mercurial Plaisters made of Cinnabar, &c. applied.

**NODE**, *Nodus*, is also used for the Tumors, or Protuberances arising on the Joints of Gouty People; call'd also *Tophi*. They are supposed to be form'd of a thick, crude, heavy, viscid indigested Matter; mix'd with a hot, sharp, bilious Juice, the grosser and more terrestrial Part whereof being detain'd, grows into a stony sort of Concretion.

**NOLI** *me tangere*, in Medicine, a kind of Cancer, or a malignant Eruption in the Face, occasioned by an extremely sharp, corrosive Humour. 'Tis said to be very dangerous touching it; for, frequently, in endeavouring to cure it, 'tis irritated the more, and the Patient's Death hastened. Hence its Name, which literally signifies, *don't touch me*.

*Noli me tangere*, is chiefly used among us for an external Ulcer in the *Alæ* of the Nose; proceeding from a Venereal Cause, tho sometimes the Effect of a

[1] Andreas Libavius, born Andreus Libau (1555 – 1616), a German physician and alchemist.

Scrophulous Constitution. It does not always confine itself to the Alæ but will spread and corrode the very Substance of the Nose. The Cure is difficult, especially when it arises from a bad Constitution.

The Botanists also describe a Plant under this denomination, which it derives from a singular Property it has, or darting out its Seed when ripe, upon the first approach of the Hand to touch its Pods.

**NON-NATURALS**, in Medicine, *Res Non Naturalis*, are the Causes and Effects of Diseases, whether near or remote. Physicians have digested all the Causes of Disease into six classes, which they call the six Non-naturals.

These are, 1. Air. 2. Meat and Drink. 3. Motion and Rest. 4. The Passions of the Mind. 5. Excretions and Retentions. 6. Sleeping and Waking.

They are usually call'd, because by their use or abuse they become either Good, *Naturals*, or Evil, *Contra-naturals*. But the Division, in effect, is of no great use; the Causes of Diseases being much more commodiously laid down otherwise.

**NUBECULA**, *little Cloud*, in Medicine, a Term sometimes used for a Disease in the Eye, wherein Objects appear as thro a Cloud, or Mist. The *Nubecula* seems to arise from certain gross Particles detain'd in the Pores of the *Cornea*, or swimming in the aqueous Humour, and thus intercepting the Rays of Light. *Nubecula* is also used for a Matter, in form of a Cloud, suspended in the middle of the Urine. This they sometimes also call *Cnæorema*.

**NUCIFEROUS**, from *Nux*, a Nut, and *fero*, to bear; Botanists call all Trees this, which bear Nuts.

**NUTMEG**, a kind of Aromatic Nut, or Spice, brought from the *East Indies*; whereof there are two Kinds, *Male* and *Female*. The *Female* is that chiefly used among us; its Form is round, its Smell agreeable, and its Taste hot and pungent. The *Male* is a wild Nut, of a longish Form, and without either Taste or Smell; yet sometimes put off, while yet in the Pod, for the Female.

The *Nutmegs* are enclosed in three different Covers : The first, thin, reddish, of an agreeable Smell and aromatic Taste, call'd *Mace*; by others, tho' improperly, *Flower of Nutmeg*. This wraps up the Shell, and opens in proportion as the Pod grows. The Shell, which makes the second Cover, is hard, thin, and blackish. Under this, is a greenish Film of no use; and in this is found the *Nutmeg*, which is properly the Kernel of the Fruit. Every *Nutmeg* has a little Hole in it, which some ignorantly take for a Defect.

The best *Nutmegs* are those gather'd in *April*. They must be chosen heavy, of a whitish brown Colour, well marbled without side, reddish within, having a fat unctuous Humour, and an agreeable Smell.

As to the Mace, it must be chosen in large Leaves of a high Colour, like the *Nutmeg* in Taste and Smell.

*Nutmegs* comfited green, are excellent to fortify the Stomach, and restore the natural Heat. They are particularly esteem'd Carminative. The Powder, *Duke*, esteem'd a Sovereign against Rheums, is only *Nutmeg* pulverized with

Sugar, and a little Cinnamon.

*Nutmegs*, by Distillation, or Expression, yield an Oil, said to have wonderful Virtues.

The *Nutmeg-Tree* is propagated after a particular manner. *Tavernier* tells us, that the Birds devouring the Nutmeg when ripe, give it back whole by Stool; and that this falling to the Ground, besmear'd with a viscous Matter, it takes Root, and produces a Tree.

**NUTRITION**, in Pharmacy, a kind of Preparation, consisting in the gradual Mixture of Liquors of different Natures, by stirring them together till they have acquired a thick Consistence; as in making *Butter of Saturn*, or *Unguentum Nutritum*.

**NUTRITUM**, a desiccative, cooling, Unguent, prepared by the Agitation and *Nutrition* of some Preparation of Lead, with Oil and Vinegar, or the Juice of *Solanum*, in a Mortar.

**NUX VOMICA**, the Fruit, or, as some will have it, the Stone of the Fruit of a Tree, growing in several Parts of *Egypt*, or in the Islands *Timor* and *Ceylon*. It is round and flat, of a grey Mouse-colour without, and various Colours within; sometimes yellow, sometimes white, sometimes brown. The largest, whitest, newest, and cleanest, are the best.

This Drug is an assured Poison for all Animals except Men. On the contrary, *Hermannus*, *Botanic* Professor at *Leyden*, who has wrote expressly on it, says that those of *Timor* and *Ceylon* are excellent Sudorifics, and to be rank'd among Diuretic Medicines.

**NUX INDIA**, the Fruit of the Tree call'd *Cacao*.

**NYCTALOPIA**, or *Nocturna Cæcitas*, a Disease of the Eyes, which prevents their seeing, when the Sun is set, and the Light begins to diminish. *Celsus* calls it *Imbecilitas Oculorum*.

Others will have the *Nyctalopia* to be properly a Disease, that prevents the seeing by Day, not by Night : which is the sense *Hippocrates* uses it in; and in which sense it is suppos'd owing to the Spirits being to much dissipated in the Day, but collected at Night.

However, in the general, any Disease which prevents the seeing at any particular time, when others see, is call'd *Nyctalopia*.

*Boerhaave* says, the *Nyctalopia* consists in this, that the *Uvea* is immovable, and at the same time very open.

The Word comes from the *Greek* νυξ, *Night*, and αλοπεξ, *Fox*; this Animal being said to see less by Day than Night.

In the *Philosophical Transactions*, we have an Instance of a *Nyctalopia*, or *Nocturna Cæcitas*, in a Youth of twenty Years of Age; who have been affected with it as long as he could remember. Dr. *Parham* assures us, he had a good Sight all Day, and distinguish'd Objects at all Distances as well as any body; but then Twilight once came, he was quite blind, and saw nothing at all; nor could make scarce any use either of Fire, Candle, or Glasses. Yet his Eyes, upon Examination, shew'd nothing at all amiss; nor had he any Vertigo, or other Disease of the Head. The Cloudiness, as he himself told the Doctor, used to come gradually on him like a Mist, as Day-light declined. He always saw alike in all Aspects of the Moon, felt no Pain, by Fire or Candle-light, and was the same in Summer as Winter.

Dr. *Briggs*[1] accounts for the Case thus : "As Vapours are raised in great quantity during the Day-time; which being condensed by the Coldness of the the Humours in the Eyes of this Youth may be affected; and, in the Evening, rendered grosser, and more turbid. As we see in Urines, which frequently grow clear, or turbid, as Heat or Cold is apply'd to them. By such Thickness or Spissitude of the Humours, the Rays being either reflected, or too much refracted, do not reach the Retina, or at least strike it too feebly."

[1] William Briggs (1642 – 1704), an English physician.

**OBESITY**, Fatness, in Medicine, the State of a Person too much charged with Fat, and Flesh; otherwise call'd *Corpulency. Etmuller* defines it to be such an increase both of the Venter and Limbs, as impedes the Actions of the Body, especially Motion and Respiration.

*Obesity, Boerhaave* observes, does not consist in the Solids of the Body being increased, but by their being distended to a greater Pitch by the abundance of Humours collected in them. Hence, *Obesity* occasions several Diseases; usually Apoplexies.

It was held Infamous among the *Lacedemonians.* History tell us of a *Spaniard* who had been so exceedingly Fat, that when he became lean again, his Skin would make several turns or folds quite around him. *Sennertus* mentions a Man that weigh'd 600 Pounds.

*Etmuller* affirms, that there is no better Remedy against *Obesity* than *Acetum Scilliticum. Borel* recommends the Chewing of Tobacco; which *Etmuller* dissuades, lest it induce a Consumption.

**OBOLUS**, in Medicine, is used for a Weight of ten Grains; or half a Scruple. *Du Cange* says it weighs three Carats, or four Grains of Wheat : Others divided the *Obolus* into six Areolæ; and the Areola into seven Minutes. Others divide it into three Siliquæ, each Siliqua into four Grains, and each Grain into a Lentil and half. Among Sicilians, *Obolus* was the Weight of a Pound.

**OBSTRUCTION**, in Medicine, a lett or stoppage of the Passage of the Humours in the Body of an Animal. *Obstructions* are supposed to arise form the gross Parts of the Blood, detain'd in the Extremities of the Vessels, and thus blocking them up.

Some Physicians doubt whether there by any such thing as *Obstructions* in the Viscera; and rather attribute the Inconveniences usually ascribed to *Obstructions*, to the Acrimonies and Crudities of the Stomach : But their Reasons are not convincing.

'Tis true, *Obstructions* may not perhaps be so frequent as is usually supposed; and many of the Symptoms ascribed to them, are doubtless owing to Disorders of the Stomach; but then there's no denying that there are any *Obstructions* at all in the Viscera, &c. Schirrus's, and other kinds of Tumours are incontestable Proofs hereof. *Obstructions* frequently prove the Causes of Dropsies.

**OCULI**, *Eyes*, in Botany, the Gemmæ, or Buds of a Plant just putting forth, or the Knots out of which the Buds arise.

**ODONTALGIA**, in Medicine, the *Tooth-Ach*; one of the most common, yet most cruel Pains the Body is subject to. The Word is form'd from the *Greek* οδος, Tooth, and αλγος, Pain.

Its Cause is a sharp Serosity, thrown on the Membrane that lines the Sockets, or *Alveoli* of the Teeth. The Liquor is sometimes so very sharp and corrosive, that it eats away the Teeth by little and little, and makes 'em fall piece-meal. Its more remote Causes are Sugars, very hot things, and very cold Acids, &c.

The Disease is frequently attended with an Inflammation, or *oedematous* Tumor of the Jaw. It is sometimes also owing to a Worm found in the Root of the Tooth.

The *Curiosi Naturæ*, Deca. II. mention an *Odontalgy* cured by a Box on the Ear given the Patient; and add an Instance of Blindness and *Odontalgy* caused by shaving a Man's Beard. The very sight of a Remedy frequently drives away the Pain.

*Animal* **OECONOMY**, the first Branch of the Theory of Medicine; or that which explains the Parts of the human Body, their Structure and Use; the Nature and Causes of Life and Health, and the Effects or Phænomena arising from them. This is otherwise call'd *Physiology*; and its Objects just enumerated are call'd Naturals, or *res secundum Naturam*.

**OEDEMA**, or Oedematous *Tumor*, a Tumor which appears whitish , soft, and lax, without any notable change of Colour, Heat, Pain, or Pulsation; and which yields to the Pressure of the Fingers so as for some time to retain the Dent or Impression thereof. *Hippocrates* uses the word Oedema for any Tumor in general.

The general Cause of *Oedematous Tumors*, is vulgarly supposed to be a *Pituita*, as it is call'd, or a phlegmy Humour in the Body. Contusions, Fractures, Luxations, &c. when of long standing, often give rise to *Oedemas*, especially in Dropsical and Aged Persons; so do irregular Living, want of Exercise, Ruptures, Disorders of the Lymphatics, Defluxions of Humours, Weakness of the Joints, &c.

Its chief Seat is the Legs : In a *Leucophlegmatia*, the whole Body is *Oedematous*. It frequently comes upon other Diseases, especially Clinics; and is familiar to Women with Child. 'Tis dangerous when it tends to an *Abcess*; when it hardens, it becomes schirrous.

There are also *Spurious Oedema's*; in which case the pituitous Humour is mix'd with other Humours; whence the Tumor becomes *Erysipelatous*, *Schirrous*, and sometimes *Gypsous*; and hence Wens, &c.

The Word comes from the Greek οεδειvm whence οιδεμα, a Tumor contrary to Nature.

**OEDEMATOUS**, in Medicine, something that is of the nature of an *Oedema*; seiz'd, or afflicted with an *Oedema*. Thus we say *Oedematous Arm, Oedematos Legs*, &c.

*Oedematous Tumors* seldom, of themselves, prove dangerous, or mortal; but when they are of long continuance, the effect of old Age, or a dropsical Habit; when they grow hard, schirrous, painful, or come to suppurate, the Cure is generally tedious and uncertain. Those which attend Wounds, Fractures, or the like, are less difficult to cure.

They are easily discuss'd in their first Formation by the external Application of Solutions of Bay-Salt, Nitre, crude Sal Armoniac, &c. in *Spanish* Wine, Urine, Lime-Water, or other lixivious Fluids; while the Patient submits to a Course of Purgatives, to discharge the Matter repell'd by such Applications.

Under the Class of *Oedematous Tumors*, are ranked *Condylomata*, *Cristæ*, *Rhagades*, *Thymi*, *Talpæ* and *Nates*, the *Ganglio* and *Psydracium*.

**OENELÆUM**, in Pharmacy, a Mixture composed of thick black Wine and Oil of Roses. In Fractures with Wounds, where the Bone is not bare, *Scultetus* orders that the Compresses, to make them stick, be drenched with *Oenelæum*, to sooth the Pain, and prevent an Inflammation; and the Bandages to be every day moisten'd with the same, till the Inflammation be out of all danger. The Word is form'd from the Greek οινος, Wine, and ελαιον, Oil.

**OESYPON**, a kind of Fatty Mucilage, of the consistence of an Unguent; of a greyish Colour, and a sickish disagreeable smell, drawn fro the greasy Wool growing on the Throats and between the Buttocks of Sheep.

This Wool they wash, boil it in Water to scower, let the Lotions or Decoctions stand for some time, and from the top skim off a fatty Substance, which being strain'd thro' a linen Cloth, and set to cool, makes the *Oesypon*, much used externally to resolve, soften, and appease Pain.

The Word is form'd from the *Greek* οις, Sheep; and σηπεσθαι, to be corrupted; the *Oesypon* being a filthy, and, as it were, corrupted Matter, drawn from Sheep.

**OFFICINAL**, in Pharmacy, a Term apply'd to such Medicines, whether Simple or Compound, as the College of Physicians requires to be constantly kept in the Apothecarys Shops, ready to be made up in extemporaneous Prescription. The *officinal Simples* are appointed, among us, by the College of Physicians; and the manner of making the Compositions directed in their Dispensatory. The Word is form'd of the *Latin Officina*, Shop.

**OIL**, a fatty, unctuous, inflammable Matter, drawn from several natural Bodies. The Word is form'd from the Latin *Oleum*, of *Olea*, Olive-Tree, the Fruit whereof abounds in such Juice.

The word Oil is sometimes apply'd to the Juices which distil naturally from Plants and Trees; as Balm, &c. but more strictly to those Juices drawn by the Expression from Plants, Fruits, Grains, or Seeds; as *Oil of Olive*, *Nut-Oil*, &c.

The Kinds of *Oils*, their Properties, manners of Expression, &c. are almost infinite: For the generality of them, the Reader is referr'd to the proper Articles; such as could not be more conveniently inserted, are as follow.

*Virgin Oil*, is understood of *Oils* express'd from Olives, Nuts, &c. fresh gather'd, without being heated, too much press'd, &c. *Granulated Oil* is that fix'd in a little Grains; this is the best, and most esteem'd, especially of *Oils* of Olives.

*Oil* frequently takes new Names from the Drugs mix'd with it; as *Oil of Roses*, which is that mix'd with Roses; *Oil of Jasmin*, that perfum'd with Jasmine.

*Plato* observes, that *Oil* is destructive to all Plants; and he adds too, to the

Life of all Animals, except those of Man, to which it is agreeable, as also to the rest of his Body. He adds further, that 'tis very useful to the external parts of the Body, but hurtful to the internal. *Fernelins* observes that *Oil* softens, moistens, and lubricates the Body, and takes off the sense of Weariness; for which reason the *Greeks* call it *Acopum*; and renders the Body prompt and agile. *Dioscorides* says it cures Leprosies, &c.

**OIL** *of Olives*, is the most popular, and most universal of all others; being that chiefly used in Medicine, in Foods, Salads, and in the Manufactures, &c.

It is drawn from Olives by Presses or Mills made for the purpose. The Fruit is gather'd when at its utmost Maturity in *December* and *January*, as it beings to redden; when 'tis put under the Mill, as soon as gather'd, it yields that *Oil* so very sweet, and of so charming an Odour, call'd *Virgin-Oil*. But, as the Olives newly gather'd yield but little *Oil*, those who rather regard Quantity than Goodness, leave them on the Ground for some time, e'er they press them.

Neither the Smell nor Taste of this second *Oil* is very agreeable; tho there is a third Kind still worse, which is the common *Oil* procured by throwing boiling Water on the Pressings, and repressing them more strongly.

The consumption of this second *Oil* is incredible; the South Parts of *France, Provence, Languedoc*, &c. as also *Candia*, some Parts of *Italy*, &c. yield vast Quantities. Its use every body knows; it being reputed one of the most universally useful things in the whole World.

**OIL** *of sweet Almonds*, cold drawn, or without Fire, is prepared various ways. Some peel the Almonds as they pound 'em; other pound 'em without peeling. Some warm 'em in luke-warm Water; others in *balneo Mariæ*; some only bruise 'em; others beat 'em into a Paste. On effect there are as many different ways of preparing this Oil, as there are Persons who make it their business to prepare it.

In this diversity, *Pomet* gives us a Method easier and less expensive than any of the rest; which, it should seem, we cannot do better than follow.

*Method of procuring Oil of sweet* Almonds *by Expression, without Fire.* Take a Pound and a half of peel'd sweet Almonds, new and dry; after pounding 'em in a Mortar, pass 'em thro' a coarse Sieve, lay 'em in a Hair-Cloth, and put 'em under the Press between two Plates of Copper, Steel, or the like; press 'em gently; and when all the unctuous and fluid Part is expressed, you will have a sweet *Oil* without any Sediments, which is scarce avoidable in any of the other manners.

*Palm* **OIL**, or *Oil of Senegal*, a thick unctuous Liquor of a yellow Colour, and a Violet-smell; so call'd because drawn, by Ebullition or by Expression, from the Fruit of a kind of Palm-Tree, growing in several Places of *Africa*, especially in *Senegal*.

The *Africans* use this *Oil* as we do Butter; and burn it when old. In Europe 'tis esteem'd a sovereign Remedy against cold Humours; and even said to give ease in the Gout.

'Tis sometimes counterfeited with Wax, *Oil* of Olives, *Iris*, and Turmeric;

but the Trick is found out either by Air or Fire. The Air alters the Colour of the Genuine, and leaves the Counterfeit unchanged; and on the contrary, Fire changes the Counterfeit, not the Genuine.

**OIL** *of Camomile*, an *Oil* made with the Flowers of this Plant steep'd in *Oil* of Olives, and exposed to the Sun in the heat of Summer : Its Colour is blueish; some add fine Turpentine. It is the most esteem'd when old. 'Tis used for the cure of several kinds of Wounds; and is reputed a kind of Balm.

**OIL** of *Petrol*, see Naptha.

**OIL** of *Aspic*, or *Spike*, an Oil drawn from the Flowers or little Leaves of a Plant of the same Name, growing in the South Parts of France, resembling our Lavender. 'Tis of a white Colour, and an aromatic Smell; and is the only Oil dissolvable in *Sandarach*; whence the genuine *Oil* is easily distinguished from the counterfeit, which is *Oil* of Turpentine mix'd with a little *Petrol*. It is used by Painters and Farriers; and is of some use in Medicine, where it males a part in several *Galenical* Compositions.

**OIL**, among the Chymists, is the second of the Elements, or Hypostatical Principles; otherwise call'd Sulphur.

All natural Bodies yield *Oil*, either by Distillation; Putrifaction; or Liquation call'd *per Deliquium* : And hence the Chymists will have it a necessary Ingredients in the Composition of all Bodies. They make it the Principle of Odours; and to the Diversities thereof, ascribe all the differences of Bodies in respect if Smells.

All Plants yield a fetid *Oil* at the end of Distillation; but Aromatic ones beside this yield another *Oil*, which rises after the Phlegm, and at the beginning of the Distillation : This they call an *Essential Oil*, because it retains the natural smell of the Plant; whereas the second *Oil*, even that of Aromatic Plants, stinks intolerably.

M. *Homberg*, from an Observation that Plants which yield the most Acid, yield likewise the most *Oil*; took occasion to think that the Acid might assist the *Oil* to disengage itself from the Body, and to rise in Distillation; which found to answer in the Experiment. Mineral Acids prov'd to have more force on the *Oils* of Plants, and put 'em in a condition of rising in Distillation, and in greater Quantity by the Action of Fire, than Vegetable ones. Accordingly, whereas the Perfumers find a deal of difficulty in raising essential *Oil* of Roses; and scarce get an Ounce out of an hundred Pounds of the Flower : M. *Homberg*, on his Principle, got at least one third more; *viz.* by laying the Roses fifteen days in Water impregnated with Spirit of Vitriol before Distillation.

The Chymists Doctrine of Principles, Mr. *Boyle* shews to be very deficient in the Article *Oils* : For the Characteristic of a Sulphur, or that which denominates a thing such, is Inflammability ; Now, there are at least three Substances manifestly different in Consistence, Texture, or both; which, according to that Notion, ought to be referr'd to Sulphurs : For sometimes the inflammable Substance obtain'd from a mix'd Body by means of Fire, appears in form of an *Oil* that will not mix with Water; sometimes in form of an inflammable Spirit, which will readily unite with that Liquor; and sometimes also in form of a consistent Body almost like common Sulphur. *Producib. Of Chym. Prin.*

Dr. *Slare* in *Philos. Transact.* gives us a Scheme, or Analysis of Oils. He distinguishes Oils into Vegetable., Animal, and Mineral. The Vegetable he divides into *Essential* and not *Essential.*

The *Essential* again, are either perfect Stillations made by the Analysis of the Chymist's Fire; where the oleaginous Particles are truly separate from all other; as those from the Seeds of Cummin, Fennel, and Dill : or light and ethereal, usually drawn from the Tops of Plants, and specifically lighter than Water, some of 'em than Spirit of Wine; as those from Thyme, Wormwood, Hysop, Lavender, Rosemary, Penny-royal, Rue, Sage, Savin, &c. Or ponderous, which commonly sink in Water.

Those *not Essential*, are imperfect, or made by Expression; which are decompounded of several Parts of the Plants; as of Almonds, Olives, Wallnuts, Lime, Rape, &c.

The *Animal* Oils are either those of the solid Parts, as Harts-horn, Human-Skull, Hoofs, &c. Or those of the Fluid, as of Human Blood. Lastly, the *Mineral* Oils are those of Amber, Petroleum, *Barbadoes* Tar, and Bees-Wax.

Of these *Oils*, there are twelve that by a Mixture of compound Spirit of Nitre, make an Ebullition, Explosion, and Flame. Eighteen that make an Ebullition and Explosion without Flame : And four that produce neither.

**OINTMENT**, in Pharmacy and Surgery, &c. See Unguent.

**OLEAGINOUS**, something that partakes of the nature of Oil; or out of which Oil may be express'd. Thus Olives, Nuts, Almonds, &c. are *oleaginous* Fruits, or Fruits out of which Oil is express'd. Pines, Firs, &c. are *oleaginous* Woods, yielding Rosin, Turpentine, &c. Of all Woods, *oleaginous* ones burn the best. An *oleaginous* Urine in malignant Fevers is a sign of Death.

**OLIBANUM**, in Pharmacy, a kind of Gum, or Resin, usually call'd male *Frankincense.* It has its name *Olibanum, quasi oleum Libani*; because distilling in form of an Oil, from a Tree on Mount *Libanon.* It is brought to us in large white Tears, bordering a little on the yellow; very heavy, of a sharp bitter Taste, and a brisk Smell.

'Tis distinguish'd from the female, or common Incense, by the largeness of the Drops. 'Tis very glutinous, consequently strengthening; and partakes enough of the Turpentine to render it somewhat detergent; 'tis more used in compound strengthening Plaisters, than in inward Compositions.

**OLIVE**, a Stone-Fruit, which yields plenty of Oil; the Produce of the Olive-Tree. There are three Kinds of *Olives*, frequently sold; different in Size and Goodness; *viz.* those of *Verona*, which a the best; those of *Spain*; and those of *Provence.*

The Olives, while on the Tree, are intolerably bitter, without any thing of that delicious Taste which procures them admittance at the richest Tables. To fit 'em for that, they must be prepared as follows.

*Manner of Preparing, or Pickling* Olives. In the month of *June* and *July*, long e'er the *Olives* are fit to yield their Oil, they are gather'd, and laid to steep some days in fresh Water; when taken out, they are put in another Water prepared with Barillia, or Kali, with Ashes of Olive Stones calcined; or at least with Lime.

They are next laid in a Liquor of Water and Salt, with which they are put in those little Barrels, wherein they are brought to us. To give 'em the Flavour, they throw over 'em an Essence usually composed of Cloves, Cinnamon, Coriander, and Fennel. This Essence, is a kind of Secret among those who deal herein; and, in effect, 'tis in this that all the difficulty of Preparation lies.

*Manner of Drawing Oil of* Olives. The *Olives* being gather'd, are laid for some time on the Ground to drain, and to ripen further; they are then ground into a Paste with a Mill-stone : The Paste is put in large Frails, and boiling Water poured over them. Lastly, the whole is press'd; by means whereof the Oil is easily separated, and swims a-top of the Water.

**OMPHACIN**, in Pharmacy, a kind of Oil, pretended to be drawn from Olives while yet green, and sour; but *Pomet* charges it as an Imposture; adding, that Olives yield no Oil at all till perfectly ripe. The Word is derived form the *Greek* ομφαξ, unripe Grape.

**ONKOTOMY**, in Chirurgery, the Operation of opening a Tumor, or Abscess; from the *Greek* ονκος, Tumor, and τεμνο, I cut.

**OPERATIONS** in Chymistry, are the Processes, or Experiments, by means whereof the proper Changes are produced in Bodies, and the Effects of the Art procured.

Now, the Changes Chymistry produces in Bodies are reproducible to two Kinds, *viz.* an Union of Parts, and a Separation thereof : Thus Chymistry either separates Spirits, Salts, Oils, &c. or compound 'em together.

A Chymical *Operation*, then, consists in changing the Situation of the Parts; particularly, either in moving some Parts, but not the Whole, which us call'd *separating*; or in adding new Parts, which us call'd *uniting*.

All Chymical *Operations*, therefore, are reducible to two Kinds, *viz.* such whereby the Parts of Bodies before join'd, or united, are separated, which the antient Chymists call'd *Solution*; and such whereby the Parts before disjoined are combined, or united, call'd *Coagulation*.

Some, however, object Digestion as a third Species of *Operation*, not reducible to either of 'em : But *Boerhaave* shews, that it is a Composition of both.

Most Chymists, however, look on this Division as scarce accurate and minute enough, and subdivide it into a number of particular, or subordinate Operations; as *Calcination, Vitrification, Distillation, Sublimation, Cohobation, Amalgamation, Fermentation, Putrefaction*, &c.

**OPERATOR**, in Medicine, &c. is a Person who operates, or works with the hand, on the human Body, to preserve, or restore its Health. Thus we say *Operator for the Stone*, meaning a *Lithotomist*, or a person who cuts.

*Operator for the Eyes*, a Person who couches Cataracts, &c.

**OPHTHALMIA**, or Opthalmia, in Medicine, a Disease of the Eyes; properly, an Inflammation of the Tunica Adnata, or Conjunctiva; accompanied with a redness, heat, and pain. The Word is form'd from the *Greek* οφθαλμος, Eye.

It sometimes happens in the *Ophthalmia*, that the two Eye-lids are so distorted, that the Eye continues constantly open, without being able to shut; which is call'd χημωσις; sometimes the Eye-lids are so fasten'd together, that the Eye cannot be open'd, which is call'd φημασις, *q.d.* closure of things that should be open.

The immediate Cause of the *Ophthalmia*, is the Blood flowing in too great abundance in the little Vessels of the *Adnata*, so as to stagnate therein, and distend them. The remote Causes are the same with those of other Inflammations. *Celsus* calls the *Ophthalmia*, *Lippitudo*, by reason of a Gum sticking to the Eye-lids in this Disease, which the *Latins* call *Lippa*.

Snow apply'd to the afflicted Eye, is reputed a good Remedy for the *Ophthalmia* : the *Ephemerides* of the *Leopoldine* Academy mention an *Ophthalmia* cured by applying Cows-dung, while hot, between two linnen Clothes, to the Eye. A Fox's Tongue, and the Fat of Gall of a Viper, are empirical Preservatives against the *Ophthalmia*.

*Pitcairn*, and some others, distinguish an external and internal *Ophthalmia*; the first in the *Adnata*, which is that hitherto spoken of; the second in the Retina. The Symptoms or Indications of the latter, are *Muscæ volitantes*, Dust seeming to fly in the Air, &c. This, when inveterate, degenerates, or ends in a *Gutta Serena*, or *Amaurosis*.

The Cure of *Ophthalmia's*, according to the modern Practice, depends chiefly on the due repetition of Purgatives. If these fail, recourse is had to Vesicatories, Issues, Setons, &c. Tho' *Pitcairn* prefers Bleeding; it being his Observation, that no Disease requires copious bleeding so much as the *Ophthalmia*. In Summer 'tis frequent to have Epidemic *Ophthalmia's*.

**OPHTHALMICS**, Medicines proper for Diseases of the Eyes; as Ophthalmic Waters, Ophthalmic Powders, Ointments, &c. There is an excellent Ophthalmic prepared of Sugar of *Saturn*.

The fifth Pair of Nerves of the Brain, dividing into three Branches; the first is call'd *Ophthalmic*, because it goes to the Eye : this again subdivides into two Branches, after sending out several Twigs which encompass the Optic Nerves, and are distributed in the *Choroides*.

**OPIATE**, in Medicine, any Composition wherein Opium is an Ingredient. The Word is frequently also apply'd to Confections, Antidotes, and Electuaries; tho some say 'tis only properly applicable to soft Compositions : In which sense it is defined an internal Remedy, variously composed of Powders, Pulps, Liquors, Sugar, or Honey, reduced into a soft Consistence.

The *Opiate of Solomon* is a Composition of great Fame, so call'd from one *Solomon*, a Physician, its Inventor; and first published by *Laurence Joubert*[1].

[1] Laurence, or Laurent, Joubert (1529 – 1582), a French physician.

There are a particular kind of *Opiates*, call'd *Incarnatives*, for the Teeth and Gums, made of Alum, Sumach, Lignum Aloes, Myrrh, Mastic, &c. reduced into Powder.

**OPIATES** is also used in the general for all Medicines given with an Intention to procure Sleep; in which sense the Word is of the same Import with Narcotics, Hypnotics, Soporifics, and Pacifics. The Operation of *Opiates*, or the manner wherein they produce their Effect in the Body, Dr. *Quincy* thus lays down :

All Pain is a Stimulus on the Part affected, and is attended with Contractions of the pained Membranes, which occasion a greater Afflux than ordinary of the nervous Juice that way : On the other hand, Pleasure, or a delightful Sensation in any part, is accompanied with a smooth Undulation, and easy Reflux of the nervous Juice towards the Brain. This is, as it were, the Entertainment of the Mind; with which being taken up, it doth not determine the Spirits to the Organs of Motion : that is, there is such a Relaxation of the muscular Fibres, and such a Disposition of the nervous Fluid, as is necessary to Sleep.

Now, 'tis shewn that an agreeable Sensation produced in the Stomach, together with a distention of its Membranes, is the immediate Cause of that Sleepiness, to which we are inclinable after Eating; the one engaging the Mind, the other acting on the Body. For Pleasure amuses the Soul, and the Fullness of the Vessels in the Brain, checks and hinders, in some measure, the derivation of the nervous Juice into the Organs.

Now, to apply this; a moderate Dose of an *Opiate*, usually transports People with a pleasing Sensation, to that degree, that, as they often express themselves, they are in Heaven; and tho they do not always sleep, (which proceeds from the presentation of pleasing Images to the Mind so strongly, that, like Dreams, they do over-engage the Fancy, and so interrupt the State of Rest) yet they enjoy so perfect an Indolence and Quiet, that no Happiness in the World can surpass the Charms of so agreeable an Extasy.

Thus we have from these Medicines, but in a far more eminent degree, all those Effects which are observed to follow upon that grateful Sense in the Stomach, which a moderate Fullness produceth. For no Bodies are so fit and able pleasingly to affect our sensible Membranes, as those which consist of volatile Parts, whose Activity is tempered and allay'd by the Smoothness of some which are lubricating and oily; for they lightly rarify the Juice of the Stomach, and cause a pleasant Titillation of its nervous Coat, whereby there is induced an agreeable Plenitude, and the Mind is entertained with Ideas of Satisfaction and Delight.

And thus, we easily see upon what Mechanism the other Virtues of *Opiates* depend; for their easing Pain, checking Evacuations, &c. proceed not only from the Mind's being taken up with a pleasing Sense, whereby it is diverted from a disagreeable one; but all Pain being attended with a Contradiction of the Part, the Relaxation of the Fibres, which they cause, eludes and destroys the Force of the Stimulus.

*Opiates* are found to abate immoderate Secretions and Evacuations, which they do by removing that Irritation of the Organs, whereby they are occasion'd. And herein lies the incrassating Quality of those Medicines, in that the twitching Sense upon the Membranes of the Lungs, Bowels, &c. being lessen'd, the sharp Humour is suffer'd to lodge there in a greater Quantity, before it is so troublesome as to be thrown off and expell'd; it being all one as if there were no Irritation of the Part, if the uneasy Sense thereof be not regarded by the Mind. And these Effects will all be heightened by the Mixture of the *Opiate* Particles with the Blood; which is hereupon rarefy'd, and distends its Vessels, especially those of the Brain; and this does still, to a greater degree, lessen the Influx of the nervous Fluid to the Parts, by pressing upon the *Tubuli*, or little Canals, through which it is derived. Whence the reason of that Difficulty of breathing, which *Opiates* occasion; this Symptom being inseparable from the Rarefaction of the Blood in the Lungs.

**OPISTHOTONOS**, in Medicine, a kind of Convulsion, wherein the Body is bent backwards, so as to form, as it were, a bow; in which sense the Word is used in opposition to Emprosthotonos, wherein the Body is bent forwards. The *Opisthotonos* arises from a tonic Motion of the Muscles of the posterior Parts of the Body; especially those on the back of the Head. The Word is compounded of the *Greek* οπισω, backward, behind, and τεινειν, *tendere*, to stretch, bend.

**OPIUM**, in Pharmacy, &c. a Juice drawn from the Head of the black Poppy, and afterwards inspissated. The Word is form'd from the *Greek* οπος, Juice. When the Juice flows of itself, thro' Incisions made in the Poppy Head, it is properly call'd *Opium*; when drawn by Expression, it assumes the Name of *Meconium*.

The differences between the Qualities and Virtues of the two Juices, is very considerable : The former is preferable on all accounts; but it is exceeding rare; the *Turks*, among whom it is produced, and who make great use of it, never allowing it to be exported : so that it is the latter that is ordinarily used amongst us, and sold for *Opium*.

'Tis mostly brought from the *Levant* and *Cairo*; generally very impure; the *Levantines*, to shorten their Labour, and to have the more Juice, drawing it equally from the Heads and the Leaves of Poppies, by Expression, and then reducing it to the thickness of an Extract by Fire.

It must be chosen dry, the smoothest, and blackest possible, of a drowsy smell, and neither rugged, nor sticky, nor all in one Mass.

'Tis a popular Error, that there is any such thing as *white Opium*; for tho' the Juice as it runs from the Heads of Poppies be of a Milk-colour, it always becomes of a very deep brown as it thickens. Wherever it is found yellowish or soft, 'tis assign the Juice has not had Fire enough.

*Prepared Opium* is call'd *Laudanum*; of which there are two Kinds : the one, *Simple*; extracted by means of Rain-Water and Spirit of Wine : The other *Compound*, call'd *Laudanum Opiatum*; wherein there enter several other Ingredients.

The Uses of *Opium* are to sooth Pain, to excite Sleep, to stop Vomiting and Looseness. Its Dose is from half a Grain to two Grains. Some Persons, who have much habituated themselves to it, can tae 50 or 60 Grains. *Charas* says, he has taken 12 Grains himself; and adds, he knew one who made no scruple of 36. And in the *Philos. Trans.* We have an instance of one Mrs. *Lovelock*, who, in a Fever, in three days time, took 102 Grains.

It raises the Spirits, occasions agreeable Sensations, and has much the same effect with Wine or strong Spirits. The *Turks* ordinarily take to the quantity of a Drachm when they go to Battel, or undertake any Affair that requires Vigour and Force.

*Opium* stops, for a time, all Overflowings of Humours, Fluxes, Hemorrhages, &c. probably from the smoothness and roundness of its Parts, which by a kind of Titillation, oblige the Intestines, and other Vessels to contract themselves.

*Willis*, *Sylvius*, and *Muller* look on *Opium* as a coagulating Poison, which fixes the Spirits in the Nerves. *Wepfer* and *Pitcairn*, on the contrary, maintain it to be a hot dissolving Poison, which subtilizes the Blood, exalts and reduces it into Vapours, which bloat up the Arteries; and the bloated Arteries compressing the Veins and Nerves, shut up the Passage of the Spirits.

By Analysis, it is found to contain a great deal of volatile Salt.

**OPOBALSAMUM**, in Pharmacy, a whitish Juice, Gum, or Resin, distilling from the Branches of a Tree call'd *Balsamum*, or the *Balm-Tree*. 'Tis whitish, pretty thick, transparent, of a Smell approaching Turpentine, but much more agreeable. 'Tis the same with the celebrated *Balsamum verum*, or Balm of the *Levant*; at least the different is not visible, nor can Authors fix it.

It obtains a Place among the Alexipharmics, and is a good Ingredient in the *Theriaca Andromachi*, and Mithridate; very ill supply'd with the expressed Oil of Mace for a Seccedaneum, which does not at all come up to the subtility and activity of its Parts, but is of a much heavier Texture. This, as all other Balsams, is Suppurative, Detersive, and Incarnating, apply'd outwardly to Tumors, Ulcers, or green Wounds.

**OPOPANAX**, or Opoponax, in Pharmacy, a Gum, yellow without-side, white within, fat, brittle, of an agreeable Taste, and a very strong Smell.

The *Latins* call it *Panaces Herculeum*, from *Hercules*, who is suppos'd to have invented it, or rather who first discover'd its specific Virtues. 'Tis one of the three celebrated *Panacea*, or universal Medicines, they attributed such wonderful Virtues to. The two others are the *Asclepian* and *Chironium*; the first found by *Esculapius*, the second by *Chiron*.

The Gum *Opoponax* flows by Incision from a Plant growing abundantly in *Achaia*, *Beotia*, *Phocis*, and *Macedonia* : while 'tis liquid, 'tis white; but as it dries and hardens, it assumes a beautiful golden yellow.

There are three Kinds imported; that in Tears, that in the Mass; and that counterfeited, or flatted. The first is the best, and the second is the better, as it has the more Tears; the third is a rank Sophistication, and good for little.

It is little used internally; tho' *Etmuller* ranks it among Cathartics. Its chief Use is in the Cure of Wounds; whence it enters the Composition of the *Unguentum Divinum*, with the *Galbanum*, *Ammoniac*, and *Bdellium*.

The Word is form'd from the *Greek* ωπος, *Juice*, and παναξ, the Name of the Tree which yields it.

**OPPILATION**, in Medicine, the Act of obstructing, or stopping up the Ducts, or Passages of the Body, by evil or peccant Humours. The Word is chiefly used for Obstructions of the Lower Belly. Viscid, heavy Foods, difficult of Digestion, are *oppilative*; don't pass off well, but stop in the Mouths of the Vessels.

**ORGASM**, *Orgasmus*, in Medicine, an Impetus, or too quick Motion of the Blood, or Spirits; whereby the Muscles convulsed or moved with uncommon Force. The Word is Greek, οργασμος, denoting violence, force, onset.

**ORPIMENT**, or Orpin, by the *Latins, Auripigmentum*, a Mineral, or Semi-Metal, usually found in Copper Mines; and supposed to contain Particles of Gold; which may be extracted by Chymistry, but which were never found to countervail the Expence.

*Orpiment* is found in Stones, or Glebes, of several Sizes, and Figures : Its Colour is always yellow, intermixed with other Shades; as green, red, orange, &c. Sometimes 'tis found almost quite red; which is the proper *Sandarach* of the Antients. But that usually call'd *red Orpiment*, or *red Arsenic*, is only the yellow *Orpiment* heated to a great degree, and put in a Crucible, with Oil of Hemp-Seed, Olives, or Nuts.

Painters, Farriers, &c. make a great Consumption of this Mineral; but as it is found a violent Corrosive, and a dangerous Poison, it must be used with a great deal of Precaution. The *Indians* use *Orpiment*, corrected with Juice of Lemons, with good success against Fevers.

*Orpiment* must be chosen of a Golden Yellow, easy to scale, and the Scales very thin, small, and shining like Gold.

Some make three Kinds of *Orpiment*; *White*, which is the same with Arsenic. *Yellow*, which is the proper *Orpiment*; and *Red*, which is *Sandarach* or *Realgal*.

**ORTHOPNÆA**, in Medicine, a great difficulty of Respiration, wherein the Patient is obliged to sit, or stand, to be able to breathe. An *Orthopnæa*, is a Species, or Degree of an Asthma. The Word is compounded of ορθος, right, and πνεειν, to respire, breathe.

It may be caused from Pus, thick, or mucilaginous Juices or Polypus's in the Bronchia; mercurial and other Fumes, hindering the playing of the Lungs; Stoppage of Evacuations; Cachexies, ill Digestions, or whatever affords viscid Chyle, or occasions the Blood to run slower through the Lungs, either by straitening the Canals, or thickening the Blood, or hindering the Motion of the Animal Spirits, so that they cannot elevate the Breast; or that causes the Blood to be more rarefy'd, or more in Quantity, so that there is not sufficient room to receive it into the Vessels of the Lungs.

**ORVIETAN**, an Antidote, or Counter-poison; so call'd, because invented and propagated by an operator from *Orvieta* in *Italy*; who made Experiments thereof in his own Person, on the public Stage, after taking several Doses of Poisons. In *Charras's Pharmacopœia* is a Method of making *Orvietan*;

where it appears that Treacle is one of the principal Ingredients.

**OSCHEOCELE**, in Medicine, a kind of Hernia, wherein the Intestines descend into the Scrotum. The Word is form'd from the *Greek* οσχεον, Scrotum, and κηλη, Tumor.

**OSTEOCOLLA**, in Natural History, *q.d. glue-bone*, a white, or ash-colour'd Stone, shaped like a Bone, and by some supposed to have a quality of uniting broken Bones; on which account it is order'd in some Plasters; but the present Practice has no such Dependence on it.

**OSTRACITES**, in Natural History, a kind of crusty Stone, reddish, and in form of an Oyster-shell, and, like that, separable into Laminæ; found in several Places in Germany; and held of good Service in the Gravel.

Dr. *Home*, in the *Philos. Transact.* says, it rather dissolves the little Stones than forces 'em out, as not being remarkably Diuretic. He adds, that he prescribes it in Powder with a third part of *Flores Chamomeli.* The Dose is from half a Drachm to a whole one in white Wine.

*Ostracites* is also the Name of a kind of *Cadmia* found at the bottom of the Furnaces where Copper is purify'd. 'Tis very heavy, and resembles an Oyster-shell, whence its Name. It is esteemed astringent and detersive; and is an Ingredient in several Unguents.

**OTALGIA**, in Medicine, a Pain in the Ear. The Word is form'd from the *Greek* υος ωτος, Ear, and αλγος, Pain.

The *Otalgia* usually arises from an Inflammation; sometimes from a sharp serous Humour, which vellicates the Membrane wherewith the Canal of the Ear is lined. It is sometimes also occasion'd by a Wound or Ulcer in that Part, or from some pun gent Matter gather'd within the Ear.

The Smoke of Tobacco convey'd to the Ear through a Pipe, *Etmuller* recommends as good to assuage this Pain; as also Millepedes in a proper Vehicle of Oil.

The *Otalgia* sometimes arises from a Worm in the Ear; which is to be drawn out alive, or kill'd within. Warm Milk tempts the Worm to come forth; Wormwood Juice destroys it within.

**OXYCRATE**, in Pharmacy, &c. a Mixture of Water and Vinegar. The usual Proportion is one Spoonful of Vinegar to five or six of Water. *Oxycrate* is proper to assuage and refresh. They male Fomentations of *Oxycrate*, Clysters of *Oxycrate*, &c. The Word is form'd from the *Greek* οξυς, sharp, sour, and κεραννυμαι, I mix.

**OXYCROCEUM**, in Pharmacy, a Preparation much used in Plaisters, for Fractures, and to form Callus's; composed chiefly of Saffron, with Gums dissolved in Vinegar. The Word is form'd from the *Greek* οξυς, sharp, sour, and κροκος, Saffron.

**OXYMEL**, in Pharmacy, a Mixture of Honey and Vinegar. There are two kinds of *Oxymels*; the one simple, the other compound. The Word is form'd from the *Greek*, οξυς, sour, and μελι, Honey.

The *simple Oxymel* is composed of two parts of Honey, and one of White-Wine Vinegar, boil'd into the consistence of Syrup; proper to incide and scour any Phlegm adhering to the Throat and Breast.

*Compound Oxymel* only differs from the simple, in that to the Honey and Vinegar, they add the Decoction of the five major aperitive Roots, with the Seeds of Smallage, Parsley, and Fennel. It is used to open Obstructions of the Liver and Spleen.

**OXYREGMIA**, in Medicine, a Sourness of Acidity of the Stomach-Liquor, occasioning Belches. From οξυς and ερευγω, *ructo*.

**OXYRRHODON**, in Mixture of two Parts of Oil of Roses, and one part of Vinegar of Roses, stirr'd together for some time. To these are sometimes added distill'd Waters. It is used for inflammations, and to dry up Tetters. *Scultet* prescribes it as follows; Two Whites of Eggs beaten, one Ounce and half of Vinegar or Roses, four Ounces of Rose-Water, and two Ounces of Oil of Roses. The Word is composed of the *Greek* οξυς, sour, and ροδον, Rose.

**OXYSACCHARUM**, a Syrup prepared with Vinegar, the Juice of four Pome-granuts, and Sugar; used to cool, refresh, and resist the malignity of peccant Humours. From οξυς, sour, and σακκαρον, Sugar.

**OZÆNA**, in Medicine, a fetid Ulcer, in one or both Nostrils; wherein the Humour is very acrid or corrosive, sanious, and sometimes mixed with a bloody Mucus. The Word is *Greek*, οζαινα, which signifies the same thing. It sometimes proceeds from neglected or ill-managed Wounds, Contusions, &c. in the Nostrils; especially in Scorbutic, Scrophulous, or Venereal Habits; and sometimes follows the Small-Pox. It often spreads and eats thro' the *Alæ*; and at other times preys into the *Septum Nasi*, *Cartilage*, and *Os Palati*; especially in Venereal Cases. Whence the great danger of the Nose in that Distemper.

**PAIN**, in Medicine, consider'd as a Symptom of a Disease, makes a considerable Article in a Palliative Cure. Pain is mitigated or asswaged divers Ways; as 1. by diluting and softening of Acrimonies, with warm Water, mix'd with Flower apply'd by way of Drink, Fomentation, Clyster, or Bath.

2. By Resolving and washing away Obstructions, by the same Means and Resolvents.

3. By relaxing the nervous Vessels, with Drinks, Fomentations, Baths, the Species of Relaxants, Anodynes and Aperients.

4. By correcting the Acrimony itself with proper Remedies.

5. By freeing the obstruent, obstructed, and acrimonious Parts from the too much Pressure of the vital Humour; and by softening, and suppurating, and depurating 'em.

6. By rebating or deadening the Sense by Narcoticks, either internally or externally.

**PALED** Flowers, in Botany, are those that have Leaves set about, or surrounding a Head, or Thrum; as in Marigolds, &c.

**PALLIATION**, the Action of mitigating, soothing, or disguising a Thing. Hence, in Medicine, *Palliation* is used for the quieting and assuaging of Pain, and providing against the severer Symptoms of a Disease, when nothing can be directly levell'd against the Cause.

**PALLIATIVE** *Indication*, is where the Symptoms of a Disease give too much Trouble, and Danger, to have their Cure deferr'd till the Disease, whereon they depend, is removed. Here, the Symptoms, themselves, are to be cured, or mitigated a-part; And hence,

**PALLIATIVE** *Cure*, is the Answering of a *Palliative* Indication; or the Removal, or Mitigation of the Symptoms of a Disease; the Cause of the Disease still remaining. The principal Symptoms which call for such a Cure are Thirst, Pain, too much Waking and Faintings. *Boerhaave* observes that every Mitigation of a Symptom takes away somewhat from the Disease itself; so that to cure all the Symptoms together, is almost to cure the whole Disease.

**PALPITATION**, in Medicine, a preternatural Beating, or Pulsation of the Heart. The *Palpitation* of the Heart, is an Irregularity in the Motions of that *Viscus*, whereby it is driven with Violence towards the Ribs, in its Contraction, attended with a great Feebleness of Pulse.

There are several Degrees of *Palpitation* : Sometimes 'tis great, sometimes moderate, sometimes small; 'tis sometimes so impetuous, as to be heard and seen.

The *Trepidation* of Trembling of the Heart differs from the *Palpitation*. In the former the Pulsations are faint, slow, and faltering; in the latter the Shakes are immoderate, violent, and convulsive.

The Cause of the *Palpitation*, according to *Boerhaave*, is usually an inordinate and violent *Impetus* of the vital Spirits into the *Villi* of the Heart; as in violent Passions, sudden Fear, hysteric Affections, violent and sudden Motions. Sometimes it is owing to an Irritation of the Fibres of the Heart, occasion'd by some sharp *Stimulus*; as an Inflammation of the Heart or *Pericardium*, or some other Disorder thereof from a Stone, Worms, Hairs, an *Aneurisma*, &c.

Sometimes it arises from a thick, copious, polypous Blood : and sometimes from the Arteries, being become cartilaginous or bony; or their Extremities obstructed therewith.

In the *Diction. De Trevoux*, an Author, himself afflicted with this Disease, makes a particular Disquisition into its Nature, and Cause. Anatomy, he observes, shews us a great Number of occasional Causes of this Disease: But Physicians are still at a Loss to determine the efficient Cause.

The Moderns, with better Reason than the Antients, seek for it in the Blood of the Pulmonary Artery, which is supposed to rebound impetuously towards the right Ventricle of the Heart; by being prevented from pursuing its Course towards the other Vessels of the Lungs, stopp'd by some Obstruction, or compressed from various Causes.

In some the Heart is extraordinarily big, and the Pulmonary Artery dilated to double, or quadruple its ordinary Capacity, with Obstructions of the Pulmonary Vein, consisting of cartilaginous Matters which cram its Cavity so close, that as *Blanchard* tells us, in his Anatomy, 'tis sometimes difficult even to get a Pin in.

From these Observations, some have concluded, that the Capillary, &c. Vessels of the Lungs, opposing an impassable Dike to the Course of the thickest Part of the Blood, driven thither by the Contraction of the Heart, so as only a small Quantity can find a Passage through them; the first must make an Effort against their Sides, and oblige them to give way and stretch them out, in Proportion to the Quantity of Blood impelled against them by the Contraction of the Heart.

But because the Pulmonary Artery cannot stretch wide enough to receive all the Blood of the right Ventricle driven thither at a Contraction; and since the Blood, by reason of Obstructions, cannot continue its progressive Motion, in Proportion to the Velocity wherewith is it impelled, by the Contraction of the Heart; the Heart at each Contraction fails to express into the Pulmonary Artery, all the Blood it contain'd in its right Ventricle.

Thus that Part of the Blood which remains, receiving the whole Shock impressed by the Contraction, returns it again to the Heart by Reflection, striking impetuously against its Sides, and making it bound and shoot towards the Ribs.

The same Consequences will arise from Obstructions of the *Aorta*, preventing the entire Evacuation of the left Ventricle; and generally, from all Obstructions or Compressions of the Vessels, as *Polypus's*, Abscesses, and Dropsies in the Parts near the Heart. As to Worms, their biting, and gnawing of the fibrous Parts of the Heart, must occasion violent Refluxes of Spirits towards the Brain, follow'd with a copious Effusion of other Spirits into the Nerves of the Lungs, by the Consent of Parts. And by such Means violent and convulsive Contractions will be occasion'd throughout the whole texture of the Lungs, which opposing the free Passage of the Blood may occasion a *Palpitation of the Heart.*

The same Disease may arise from a Compression of the Lungs, occasion'd by the extraordinary Rarefaction of the vicious and fermentative Juices, sojourning the Stomach and Intestines; which dilate those Parts to that Degree, that the Diaphragm and Lungs, being extremely straightened, the Blood cannot circulate without Abundance of Difficulty; a *Palpitation* therefore must ensue; which will last as long as that Rarefaction in the first Passages.

Such, according to modern Physicians, are the immediate Causes of the *Palpitation* of the Heart : The remote or occasional Causes are whatever may occasion such Obstructions of the Pulmonary Artery, &c.

In the same Work, another Physician lays down Winds or *Flatus's*, as a Cause of the *Palpitation*; he adds, that the Ancients, to a Man, look'd on that as the most ordinary Occasion thereof : In Effect, says he, from this Source may be deduced a Multitude of Causes of sympathetic *Palpitation*, by Means of the Ventricle, the Diaphragm, Mediastin, &c.

Others will have the sole Cause of *Palpitation* to be a viscid Blood; which, by its extraordinary Rarefaction, dilating the Pulmonary Artery, and, by that means, opening the Cavity of its Capillary Vessels towards their Extremes; or, by this Dilatation, compressing the other little Vessels of the Lungs, prevents the Blood from continuing its circulating Motion with Freedom : and, thus occasions a *Palpitation of the Heart.*

All these Authors hold the *Palpitation* a dangerous Disease, and *Galen* observes, that those troubled with it, when young, never live to grow old.

According to M. *Pison*[1], a Doctor of the Faculty of *Paris*, the *Palpitation* of the Heart may arise, either from a too abundant Serosity, swelling the proper Membrane of the Heart; as *Galen* found to be the Case in opening a Monkey; or from too great a Quantity of Water contained in the *Pericardium*; by which means, the Heart being straighten'd, and disabled from moving with its usual Freedom, is obliged to make several Jerks or half Beats, instead of the regular Motions it had before; or, again, from a Serosity thrown into the Ventricles of the Heart, either form the grand Vessels which furnish the Blood, or from the Lungs, or from the Brain.

Of these three Causes, the most ordinary seems to be the great Extension of the *Pericardium*, by Water, as it is found to be in the Bodies of most of those open'd after this Disease.

The different Causes have their different Symptoms. The boiling Serosity, thrown out of the Blood-Vessels into the Heart, shews itself by sudden Beatings of the Temples, Whizzings in the Ear, dim Sight, wandering Pains in various Parts of the Body.

In that produced by the Abundance of Water in the *Pericardium*, or from the Humour swelling the proper Membrane of the Heart; the Heart seems as if suffocated with Water; the Pulse weak, the *Palpitation* continual, or nearly so, together with a Feverishness, and a Difficulty of Breathing. To which may

[1] Charles Pison (1563 – 1633), a French physician.

be added, that the Disease comes by little and little.

The *Palpitation* arising from the Serosity is cured by bleeding, the other by purging.

**PALSY**, *Paralysis*, in Medicine, a Disease, wherein the Body or some of its Parts, lose their Motion, and sometimes their Sensation. The Causes of the *Palsy* are in impeded Influx of nervous Spirits into the *Villi* of the Muscles; or of the arterious Blood into their Vessels, which may happen from some Fault, either in the Brain, the Nerves, Muscles, or their Vessels.

The *Palsy* is said to be *perfect* or *compleat*, when there is a Privation of Motion and Sensation at the same Time. *Imperfect*, when one of the two is destroy'd, the other remaining.

The *Palsy* is either Universal, Lateral, or Particular. The first, call'd *Paraplegia* or *Paraplexia*, is a general Immobility of all the Muscles that receive Nerves from the *Cerebrum* or *Cerebellum*, expect those of the Head : Its Cause is usually supposed to reside in the Ventricles of the Brain, or in the Root of the spinal Marrow.

*Etmuller* makes this a different Disease form the *Paralysis*, which he supposed to consist in a Relaxation of the Ligaments and Membranes serving for Motion; but the *Paraplegia* in a mere Obstruction of the Nerves.

The *Paraplegia* is seldom a primary Disease, usually a secondary one, attending or following an Apoplexy, *Scorbutus, Carus, Arthritis*, &c.

The second, call'd *Hemiplegia* is the same Disease with the *Paraplegia*; only it affects but one Side of the Body : Its Cause is the same, only restrained to one Side of the Brain, or spinal Marrow.

The third, call'd *particular Paralysis* or *Palsy*, is where some particular Part or Member alone is affected; *e.gr.* where the Motion of the Arm or Leg is destroy'd.

Dr. *Quincy* observes, that a *Paralysis* where Motion is destroy'd, Sensation remaining, may be produced, first, by too much Humidity, stretching the muscular Fibres in Length. Secondly, from cold Things, which thicken the Juices. Thirdly, from external Compression. Fourthly, from hot Things, which straighten the supple Membranes and Vessels. All these Causes affect either the Blood, or Muscles; the former, by thickening that Tumour so that it cannot suddenly rarify; and the latter, by relaxing the Muscles into a too great a Length, by too much Moisture, or contracting them into too narrow Dimensions by too much Heat. But the Sensation may yet be preserv'd, because, notwithstanding all these Hindrances, the animal Spirits and Nerves may not be at all affected.

The Causes of the *Paralysis* where Sensation is destroy'd, Motion remaining, he observes, may be all those Things which so far Thicken the animal Spirits in the Nerves, arising below the *Cerebellum*, that tho' indeed they may flow into the Muscles thro' the Nerves, and there, by the Occursion of some Liquor secreted from the Blood, rarify; yet they cannot alone flow in such Quantities into the Nerves, as from a very slight Cause to be made to undulate; whence Sensation will cease without losing the Motion of the Part.

The Causes of this Kind are also whatsoever render those Nerves more lax and moist, and so less apt for lively Vibrations; the animal Spirits flowing in the mean time into the Muscles, from whence Motion is perform'd without Sensation.

The Cure of the *Palsy*, according to *Waldschmid*[1], does not differ much from that of the venereal Disease. Internally, Mercurials, Sudorifics, and Decoctions of the Woods are good : Externally, Unctions, particularly of spirituous and penetrating Things, not on the Part affected, but on the *Spina Dorsa.*

**PANACEA**, an universal Medicine; or a Remedy for all Diseases. The Word is from the *Greek* παν all, ακεομαι, I cure. The accurate *Boerhaave* overturns the Notion of *Panacea's*; and shews, from the different Causes, Natures, Effects, Seats, &c. of Diseases, that several may be cured by one Medicine; but, all, by none. He observes, that the most universal Remedies known are *Water, Fire, Mercury,* and *Opium*; and adds, that by these alone, cautiously disguised, some have acquir'd the Reputation of universal Physicians.

**PANACES**, or Panaceous, a Name applied to several Plants, by reason of the extraordinary Virtues ascribed to them. There are three of these *Panaces*; the *Heraclean, Asclepean,* and *Chironian*; so called from their Inventors, *Hercules, Asclepias,* and *Chiron.* The first is the *Sphondilium majus* of *J. Bauhin*[2]; from the Root and Stem of this is drawn, by Incision, the Gum *Opoponax.* The *Asclepian*, according to some Botanists, is a Kind of *Ferula*, which *Gas. Bauhin*[3] calls *Libanotis Ferulæ folio & femine.* The *Chironian*, according to some is a Kind of *Helianthemum.*

**PANADA**, or *Panatella*, a Diet, consisting of Bread boil'd in Water, to the Consistence of a Pulp; given to sick Persons whose Digestion is weak, or to whom stronger Foods would be improper. 'Tis sometimes made thin; to serve as a Drink; and sometimes likewise sweetened, &c. to render it more palatable. The Word is form'd from the principal Ingredients *Panis* Bread.

**PANARIS** or Payorchia, in Medicine, a painful Tumour or Inflammation, arising on the Extremities of the Fingers or Toes, popularly called, among us, *Whitloe.* It is occasion'd by a sharp or saline Humour, lodg'd between the Bone and the *Periosteum*, and the Nerves and Tendons. An infallible Remedy for it, is to open it either with the Point of a Lancet, or with some Unguent, and then to dip the Finger in a Lixivium of Vine Ashes.

The *Panaris* is exceedingly restless. Beside the mild Kind call'd *Whitloe*, there is also a malignant Kind, called a *Fellon.* It sometimes tends to an Imposthume, but more usually Gangrenes. For the *Panaris*, after bleeding, and the universal Remedies, Dr. *Burnet* orders the Patient to hold his Finger a good while in a rotten Egg, or a putrify'd Mouse. *Helmont* adds, he has seen a Finger as big as an Arm, by means of *Panaris*, cured by rubbing it with

1 Johann Jacob Waldschmidt (1644 – 1689), a German physician.

2 Johann Bauhin (1541 – 1613), a Swiss physician and botanist.

3 Gaspard Bauhin (1560 – 1624), a Swiss physician, anatomist and botanist, and brother to Johann.

4 This may be Thomas Burnet (b. 1670), a Scottish physician and author.

Blood, then wrapping it up in a Mole-Skin. *Riverius* adds, that to hold the Finger affected in a Cat's Ear, cures a *Panaris* in two Hours.

The Word is form'd from the Latin *Panaricium*, which we find in *Apuleius*; and that from the *Greek* παρωνυκια, *i.e.* an Abscess at the Root of the Nails.

**PANCHREST**, *Panchrestos*, in Medicine, a *Panacea*, or Remedy for all Distempers. The Word is form'd of the *Greek* παν, all, χρεστος, *Utilis*, useful.

**PANCHYMAGOGUE**, in Pharmacy, an Extract of Aloes, Rhubarb, Senna, Scammony, Jalap, Agaric, Coloquintada and Black Hellebore. Its Name arises hence, that being a Composition of all the Kinds of Purgatives, it has the Virtue of purging all the Humours of the Body at once. The Word is form'd from the *Greek* παν, all, χρεστος, *Succus*, Juice; and αγειν, to draw off.

**PANDICULATION**, that Restlessness, Stretching, and Uneasiness, which usually accompany the cold Fit of an Intermitting Fever. It is supposed to arise from a convulsive Dilatation of the Muscles, whereby Nature endeavours to throw off something that disturbs her.

**PANICULA**, Panicle, in Botany, called also *Juba*, a soft woolly Beard, or String, whereon the Seeds of some Plants hang, pendulous, as in Reeds, Millet, &c. Such are hence called *Paniculated Plants*.

**PANNUS**, in Medicine, &c. a Disease of the Eye, popularly call'd the *Web*; and by the *Arabs*, *Zebel*. The *Pannus* is an Excrescence arising on the *Adnata* or *Conjunctiva*; less hard and membranous than the *Unguis*; and representing a Web, or Tissue of little Veins swell'd with Blood.

Its Cause is an Obstruction of the Blood in the minute Vessels of that Tunic. Its Cure is almost the same with that if the *Pterigium* or *Unguis*; between which, and the *Pannus*, there is a great Affinity.

The chief Difference is, that in the *Unguis*, the membranous Excrescence only cover Part of the Eye, after the manner of a Nail; whereas in the *Pannus* it covers the whole.

**PAPILIONACEOUS**, in Botany, the Flowers of some Plants are thus called, by Botanists, as representing something of the Figure of a *Papilio* or Butterfly, with its Wings display'd. They have four such Leaves, joined together at the Extremities; on in the Middle of the Flower is larger than the rest, and by some called *Vexillum*. The Plants, that have this Flower, are of the leguminous Kind, as Pease, Vetches, &c.

**PAPPUS**, in Botany, that soft light Down, which grows out of the Seeds of some Plants, as Thistles, Dandelion, Hawkweed, &c. and which buoys then up so in the Air, that they may be blown any where about with the Wind. This distinguishes a Class or Kind of Plants, which are hence denominated *Papposa*, or *Pappi Flore*.

**PARACENTESIS**, in Chirurgery, an Operation in Chirurgery, popularly call'd *Tapping*. It consists in the opening a little Hole in the lower Venter, or

Belly, to let out Waters collected in the Capacity thereof, or between the Teguments, in an *Ascites* or *Water-Dr*opsy. The Word is form'd from the *Greek* παρα, with, and κεντειν, *pungere*, to prick.

The Antients cut the Aperture with a Lancet; but the Moderns punch it with a Kind of Scillet or Bodkin; clapping a *Cannula* or Tap into the Hole when made, to carry off the Water. The Operation is usually perform'd two or three times. Fingers Breadth on one Side of the Navel, sometimes a little lower, but always so as to avoid the *Linea Alba*. The Water is usually draw off at several Times, as the Patient's Strength will allow; and a new Puncture is made, every Time the Belly is thus to be emptied.

The *Paracentesis* does not often succeed, tho' often repeated; because the Root of the Disease, notwithstanding the carrying off the Water by this Means, is still left behind.

Some Authors give the Name *Paracentesis* to all Operations with the Lancet, Needle, or Punch; not excepting the Operation of Couching for Cataracts; founded on the Etymology of the Word : others restrain it to Apertures made in the Head, Breast, Belly, and Scrotum; and others to the single Operation of *Tapping in Dropsies*.

**PARAGORICKS**, Medicines prescrib'd with an Intention to assuage Pain. They are thus call'd, from the *Greek* παραγωρεω, I mitigate, abate; but are more ordinarily denominated *Opiates*.

**PARAGUAY**, or Paragoue, in Nat. History, a celebrated Plant, of the Shrub Kind, growing in some Provinces of *South America*, especially at *Paraguay*, whence its Name; tho' better known, of late, among us, under the Denomination of *South-Sea Tea*.

This Plant, which does not rise above a Foot and half high, has very slender Branches, and Leaves like those of Senna; it may be look'd on as a Kind of Occidental Tea, which, like the Oriental, is taken infused in hot Water, to which it communicates a Colour and Smell nearly kike those of the best Teas seen in Europe.

There are two Kinds of *Paraguay*, the one call'd simply *Paraguay*; the other *Camini*, by the *Spaniards*, *Yerva-Camini*; which last is most esteem'd, and sold for a Third more than the other.

The first the *Spaniards* call *Yerva-Conpalos*, *i.e.* Herb with little Sticks, because full of broken Branches, and is chiefly used by Domesticks and Slaves : The latter is the Drink of the richest. But both are of so much Use, and esteem'd of such absolute Necessity, that no body in that Part of America will live without 'em. The Works of the Mines of *Potosi* wou'd stand still, but that the Masters take care to supply the poor Slaves that labour therein, with *Paraguay*. Nor will a Servant engage himself with any Master, but upon this among other Conditions, that he have nothing but *Paraguay* for Drink.

The *Paraguay* makes one of the most considerable Articles of the *South America* Commerce. At *Peru*, *Chilly*, and *Buenos Aires*, there are above two Millions Worth sold *per Annum*; which passes almost altogether thro' the Hands of the Jesuits. The Use of *Paraguay* began lately to obtain in *England*; where many People seem'd to like it as well as Tea. But Foreigners say, that their Approbation flow'd as much from their Interest as their Taste; in regard they come so easily by it, by reason of their Commerce with the *Spaniards* of *S. America*, and *Buenos Aires*, since the Treaty of *Utrecht* in 1713.

The Preparation of the Plant, and the making it into a Drink is much the same with that of Tea, except that they infuse both Leaves and Wood, that they drink it immediately out of the Vessel 'tis made in; without letting it have Time to infuse, by reason of the black Tincture it gives; and that to prevent Leaves and all from coming, they suck it thro' a silver, or glass Pipe, which goes round the Company one after another.

Beside all the Virtues which the Eastern People ascribe to their Tea; as to be good in Diseases of the Head, Breast, Stomach, against Phlegm, and to restore Sleep; the *Americans* attribute to theirs this further of purifying all Kinds of Water, how foul and corrupted soever, by only infusing it therein, either hot or cold. Thus, having always some of it with 'em, if they meet with none but the worst Waters in the vast Desarts to be cross'd in going from *Buenos Aires* to *Peru* and *Chilly*, they are not afraid to drink it, after steeping some of the plant a little while therein. It is also held sovereign against the Scurvy, and putrid Fevers.

**PARALYSIS**, in Medicine, a Disease popularly call'd *Palsy*. The *Paralysis* only differs from the *Paresis* as the greater from the less. Authors distinguish the *Paralysis* into a *Paraplegia*, or *Paraplexia*, *Hemiplegia*, and, particular *Paralysis*. The first is a Palsy of the whole Body. The second, of one Side of the Body. The third of some particular Member, which is the proper Palsy. The Word Paralysis is form'd from the Greek παραλυω, I unbind; This Disease being supposed to unbend the Nerves, and Muscles.

**PARAPHRENESIS**, or Paraphrenetis, or Paraphrenitis, in Medicine, a Kind of Phrenzy, the Cause whereof was attributed, by the Antients, to an Inflammation of the Ventricle, the Liver, and especially the Diaphragm.

They also called it a *Pseudo Phrenesis*, false Phrenzy, to distinguish it from the true one, which they made to consist in an Inflammation of the Brain and its *Meninges*. The Moderns don't make any such Distinctions in Phrenzies : They all come form the same Cause; but that Cause is neither an Inflammation of the Brian , nor of the Diaphragm.

*Paraphrenitis*, among the modern Physicians, is an Inflammation of the *Mediastinum*, or *Pleura*, about the Diaphragm, attended with a continual Fever, and exquisite Pain in the Parts affected, on contracting the abdominal Vessels, as also a *Delirium* and arising of the *Hypochondria*.

**PARASITES**, or Parasitical Plants, in Botany, a Kind of diminutive Plants, growing on Trees, and so called from their Manner of living and feeding, which is altogether on others.

Such is Moss, which was antiently supposed the Effect of a Derangement of the Texture of the Bark; or a Kind of Rust; or, at most, little Filaments arising from the Bark : But from many Observations of the Moderns, it appears, that Mosses are real Plants, whose Seed is exceedingly fine, and inclosed in very little *Capsulæ*; which bursting of themselves, the Seed is driven by the Wind, and, at length, detained in the Inequalities of the Barks of Trees; where it takes Root and is fed at the Expence thereof. Of these Mosses M. *Vaillant* reckons no less than 137 Species, all in the Neighbourhood of Paris; which, with the Lichens and Mistleto's, make the Genus of the Parasite Plants.

The most pernicious of these *Parasites*, to the Trees that support 'em, are the Lichens; which appear on the Barks of Trees, in Form of a Crust, mix'd with Yellow and a dirty White.

M. *de Ressons*[1] gives is a Remedy for this Disease, in the French Memoirs of the *Acad. Roy.* It consists in making an Incision thro' the Bark to the very Wood, from the first Branches to the Earth; the Bark closes again in a little Time; and always preserves itself clean and free from Mosses for the future.

This Aperture renders the Course of the Sap more free, and prevents the Forming of those Inequalities so favourable to the Production of Mosses. The Incision, he adds, is to be made from *March* to the End of *April*; and on that Side turn'd most from the Sun.

**PARASYNANCHE**, in Medicine, a Kind of Angina or Squinancy, wherein the exterior Muscles of the Throat are inflamed. The Word comes from παρα, συν αγκειν to suffocate.

**PARBOILING**, in Pharmacy, &c. a Term applied to Fruits, Herbs, &c. which are boiled a little while, to draw out the first Juices, to be afterwards inspissated or thickened.

**PAREGORICKS**, in Medicine, Remedies which asswage Pain; the same with what we otherwise call Anodynes, and Opiates. The Word is Greek παραγεινα.

**PAREIRA BRAVA**, the Root of a Plant growing in the *West-Indies*; chiefly *Mexico* and *Brazil*; esteem'd a Specific for the Cure of the Stone and Gravel.

The Name, which in the original *Portuguese*, signifies *Wild-Vine*, or *Bastard Vine*, bears a good deal of Analogy to the Plant, which bears Branches loaden with Leaves perfectly like those of the Vine; and which, like them, creep along Walls and Trees.

The *Portuguese* value this Root on an equal footing with the *Ipecacuanha*. Some Druggists call it, by Corruption, *Parada Brava*.

M. *Geoffroy* attributes the Efficacy of this Root, in Nephritic Cases, to its dissolving the viscid Matters, whereby the Particles of the Sand, &c. were cemented together : And hence, he gives it with the same Intention in Jaundice, Asthma's, &c. it is given in Decoction. The *Portuguese* hold it also a Remedy for Dysenteries, Quinzies, Bites of venomous Beasts, &c.

**PARENCHYMA**, or *Parenchymous Flesh*, in Anatomy, a Term used for the peculiar Substance of several Parts of the Bodies of Animals, as the Heart, Lungs, Liver, Spleen, Kidneys, &c, thus called from the *Greek* παρεγχυμα,

[1] This may be Jean-Baptiste Deschiens de Ressons (1660 – 1735), a French soldier and scientist.

Effusion, *q.d.* generated by a Collection and Condensation of Juice.

*Erasistratus* first gave the Name; as imagining the Substance of these Parts not to be Vascular like the rest, but to consist of a mass or *Coagulum* of Blood, stagnated in the Vessels of the Parts : But the Moderns reject this Opinion : The Observations made by Microscopes, Injections, &c. clearly shewing, that the Heart is a true Muscle, the Lungs and Spleen, Clusters of membranous Vesicles, and Vessels and the Liver and Kidneys, Compositions of Glands, thro' which the Bile and Urine are filtrated.

**PARENCHYMA** *of a Plant.* Dr. *Grew* gives the Name *Parenchyma* to the *Pith* or *Pulp*; or that inner Part of the Plant, thro' which the Juice is supposed to be distributed.

This, when view'd with a Microscope, appears to resemble Marrow; or rather a Spunge; being a porous flexible dilatable Substance.

Its Pores are innumerable, and exceedingly small; receiving as much Humour as is requisite to fill and extend them; which Disposition of Pores it is, that us supposed to fit the Plant for Vegetation and Growth.

The *Parenchyma* is white, at first, but changes its Colour, in Proportion as the Root grows thicker. Thus it becomes yellow in the Root of the Bastard Rhubarb, and red in that of the Snake-weed.

**PARESIS**, in Medicine, a Disease call'd also *Paralysis* and *Palsy*.

**PAROXYSM**, in Medicine, the sever Fit of a Disease which grows higher, or exasperates as the Gout, &c. It is sometimes also used for the Access or Return of a Disease that intermits, as an Ague. The Word is form'd form the *Greek* παρα, much, and οξυς, acute.

**PARTICLE**, in Physicks, the minute Part of a Body; of an Assemblage or Coalition of several whereof Natural Bodies are compos'd. *Particle* in the new Philosophy, is frequently used in the same Sense with *Atom* in the antient *Epicurean* Philosophy; and *Corpuscle* in the later.

Some of the more accurate Writers, however, distinguish 'em; making *Particle* an Assemblage or Composition of two or more primitive, and physically indivisible Corpuscles or Atoms; and *Body*, an Assemblage or Mass of several *Particles* or secondary Corpuscles.

Indeed, the Distinction is of no great Moment; and, as to most Purposes of Physicks, Particle may be understood as synonymous with Corpuscle. Particles, then, are, as it were, the Elements of Bodies : 'Tis the various Arrangement, and Texture of these, with the Difference of the Cohesion, &c. that constitute the various Kinds of Bodies, *hard, soft, liquid, dry, heavy, light*, &c.

The smallest *Particles* or Corpuscles cohere with the strongest Attractions, and compose bigger *Particles* of weaker Cohesion; and many of these cohering compose bigger *Particles* whose Vigour is still weaker; and thus on for divers Successions till the Progression end in the biggest *Particles*, whereon the Operation in Chymistry, and the Colours of natural Bodies depend, and which, by cohering compose Bodies of sensible Bulks.

*The Cohesion of the Particles of Matter*, the *Epicureans* imagined was effected by Means of hooked Atoms; the *Aristotelians* by Rest, that is, by nothing at all. But Sir *Isaac Newton* shews it is done by means of a certain Power whereby the *Particles* mutually attract or tend to each other.

By this Attraction of the *Particles* he shews that most of the *Phænomena* of the lesser Bodies are effected; as those of the heavenly Bodies by the Attraction of Gravity.

All Bodies, the same great Author shews, consist of the same solid perfectly hard *Particles* or Corpuscles.

**PARTING** or Departing, a Method of separating Gold and Silver by Means of Aqua Fortis.

**PARTUS**, in Medicine and Law, the Delivery of a Woman, or the Birth of a Child. *Ceasareus Partus*, is that where the Mother is cut open, and the Child taken out at the Side.

**PARULIS**, in Medicine, an Inflammation of the Gums, attended with a violent Pain, and an Aposthume; sometimes ending in an Ulcer, and sometimes in a Cancer, Fistula, Gangrene, &c. *Sennertus* orders it to be cured by Revulsion, Derivation, and proper Gargarisms. Care is to be taken in the Beginning to prevent an Aposthume. The Word is *Greek*, form'd of παρα, near, and ουλον *Gingiva*, Gum.

**PASSA**, or *Passa Uva*, in Pharmacy, a Term applied to those dried Grapes, which we call *Raisins*. *Uvæ Passæ* is sometimes also used, with less Propriety, for Figs.

**PASTIL**, is also us'd for a dry Composition, yielding a fragrant Smell when burnt in a perfuming Pan, to clear and scent the Air of a Chamber. It is composed of odorous Resins, mixt with Aromatic Woods, or Drugs pulveriz'd, and incorporated with Mucilage of Gum Tragacanth. Some call 'em *Osselets of Cyprus*. There are also *Pastils* for the Mouth, eaten to procure a sweat Breath. These have several Names, and consist of several Preparations, as Muscadines, Conserves, &c.

**PASTIL**, is sometimes also us'd for the Plant otherwise call'd Woad or Glasswort.

**PASTIL** in Confectionary, is a Preparation of Sugar with Lemon-Water, &c. boil'd up with Gum-Water, strain'd, beat up, and by the Addition of more dry Sugar, work'd into a plyable Paste, and thus form'd into round or oblong Figures and dry'd in the Stove.

**PATHOGENOMIC**, in Medicine, an Essential Sign or Characteristic; or a Symptom peculiar to, and inseparable from some Disease; and every Stage thereof. Thus *Blanchard*, and after him *Harris*, &c. But the Truth is, there is nothing in all Medicine that Answers to the Idea of a *Pathogenomic*; Disease and Symptoms are too complicated.

**PATHOLOGY**, that part of Medicine which considers Diseases; both those of the Body, and the Mind; their Natures, Causes, Symptoms, &c. The Word is form'd from the *Greek* παθος Passion, Suffering, and λογος, Discourse.

**PEARL**, Pin, or Web in Medicine, an unnatural Speck, or thick Film over the Eye.

**PECCANT**, in Medicine, an Epithet given to the Humours of the Body, when they offend either in Quantity or Quality, *i.e.* when they are either Morbid, or in too great Abundance. Most Diseases arise from *Peccant* Humours, which are either to be corrected by Alteratives and Specificks, or evacuated.

**PECTEN** *Arboris*, in Botany, is the Grain of the Wood of any Tree.

**PEDICLE**, in Botany, the little Stalk or Tail, whereby the Leaf, Fruit, or Flower is connected to its Branch or Stem. The Pistil of the Flower frequently becomes the *Pedicle* of the Fruit. Flowers will keep fresh a long Time after gathering, by immerging their *Pedicles* in Water. The great Secret of preserving Fruits for the Winter, is to seal up their *Pedicles* with Wax. Cherries with the shortest *Pedicles*, are esteem'd the best.

**PEDICULARIS** *Morbus*, in Medicine, the *lousy Distemper*; a Disease arising from some uncommon Corruption in the Body, which generates infinite Quantities of Lice on the Skin. *Herod* died of the *pedicular* Disease. The Word comes form the Latin *Pediculus*, Louse.

**PELLUCID**, a Term of the same Import as *Diaphanous* or *Transparent*. Pellucid, stands in opposed to *Opake*. The Word is form'd of the *Latin Pelluceo* or *Perluceo*, I shine thro'.

**PENECILLA**, in Pharmacy, a *Lozenge*, made round by rolling; the same as *Turundula*; thus call'd from *Penecillus* a Pencil, which it resembles in shape.

**PENECILLUS**, among Chirurgeons, is used for a Tent, to be put in Wounds or Ulcers.

**PENIDIUM**, in Pharmacy, Barly-Sugar; a Preparation of Sugar, made by boiling it up with a Decoction of Barley, till it becomes Brittle; which done, it is turn'd out upon a Marble, anointed with Oil of Sweet Almonds, kneaded with the Hands like past; and while yet hot, drawn out into Sticks twisted like Cords. *Penidia* are very good against Colds, to moderate the Acrimonies of the Breast, promote Expectorations, &c. Dr. *Quincy* uses the term *Penidium*, for a kind of clarified Sugar, with a Mixture of Starch, made up into Bolus's.

**PENNATA** *Folia*, winged Leaves; amongst Botanists, are such Leaves of Plants, as grow directly one against another, on the same Rib, or Stalk as : those of Ash, Walnut Trees, &c.

**PEPPER**, an Aromatic Fruit, or Grain of a hot, dry Quality; chiefly used in the seasoning of Meat. It is the Product of a Shrub growing in several Parts of the *East-Indies*, chiefly *Java, Sumatra, Malacca*, and the Coasts of *Malabar*. The Plant is very weak and of the reptile Kind, and for that Reason usually planted at the Foot of the larger Trees, as the *Areca, Cacoa*, &c.

The *Pepper* grows in Grapes or Clusters; at first green, as they ripen they grow red; and at last, after being exposed a While to the Sun, become black, in the Condition we see 'em.

The Fruit is gather'd in *November*. It must be chosen large, well fed, not wrinkled, without Dust, with a good many white Grains in it; and Care be taken the largest Grains hasn't been pick'd out to make white *Pepper*.

*White* Pepper is the Fruit of the same Plant with the Black, and is prepared from it moistening it with Sea-Water, and exposing it to the Sun, and casting away the outer Bark, which abandoning the Grain, leaves it white. Indeed, M. *Dellon*[1], a late Traveller, says, they strip off the Skin, by beating it before it be quite dry; or by soaking it in Water after it has dried, and then beating it.

Many Authors, and among the rest *Pomet*, will have the white *Pepper* to be natural, and the Fruit of a different Plant from the Black; but M. *Dellon*, who expressly declares the contrary from his own long Experience, seems to put the Matter past doubt.

White *Pepper* must be chosen after the same manner as black; with this further Care, that it hasn't been whiten'd.

*Pepper* that is sold ground, is very apt to be sophisticated; the Black with burnt Crust of Bread, &c. the White with beaten Rice.

*Long* Pepper is a kind of *Pepper* denominated from its form, which in Length and Thickness equals a Child's Finger; it consists of an assemblage of Grains join'd close to one another, of a brownish Colour, bordering on red, and within on black; and grows by a long Pedicle to a Plant, like that of the black *Pepper*, but lower, and its Leaves smaller and greener. Its Taste resembles that of the former, but less sharp.

There are three kinds of Pepper, that of the *East-Indies*, that of *America*, and that of *Ethiopia*, call'd also Grain of *Zeilon* : Tho' the first alone is the proper long *Pepper*; the rest resembling it but little.

It must be chosen new, large, heavy, well fed, hard to break, without Dust or Mixture; its chief Use is in Medicine, where it enters several Galenical Compositions, among the rest Treacle.

*Guinea* Pepper, is a red *Pepper*, of a Coal Colour, much esteem'd by the *Americans*, from among whom 'tis brought, and by them call'd Chile, by the *Spaniards* Pimenta, and the *French*, Garden Coral.

'Tis now cultivated pretty commonly in *France*, especially in *Languedoc*; used in making Vinegar, and likewise confected with Sugar. It must be chosen new, in large Pods, dry, entire, and red.

There are four Kinds, the first call'd by the *Americans Chilchotes*; the second very small *Chilterpin*, both of a very pungent Taste; the third *Tonalchiles*, moderately hot, and eaten by the Natives like other Fruit with Bread; the fourth *Chilpelagua*, moderately pungent, much used by the

[1] Charles Dellon (1649 – ca. 1709), a French physician and traveller.

*Spaniards* in the Preparation of Chocolate; there is also a fifth Kind call'd *Agy*, growing in *Peru*.

*Jamaica* Pepper, call'd by the *Dutch Amomi*, is the Fruit of the Tree that yields the *Indian* Wood, growing plentifully in *Jamaica* and other *American* Islands. It is a real Aromatic, and may supply the *Dutch* both of Cloves, Nutmeg, and Cinnamon; the *French* call it the *round Clove*, from its Taste resembling that Spice.

**PEPASTIC**, or Peptic, in Medicine, a kind of Medicament, of the Consistence of an Emplaster; proper to bring vitious and corrupt Humours to a Head, and dispose 'em for Suppuration. Butter, Roots of Mallows, of Flowers-de-lis, Onions and Leaves of Oxylapathum are esteem'd good *Pepasticks*, or Maturatives. The Word is form'd from the Greek πεπαινειν to digest or ripen.

**PER** *Minima*, in Pharmacy, an intimate and perfect Mixture of natural Bodies; wherein their very *Minima, i.e.* their Atoms, or first component particles are supposed to be accurately blended together. If Silver and Lead be melted together, they will mingle together *Per minima*.

**PER-SE**, in Chymistry. When a Body is distill'd singly, and without the usual addition of any other Matter to raise it; it is said to be *distill'd Per-se*. The genuine Spirits of Harts-horn, are those rais'd *Per-se*, in opposition to those distill'd by the addition of Chalk.

**PERCOLATION**, in Medicine, &c. the Action of Filtrating.

**PERIANTHEUM**, in Botany the little green Leaves which compass the Bottom of a Flower; call'd by Dr. *Grew* the *Empalement*, and by others the *Calyx*. The Word is form'd from the *Greek* περι, about, and ανθος, Flower.

The Use of the *Perianthеum* is to be a Support, Security, and as it were Bands, to the other Parts of the Flower.

Mr. *Ray* observes that Flowers, whose Leaves or Petala, are strong, as Tulips, have no *Periantheum*, as needing none. Carnations, &c. whose Petala are long and slender, have their *Periantheum* of one piece; others, as the Knap-weed, &c. have it of several Pieces, and in divers rounds, and all with a counterchangeable Respect to each other, for the greater Strength and Security of 'emselves, and the Petala, &c. they include.

**PERIAPTA**, a kind of Medicines, otherwise call'd *Periamma*, *Appensa*, and *Amulets*; which being tied about the Neck, are supposed to prevent, or cure Diseases.

**PERICARDIARY**, an Epithet given to Worms generated in the Pericardium, or Capsula of the Heart. M. *Andry* makes these one of the twelve Kinds of Worms engender'd in the human Body : They sometimes occasion Convulsions; the Paroxysms whereof last but a little while, but return incessantly. These Worms are accompanied with a frightful Paleness of the Face, a low Pulse, violent Pains of the Stomach and Breast. They sometimes occasion a Palpitation of the Heart. M. *Andry* adds, that they have been known to occasion sudden Death.

**PERICARPUS**, in Botany, a Pellicle, or thin Membrane, incompassing the Fruit or Grain of a Plant. The Word is form'd of the *Greek* περι about and καρπος Fruit.

**PERIODUS** *Sanguinis*, the Circle of the Blood, or the Tour it makes round the Body, for the Support of Life.

**PERIPNEUMONIA**, in Medicine, an Inflammation of some Part of the Thorax, properly of the Lungs; attended with an acute Fever, and a Difficulty of breathing. The Word is form'd from the *Greek* περι about, and ϖνευμων, Lungs.

The *Peripneumonia* is distinguish'd into *vera, true*; and *notha, spurious*. The *first* is a real Inflammation of the Lungs, attended with a symptomatical Fever, and a Cough; by the Former of which it is distinguish'd from an Asthma; and by the latter form a Pleurisy. Its usual Cause are, want of Exercise, hard Study, Suppression of natural Evacuations, a moist Air, or the like.

When it arises from a Phlegmon, the Patients spits pure Blood; when it is Eresipelatous, the Sputum is yellow, and not much tinged with red. In this last, the Breast is no so much contracted, but the Fever more violent.

The *Peripneumonia* is more dangerous, tho' less painful than a Pleurisy : Its usually way of going off is by Expectoration of well concocted reddish, yellow, or white Matter. The slowing of the Menses, or any Hæmorrhage, a Diarrhæa, Abscesses about the Ears, or other Parts, are also good Prognosticks.

The Medicines prescribed are mostly the same that obtain in Asthmatick and Pleuritick Cases.

**PERIPNEUMONIA** *Notha* or *Spuria* is a Disease of the Lungs, arising from a heavy pituitous Matter generated throughout the whole Mass of Blood, and discharged upon the Lungs.

'Tis known by the Viscidity, Paleness, and Slowness of the Blood, Ropiness of the Saliva, Paleness and Want of Scent of the Urine, Swellings and Obstructions in the minuter Vessels, short Breath, Oppression in the Thorax, &c. worn out, phlegmatic, cold, phthisical, catarrhous, Constitutions, are most liable to it. It begins with a Feebleness, Indolence, Weariness, Difficulty of Breathing, Oppression of the Breast, Feverishness; and goes on without any great Appearance of danger to Death itself, without any Prognostic thereof in the Urine, Pulse, &c. It is cured by Blood-letting, Clysters, thin Diet, Dilutents, Abstergents and Aperients.

**PERISTALTIC**, in Medicine, a Motion proper to the Intestines, wherein the several Parts are successively contracted from above downwards, in a manner resembling the creeping of a Worm; whence it is also call'd the *Vermicular Motion*. The Word is form'd from the *Greek* πριστελλω; and literally implies something *sent all a-round*.

The *Peristaltic* Motion is perform'd by the Contraction of the circular and longitudinal Fibres, whereof the fleshy Coat of the Intestines is composed. 'Tis by Means hereof, that the Chyle is driven into the Orifices of the lacteal Veins, and the Excrements press'd downwards, and at last expell'd.

When this Motion comes to be depraved, and its Direction changed, so as to proceed from below upwards, it produces what we call the *Iliac Passion*.

M. *Perrault*, in an express Treatise on the *Peristaltic Motion*, observes, that tho' 'tis ordinarily, only attributed to the Intestines; yet, it is really an Action common to all the Parts of the Body which alter, prepare, concoct the several Humours and Spirits, which are the Matter and Instruments of animal Action. In effect, he gives the Name to all the Motions whereby the Cavities of the Body are press'd and compress'd.

**PER MINIMA**, in Medicine, denotes a perfect Mixture of the smallest Particles of several Bodies, or Ingredients.

**PERNIO**, in Medicine, a Disease afflicting the Hands and Feet in Winter-time, popularly call'd a *Kibe* or Chilblain. The Parts affected swell, inclining from a white to a bluish Colour, itch and ake; yet, the Tumour vanishes without any Exulceration, upon anointing the Part with Petrol.

**PERPETUAL** *Pills, Pilulæ perpetuæ*, among Physicians, are Pills made of Regulus of Antimony; which being swallow'd, and voided 50 Times, will purge every Time, with undiminish'd Force.

**PERSPIRATION**, in Medicine, the Action of evacuating the Juices of the Body, through Pores of the Skin. When this Evacuation is copious enough to be perceiv'd by the Senses, as in sweat, the *Perspiration* is said to be *sensible*; where it escapes the Notice of the Senses, as is the case in the ordinary State of the Body, the *Perspiration* is said to be *insensible*.

The Word *Perspiration* used simply, and without any Adjective, is understood of *insensible Perspiration*. *Sanctorius*[1], the great *Paduan* Physician, was the First who took Notice of this Evacuation : To him we owe both the Invention and Perfection of the Doctrine of *insensible Perspiration*.

The Vessels thro' which the *Perspiration* is perform'd, lye obliquely open under the Squamæ or Scales of the Cuticle or Scarf-skin. They are inconceivably small : From a Calculation of *Leewenhoeck*, it appears that the Mouths of 125000 of 'em may be cover'd with a common Grain of Sand. Thro' these Vessels is continually transuding a subtile Humour, from every Point of the Body, and throughout the whole Expanse of the Cuticle.

The Matter evacuated this way, is found by sure Experience to be more than equal to that evacuated all the other Ways, *i.e.* by Stool, Urine, &c. *Sanctorius* found in Italy, under the Circumstances of a moderate Diet, middle Age, and easy Life, that the Matter insensibly perspired was 5/8 of that taken in for Food: so that there only remain'd 3/8 for Nutrition, and the Excrements of the Nose, Ears, Intestines, Bladder, &c.

[1] Sanctorius of Padua, born Santorio Santorio (1561 – 1636), an Italian physician.

The same Author shews, that as much is evacuated by insensible *Perspiration* on one Day, as by Stool in fourteen Days; particularly, that in a Night's Time, about sixteen Ounces is ordinarily sent out by Urine, four Ounces by Stool; and above forty Ounces by *insensible Perspiration.*

He also observes, that if a Man eat and drink 8 l. in a Day, 5 l. of it is spent in insensible Perspiration, and adds as to the Times, that within, 5 Hours after eating there is perspired about 1 l. from the 5th to the 12th Hour about 3 l. and from the 12th to the 16th scarce half a Pound.

The Benefits of insensible *Perspiration* are so great, that without it, *Borelli* says, animal Life cou'd not be preserv'd.

The great Subtility, Equability, and Plenty of the Matter thus perspired, its Increase after Sleep, &c. constitute the grand Symptoms of a perfect State of Health; and the chief Means of preserving the same. On the contrary, the departing from these is the first sure Sign, and perhaps Cause, of Diseases.

*Perspiration* is performed, preserved, and encreased by the Viscera, Vessels, Fibres; by Motion or Exercise as far as the first Appearance of Sweat, by moderate Use of Venery; Sleep of 7 or 8 Hours, the Body well cover'd yet not loaden with Bed-cloths, Cheerfulness, light fermented yet solid Food, not Fat; pure, cold, heavy Air, &c. The contraries of all these, as also the Increase of the other Excretions, diminish, prevent, deprave it.

Hence we see the Cause, Effect, &c. of this perspirable Matter, its Use is preserving the parts soft and flexible, in supplying what's lost, but chiefly in preserving the nervous Papillæ moist, fresh, lively, fit to be affected by Objects, and to transmit their Impressions.

To determine the State and Conditions of the Perspiration, so necessary for judging of those of the Body, *Sanctorius* invented a *weighing* Chair, whereby he examin'd Quantity, Degree, &c. of *Perspiration* in several Circumstances of the Body, under several Temperatures of the Air, in the several Intervals of eating, drinking, sleeping, &c.

Some of the more extraordinary Phænomena observ'd herewith, are; that for some time after eating the *Perspiration* is least of all. That between the 5th and 12th Hour after Meals *Perspiration* is greatest. That riding either on Horseback, in a Coach, or Ship, &c. brisk Motion on the Ice, &c. but above all, a brisk Friction of the Skin; promote *Perspiration* surprisingly. That in sweating the *Perspiration* is much less than at other Times : And that *Perspiration* is always much less in Women than Men.

**PESSARY**, in Medicine, a solid Medicament of the Length and thickness of the Finger, but a Pyramidal Form; convey'd into the natural Parts of a Women to provoke, or put a Stop to the Menses, or to prevent a Descent of the Matrix, or on other Occasions of those Parts. At one End 'tis fasten'd to a little Ribbon, by which it may be drawn out at pleasure. It consists of Cork, or other light Wood, or of a little Linnen Bag, full of Pouders, incorporated with Wax, Oil, and Cotton; cramm'd close together to make it solid enough for intromission. The Word is form'd from *Greek* πεσσος, which signifies the same Thing.

**PESTILENCE**, in Medicine, a contagious Disease, usually mortal; popularly known under the name of Plague. The Word is form'd from the *Latin Pestis*.

**PESTILENTIAL** *Fevers*, among physicians, are such as do not only afflict the Patient with a vehement Heat, but also a malignant and venomous Quality.

**PETALA**, in Botany, the Leaves of a Flower; so call'd to distinguish 'em from the Leaves of the Plant. By Flower is properly meant, That assemblage of Parts call'd *Stamina* and *Pistil*, which serve for the propagation of the Kind. The Calyx or Perianthium sometimes serves in lieu of *Petala*.

The colour'd Leaves which incompass those Parts, are in reality no more than Cases or Covers to secure and screen the generative Parts; unless, as Mr. *Bradley* conjectures, they may serve to secrete some fine Juice for the Nourishment of the Seed.

The most easy Division of Flowers is into simple Flowers, *i.e.* those form'd of *Stamina* and *Pistils* only; and compound Flowers, whose *Stamina* and *Pistils* are incompass'd with *Petala*, call'd by Dr. *Grew* the *Foliation*, and by Mr. *Ray Folia*.

Compound Flowers again, are either incompass'd with a single *Petalum*, or Piece; or with several Pieces; the first of which are call'd *Monopetalous*, the second *Polypetalous* Flowers.

Again, from the regular or irregular Configuration of the *Petala*, M. *Jussieu*[1] makes another Division of into Classes; as regular and irregular *Monopetalous*; regular and irregular *Polypetalous*, &c.

Nature shews a World of Art in the folding up of the *Petala*, in the Perianthum, before they begin to blow or expand : Of these Foldings Dr. *Grew* notes the following Varieties, *viz.* the close Couch as in Roses; the concave Couch, as in *Blattaria flore albo*; the single Plait as in Pease-blossoms; the double Plait as in Blue-bottles. The Couch and Plait together as in Marigolds, &c. The Rowl as in Ladies Bower; the Spire as in Mallows; and lastly the Plait and Spire together as in *Convolvulus Doronici Folio*.

The Word is form'd from the Greek πεταλον a Leaf; And in that Language serves indifferently for the Leaves of the Plant and the Flower.

**PETALOIDES**, a Name sometimes given to Urine, when it seems to have little Leaves or Scales in it.

**PETECHIÆ**, are Spots in the Skin, like Flea-Bites, which come out in some Fevers. Hence *Petechial* Fever is the spotted Fever, commonly so called.

**PETRIFACTION**, or Petrification, in Physiology, the Action of converting Fluids, Woods, and other Matters into Stone. The Word is form'd from the *Greek* πετρα Stone, and the *Latin fio* or *facio* to become, to do.

The Faculty of *petrifying* Wood is ascribed to several Springs, Lakes, &c. The ancient Naturalists mention a River whose Waters turn'd Bodies into

[1] This may be Antione de Jussieu (1686 – 1758), a French physician and botanist.

Marble, by mere contact; nay, which being drunk *petrified* the Viscera of the Drinker.

*Seneca* relates, that the Mud of this River is of such a Nature as to harden and glue together the Parts of Bodies. As, says he, the Dust of Puzzuoli, by barely touching Water becomes Stone; so this Water by touching any Solid, sticks, and grows to it : Whence Things cast into it, are immediately taken out Stones. *Pliny* adds very well, that Wood cast into this River, is presently found cover'd with a stony Bark or Rind; and subjoins the Names of several other Rivers which do the same; particularly the River *Silarus* near *Tarentum*, whose Waters are yet found vey wholesome. To *Pliny's* List, we might add many more among ourselves; particularly the Lake *Lohmond* in *Scotland*, &c.

But, in effect, there does not seem any real Transmutation of the woody Nature into the Nature of Stone, in ay of these Cases; all that is done is this, the Stony Particles which before floated in the Liquor are now lodged, and deposited in the Pores of these Substances, in such manner, and in such Plenty as to leave little else, but the appearance of Stone.

*Petrifications* too, are frequently nothing else but incrustations of stony Particles, which surround the Bodies immerg'd, as Salts shoot upon and adhere to them. *Varenius*[1] has a Conjecture that Waters only petrify Woods by means of certain minute, sharp, and pointed Particles lodg'd therein, which cut the longitudinal Fibers of the Wood in an infinite Number of Points, and thus destroy the Form they were distinguish'd from Stone.

Near *Nacsivan* is a little River, whose Water the People turn off into little Canals; where, in a little Time it *petrifies*; and of this *petrified* Water is built a large *Caravansera* in the Neighbourhood.

*Petrifications* of Waters, or Juices of the Earth are incontestable. In the Place call'd *les Caves Goutieres* in *France*, the Water falling from the Upper-parts of the Cave to the Ground, immediately hardens into little Stones, of such Figures as the Drops falling either singly, or upon one another chance to exhibit.

Of this Kind of Caves we have several in England; Mr. *Derham*[2] mentions one on the Top of *Bredon* hill in *Worcestershire*; to which we may add an other call'd the *Elve-hole* in *Withersack* in *Westmoreland*; lin'd a-top with these stalactical Stones, hanging like Icicles; which are manifestly nothing else but Exsudations or Extillations of some petrifying Juices of the rocky Earth there.

**PETROL**, Petroleum, *q.d. Petræ-oleum*, Oil of Rock; an Oleaginous Juice, issuing out of the Clefts of Rocks.

Beside artificial and vegetable Oils, *i.e.* those drawn from Plants, &c. by Expression; there are also natural and mineral Oils issuing of themselves from the Entrails of the Earth; call'd by a common Name *Petrols* or *Petrolea*.

These, according to all Appearance, must be the Work of subterraneous

[1] Bernhardus Varenius, born Bernhard Varen (1622 – 1650), a German physician and geographer.

[2] This is probably William Derham (1657 – 1735), an English theologian and astronomer.

Fires, which raise, or sublime the more subtile Parts of certain bituminous Matters that lie in their Way. These Parts being condens'd into a Liquor by the Cold of the Vaults of Rocks, are there collected, and Ooze thence through Clefts and Apertures, which the Disposition of the Ground furnishes 'em withal.

*Petrol*, then, is a Liquid Bitumen; only differing by its Liquidity from other Bitumens, as Asphaltum, Jet, &c. The Naptha, which is either a Liquid, or at least a very soft Bitumen, is much the same with the *Petrol*.

Hitherto there has been little *Petrol* found, except in hot Countries. *Olearius* says he saw above 30 Springs of it near *Scamachia* in *Persia* : There are *Petrols* in the Southern Provinces of *France*; but the best are those in the Duchy of *Modena*, first discover'd by *Ariosto*[1] a Physician, in 1640, in a very barren Valley, 12 Leagues form the City of *Modena*.

There are three Canals dug with great Expence in the Rock; by which three Kinds of *Petrol* are discharg'd into little Basons or Reservoirs : The first, as white, clear, and fluid as Water, of a brisk penetrating Smell, and not disagreeable; the second of a clear Yellow, less fluid, and a less brisk Smell than the White; the third a blackish Red of thicker Consistence, and a Smell more approaching that of Bitumen.

M. *Boulduc* has made several Experiments in the *Petrol*, describ'd in the *Hist. of Acad. of Sciences* M. DCC. XV. He observes, that he cou'd not raise any Phlegm or saline Spirit by any Distillation, either in *Balneo Mariæ*, or in a Sand heat : All that wou'd rise was Oil; at the Bottom of the Pellican remain'd an exceeding small Quantity of a thickish brownish Matter.

Hence, to use *Petroleum* in Medicine, it must be prescrib'd just as it is. 'Tis a remedy Nature has prepar'd to our Hands; it is found very warm and penetrating; and commended in many outward Complaints, Rheumatick and Arthritick Pains, and paralytick Limbs.

**PHAGEDÆNA**, in Chirurgery, &c. a deep, bloated Ulcer, which eats and corrodes the neighbouring Parts; so call'd from the *Greek* φαγεδαινα of φαγομαι I eat. Hence, *Phagedænic* Medicines; such as are used to eat off fungous, or proud Flesh.

**PHAGEDÆNIC** Water, in Chymistry, a Water drawn from quick Lime; so call'd from its Efficacy in the Cure of *Phagedænic* Ulcers.

To prepare this Water; they put two Pounds of fresh quick Lime in a large Earthen-pan, and pour upon it about ten Pounds of rain Water; these they let stand together two Days, stirring 'em frequently : At last, leaving the Lime to settle well, they pour off the Water by Inclination, filtrate it and put it well up in a Glass Bottle, adding to it an Ounce of Corrosive Sublimate in Powder; which, if white becomes yellow, and sinks to the Bottom of the Vessel.

The Water being settled, is fit for Use, in the cleansing of Wounds and Ulcers, and to eat off superfluous Flesh : Especially in Gangrenes; in which Case may be added a third or fourth Part of Spirit of Wine.

The Ephemerides of the Academy of the *Curiosi Naturæ*, relate that

[1] Francesco Ariosto (d. 1492), an Italian professor of philosophy and civil law.

*Phagedænic* Ulcers have been frequently cured with Sheeps Dung.

**PHANTASY**, or Fancy, the *Imagination*; the Second of the Powers, or Faculties of the sensitive or rational Soul, by which the Species of Objects receiv'd in by the common Sense, are retain'd, recall'd, further examin'd, and either compounded or divided.

The Organ of this Sense is vulgarly suppos'd to be the middle Part of the Brain; and its objects, all the Species communicated to it by the common Sense, by the comparing of which it frames infinite others to itself.

In Melancholic, and mad Men this Faculty is very strong, representing many extravagant and monstrous Things; and framing its Images as lively as those of Sensation; whence the Visions and Deceptions those Persons are liable to.

In Poets and Painters, that same Faculty is to be the Predominant one; to enable 'em to feign, and pursue and execute their Fictions or Fables with more Strength, Consistency, &c. In Men it is suppos'd to be subject to Reason, but in Brutes it has no Superior; this being the *Ratio Brutorum*, or what we call Reason in Brutes.

The *Phantasy* is free from the Ligature or Suspension of Sleep, witness our Dreams, &c. Some Philosophers use the Word *Phantasy*, in a more general Signification, *viz.* for what we usually call *Sensus Communis*, the common Sense.

**PHARMACUETICA**, that part of Physick which directs the Use, Preparation, &c. of Medicines.

**PHARMACOLOGY**, a Treatise of Medicines; of the Art of preparing 'em, judging of 'em, &c.

**PHARMACOPOEIA**, a *Dispensary*; or a Treatise containing the Preparations of the several Kinds of Medicines, with their Uses, manner of Application, &c. The Word is form'd form the *Greek* φαρμακον, Remedy, and ποιειν *facere*, to make. We have various *Pharmacopœia's*; as those of *Bauderon*[1], *Quercetan, Zwelfer, Charras, Bates*[2], *Salmon*[3], *Lemery*, &c. The latest and most rational, and that in most Esteem, is *Quincy's Pharmacopœia officinalis & extemporanea.*

**PHARMACAPOLA**, an *Apothecary*; or a Person who prepares and sells Medicines. The Word is seldom used but by way of ridicule. It is form'd from the *Greek* φαρμακον and πωλειν *vendere*, to sell.

**PHARMACUM**, a Medicament, or Medicine.

**PHARMACY**, that Branch of Medicine which teaches the Choice, Preparation, and Mixture of Medicines. *Pharmacy* is divided into *Galenical*

[1] Brice Bauderon (1540 – 1623), a French physician.

[2] This is probably George Bate (1608 – 1688), an English physician.

[3] William Salmon (1644 – 1713), an English empiric doctor (i.e. not a qualified physician).

and *Chymical*. The Word is deriv'd from the Greek φαρμακον, *Remedy*.

*Galenical* Pharmacy, call'd also simply *Pharmacy*, is that deriv'd to us from the Ancients; consisting in the Knowledge and Management of the several Parts of the *Materia Medica*, now in the Hands of the Apothecaries. The chief Obstacle in the Way of the Improvement of Phsyic, is the Physicians neglecting of *Pharmacy*.

*Chymical* Pharmacy, call'd also *Spagyrical* and *Hermetical*, is that introduced by *Paracelsus*, who calls it *Ars distillatoria*; consisting in the resolving of Bodies, into their component Parts, in order to separate the useless and Ill, and collect and exalt the Good.

Simples, vulgar, familiar, easily prepar'd, readily procur'd Simples, *Pliny* well observes, were the only Remedies intended by Nature : so soon as Fraud was got into the World, and Men began to live by their Wits; Shops were soon set up; and Life offer'd every Man to Sale. Straight, innumerable Compositions; endless, inexplicable Mixtures, are cri'd up; *Arabia* and *India* are crouded into a Draught; and a Plaister for a little Ulcer fetch' from the red Sea. When as the proper Remedies are those the Poor every Day feed on. – *Hist. Nat. Lib.* 24. c. 1.

**PHIAL**, *Phiala*, a little Glass-bottle, popularly call'd a *Vial*. The Word is form'd of the *Greek* φιαλη which signifies the same Thing.

**PHILONIUM**, in Pharmacy, an Opiate, where there are two Kinds; the *Roman* and the *Persian Philonium*. The *Roman*, call'd also the great *Philonium*, took its Name from the Physician *Philo* who invented it. It consists of the Seeds of Jusquiamus, Poppy, and other Ingredients. 'Tis used to promote Sleep, against Colds, Colicks, &c. The *Persian* Philonium consists of several Ingredients, among which are Opium, Terra sigillata, Lapis Hematites, Castor, and Saffron. 'Tis used to stop Hæmorrhages, Dysenteries, &c.

**PHILOSOPHERS STONE**, the great Object of Alchymy, is a long sought-for Preparation, which shall transmute impurer Metals, as Tin, Lead, and Copper into Gold and Silver.

There are three ways whereby the Alchymists have attempted to arrive at the making of Gold : The first by *Separation*; for every Metal yet known, contains some Quantity of Gold : Only, in most, the Quantity is so little that it wont defray the Expence of getting it out.

The second by *Maturation*; for the Alchymists hold Mercury to be the Basis and Matter of all Metals; that Quicksilver purg'd from all heterogeneous Bodies wou'd be much heavier, denser and simpler than the Native Quicksilver; And that by subtilizing, and purifying and digesting it with much Labour, and long Operations, it may be converted into pure Gold. This Method of *Maturation* is only for Mercury. The other Metals it is ineffectual for, on two accounts : 1°, Because their Matter is not pure Mercury, but has other heterogeneous Bodies adhering to it. And 2°, by reason the Digestion whereby Mercury is turn'd into Gold wou'd not succeed in other Metals, in regard they had not been long enough in the Mines. Weight is the individual and inimitable Character of Gold, &c. Now Mercury has ever some Impurities in it; and those Impurities are lighter than Mercury. Cou'd those be purged quite out, as it does not appear impossible but they might, Mercury wou'd be as heavy as Gold; and what is as heavy as Gold is Gold, or at least is very easily made Gold.

The third Method is, that of Transmuting; or of turning of all Metals readily into pure Gold, by melting 'em in the Fire, and casting a little Quantity of a certain Preparation into the infused Matter; upon which, the Fæces immediately retire, are volatiz'd and burnt, and so carried off; and the rest of the Mass turn'd into pure Gold. Now, that which works this change in the Metals is call'd the *Philosophers stone.*

Whether this third Method be possible or not is very hard to say. We have so many Testimonies of Persons, who on all other Occasions speak perfect Truth, that 'tis somewhat hard to say they lye in this, that they have been Masters of the Secret. All required is to do that by Art which Nature does in many Years and Ages. For Lead and Gold do but differ little in Weight. Therefore there is not much in Lead besides Mercury and Gold. Now, if I had any Body which wou'd so agitate all the Parts of Lead, as to burn all that is not Mercury therein; and has some Sulphur to fix the Mercury; wou'd not the Mass remaining be converted into Gold? There is nothing in Nature so heavy as Lead; Gold and Mercury only excepted. 'Tis evident, therefore, there is something in Lead that comes very near to Gold. If now 19 Ounces of Lead be dissolved by the Fire, and 8 Ounces be thus destroyed; we shall have good Gold; the Ratio of Lead to Gold being as 11 to 19. If then the *Philosophers-stone* can purify the mercurial Metal in Lead, so as nothing shall remain but the pure mercurial Body; and you can fix and coagulate this, by means of Sulphur; out of 19 Ounces of Lead you will have 11 of Gold. Or, if you reduce the Lead from 11 to 14, you will then have converted it into Mercury; and if you further purify this Mercury from 14 to 19 you will have Gold; provided you have but a Sulphur to fix and coagulate withal.

Such is the Foundation of the *Philosophers-stone*; which the Alchymists contend to be a most subtile, fix'd, concentrated Fire, which assoon as it melts with any Metal, does by a magnetick Virtue immediately unit itself to the mercurial Body of the Metal, volatilizes and cleanses off all that is impure therein, and leaves nothing but a Mass of pure Gold.

**PHILOSOPHERS TREE**, a Chymical Preparation, call'd also *Arbor Dianæ, Diana's Tree.*

**PHILOSOPHICAL EGG**, among the Chymists, is a thin Glass Vessel, or Bubble, of the Shape of an Egg; with a long Neck or Stem; used in Digestions.

**PHILTRATION**, or Filtration, the Separation of the finer Part of a Fluid from the Coarser; by passing it through a *Filtre, viz.* a Linnen Cloth, Shammy Skin, Brown Paper, or the like.

**PHILTER**, Philtre, Philtrum, in Pharmacy, &c. a Strainer, or Filtre.

**PHILTER**, or Filtre, is also used for a Drug, or Preparation, which 'tis pretended will excite Love. The Word *Philtre* is form'd from the *Greek* φιλεειν, to love.

*Philters*, are distinguish'd into *true* and *spurious* : The Spurious are Spells or Charms, supposed to have an Effect beyond the ordinary Laws of Nature, by some magick Virtue; such are those said to be given by old Women, Witches, &c. The true *Philtres* are those supposed to work their Effect by some natural and magnetical Power.

There are many grave Authors who believe the Reality of these *Philtres*; and alledge matter of Fact in Confirmation of their Sentiments : among the rest, *Van Helmont*, who says, that upon holding a certain Herb in his Hand for some time, and taking afterwards a little Dog by the Foot with the same Hand; the Dog follow'd him wherever he went, and quite deserted his former Master.

He adds that *Philtres* only demand a Confirmation of Mumia; and on this Principle accounts for the Phænomena of Love transplanted by the Touch of an Herb; for, says he, the Heat communicated to the Herb, not coming alone, but animated but the Emanations of the natural Spirits; determines the Herb towards the Man, and identifies it to him : Having, then received this Ferment, it attracts the Spirit of the other Object magnetically, and give sit an amorous Motion. But this is mere Cant; and all *Philters*, whatever Facts may be alledg'd, are mere Chimera's.

Naturalists ascribe an Effect somewhat of Kin to that of a *Philtre* to *Cantharides*, taken inwardly; these, 'tis true, tend to excite Love, or rather Lust : but 'tis Lust in the General, not determin'd by any particular Object; and they do it no otherwise than by irritating the Fibres of the Nerves and Muscles, by whose Action the *Emissio Seminis* is effected.

**PHLEBOTOMY**, in Medicine and Chirurgery, *Bleeding*; or the Art or Operation of letting Blood. The Word is compounded of the *Greek* φλεψ, Vein, and τεμνειν, to cut. *Phlebotomy* is a Manner of Evacuation of the utmost Importance in Medicine, an Idea of its Effects, with the Reason of its Use may be conceiv'd from what follows.

'Tis evident the Blood thrown out of the Heart, while it strikes upon the antecedent Blood, and drives it forwards, transfers to it Part of its own Motion, and is therefore so much retarded in its own Motion. Hence, if Blood be drawn out of the Basilic Vein of the right Arm; the succeeding Blood, or that carried by the axillary Artery, or right Subclavian, will be less hinder'd in its Motion, than it was before that Vein was open'd; for Part of the Blood being taken away by the opening of that Vein, there remains behind a lesser Quantity in the axillary Vein, or less is contained between the farther Extremity of the axillary Artery and the Heart, than was before : therefore the Blood being let out by the Vein, the Remainder in the Artery will be less impeded in its Motion than before.

Hence the Blood of that Artery which communicates with the Vein that is opened, will flow with a greater Velocity after the Aperture is made than before. Consequently, while the Blood is flowing out of the Vein in the Arm, that thrown out of the Heart into the Aorta, will find less Resistance in the ascending Trunk, than in the Descending; and will therefore flow faster in the Ascending, than in the descending Trunk : And thence too it will find less

Resistance in the right Subclavian Artery than in the left.

Lastly, it hence appears, that the Blood being let out of a Vein in the right Arm, the remaining Blood in the right axillary Artery runs with a greater Velocity into the Artery of that Arm, or the right Scapulary, which is likewise contiguous to it; because, when the Blood is not supposed to be drawn out from any Vein corresponding to the thoracic Artery, or into which this discharges itself, there is proportionally a greater Impediment to the Motion of the Blood in the thoracic Artery, than in that of the Arm. But because the Velocity of the Blood in the subclavian Artery, or the right Axillary, is greater than in the Left; the Velocity in the right Thoracic will also be greater than in the left thoracic Artery. Hence it is manifest, that the Blood being let out of a Vein in the right Arm; the greatest Velocity of the remaining Blood will be in the Artery of that Arm, because it immediately empties its Blood into the Vein that is opened; and the next greatest Velocity will be in the thoracic Artery, or Scapulary of the same Side, going out from the axillary Artery. But the Velocity of the Blood will be far less in the brachial Axillary, and thoracic Artery on the left and opposite Side; and least of all in the Arteries arising from the descending Trunk of the Aorta.

On this View it may easily be gathered, what is to be done in the several Circumstances of Blood-letting : For instance, if we would prevent the Increase of any Humour from the Blood stagnating in the left Leg, or bring it about, that as little Blood as possible, should flow to that Leg in any given space of Time; first, Blood is to be taken from the Arm or Leg of the right Side, because this is truly making what is call'd a *Revulsion*.

Again, if Blood be drawn away on the same Side, and from some Vein that receives blood from a Branch of that Trunk which transmits it to the swell'd Part; it will occasion a greater Derivation of Blood to that Limb.

As to what relates to the whole Habit; in all Lentors and Viscidities, if there by a due Strength and Elasticity remaining in the Solids, *Phlebotomy* will make the remaining Blood circulate the faster, and become thinner and warmer; but in a Plethora, from Debauch, and too large Quantities of spirituous Nourishment, or from a Diminution of Perspiration, where the Blood yet retains its natural Fluxility, *Phlebotomy* will make the remaining Mass circulate slower, and become cooler.

In the former Case, a Diminution of the Resistance in the Blood-Vessels, will increase the contractile Powers of those Vessels, and make them beat faster, and circulate their Contents with greater Velocity; but in the latter Case a Diminution of the Quantity of Spirit secreted in the Brain, the Consequences of which will be that the Heart and Arteries will not contract so often nor so strongly as before, and therefore the Blood will move slower, and become cooler.

**PHLEGM**, in Chymistry, is an aqueous and insipid Fluid, supposed to be found in all natural Bodies; coinciding with what the other Philosophers call Water. *Phlegm* makes the 4th of the Chymical Elements, or Elementary Principles.

In the Distillation of Vinegar, as also of all Minerals and inodorous Vegetables, *Phlegm* comes out first; in that of Wine last.

This *Phlegm* is supposed to be the common Vehicle and Diluter of all solid Bodies; and in proportion to its Quantity in the Mixture, are the other Parts more languid and disabled in their Attractions; yet, in the Chymists Principles, *Phlegm* shou'd be a Principle of Action; as being necessary to the Dissolution of the Salt in Bodies, without which the Salt must remain inactive.

It is much to be question'd whether this *Phlegm* can ever be procured without any Mixture of other Matters; that which has the least must come nearest to the Nature of a Principle; and on that account Rain-water shou'd afford it most.

*Phlegm*, *Boerhaave* observes, drawn by Distillation from Vegetables, does always carry with it some what of the Smell of the Vegetable, which it derives partly from the Oil, and partly from the Spirit residing therein. The same *Phlegm*, by frequently reiterated Distillations, lays aside most of this Smell, and approaches nearer to pure Water, but never becomes perfectly such. Add, that the purest distill'd Water, if exposed a few Days to the Sun, is much changed, and render'd turbid.

That *Phlegm* is not an elementary Body, Mr. *Boyle* argues from its different Powers and Properties; the *Phlegm* of Wine, and most Liquors, have Qualities that make them different from mere Water, and from one another; the *Phlegm* of Vitriol that Author observes is an effectual Remedy against Burns; and a valuable Nostrum for discussing hard Tumours; that of Vinegar will extract a Saccharine Sweetness out of Lead, and even dissolve Corals with long Digestion; and that of Sugar of Lead, is said to dissolve Pearls.

In Effect, the Characters which serve to denominate a Fluid, *Phlegm*, or Water, among the Chymists, are Insipidity and Volatility; yet, Quick-silver has all these, which no Body pretends to be *Phlegm*. Add, that it appears from several Experiments, that Water itself, by repeated Distillations, may be converted into Earth. Yet Water, the same Author observes, has a much fairer Pretence to be an Element, than any of the *tria prima*.

Add, that as to the Qualities which occasion that name to be given any visible Substance, *viz.* its being Fluid, Insipid, and inodorous; we have never yet seen any of these separated Substances, which the Chymists call *Phlegm*, perfectly destitute both of Taste and Smell.

Common Salt, and several other saline Bodies distilled every so dry, will each yield a large Quantity of *Phlegm*; which can no other way be accounted for, but from this, that among the various Operations of the Fire, on the Matter of a Concrete, several Particles of that Matter are reduc'd to a Shape and Size, requisite to compose such a Liquor as the Chymists call *Phlegm*, or Water.

**PHLEGM**, in the Animal Œconomy, is one of the four Humours, where the Ancients supposed the Mass of Blood to consist. *Phlegm* is the same that is otherwise call *Pituita*.

**PHLEGMAGOGUE**, a Medicine proper to purge Phlegm, or Pituita. Agaric, Hermodactyls, Turbith, &c. are *Phlegmagogues*. The Word is form'd from the *Greek* φλεγμα, *pituita*, and αγειν, *to drive*.

**PHLEGMATIC**, a Temperament wherein Phlegm, or Pituita, is the prevailing Humour. *Phlegmatic* Constitutions are subject to Rheums, Defluxions, &c.

**PHLEGMON**, in Medicine, a general Name for all Tumors form'd of the Blood. An Inflammation, attended with a considerable swelling of the Part, constitutes a *Phlegmon*. The Word is form'd from the *Greek* φλεγειν, to cause an Inflammation.

If the Blood be good, and laudable, and only peccant in Quantity, 'tis call'd a *true Phlegmon*. When corrupted and adulterated with Bile, or Pituita, 'tis call'd a *bastard Phlegmon*; in which case it participates of the *Eresypela*, *Oedema*, or *Schirras*. The Blood here extravasated produces a Heat, Redness, Tension, Renitency, Pulsation, and great Pain.

The Bubo, Carbuncle, Furuncle, Pustles, and other Tubercles arising from the Blood, are all reducible to the *Phlegmon*. The Ophthalmia, Parotides, Squinancy, and even Pleurisy and Peripneumony, are Species of the *Phlegmon*.

**PHLOGOSIS**, in Medicine, a Degree of the *Ophthalmia*. When the Inflammation of the Eye is light and gentle it is call'd a *Phlogosis*; when very severe, *Chemosis*.

**PHLYCTÆNÆ**, or Phlyctenes, little white itching Vesiculæ, arising on the Skin, chiefly between the Fingers, and about the Wrist, and full of a limpid Serum. They sometimes degenerate into the Itch, and sometimes into Tetters. They are cured like other cutaneous Eruptions.

**PHLYCTÆNÆ**, are also little ulcerous Vesicles, arising sometimes on the Adnata, sometimes on the Cornea, of the Eye, like so many little Bladders full of Water; popularly call'd *Blisters in the Eyes*. They shew like Grains of Millet; and when produced by a sharp corroding Humour, occasion violent Pain : The Pustles on the *Adnata* are red; those in the *Cornea* blackish, if near to the Surface, but whiter if deeper. They are cured by Excutients and Exsiccants.

**PHLYSTENE** or Phlystæna, in Medicine, a Disease which produces Bubo's, full of a serous Humour. The Word is form'd from the *Greek* φλυω, φλυζω of φλυσσο, *ebullio*, I boil, bubble, &c. The *Phlystene* is a kind of Pox. The Bubo's it occasions are sometimes big, livid, pale, black, or any Colour different from that of the natural Flesh. When pierc'd, the Flesh frequently appears ulcerated under 'em. They are usually occasion'd by a hot, sharp Humour, and arise on all Parts of the Body; but are most dangerous on the *Cornea* of the Eye.

**PHOENIGMA**, a Medicine which raises Redness, with Blisters, on the Place it is applied to. Such are Mustard-Seed, Pepper, Vesicatories, &c. *Phœnigma's* are applied to draw the Humour to the Part they are applied on, and divert it from the Part affected. The Word is form'd from the *Greek* φοινιξ, red.

**PHRENITIS**, *Phrenesis*, Phrensy, in Medicine, a constant and vehement Delirium, or Distraction; accompanied with an acute Fever, raving, waking, &c. It differs from the *Mania*, and Melancholy, in that these are without Fevers. It has its Name from φρην, *Mens*, the Understanding; or as some will have from φρην, the Diaphragm, in regard the Ancients supposed it to have its Seat in that Part.

Physicians generally make the *Phrenitis* to consist in an Inflammation of the Meninges of the Brain; and distinguish it from the *Paraphrenitis*, which they suppose to be an Inflammation of the Diaphragm.

*Willis* will have them the same Disease, and both to consist in an Inflammation of the Animal Spirits. He only distinguishes them as the Inflammation arises from the *Cerebrum* alone, or from the *Cerebrum* and *Cerebellum* together; and concludes, that they both arise after a Fever, from the boiling Blood's throwing its adjust Recrements into the Brain.

*Boerhaave* makes the *Phrenitis* either *true*, wherein the *Cerebrum*, or Meninges, or both, are inflamed; or *symptomatic*, where the Matter of a Fever is translated into the *Cerebrum*.

The true one either kills on the third, fourth, or fifth, or seventh Day; or changes into a Mania, Lethargy, Comus, &.c Tremors, Gnashing of the Teeth, grumous Blood distilling form the Nose, are Prognosticks of Death.

The Disease is oftenest the Effect of Inflammatory or Malignant Fevers; tho' it sometimes also arises from a Suppression of the natural Evacuations, as the *Menses*, &c.

The Cure is the same as of an Apoplexy; but where the Evacuations are concern'd, they must be rectified.

**PHTHIRIASIS**, in Medicine, the *Morbus Pedicularis*, or Louzy Disease, wherewith Children, and even sometimes Adults are afflicted. The Word is form'd from the *Greek* φθειρ, Louse. Its Cause is in the Seeds of that Vermin laid in the Cuticle, which here happening to prove a proper *Nidus*, cherishes and fosters the Seed so as to hatch it. The Linnen Cloths used by Goldsmiths to wipe their Vessels with after gilding, are excellent against the *Phthiriasis* by reason of the Mercury they contain, when applied by rubbing the Child's Head.

**PHTHISIS**, in Medicine, in its general Sense, is any kind of Consumption of the Body, in what soever it be seated, or from what Cause soever it arise. Thus we have a *Nervous Phthisis, Renal Phthisis, Dorsal Phthisis, Pulmonary Phthisis*, &c. The Word is form'd from the *Greek* φθισις, Corruption, Attenuation, &c.

But in its proper Sense, *Phthisis* is restrain'd to a *Pulmonary Consumption*, or a Consumption arising from an Ulcer or other Disorder of the Lungs, accompanied with a slow hectic Fever, which wastes, extenuates, and consumes the muscular Flesh.

*Sydenham* observes, that the hectic *Phthisis* usually has its Origin in the Winter's Cold; from a sharp Humour trickling down upon the Lungs, where, like a Catarrh, it irritates them so as to raise a Cough. This by degrees brings on other Symptoms; as a spitting, first of a viscid *Pituita*, then a heavy fetid

*Pus*, then of pure Blood, and sometimes of the very Substance of the Lungs rotted by a long Exulceration; with Night-Sweats, falling of the Hair, and a colliquative Flux which is soon followed by Death. The same Author adds, that Phthisis kills two thirds of those that die of Chronic Diseases.

In the last Stage of the *Phthisis* the Nose appears sharp, the Eyes hollow, the Temples fallen, the Ears cold and contracted, the Skin about the forehead hard and dry, and the Complexion greenish, or livid, &c. which is call'd the *Facies Hippocratica*.

Among the Causes of the Disease may also be reckon'd Intemperance as it brings on a Plethora or Cacochymia, Peripneumonies, Asthma's, Pleurisies, &c. *Morton* adds, that the *Phthisis* frequently arises form an ill Conformation of the Breast; which is either *Natural*, as when the breast is too narrow, the Neck too long, &c. or *Accidental*, where there happens a Curvity or Distortion of the Breast; among the Symptoms he reckons a *Nausea*, or Reaching, with a Heat in the Palms of the Hands, and Redness in the Cheeks, all after Eating.

For the Cure; *Sydenham* orders the Defluxion on the Lungs, in the first Stage, to be abated by Blood-letting, &c. and Pectorals to be used, accommodated to the various States of the Diseases, *viz.* with Emulsions, Asses-Milk, &c. and Balsamicks, to cure the Ulcer.

But the chief Assistance in this Disease is from riding constantly on Horseback, where the Patient need not confine himself to any Laws of Diet, &c. This alone, he adds, is almost as sure a Cure for a *Phthisis*, as the Cortex for an Intermitting Fever.

Dr. *Baynard* recommends Butter-Milk as an admirable Succedaneum to Asses-Milk. *Sylvius* says, he knows of no Medicine, either internal or external, so good against fresh Ulcers of the lungs, as Balm of Sulphur, especially when prepare with Oil of Anise.

*Etmuller* observes, that the Cough of *Phthisical* People is at first only Stomachal; at length it becomes Pulmonary. He adds, that Vomitories are good in a beginning *Phthisis*, Purgatives by all means to be avoided; and commends the use of Medicines made of Tobacco, not only as they promote Expectoration; but as Vulnerary.

'Tis a common Observation, that in those Countries where they burn Turf, People are rarely afflicted with the *Phthisis*; which *Willis* ascribes to the Sulphur abounding therein, and recommends Tincture of Sulphur as the best Remedy he knows of in any Cough without a Fever; adding, that a Suffumigation, or Smother, of Sulphur and Arsenic has frequently proved a Cure in the most desperate *Phthisis*.

*Bonetus*[1] holds the *Phthisis* to be contagious; and that there are frequently Instances of its being communicated by Cloaths, Linnen, Beds, &c.

*Pitcairn* recommends *Mercurius Dulcis*, in the Beginning of a *Phthisis*. And *Barbette* and *Colbatch* assert, that, contrary to the Opinion of most Authors, they have frequently used Acids with Success in *Phthisics*.

**PHYGETHLON**, in Medicine, is defined by *Celsus*, a hard flat Tumor, somewhat resembling a Pustle; occasioning an intense Pain, and sometimes a

[1] Theophilus Bonetus, born Theophile Bonet (1620 – 1689), a Swiss physician.

Fever. The Word is derived form the *Greek* φυω, I engender.

The *Phygethlon* only differs from the *Phyma*, in that it does not rise so high; it ripens very slowly, and produces but little Pus.

The *Latins* call it *Panis*, or *Panus*, and sometimes *Panicula*. *Gorræus* defines the *Phygethlon*, a *Phlegmon* arising on the glandulous Parts, especially about the Neck, Armpits, and Inguen; which last is call'd a Bubo.

The *Phygethlon* has the same Causes, and the same Symptoms with the common Bubo. It frequently arises after Fevers, and Pains of the Belly, and is cured like other Inflammations.

**PHYMA**, or Phymus, in Medicine, a roundish pointed Tumor, arising on the Glandular Parts, especially under the lower Jaw. The *Phyma* is smaller and smoother, less red and painful, than the Phygethlon.

It is easily cured in Children; more difficulty in Adults, but in those it is more rare. It is remedied by assisting Nature in the Work of Maturation; as, by a suppurating Cataplasm, &c. It is supposed to have its Rise from a pituitous Blood; and is most common in Children, where it frequently arises from too tight Bandages.

*Gorræus* observes, that some make *Phyma* a general Name for all Tumors, or Aposthumes, that maturate and suppurate readily, of what kind soever, or in whatsoever glandulous Part they arise.

**PHYSIC**, or Physick, the Art of Healing; properly called *Medicine*. For the Rise, Progress, Division, &c. of *Physic*. The Word is form'd from the Greek φυσις, Nature; in regard Medicine consists principally in the Observation of Nature.

**PHYSICIAN**, a Person who professes Medicine, or the Art of Healing. The Ancients distinguished their *Physicians* into various Classes or Sects : As, *Methodical Physicians*, those who proceeded in a certain regular Method, founded upon Reason; deducing Consequences therefrom, to particular Cases.

*Dogmatical Physicians*, those who laid down Principles, and reason'd from those Principles, and from Experience. *Empirical Physicians*, those who kept wholly to Experience, and excluded all Use of Reason in Medicine. Such was *Serapim, Apollonius, Glaucus*, &c.

Again, *Clinical Physicians* were those who visited their Patients a-bed, to examine their Cases. In opposition to the *Emperists*, who sold their Medicines in the Streets, &c.

They also had their *Astrological Physicians*, *Botanic Physicians*, *Anatomical Physicians*, Chirurgeons, Iatraliptes, or those who applied external Unctions and Frictions, &c. *Cosmetick Physicians* for the Complexions; Ophthalmic *Physicians* for the Eyes; Vulnerary *Physicians* for Wounds, &c.

Among the Moderns, a *general Physician* includes almost all these several Kinds : *Regular Physicians* are contra-distinguished from *Emperical Physicians*, who prescribe at random; having one or two Remedies which serve in all Diseases.

*Galenical Physicians* are those who prescribe gentle, natural and ordinary Medicines. *Spagyrical* or *Chymical Physicians* are those who prescribe violent Medicines drawn fro Minerals, &c. by Fire.

**PHISIOGNOMICKS**, a Term used by some Physicians and Naturalists, for such Signs as are taken from the Countenance to judge of the State, Disposition, &c. of the Body and Mind.

**PHYSIOGNOMY**, the Art of knowing the Humour, Temperament, or Disposition of a Person, from Observation of the Lines of the Face, and the Characters of its Members, or Features. The Word is form'd from the *Greek* φυσις, Nature, and γινωσκω, I know.

*Baptista Porta* and *Robert Fludd*[1] are the top modern Authors on *Physiognomy*. The ancient ones are the Sophist *Adamantius*, and *Aristotle*; the Physiognomy of which last we have translated into *Latin* by *de Lacuna*.

There seems to be something in *Physiognomy*; and it may perhaps bear a much purer Philosophy than what these Authors were acquainted withal. This, at least, we dare say, that of all the fanciful Arts of the Ancients, disused among the Moderns, there is none has so much Foundation in Nature as this.

There is an apparent Correspondence between the Face and the Mind; the Features and Lineaments of the one are directed by the Motions and Affections of the other : there is even a peculiar Arrangement of the Members of the Face, a peculiar Disposition of the Countenance, to each particular Affection; perhaps to each particular Idea of the Mind.

In effect, the Language of the Face, *Physiognomy*, is as copious, nay, perhaps, as distinct and intelligible, as that of the Tongue, *Speech*. Thanks to bounteous Nature, she has not confined us to one only Method of conversing with each other, and of learning each other's Thoughts; we have several : We don't wholly depend in the Tongue, which may happen to be bound; and the Ear, which may be deaf; but in those Cases we have another Recourse, the Countenance and the Eye; which affords us this further Advantage, that by comparing the Reports of the Tongue, (a Member exceedingly liable to deceive) with those of the Face, the Prevarications of the former may be detected.

The Foundation of *Physiognomy* is this : The different Objects that present themselves to the Senses, nay, the different Ideas that arise in the Mind, do each make some Impression on the Spirits; and each Impression correspondent or adequate to it's Cause; therefore each a different Impression.

If it be ask'd how such an Impression should be effected; 'tis easy to answer, that it follows from the Œconomy of the Creator, who has fix'd such a Relation between the several Parts of the Creation; to the end we may be apprized of the Approach or Recess of things useful or hurtful to us.

If this be'nt philosophical enough, take the manner in the *Cartesian* Language, thus : The Animal Spirits moved in the Organ by an Object,

[1] Robert Fludd (1574 – 1637), an English physician and philosopher.

continue their Motion to the Brain; whence that Motion is propagated to this, or that particular part of the Body, as is most suitable to the Design of Nature; having first made a proper Alteration in the Face, by means of its Nerves, especially the Pathetici and *Oculorum Motorii.*

The Face, here, does the Office of a Dial-Plate; the Wheels and Springs within-side the Machine actuating its Muscles, shew what is next to be expected from the striking Part. Not that the Motion of the Spirits is continu'd all the Way by the Impression of he Object; the Impression probably terminates in the Medulla of the Brain, the common Fund of Spirits; the rest Dr. *Gwither* imagines may be effected much after the same manner as the Air is convey'd into the Pipes of an Organ, which being uncover'd, the Air rushes in, and when the Keys are let go stopp'd again.

Now if by repeated Acts, or the frequent entertaining of a favourite Passion, or Vice, which natural Temperament has hurried one to, or Custom dragg'd; the Face is often put in that Posture which attends such Acts; the Animal Spirits will make such patent Passages thro' the Nerves, (in which the Essence of a Habit consists; see Habitude;) that the Face is sometimes unalterably set in that Posture; (as the *Indian* Religious are by a long continued sitting in strange Postures in their Pagods) or at least falls insensibly and mechanically into that Posture, unless some present Object distort it therefrom, or Dissimulation hide it.

This Reasoning is confirm'd by Observation : Thus we see great Drinkers, with Eyes generally set to the Nose; the adducent Muscles being oft employ'd to put 'em in that Posture, to view their lov'd Liquor in the Glass in the time of Drinking; whence those Muscles are also denominated the *bibitory Muscles*. Thus also lascivious Persons remarkable for the *Oculorum morbilis petulantia*, as *Petronius* calls it.

Hence we may account for the Quakers expecting Face, waiting the Spirit; the melancholly Face of most Sectaries; the studious Face of Men of great Application of Mind, &c.

Were our Observations a little more strict and delicate, we might doubtless not only distinguish Habits, and Tempers but even Professions. In effect does there need much Penetration to distinguish the fierce Look of the veteran Soldier, the contentious Look of the practis'd Pleader, the solemn Look of the Minister of State, &c.

**PHYSIOLOGY**, the Doctrine of Nature, or Natural Bodies; call'd also *Physicks*, and *Natural Philosophy*. The Word is form'd of φυσις, Nature, and λογος, Discourse, Reason.

It is to be observ'd, that the Word *Physiology* properly denotes only an internal reasoning or discoursing, which stops or terminates in the Speculation, or abstract Contemplation of its Object, *viz.* Natural Appearances, their Causes, &c. and does not direct or prescribe Rules for the making of natural things, *e.gr*. Stones, Plants, &c.

In this View Chymistry does not properly belong to *Physiology*, but is a kind of a counter-part thereto, as imitating or mimicking Nature, rather than considering and explaining her.

*Physiology* is particularly used for a Branch of Medicine, which considers

Nature with Regard to the Cure of Diseases; particularly the human Body, its Parts, Structure, Health, Life, Functions, Œconomy, &c.

*Physiology*, in this Sense, is the same with what we otherwise call the Doctrine of Animal Œconomy.

**PHYTOLOGY** a Discourse upon Plants; or a Description of their Forms, Kinds, Properties, &c. See Plant. The Word is compounded of the *Greek* φυτον, Plant, and λογος, Discourse, or λεγω, scribo, I describe, rehearse.

**QUARTAN**, in Medicine, an intermitting Fever, or Ague, where the Fit returns every third day. It is call'd *Quartan*, q.d. *fourth*, by reason the two sick days are reckon'd, which with the two intermitting ones, make four.

**QUID PRO QUO**, or *Qui pro quo*, is also used in Physic to express a Mistake of an Apothecary, in administering one Medicine for another; or in using an Ingredient in a Composition different from that prescribed.

In Propriety, the *Quid pro quo* is a Mistake in the Physician's Bill, where *quid* is wrote *quo*, one thing for another; or of the Apothecary in reading *quid* for *quo*, and giving the Patient the wrong Medicine.

Hence the Term is in the general extended to all Mistakes committed in Medicine, either in the Prescription, the Preparation, or Application of Remedies.

A Northern Physician in a printed Thesis on *quid pro quo's* owns ingeniously, that they are very frequent. He distinguishes very accurately a great Variety of Kinds of *quid pro quo's*; some with regard to the Operation, others with regard to the Subject, and others with regard to their Form, or their Effect. The first comprehends the *quid pro quo's* of the Physician, the second those of the Patient, the third those of the Apothecary.

He adds *quid pro quo's* of the Chirurgeon, and of the Cook; quid pro quo's of the Nurse, &c. Nor does he omit that there are salutary *quid pro quo's*, dangerous *quid pro quo's*, indifferent, &c. God preserve us from *quid pro quo*.

**QUINQUINA**, Quinaquina, call'd also *China China*, and *Kin-Kina*, a Medicinal Bark brought from the *West-Indies*; call'd also, by way of Eminency, the *Bark*; and *Cortex Peruvianus*, the *Peruvian Bark*, from the Country whence it is brought; and popularly the *Jesuits Bark*, because at its first Introduction chiefly sold and administered by the Jesuits.

The Tree which yields this Bark grows in the Province of *Peru* call'd *Quito*, on the Mountain near the City of *Loxa*. The Natives call it *Ganaperide*, and the Spaniards *Palo de Calenturas*, *i.e.* Fever-Wood. There are two kinds – the one wild, the other cultivated; whereof the latter is much the best.

The *Quinquina* was but little known in *Europe* till the Year 1640. The Jesuits of *Rome* first brought it in vogue in *Spain*, and *Italy*, in 1649; and in 1650, the Cardinal *de Lugo*, of that Order, brought it into *France*. It was at first sold for its Weight in Gold : when reduced into a Powder, it is by Foreigners call'd the *Cardinals Powder*; among us usually, the *Jesuits Powder*, *Pulvis Pastrum*. It met with a world of Opposition at first. *Chiflet*[1] and *Plempius*[2] distinguish'd themselves against it. But is now almost universally allow'd one of the greatest and best Remedies within the whole Province of Medicine.

[1] Jean-Jacques Chiflet (1588 – 1660), a French physician.

[2] Vopiscus-Fortunatus Plempius (1601 – 1671), a Dutch physician.

**QUINSET**, or Quinzy, or Quincy, in Medicine, the *Squinancy*, or *Angina*.

**QUINTESSENCE**, *Quinta-Essentia*, in Chymistry, a Preparation consisting of the Essential Oil of some Vegetable Substance, mix'd and incorporated with Spirit of Wine.

Thus, on a proper quantity, *e.gr.* of Essential Oil of Fennel, pouring twelve times the quantity of pure Alcohol prepared per se; they instantly unite into one similar Liquor, which is the *Quintessence* thereof.

The Antients were perfectly unacquainted with the Method of dissolving Oil in Spirit of Wine; and even some of the Moderns question'd its Reality : But the Certainty of the thing is easily proved from the Instance above.

If such *Quintessence* be several times digested, cohobated, &c. an Oil will at length be broke so fine, as, like the Spirit itself, perfectly to mix with Water; which is one of the most extraordinary Effects in all Chymistry.

After the like manner is made a *Quintessence* of Camphor, by only reducing it into a Powder, and pouring on Spirit of Wine.

*Quintessences* thus prepared are of great Medicinal Virtue; as may appear from the pure and potent Ingredients used in the Composition, which retain, in a great degree, all the Virtues of the Plants they are procured form : And hence their Denominations.

*Boerhaave* thinks they might properly be call'd Vegetable Sulphurs made potable, and rais'd to their utmost degree of Power and Efficacy.

Dry *Quintessences* may be made from the Liquid ones, by adding to 'em some Essential Oil of the same Vegetable from whence the liquid *Quintessence* was procured, with a little Sugar; all mix'd together, and distill'd by a gentle Heat till all the Moisture is come over : The Matter remaining is a dry *Quintessence*.

This Form is principally useful to Travellers, Sailors, &c. in as much as it renders the *Quintessence* portable; so that the Quantity, *e.gr.* of a Pin's Point, shall be an efficacious Medicine.

**QUINTESSENCE**, in Alchymy, is a mysterious Term signifying the first, or last and highest Essence, or Power of a natural Body.

This is supposed to be, as it were, the Soul drawn from the gross Body and its four Elements, by a most perfect Distillation; and by means hereof, the thing is said to be spiritualiz'd, *i.e.* render'd exceeding pure, spirituous, and, as it were, incorruptible. *Dict. Hermetique.*

The Antients, who allow'd of nothing real but what has a Body; would have the Soul of Man to be fifth Element, a kind of *Quintessence* without a Name, unknown here below, indivisible, immovable, all cœlestial, and divine.

**QUOTIDIAN**, in Medicine, an intermitting Fever, or Ague, the Access whereof returns every day.

**RADIATED**, in Botany, an Epithet applied to round flat Flowers, consisting of a Disk, and a single row of longish pointed Leaves, ranged all around in manner of Rays, or Spokes. The Word is also used in speaking of Medals, and in Heraldry; where the ancient Crowns are called *radiated Crowns, Coronæ Radiatæ.*

**RADICLE**, *Radicula, little Root*; in Botany, is a little Point discovered by the Microscope in all Seeds, which in the growth of the Pant becomes the Root. When, in sowing, the *Radicle* happens to light lowest; 'tis no wonder the Root should spread it self under Ground, and the Stem of the Plant rise up perpendicularly : But when the *Radicle* falls uppermost, by what means it is, that it changes its Position to favour the Ascent of the Stem, is one of the Wonders of Vegetation.

**RAMIFICATION**, the Production of Boughs or Branches; or of Figures resembling Branches.

**RAMIFICATIONS**, in Anatomy, are the Divisions of the Arteries, Veins, and Nerves, arising from some common Trunk.

**RANULA**, in Medicine, a Tumour under the tongue, which like a Ligament hinders a Child from speaking or sucking. The *Ranula sub Lingua* is the same with what we otherwise call being *Tongue-tied.*

The *Ranula* is usually caused by a short Frænum not permitting the Tongue to perform its proper Motions : At other Times, though rarely, there is a string Concretion in that Part. Sometimes it is *oedematous*, as others *melicerous, scirrhous, black, livid*; in which Cases the Operation of Cutting is dangerous; and it grows to the Magnitude of a Bean or Chestnut.

If a short *vinculum* be the Cause, it is to be cut asunder with a Scalpar, and the Part gently touched with *Mell. Rosat.* And *Tinct. Myrrh*; being very careful not to cut the Arteries, Nerves, or Salival Glands in the Operation.

**RARE**, in Physicks, a Body that is very porous, whose Parts are at a great Distance from one another, and which contains but little Matter under a great deal of Bulk. In this Sense *Rare* stands opposed to *Dense.*

The Corpuscular Philosophers, *viz.* the *Epicureans*, Gassendists, *Newtonians*, &c. assert that Bodies are rare, some than others, in virtue of a greater Quantity of Vacuity included between their Pores. The *Cartesians* hold, that a greater *rarity* only consists in a greater Quantity of *Materia Subtilis*, included in the Pores. Lastly, the *Peripateticks* contend, that *Rarity* is a new Quality super-induced upon a Body, without any Dependance, either on Vacuity, or subtle Matter.

**RAREFACTIVES**, or *Rarefacientia*, in Medicine, Remedies which open and enlarge the Pores of the Skin, to give an easy vent to the Matter of Perspiration. Such are Anise, Mallows, Pellitory, Camomile-Flowers, Line-Seed, &c.

**REALGAL**, or Risalgal, a Mineral; a kind of red Arsenic, differing from the common Arsenic, which is white; and from Orpiment, which is yellow. There are two Kinds or *Realgal*, the one *natural*, and the other *factitious* : The Natural is calcined in the Mine by the subterraneous Fires : The Factitious, which is the more common, is calcined by a common Fire.

Some able Druggists doubt whether there be any such thing as a native *Realgal*. The *Realgal* is a violent Poison; yet less Caustic than the common Arsenic. 'Tis of some use in Chirurgery.

In the History of the *French* Academy, we have an account of a Cup brought to *Paris* by the Embassadors of *Siam*, and presented there, as a Remedy used by that People against all Diseases. Upon an Examination, which had like to have cost M. *Homberg* dear, he found it to be a kind of *Realgal*, or red Arsenic, more Caustic than ours.

Its use among the *Siamese*, he takes to have been the same with that *Regulus* of Antimony; *viz.* to give an emetic Quality to the Wine drunk out of it.

As the Dose of Medicines is much stringer in the torrid Zones than among us, (the Quantity of Ipecacuanha, *e.gr.* ordinarily taken by the *Indians*, being twenty times as great as that among us) 'tis very possible a Cup of *Realgal*, though enough to Poison an European, may prove a gentle Medicine to a *Siamese*.

**RECIPE**, in Medicine, a Prescription, or *Formula* of a Remedy, appointed to be administered to a Patient. 'Tis thus call'd, because always beginning with the Word Recipe, Take; ordinarily express'd by $R_x$.

**RECIPROCAL**, Receiver, in Chymistry, an Appendage of an Alembic, Retort, &c. being a Vessel luted to the Beak thereof, to receive the Liquor rais'd in Distillation, &c. *Recipient* is also Part of the Apparatus of an Air Pump; being a Glass Vessel placed a-top of the Plate, for the Air to be exhausted from. To an Air-Pump belong various *Recipients*, of various Forms and Sizes, and serving for various Purposes.

**RECREMENT**, *Fæces*, in Medicine, &c. some superfluous Matter mixed with other that is useful. Sometimes it also signifies such secreted Juice in the Body, as are afterwards of use to the Œconomy; as the Lympha, Gall, &c. which are thus called in contribution to Excrements, which are expell'd out of the Body, as of no further use.

**RECRUDESCENCE**, in Medicine, is when a Disease that was gone off returns again.

**RECTIFICATION**, the Act of Rectifying, *i.e.* of correcting, or redressing some Defect or Error, in respect either of Nature, Art, or Morality. The Word is compound of *rectus*, right, direct, and *fio*, I become.

**RECTIFICATION**, in Chymistry, is the repeating of a Distillation or Sublimation several times; in order to render the Substance purer, finer, and freer from Aqueous, or Earthy Parts. *Rectification* is a reiterated Depuration of a distill'd Matter, *e.gr.* Brandy, Spirit, or Oils; by passing them again over their Faeces, or Marc, to render them more subtile, and exalt their Virtues. Fix'd Salts are *rectified* by Calcination, Dissolution, or Philtration. Metals are *rectified, i.e.* refined, by the *Couppel*; Regulus's, by repeated Fusions, &c.

**RECTIFIED SPIRIT**, &c. are such as have undergone the Operation of Rect-ification, or have been distill'd over and over, to separate from them any heter-ogeneous Matter, which might have arisen with them in the former Distillations. Hence we say, *Spirit of Wine twice rectified, thrice rectified,* &c. 'Tis the *Rect-ification* that makes the Difference between Brandy and *rectified* Spirits of Wine.

**REDINTEGRATION**, in Chymistry, the restoring of any mixt Body, or Matter, whose Form has been destroyed by Calcination, Sublimation, or the like; into its former Nature and Constitution. The *Redintegration* of Mercury is properly call'd *Revification.*

Mr. *Boyle* has an express Treatise on the *Redintegration* of Salt-Petre; where he shews that after reducing it by Fluxion into fix'd Nitre, which is next of-kin to Salt of Tartar in all its Properties; he could presently *Redintegrate* it by pouring a sufficient Quantity of Spirit of Nitre to it; *i.e.* he could re-produce true Crystals of the usual Form and Value.

'Tis a strong Objection against the Chymical Principles that you cannot *redin-tegrate* the Body they were procured from, by re-mixing them. This seems to argue that the Body did not properly consist of such Elements. Or that they were not originally contain'd in it, but were rather produced by the Fire.

**REDUCT**, among Chymists, is a Powder by which calcin'd Metals and Minerals are reduced again to their *Regulus*, or pure Substance.

**REDUCTION**, in Chirurgery, is an Operation whereby a dislocated, luxated or fractured Bone, is restored to its former Place.

**REFRIGERATIVE**, in Medicine, a Remedy or Diet which refreshes the inner Parts by cooling them. Such, usually, are Ptisans, Clysters, Potions, &c.

**REFRIGERATORY**, in Chymistry, a Cooler; or a Vessel filled with cold Water, placed about the Head of an Alembic, to cool and condense the Vapours rais'd thither by the Fire, and to convert them into a Liquor, to be discharg'd thence through the Beak. The Water in the *Refrigeratory* is to be changed from time to time, as it begins to grow warm.

Sometimes they content themselves with wrapping a wet Cloth about the Head of the Alembic, instead of a *Refrigeratory* : But the more usual Method now used to supply the Place of the *Refrigeratory,* is by a Worm, or spiral Pipe running through a Tub of cold Water. Distillation is perform'd by Evaporation and *Refrigeration.*

**REGALIS** *Aqua*, or *Aqua Regia*, an Acid corrosive Spirit or Water, serving, as a Menstruum, to dissolve Gold. The Basis or essential Ingredient of *Aqua*

*Regia*, is common or Sea Salt; which is the only Salt in Nature that will operate on Gold. There are divers Ways of preparing it; for, in effect, the Salt will not fail at its End, in what form soever applied. The common Way is by mixing common Salt, or Sal Armoniac, with Spirit of Nitre; or with common Aqua Fortis, which is made of Nitre and Vitriol. It has its Name from its dissolving Gold; reputed among Chymists, the *King* of Metals. *Aqua Regalis* dissolves Gold, but not Silver; *Aqua Fortis* Silver, but not gold.

**REGIMEN**, in Medicine, a Rule or Course of living, with regard to eating, drinking, cloathing, and the like; accommodated to some Disease, and to the particular Course of Medicine the Patient is under. 'Tis doubted whether hot or cold *Regimens* be most convenient in Fevers. The hot *Regimen* which antiently obtained in the Small-Pox, begins to be disused. The *Regimen* is very different in different Countries : *Bartholin* says, a Slice of *Bacon*, in *Denmark*, is an usual Dish for a Person in a high Fever. The Word is pure *Latin*, and signifies Government and Rule.

**REGIMEN**, in Chymistry and Alchymy, is the Method of ordering and conducting any thing, that it may answer its Intention. Thus, *Regimen of the Fire*, is the manner of making and ordering a Fire, and the Degrees thereof.

*Regimen of the Work*, that is, *of the Philosopher's Stone*, call'd the *Work of Patience*, is the Rule and Conduct to be observ'd to attain Projection. There are three things to be chiefly regarded in the *Regimen of the Work*. The first to administer a gently, easy Heat, at the beginning of the Coction.

The second to continue this external Heat according to the Season of the Work; always observing four Seasons, as in the common and astronomical Year: The beginning being the Winter, the Progress the Spring, then Summer, and lastly Autumn, which is the time of Maturity and Perfection of the Stone : In all which the Heat is to be augmented in proportion to the Augmentation observ'd in Nature.

It is to be added, that the Work may not be begun in any Season, but regard is to be had to the Seasons of Nature; least the Winter of the Work be found in the Summer of the Year, &c. Which, however, is to be understood of the Day wherein the Mercury is put in the *Ovum Philosophicum*; not of that when it is begin to be set at Liberty from the Prisons Mature had inclosed it in.

The third is that in augmenting the Fire, the Augmentation be not of a whole Degree at once; the Spirits being unable to bear such Violence; but a Degree is to be divided into four Parts, and one Part to be taken at a time.

All the Operations of the first *Regimen*, are occult and invisible : In the second *Regimen* comes Putrifaction, which is the first sensible Change; shewing it self by its black Colour.

**REGULUS**, in Chymistry, is the finest and purest Part of a Metal or Mineral, which sinks or precipitates to the bottom of the Crucible or Furnace, in melting a Mineral, or metallic Ore.

To procure the *Regulus's* of Metals, &c. Flux Powders are commonly used; as Nitre, Tartar, &c. which purge the sulphurous Part adhering to the Metal, by attracting and absorbing it to themselves.

*Regulus* is principally used for that of Antimony, which is a ponderous metallic Powder, that upon fusing some of that Mineral in its crude State, sinks to the bottom, leaving the Scoria or Impurities a-top.

The Alchymists will have this matter called *Regulus.*, *i.e.* little King, as being the first born of the Royal metallic Blood; which is really a Son, but not a perfect man, *i.e.* not yet a perfect Metal for want of Time and proper Nourishment.

Antimony purified by simple Fusion, is call'd *Regulus of Antimony*; or *Regulus Antimonii stallatus Philosophorum*. But the more common way of reducing it into a *Regulus* is with the Addition of Flux Powders, as Tartar and Nitre. The Scoria found at the top of this *Regulus* is violently emetic, as well as the *Regulus* itself, whereof if Cups or drinking Vessels be cast, the Wine put into them will be become vomitive.

Of this *Regulus* cast in Moulds are made those commonly called the *Antimonial Pills*, weighing about eight or ten Grains each, one of which being swallowed, will operate considerably both by Vomit and Stool.

These Pills having thus performed their Office, and being discharge the Body, will serve the same Purpose again and again; whence they have obtained the Name of *perpetual Pills*. The Virtue of this *Regulus* is not however inexhaustible, as has been imagined; for by repeated Infusions in Wine, though the Liquor be made violently Emetic at first, yet by Degrees it loses its Force, and at length ceases to be Vomitive.

*Martial Regulus of Antimony* is a Mixture of the Nails of Horse's Shoes, melted with the *Regulus*. In this Operation the Iron dissolving and absorbing the sulphurous Parts of the Antimony, more strongly than the Fluxes in the former Case; and turning it into a Crocus; the Antimony is hereby brought to a greater Degree of Purity, and render'd more efficacious than in the common *Regulus*. This *Regulus* is sometimes further purified by repeated Fusions and Detonations, with the Addition of fresh Antimony, and more Nitre, respectively.

**REINS**, in Anatomy, the Kidneys; or that Part of an Animal whereby the Urine is separated from the Blood. The Word, according to *Varro*, is form'd from the *Greek*, απο του ρειν, *Quasi Rivi obsceni humoris ab iis oriantur*. The *Greeks* call the *Rein*, νεφρος, from the Verb, νεφρειν, to Snow, Rain.

**RELAPSE**, a return or back-sliding into a Danger, or Evil; out of which a Person had escaped. Fevers, Dropsies, &c. are Diseases into which Relapses are very frequent and dangerous.

**RELAXATION**, in Medicine, &c. the loosening or slacking of the Tone or Tension of the Fibres, Nerves, Muscles, &c. The *Relaxation* of a Muscle is supposed to be effected, either by the Perspiration of the nervous Spirits, or the Regress of the Spirits, Blood, &c. which inflated its Fibres; or by the contraction of the Air, in the Globules of Blood before expanded by the sudden influx and admixture of the Spirits, &c.

**REMEDY**, *Remedium*, in Physick, a Medicine, or Preparation applied either internally or externally, for the Cure of a Disease. Emplasters, Unguents,

Cataplasms, &c. are *Topical Remedies.* Mercury and the Bark are *Specific Remedies.* Mineral Waters, and Asse's Milk, and Country-Air, are usually the *last Remedies.* Salivation is sometimes call'd by way of Eminence, *the Remedy.* When *Remedies* are stuff'd with too many Ingredients, they load the Stomach with a slimy Mucilage, which swelling does more hurt than good.

**REPELLENT**, *Repellens,* in Medicine, a Remedy which *repels* or drives back a morbid Humour into the Mass of Blood, from which it was unduly secreted. Or, Repellents are Medicines which prevent such an afflux of the Fluids to any particular Part, as will raise it into a Tumour; or drive them back when they are collected.

To form an Idea of the Manner of their Operation, it may be observ'd, that all Tumours arise either from an increase in the Velocity or Quantity of the Fluids, or a Weakness in some particular Part; though sometimes both concur. Now an increase in the Velocity of the Fluids makes them more forcibly push against, and distend all the Parts in their Circuit; if therefore any Part be unequally pressed or relaxed by external Injuries, that will be more elevated than any other; and for want of equal Resistance with the rest of the Body, will at length receive such a Quantity of Fluids, as will raise it to a Tumour, especially if any of its Vessels be obstructed : Because the Protrusion of fresh Matter, *a tergo,* will continue to add thereunto, till the Part is on the utmost stretch, and can hold no more.

In this Case all those Means are said to be *repellent,* which check the growth of the Tumor, and assist the refluent Blood in taking up the obstructed Matter, and washing it again into the common Stream.

This Intention is chiefly favoured by Evacuation and Revulsion; for whatever lessens the Quantity of the Fluid, will diminish the force upon the tumified Part. But it concerns us most to know how external Application to the Part itself, helps this Affair.

Herein a Medicine comes to be *repellent,* by consisting of such subtile Parts, as may transmit some of them through the Pores, and help to render the obstructed Matter more fluid, so that it comes the more easy to be loosened, and fall again into the circulating Current. But in this Case there is a Hazard of such things likewise putting the obstructed Humour into a Ferment, whereby it sooner turns into Pus, and then they come under the Denomination of Suppuratives or Ripeners.

What, therefore, in the most strict Sense, is to be reputed a *Repeller,* is that which astringes and strengthens the Part, so as to make it resists any such Lodgment.

These are such whose Qualities are most manifest in their Coldness, and drying Properties : But there are so few Instances wherein Bandage is not better than such Application, that very little comes to be used for that purpose. In Hemorrhages, and Ouzings out of Serum, so as to deform the Skin; Simples of this Nature mostly take place; which answer their Ends in astringing the Fibres, whereby those Apertures are so closed, as not o admit through them afterward any such fluid.

Some things also answer this End only by stimulating the Fibres of the tumefied Part, so as to give them sudden and forcible Twitches, whereby the obstruction is sometimes loosened and shook away, as it were, into the refluent Current. Such a sort of Motion will be occasioned by the sudden Application of any thing extremely cold, as common Water; but the Practice is seldom safe, because if the first Efforts which the Fibres are put upon by those means, do not succeed in breaking away the inclosed Matter, they will be strained, and not able afterwards to repeat their natural Vibrations : The Consequence of which is weakening the Part, which will render the Tumor more obstinate.

**REPLETION**, in Medicine, a *Plenitude*, or *Plethora*. *Repletion* is more dangerous than Inanition. Bleeding and Diet are the great Recourses when a Person is incommoded with a *Repletion*.

*Repletion* is sometimes also used where the Stomach is over loaden, with too much eating or drinking. The Physicians hold all *Repletion* prejudicial; but that of Bread the worst.

**RESIN**, *Resina*, a fat, viscid, sulphurous Juice, oozing either spontaneously, or by Incision, from several kinds of Trees, particularly the Pine, Fir, &c. Mastic is the *Resin* of the Lentisk. Camphor is also a kind of *Resin*. The best of all the Class of Resins is Turpentine. The Coarsest is what we commonly call *Rosin*. *Resin* is properly a Juice of the Bark only.

*Boerhaave* will have it to be the Oil of the Bark further inspissated by the Heat of the Sun, &c. so as to become friable. He adds, that it may be produced from any vegetable Oil, by boiling it much and long.

If Turpentine be set over a gentle Fire, it first dissolves and becomes an Oil, then a Balsam, then Pitch, and then *Rosin*; in which State it is friable in the Cold, fusible by Fire, and withal inflammable and combustible, and dissoluble in Spirit of Wine, but not in Water, which are the Characters of a *Resin*.

There are two kinds of *Resins*, the one *liquid*, the other *dry* and hard. The first is the natural *Resin* as it flows from the Tree. The second only differs from the first in that it is condensed by the Heat of the Sun, or by that of a culinary Fire.

*Resins* will incorporate with Oil, or rectified Spirits, but not with an aqueous Menstruum.

The Difference between *Resins* and Gums consists in this, that *Resins* are more sulphurous, and Gums more aqueous; so that the first dissolve in Spirit of Wine, and the last in Water. See Gum.

M. *Tournefort* makes a kind of intermediate Class of vegetable Juices, which he calls *Gum-Resins*; which dissolve partly in Spirit of Wine, partly in Water. Such are *Galbanum, Bdellium, Oppoponax, Sagapenum*, &c.

The *Resin* of several Vegetables which abound with Resinous Particles, but not so as to yield any by Incision, as Jalap, Benjamin, Scammony, Turbith, &c. is thus obtained. The Vegetable being grossly powder'd, is put into a Matrass, and rectified Spirit of Wine pour'd on it, to the height of four Fingers above the Matter. Then the Neck of another Matrass being luted into the former to make a double Vessel, the Matter is digested 3 or four Days in a Sand Heat, till it have given a good Tincture to the Spirit of Wine. Then the

Dissolution is filtrated, and two thirds of the clear Liquid evaporated off, and the remainder pour'd into a large Vessel of Water, where it turn into a kind of Milk; whence, the *Resin*, in Time precipitates to the Bottom in a white Powder. This when wash'd and dried in the Sun, grows into the Consistence of a *Resin.*

**RESOLUTION**, in Chymistry, is the Reduction of a Mass or mix'd Body into its component Parts, or first Principles; by a proper Analysis. The *Resolution* of Bodies is perform'd variously; by *Distillation, Sublimation, Dissolution, Fermentation*, &c.

**RESOLUTION**, in Medicine, the Coction or Alteration of the Crude peccant Matter of any Disease, either by the natural Strength of the Patient, or of its own accord, or by the Application of Remedies; whereby its bulk, Figure, Cohesion, &c. are so far chang'd as that it ceases to be Morbid, and becomes laudable. This, the learned *Boerhaave* observes, is of all others the most perfect Cure, where 'tis effected without any Evacuation; as supposing the Matter favourable, the Constitution excellent, and the Medicines good.

**RESOLVENTS**, *Resolventia*, in Medicine, remedies proper to resolve and dissipate Tumors and Gatherings; to soften Hardnesses; and by their Tenuity and Warmth, evacuate redundant or peccant Humours through the Pores. Under this Class come various Unguents, Emplasters, &c.

**RESTINCTION**, in Chymistry, the quenching of a Metal or Mineral in some Liquor; in order either to correct, or give it some new Quality, Power, &c.

**RESTORATIVE**, in Medicine, a Remedy proper for the restoring and retrieving of Strength and Vigour. Restoratives belong to the Class of Balsamicks. The Medicines that come under this Denomination are of an emollient, softening Nature, but nutritive withal; and are rather administered to repair the Wastes of the Constitution, than to alter and rectify its Disorders.

Such are the Leaves of white Maiden-hair, Adianthum Nigrum; black Hellebore; Rocket, Eruca; Scabious; Tusilago; Colts-Foot; Bohea-Tea; Chich-peas; Hops; Chocolate; Pistach-Nuts; Balsom of Tolu; Bdellium; Benzoin; Storax; Eryngo; Iris; Satyrion, &c.

**RESUMPTIVE**, in Pharmacy, an Epithet give to a kind of Unguent, used to recruit and restore arid languishing Constitutions, and to dispose the dry Body to receive Nourishment. 'Tis called in Latin, *Unguentum resumptivum.*

**RETENTION** is also used in Medicine, &c. for that State of Contraction in the Solids, or vascular Parts of the Body, which makes them hold fast their proper Contents. In this Sense *Retention* stands opposed to *Evacuation*, or *Excretion*. *Retention* and Excretion make one of the six Non-Naturals.

*Retention* is frequently considered as a Disorder; and defined the Act of retaining the Excrements, Humours, &c. so as they cannot be voided out of the Body. A *Retention* of Urine is very painful and dangerous. 'Tis a *Retention* of peccant Humours which Causes such a Disease.

**RETORT**, in Chymistry, a kind of crooked Matrass, or a round, bellied Vessel, either of Earth or Glass, with a slender crooked Beak, or Nose, to which the Recipient is to be fastened. The *Retort* serves to draw the Spirits and Oils from Woods, Gums, Minerals, Earths, and other Matters which require a strong Fire.

The *Retort* is a kind of Compendium or Improvement of the Cucurbit and Bolt-head; answering all the Purposes of both, without the Assistance of a Capital or Head, which the other frequently require. When the *Retort* is of Glass, 'tis usually lin'd with a Lute or Past an Inch thick; to enable it to bear the Fire the better.

**REVERBERATION**, in Chymistry, a kind of Circulation of the Flame, by means of a *Reverberatory*; or the return of the Flame from the top of the Furnace, back to the Bottom.

*Reverberation* is of two Kinds. The first which a close Fire; that is, in a *Reverberatory* Furnace, where the Flame has no vent a-top; being cover'd with a Dome, or Capital, which repels its Action back on the Matter, or the Vessel that contains it, with increased Vehemence. After this Manner are Refining, the Distillation of acid Spirits, &c. perform'd.

*Reverberation* with an open Fire, is that performed in a Furnace or *Reverberatory* whose Registers are all open; chiefly used in Calcination.

**REVERBERATORY**, or Reverberating *Furnace*, is a Chymical Furnace built close all around, and cover'd a-top with a Capital of Bricks or Tiles, so as not to give any Vent to the Heat or Flame, but to determine it to Reverberate or turn back from the Brick Work with new Force, upon the Matters placed at the Bottom.

When the Fire has no vent or Passage a-top, 'tis a whole *Reverberatory*; when the middle of the Capital is open, and only the Sides close to, so that there is only half Circulation of the Flame, 'tis call'd a *half Reverberatory*.

The *reverberating* Furnace is chiefly used for the Fusion of Metals, and Minerals, and other Occasions where the most intense Heat is required, as in Assaying, &c. Whence it is also called the *Melting Furnace*, and *Assaying Furnace*.

**REVIVIFICATION**, or Resuscitation, in Chymistry, the Art of restoring a mix'd Body to its first State, after it had been alter'd and disguis'd by Dissolution, Calcination, or the like.

Thus Cinnabar and other Preparations of Mercury, are *revived*, or *revivified* into fluid Mercury. *Olaus Borrichius* assures us, that having tormented Mercury with several Fires, for the Space of a whole Year; having reduced it into Water, Turbith, into Ashes, &c. it revivified, and resumed its first Form in the middle of the Flames, by the Attraction of Salt of Tartar.

Gold, and other Metals, 'tis said, may be recovered or *revivified* into running Mercury, by the use of certain Salts, which penetrating the Substance of the Metals, absorb the fixing Sulpher or Cement, by which the Mercury was before bound into a malleable Mass.

**REVULSION**, in Medicine, the turning of a violent Flux of Humours, from one Part of the Body to another, either neighbouring or opposite Part.

In very dangerous Wounds, where the loss of Blood is great, and the stopping it speedily enough impracticable; 'tis usual to open a Vein in some remote Part, to cause a Revulsion; that is, to turn the Course of the Blood from the former Part. *Revulsions* are also caused by Cupping, Friction, &c.

The Term *Revulsion* is also used for a great Turn or Revulsion of Humours in the Body. Sudden Diseases are occasioned by great Revulsions of Humours, which fall all at once on certain Parts.

**RHAGADES**, in Medicine, a *Greek* Term used for the Chaps or Clefts in the Lips. *Rhagades*, are also a sort of little chap'd Ulcers of the Oedematous Kind; form'd of a sharp, saline Humour, and occasioning a great Contraction, and streightening of the Part, which is by this means shrivell'd up like a wet Parchment when held to the Fire.

They arise chiefly on the Fundament, the Neck of the Womb, the Preputium, and even the Mouth; in which last Case the Patient is not able to speak, chew, or the like.

They are sometimes moist, and of a cancerous Nature, eating deep, and difficult of Cure; but are more commonly of a less malignant tendency, being the Consequences of a Diarrhæa, Dysentery, or the like.

**RHAPONTICUM**, a medicinal Root, in form resembling Rhubarb; and nearly of the same Virtues. 'Tis frequently mix'd with Rhubarb by those who send that Drug into *Europe* : They are distinguish'd by this, that the Rhubarb is usually in roundish Pieces, the internal Streaks or Lines whereof run transverse : And *Rhaponticum* in longish Pieces, having its Streaks running length-wise. Besides, that *Rhaponticum* chew'd in the Mouth, leaves a Viscidity behind it, which Rhubarb does not.

The scarcity of the *Rhaponticum* of the *Levant*, occasions the *Mountain Rhaponticum*, or *Monk's Rhubarb*, to be frequently substituted for it, which is a wild *Hypolapathum*. They are distinguish'd by this, that the former is yellow without, and reddish within; but the latter blackish without and yellow within.

Dr. *Quincy*, however, confounds the two, when he says, the *Rhaponticum* grows plentifully in *England*; and that 'tis only used as an Alterative, and does not come up to a Cathartic.

'Tis certain, what now obtains in the Shops, under the Name of *Rhaponticum*, is no other than the Mountain *Rhaponticum*, or Monk's Rhubarb; and is much inferior in Virtue to the *Rhaponticum Verum*.

**RHEUM**, a thin serous Humour, occasionally oozing out of the Glands about the Mouth and Throat. The Word is form'd from the *Greek*, ρεω, *fluo*, I flow.

A Fluxion of *Rheum* usually happening after taking Cold, occasions Excoriations and Inflammation of the Fauces, Lungs, &c. *Rheum* is also used for a *Catarrh*, or a Defluxion of such Humours on the Trachea, and the neighbouring Parts; occasioning a Coughing, Spitting, Hoarseness, Running at the Nose.

The *Rheum* is not caus'd by a Pituita falling from the Brain on these Parts, as the Antients imagined, there being no Passage from the Brain thither; but from a thin, sharp, serous Humour, oozing out of the Extremities of the Glands of these Parts. The most ordinary Occasion of *Rheums*, is external Cold; especially the being exposed to it, when the Body is much heated. And hence the Disorder it self is popularly call'd a *Cold*.

*Rheums* falling on the Breast, Lungs, &c. are dangerous; others, not very violent, serve to clear the Head, &c. The usual Remedies are Astringents, Agglutinants, and Absorbents.

**RHEUMATISM**, in Medicine, a painful Disorder felt in various Parts of the external Body, accompanied with Heaviness, Difficulty of Motion, and frequently a Fever. Or, a *Rheumatism* is a Pain usually wandering, but sometimes fix'd in the muscular and membranous Parts of the Body; happening chiefly in Autumn. The proper Seat of the *Rheumatism* is supposed to be in the *Membrana Communis* of the Muscles; which it renders rigid and unfit for Motion without great Pain.

*Particular Rheumatism* is that which is confined to particular Parts : In which Case the Pains are usually erratic, passing from one Side to another; but sometimes fix'd, call'd also a *windy* and *scorbutic Rheumatism*. The *Rheumatism* bears a great Analogy to the Gout; whence some call it the *universal Gout*. The Difference between them consists in this, that the *Rheumatism* not attacks only the Joints, as Gout does, but also the Muscles and Membranes between the Joints.

A Fit of *Rheumatism* is frequently preceded by a Fever of two or three Days; and some-times by a Shivering. The Attack happens in various Parts of the Body, as the Hands, Arms, Thighs, Legs, Feet, &c. a Redness, Swelling, and Lameness often succeeding.

The Pain sometimes fixing on the Loins, and reaching as far as the *Os Sacrum*; the Disorder is call'd *Lumbago*; and bears a near resemblance to the *Nephritis*; being only distinguishable therefrom by this, that the latter is attended with a Vomiting, which the former is not.

The *Rheumatism* is supposed to arise from a sharp serous Humour thrown on the sensible Parts, and occasioning a Pain by its Vesication. Dr. *Quincy* says, it proceeds from the same Cause, as that whereby the mucilaginous Glands become stiff and gritty in the Gout.

Dr. *Musgrave* takes it to be occasioned from a sharp alkaline Salt, rather than an acid one; from this Consideration, that the Urine of *Rheumatic* People does not afford above a thirtieth Part of the Alcaline Salt founding that of healthful People.

Hence, he conjectures, that the Salt is retain'd in the Blood, implicated and embarrass'd in the Pituita; by which means it forms a Viscidity which occasions all the Pains and Tumours of the *Rheumatism*.

The exposing the Body too suddenly to the cold Air, after having heated it to a great Degree; is the most usual remote Cause. The Cure is by Evacuation, with a plentiful Use of Volatiles and Diluters. *Schmitzius*[1] recommends

[1] This is probably Johann Andreas Schmitz (1621 – 1652), a German physician.

Sudorificks, and *Musgrave*, Catharticks, and Emeticks.

It usually proves a tedious, lasting Disease; holding for several Months, sometimes Years; not continually but by Paroxisms. In aged Persons, and those of weak Constitutions, and decay'd Viscera, it sometimes seizes the Head.

**RHEXIS**, or *Rhegma*, among Occulists, a Rupture of the Cornea of the Eye. The Word is form'd from the *Greek* ρηξις, rupture, of ρηγνυμαι, *frango*, I break.

**RHODIUM LIGNUM**, *Rhodian-Wood.* See Aspalathum.

**RHODON**, in Pharmacy, from ροδον, *Rosa*; a Name given to some Compositions wherein the Rose is the chief Ingredient; as *Diarrhodon.* Hence also *Rhodoseccharum, q.d. Sugar of Roses*, &c.

**RHUBARB**, a medicinal Root, compact, and heavy; yellow without, of a Nutmeg Colour within; an astringent, bitterish Taste; and an agreeable, aromatic Smell : Of great Use in Medicine, as a Purgative.

Considering the mighty Use of this Drug, 'tis surprizing we should know so little of the Place where the Plant grows that produces it. Some say it comes from the Kingdom of *Boutan*, in the Extremities of *India*; others, that 'tis founding the Provinces of *Xensi* and *Suchen* in *China*. Others will have it only grow in *Persia*; and others on the Confines of the *Muscovy*; deriving its Name from *Rha*, the River among us call'd the *Volga*, and *Barbarum, q.d.* Root found by the Barbarians on the River *Rha.*

*Rhubarb*, in Latin, *Rhabarbarum Officinarum*, was not known of the Antients; and their *Rhaponticum*, which indeed resembles it, is not the real *Rhubarb.*

Good *Rhubarb* steep'd in Water gives it a Saffron Colour; and when broke looks bright, with somewhat of a Vermillion Cast. Some Druggists have the Art of renewing their Old Roots, by giving them a yellow hue; but the Cheat is easily known by handling them; the Powder wherewith they colour them sticking to the Fingers.

*Rhubarb* is esteemed an excellent Cathartic; proper for a Diarrhæa, to fortify the Stomach, and to create an Appetite.

M. *Boulduc* informs us, in the Memoirs of the *French* Academy, that hew drew Extracts from *Rhubarb* both with Water and Spirit of Wine; but the purgative Virtue, he says, was much more visible in the former than the latter; which shews that it consists more in a Salt than an Oil. He observes, however, that *Rhubarb* taken in Substance, has a still better effect; and adds, that of all the Operations he could make with it, none gave any Credit to the common Opinion, which ascribes an astringent Quality to it.

**RHYAS**, in Medicine, a Diminution or Consumption of the *Caruncula Lachrymalis*, situate in the great Canthus or Angle of the Eye. The *Rhyas* is used in opposition to the *Encanthis*, which is an excessive Augmentation of the same Caruncle. The Cause of the *Rhyas* is a sharp Humour falling on this Part; and gnawing and consuming it by Degrees; though it is sometimes also produced by the too great Use of Cathereticks in the *Fistula Lachrymalis*. It is cured by Incarnatives.

**RIGOR**, in Medicine, a convulsive Shuddering, from Cold, or an Ague Fit.

**ROB**, in Pharmacy, a Preparation antiently much used, consisting of the Juices of Fruits, purified, and boil'd to a Consumption of two thirds of their Moisture.

There are *Robs* made of Quinces, Mulberries, Elderberries, Aloes, Acacia, Liquorice, Barberries, Gooseberries, and other Fruits, for various Disease. The Juice of Grapes thus prepared, is particularly call'd *Sapa*; which *Sapa* is almost of the Consistence of a Syrup.

When only one third of the Humidity is boil'd away, 'tis call'd *Defrutum*; and when only boil'd to the Consistence of a soft Electuary, a *Resin*.

The Word *Rob* is pure *Arabick*; and signifies, originally, a Juice dried in the Sun, or over a Fire; that it may keep the longer with Damage. Sometimes it also denotes a Composition of some Juice made up with Honey or Sugar; in which Sense it is confounded with *Loche* or *Lohoc*.

The *Rob* is a Form now much out of use; though there are several directed in the College Dispensatory; as *Robs* of black Cherries, of Sloes, of Quinces, &c.

**ROBORANTIA**, in Medicine, *Strengtheners*; or such Medicines as strengthen the Parts, and give new Vigour to the Constitution.

**ROOTS**, in Medicine. The Principal *Roots* used in the Practice of Medicine, are, *Rhubarb, Rhaponticum, Sarsaparilla, Ipecacuanha, Jalap, Zedoary, Galangal, Cassumenar, Gentian, Turmeric, Liquorice, Madder*, &c.

**ROS VITRIOLI**, among Chymists, is sometimes used for the first Phlegm distill'd from Vitriol in *Balneo Mariæ*.

**ROSADE**, a kind of Liquor, prepared of pounded Almonds and Milk, mix' with clarified Sugar.

**ROSE**, *Rosa*, a medicinal Flower, produced by a Shrub of the same Name; which gives the Denomination to several Preparations in Pharmacy. The Kinds of *Roses* are various : Those used in Medicine are the Red and Damask *Roses*. The *Damasks* are a good and safe purgative, administered in infusion, or by way of Syrup. The *Red* are astringent; and the Conserve thereof used with success against Distempers of the Breast and Lungs, and Disorders of the Eyes. *Sugar of Roses*, is made of Red-*Rose* Leaves, dried in an Oven, pulverized, and put into a proper Quantity of Sugar dissolv'd with a little Water in a Chafing-dish, over the Fire.

**ROSE**-*Water*, a Water drawn by Distillation from Red or Damask-*Roses*. It is a good Cordial, and was formerly highly esteemed; but is since fallen from its Reputation, and is little used but in Diseases of the Eyes, and in Perfumes and Washes. 'Tis, however, in great esteem in the *East*, particularly in *China* and *Persia*, where the Trade thereof is very considerable. The *Rose* Leaves remaining at the Bottom of the Still, have the natural cathartic Quality; and are also kept for a Perfume.

**ROSE-WOOD**, *Lignum Rhodium*, or *Aspalathum*.

**ROSEMARY**, *Rosmarinus*, a medicinal Plant, whose Flowers are of considerable use in the present Practice. They abound with a subtle detergent Oil, which makes them deobstruent and opening, whence their use in uterine Obstructions, the Jaundice, &c.

They are the Basis of the celebrated *Hungary* Water; with a small Quantity of which, diluted in common Water, the Confectioners make the Conserve of *Rosemary* Flowers, Essence of *Rosemary*, *Rosemary*-Water, &c.

Dr. *Quincy* speaks of them as good in most nervous Complaints, especially such as arise from too great Moisture and Cold, as they are hot and drying. In Epilepsies, Apoplexies, Palsies, &c. they are rarely omitted in Prescription, under one Form or other.

**ROSOLIS**, popularly, *Rosa-solis*, *Sun-Dew*, an agreeable spirituous Liquor, chiefly taken after Meals, by way of Dram, to aid Digestion. It had its Name because antiently prepared wholly of the Juice of the plant *Ros solis*; but that Plant is no longer any Ingredient therein.

'Tis composed of burnt Brandy, Sugar, Cinnamon, and Milk-Water, and is sometimes perfumed with a little Musk. The best is that of *Turin*. The *French* have a particular Kind not called *Ros solis*, but *du Roy*; because used with good Effect by the late King *Lewis* XIV. 'Tis composed of *Spanish* Wine, wherein are infused Anis, Fennel, Aneth, Coriander, &c. for three weeks.

**ROSTRUM**, in Chymistry, signifies the Nose, or Beak which conveys Liquor distill'd, into its Receiver; in the common Alembicks.

**ROSTRUM**, is also a crooked Scissars, which the Surgeons in some Cases make use of for the Dilatation of Wounds.

**RUBIFYING**, in Chymistry, &c. the Act of turning a thing Red by the Force of Fire, &c. Red Arsenic is supposed to be no more than the common yellow Arsenick *rubified* by Fire, with the addition of Nut or Olive Oil. The Word is form'd from the *Latin*, *rubens*, ruddy, and *fio*, I become.

**RUBY**, in Chymistry, is a Name given to several Preparations of natural Bodies, because of their red Colour; as, *Ruby of Arsenick*, &c.

**RUCTATION**, Belching, a Ventosity arising from Indigestion, and discharging it self at the Mouth with a disagreeable Noise. There are Belches owing to Repletion, and others to Inanition, or Emptiness. Dr. *Quincy* says, Hypo-chondriac, and Hysteric People are particularly liable to this Disorder. They are rather to be cured with proper Stomachicks, than Carminatives and hot Liquors. *Burnet* recommends the Iliac Pills of *Rhasis* against *Ructification*.

**RUE**, *Ruta*, a medicinal Plant, much used in the present Practise. *Schroder* commends it as an Alexipharmic, and Cephalic; says it resists Poisons and Malignities, and is therefore to be used in Fevers; and that it is good in all convulsive Cases.

It is replete with a fat viscous Juice, and by that means yields little to any Purpose in Distillation, unless where first digested in a spirituous Menstruum. Hence its simple Water in the Shops, according to Dr. *Quincy*, is nothing worth. It ought to be raised with a spirituous Liquor, or used in Conserve; or, which is best of all, eat alone fresh gathered, with Bread and Butter. It is of Service in nervous Cases, particularly such as arise from the Womb, as it deterges the Glands, and by its Viscidity, bridles those inordinate Motions, which frequently begin there, and affect the whole Constitution.

**RUPTURE**, in Medicine, call'd also *Hernia*, and popularly *Burstness*; is when the Rim or thin Film or Caul, which holds up the Intestines, is broken or over-strained or stretch'd, so as the Guts fall down either into the Groin, Cod, or Flank. According as the Rupture happens in the Abdomen, Inguen, or Scrotum, it is call'd *Exomphalus*, *Hernia Inguinalis*, or *Hernia Scroti*.

**RUST** of a Metal, the Flowers or Calx thereof; procured by corroding and dissolving its superficial Parts by some menstruous Fluid. Water is the great Instrument or Agent in producing *Rust*; the Air apparently *rusts* Bodies, but 'tis only in Virtue of the Water it contains.

Hence, in a dry Air, Metals remain a long time without contracting *Rust*; and hence Oils and other fatty Bodies secure metals from *Rust*; Water being no Menstruum to Oil, &c. And therefore not able to make its Way through it.

All Metals are liable to *Rust*; even Gold it self, though generally held incapable thereof, grows *Rusty* if exposed to the Fumes of Sea-Salt.

The reason why it is so rarely found to *rust*, is that Sea-Salt, which is the only Salt that will prey upon it, is of a very fix'd Nature, and therefore little of its Effluvia or Exhalations are found floating in the Air.

*Rust* is usually supposed a Corruption of the Metal, but without much Foundation : 'Tis the very Metal itself only under another Form; and accordingly we find that *Rust* of Copper may be again turned into Copper.

Ceruss is made of Lead converted into *Rust* by Vinegar. Iron, in time, turns wholly into *Rust*, unless preserv'd from the Air by Paint or Varnish.

**RYPTICKS**, in Medicine, detergent Remedies. The Word is form'd of the *Greek* ριπτειν, to wipe, cleanse.

**SAFFRON**, or *Saffran*, a Plant which produces a Flower of the same Name; whence, also a Drug called *Saffron* or *Crocus* is gathered. The Root which produces the *Saffron*, is a kind of Onion, covered with several bulbous Cartilages. Its Leaves are long, narrow, thick and soft to the Hand. Its Flower, which appears a long Time before the Leaves, is a faint Blur, tinged with a little Yellow at the Extreme towards the Stalk. From the Middle of the Flower arise three reddish Filaments or Chives, which are properly the *Saffron*; the rest of the Flower being of no use. Assoon as the Flower is gathered, they separate the Chives, and lay them on Hurdles, or in large Sieves, or on a little Kiln for that Purpose, with a little Coal-fire underneath to dry them. When dry, the Saffron is in its Perfection, and fit for Use.

'Tis observed that five Pounds of fresh Chives only make one Pound of dry *Saffron*. The good Qualities of *Saffron* are, That its Chives being and broad, that they be velveted over with a fine Red, of an agreeable Smell, free of yellow Threads, and very dry. The best *Saffron* in *Europe* is that of *England*. That brought from *Spain* is good for nothing; because of the Oil the Spaniards mix it with to keep it.

'Tis used in both Foods and Medicines, to chear, fortify, and resolve. 'Tis also used by Illuminors, to make a golden yellow Colour. The Word is formed from the *Arabic*, *Zephran*, which signifies the same Thing.

**SAFFRON**, is also a Name given to several Chymical preparations from the Resemblance of their Colour to that of *Saffron*, but more usually called *Croci*: Such is *Saffron of Venus*.

**SAGAPENUM**, or *Serapinum*, a Gum whose Smell comes very near that of the Pile, whence its Name. It flows by Incision from the Trunk of a ferulaceous Plant growing in *Persia*. The best is in bright transparent Tears, of a string Smell; and the whiter, and freer of Dirt, the better. Sometimes 'tis found as white, both within and without Side, as Milk; tho' this is very rare. 'Tis esteemed operative and purgative, proper in the Epilepsy, Asthma, and Palsy, and is also used externally to assuage Pains, and resolve Tumors.

**SAGE**, *Salvia*, a Medicinal Herb of an agreeable, aromatic Taste; esteemed an excellent Cephalic of the detergent Kind; and on that Score likewise used as a Vulnerary and Diuretic.

There are several Kinds of *Sage*; those used and cultivated by us are the *Tea-Sage*, or *Sage of Virtue*, the *Red Sage*, and the *Wormwood Sage*. The first has the most agreeable Flower; and on that Score is cut when young and full of Sap, dried, and kept for Tea. The *Dutch* dry and prepare their *Sage* like other Teas, and carry it to the *Indies* as a very precious Thing. They there find a good Market for it; the *Chinese* preferring it to the best of their *Indian* Teas; and for every Pound of *Sage* Tea, giving, in Exchange, Four Pounds of theirs, which they sell again very dear in *Europe*.

But the Wormwood *Sage* is esteemed of the most efficacy in Medicine, and is that alone used in the Shops. It makes an excellent Gargarism, especially if sharpened with a little Acid. Its Decoction is very grateful and cooling, with the addition of a little Lemon-juice. 'Tis both detergent and absorbent, and as such, finds a Place in Diet-drinks, and medicated Ales, intended for Sweetners and Cleansers of the Blood. The School of *Salernum* recommend Sage as a Remedy in all Diseases.

*Sage* when viewed with a Microscope, appears covered all over with little Spiders, which are seen to walk, &c,. about. It yields, by Distillation, a very agreeable, aromatic Oil, of some Use in the Shops.

**SAL** *Volatile Oleosum*, an Aromatic *Volatile Salt*, first prepared by *Sylvius de la Boe*, and found a very notable Medicine, chiefly as a Cephalic and Cordial.

'Tis made thus : To an Ounce of *Volatile Salt* of *Sal Ammoniac*, distill'd with *Salt of Tartar*, and dulcified with Spirit of Wine, put a Dram and a Half of some aromatic Oil, or Essence, drawn from some generous Aromatic Vegetable, as Cinnamon, Cloves, Rosemary, Balm, &c. And when the Spirit and Oil are well stirred and incorporated together; draw off the *Volatile Salt* and Spirit in a Cucurbit. Some, instead of this, mix all the Ingredients together at first, *viz.* the *Sal Ammoniac*, *Sal Tartari*, Spirit of Wine and Powder of Cinnamon or Cloves, &c. and distill off the Volatile Spirit and *Salt* at once; but the former Way is preferred.

**SALAMANDER'S BLOOD**, a Term the Chymists give to Red Vapours, which in Distillation of Spirit of Nitre, towards the latter End do fill the Receiver with red Clouds; they are the most fixed, and strongest Part of the Spirit; and nothing but Nitre yields a Red Vapour in Distillation.

**SALIVA**, *Spittle*, a thin pellucid Humour, separated by the Glands about the Mouth and Fauces; and conveyed by proper *Salival Ducts* into the Mouth, for several Uses. It consists of a great deal of Water or Phlegm, and a volatile Salt; some add, a sulphurous Spirit.

The *Saliva*, *Boerhaave* observes, is void both of Taste and Smell; does not harden by Heat; is more copious, fluid, sharp, penetrating, and detergent, as a Person has fasted longer; and is separated from the pure Arterial Blood. The Glands wherein the *Saliva* is separated from the Blood, are the *Parotides*; the *Maxillary Glands*; the *Sublinguals*, or those under the Tongue; the *Amygdalæ*, or Almonds of the Ears, and the *Palatinæ*, or Glands of the Palate.

The great Use of the *Saliva*, is in masticating and diluting the Food, and making the first Digestion thereof. The other Uses are to moisten the Tongue, to render its Motion more quick and easy; to lubricate the Throat and *Oesophagus*, in order to facilitate Deglutination, to prevent thirst, and to assist in the Sensation of Tastes, by dissolving the Salts. Some imagine it to do the Office of a *Menstruum* to mix the oily and aqueous Parts of the Food more intimately, to dissolve the Saline Parts, and to procure a Fermentation in the Stomach.

But Dr. *Drake* will not allow it fit for that Purpose. Were the *Saliva*, says he, acrimonious enough for this, 'twould be impossible but it must offend the Stomach; especially, considering Quantities of it that many swallow, even upon an Empty Stomach.

M. *Gastaldy*[1], who has a Medical Thesis on the Subject of the *Saliva*, observes, That it takes its Name from the *Salt* it contains; which Salt he will have to be partly a Volatile Acid and partly Alcalious. He adds, That it contains some Oleaginous Parts, and a little Earth. By being Compounded of so many different Kinds of Parts, it becomes a Dissolvent proper for all the different Kinds of Foods whereof we live. Its natural and laudable State, is to be a little more Viscid than common Water, and much less so than Milk. 'Tis preserved in this State by the Application of the Spirits, and of the Particles of Air which insinuate into it. According to all Appearance, the *Saliva* is derived from the Blood of the Arteries. Part of the Arterial Blood brought to the *Salival Glands*, serves to feed them; another Part is returned into the Veins, and continues the Circulation, and a third Part, which is the *Serum*, receiving a sub-acid Quality from them is converted into *Saliva*. Some Authors have imagined, that the Nervous Juice contributed to the composition of the *Saliva*; the rather because larger and more numerous Twigs of Nerves are communicated to these Glands, than to most other Parts, which yet have a more exquisite feeling than these. Dr. *Nuck* has refuted this Opinion by several Experiments.

Too great an Excretion of *Saliva*, *Boerhaave* observes, disorders the first Digestion; and hence causes Thirst, Dryness, a black Bile, Consumption, Atrophy : On the contrary, if no *Saliva* be discharged into the Mouth, or less than ordinary, it spoils both the Manducation of the Food, and its Taste, Swallowing, and Digestion; and withal, occasions Thirst.

**SALIVAL**, or *Salivary Ducts*, in Anatomy, certain little Canals lately discovered; whereby the Saliva falls into the Mouth. The *Lower Salival Duct* comes from the *Maxillary* Glands, situate under the lower Jaw, and terminated behind the *Dentes Incisores*. It was first described by out Dr. *Wharton*, in his Treatise of the *Glands*, in 1656. It comes from the Parotid Glands; whence perforating the *Buccinator*, it terminates near the third Upper Grinder. *Casp.*

*Bartholine*, in 1682, discovered another *Salival Duct*, coming from the Glands situate on the Side of the Tongue; tho' *Rivinus*[2], a Physician of *Leipsic*, had mentioned it before, in a Dissertation printed in 1679. *Anth. Nuck*, Professor at *Leiden*, discovered a fourth *Salival Duct*, arising from a Gland situate in the Orbit of the Eye, between the *Musculus Obductor*, and the Upper Part of the *Os Jugale*. These Ducts are all double, there being one of each Kind on either Side. But 'tis pretended, the Two last are only found in some Brutes, and not in Man.

As the Demand of *Saliva* is greatest in Mastication, Deglutition, Talking, &c. so, Dr. *Drake* observes the Disposition of the *Salival Ducts*, to favour the Discharge on those Occasions, is very remarkable : Thus the Ducts of the *Parotides* pass close over the *Musculi Masseleres*, and tho' the *Buccinators*. The *Salival Ducts* of the *Maxillary Glands* pass close under the *Mylohyiodeus*, where the *sublingual* Glands are placed; by means whereof,

[1] This is probably Jean Baptiste Gastaldi (1674 – 1747), a French physician.

[2] Augustus Quirinus Rivinus, born August Bachmann (1652 – 1723), a German physician and botanist.

the Intumescence of the *Masseters*, in Chewing, accelerate the Spittle in the *Parotid Salival Ducts*; as the *Mylohyiodeus* does in the Action of Deglutination, in drawing the *Hyiodes* upwards. The agitation of the Cheeks and Lips, is Sufficient to promote the Discharge from the Glands of the Lips, &c.

**SALIVATION**, in Medicine, a promoting of the Flux of *Saliva*, by Means of Medicines; chiefly Mercury. The chief Use of *Salivation* is in Diseases adhering to the Glands, and the *Membrana Adiposa*; principally in the cure of the Venereal Disease. 'Tis sometimes also used in Epidemic Diseases.

The Body is prepared for *Salivation* by a copious and continued Use of attenuating, diluting, softening Decoctions; as of Scabious, Pellitory, China, Sarsparilla, Sassafras and Santal.

*Salivation* is either *Partial* or *Universal*. By the first, only, the Humours of some Part of the Body are to be discharged; as in *Catarrhs, Tooth-ach*, &c. By the second, the whole Mass of Blood is to be purged. The first is raised by a flow continued Chewing of some tenacious Matter, as Mastich, Wax, Myrrh; especially if other sharp Things be mixed with them, as Pyrethrum or Bartram, Ginger, or Pepper. Or by drawing in sharp irritating Vapours, as those of Tobacco, Rosemary, Thyme, Marjoram, &c.

The latter is affected by the Action of such Medicines as create some slight but constant *Nausea*; as *Stibium* not quite fixed, nor yet quite Emetic; a little common Vitriol, &c. but chiefly such as dissolve all the Parts of the Mass of Blood, turn them into *Lympha*, and thus cause a *Ptyalism*. Such is crude Quicksilver, Cinnabar, a Solution of Quicksilver in *Aqua-fortis*, White and Red Precipitate, Turbith Mineral, sweet Sublimate of Mercury, &c.

*Mercurial Salivation*, is now a very usual Method of Cure; especially in Venereal Scrophulous, and Hypochondriac Cases. In Effect, it proves the surest Remedy yet discovered for the *Lues*; tho' the Discovery hereof, as that of most other Remedies, is owing to Chance. *Jac. Carpi*, a Physician of *Boulogne*, having reading *Avicenne* and *Mesue*, Two *Arab* Authors, that Mercury applied externally, was proper for the *Lepra*, and some Kinds of Pustules, particularly in the *Scabies* or the Itch; had a Mind to try it in a Pocky Itch : A *Salivation* was hereupon unexpectedly raised, and the Patient was cured not only of his Itch, but of his Pox. The same Method he afterwards used for the Pox itself; and meeting with great success therein, others were induced to follow him; and thus did it arrive at its present Height.

There are two Manners of applying Mercury to raise a *Salivation* : The one *external*, by mixing it up with some Unguent, Plaister, or Perfume, and then rubbing it on the Joints, &c. The other *internal*, where 'tis taken at the Mouth. In each Case the Mercury insinuates it self into the Mass of Blood, and mixing with the Venereal Poison, the Two Bodies thus locked together, are drawn, with the Serosity, into the *Salival* Glands, where they are separated and discharged, as finding the Pores of the Glands proportioned to their Figures, and proper to receive them.

Dr. *Quincy*, will have the internal to be much the safer, and better Method. The Mineral Globules, he thinks, being intimately combined with Salts, in the Preparations given inwardly, will, by the Irritation thereof, be easily and fully thrown off by the Secretory Organs, 'till the Blood is quite discharged of its Load: Whereas, in Mercurial Frictions, some of the heavy Particles may be left lodged in the Interstices of the Fibres, or Cells of the Bones. Add to this, that by computing the Proportion of Mercury in all the Doses necessary to promote a Spitting, internally; and the Weight of the same Mineral used when 'tis done by Unction; the Quantity used in the latter Case, far exceeds that in the former; consequently, the ill Effects apprehended from that dangerous Medicine, must be vastly more sensible in the one Case than the other. The external Application, therefore, is only to be allowed of, where either the Case will bear the Violence of such a Management, or outward Ulcers and Tumours, require a particular Cure by Linements.

Indeed, a great *French* Physician, M. *Chicoyneau*[1], Chancellor of the University of *Montpellier*, has lately done some Discredit to the Practice of *Salivating* in any Manner; And that, in a little Treatise lately published, where he endeavours to prove, That the *Salivation* it self contributes nothing to the Cure, but is rather prejudicial thereto : That the Salutary effects of the Mercury are independent of any Evacuation at all; and that it acts purely as a Specific. 'Tis without Reason, therefore, he urges, that Venereal Patients are put to the Torture of a *Salivation*, since the full Effect of the Medicine is had without carrying Matters that extremity. The *Salivation* is only an Accident to the Cure; which is effectually obtained by a Mercurial Unguent rubbed on the Joints in such Quantities, and at such Intervals, as no to raise any *Salivation*. He supports the whole by the Experience of Forty or Fifty Cures wrought in one Year, by the New Method. This Method, it seems, has been lately, too, tried in *England*, and with Success; as appears from a Translation of *Chicoyneau's* Piece just published with Notes.

**SALT**, *Sal*, in Chymistry, a simple, acid Substance which enters the Composition of all Bodies, and is held one of the Five *Principles*, or Elements thereof; only to be extracted by Fire. *Salt*, M. *Homberg* observes, is an Ingredient in all Animal, Vegetable, and Mineral Bodies, excepting perhaps some Metals, and Stones. In Vegetables and Mineral Bodies, that have undergone a Fermentation, the *Salt* rises first in the Alembic, then the Phlegm : If the Mixt have undergone a Fermentation, the Salt rises after the Phlegm.

*Salts* are distinguished, with Regard to the Manner of extracting them, &c. into *Volatile*, *Fixed*, and *Essential*. *Volatile Salts*, are those light, subtle ones, which rise easily on Distillation, or are even exhaled by the Nose, and rendered sensible to the Smell. *Fixed Salts* are such as, being more Gross, and Material, resist and sustain the Fire; and are not raised by it, but remain, after Calcination, or Distillation, in the Earthy Part, at the Bottom. *Essential Salts* those drawn from Vegetables, without the use of Fire, as by Crystallization, and other easy, natural Means. *Volatile Salts* become distinguishable to the Nose, Tongue, and Brain, by their Tenuity and Briskness; *Fixed Salts* by their Bitterness, and Heat in the Mouth. To these may be added an intermediate Kind of Salt, under the Title of Mixed Salts; which are those resulting from a Mixture of a *Volatile* with *Fixed Salt*.

[1] Francois Chicoyneau (1672 – 1752), a French physician.

*Salts* of different Kinds, according to the different Matters wherewith they are found mixed: Some are mixed Bodies themselves, and their Mixture separable by Fire, and Lixiviation; such are all Essential Salts of Plants, and all Fossil Salts, &c. but these are no proper Chymical Principles. There are other which we are sensible are mixed, and whose Mixture we know pretty nearly, though we are not yet able to decompound them : 'Tis these make the Chymical Principle Salt; for our Analyses will not render them more Simple, which is the Character of a Principle : And in this Sense Salt is defined, *A Matter dissoluble by Water*, and unchangeable by Fire; to which some add, *Of a pungent Taste.*

There are three Kinds, or Classes of *Salts*, which come under this Definition; Two whereof are *Volatile*, and the Third *Fixed*. The *Volatile* ones, are *Acid Salts*, and *Urinous Salts*; the *Fixed*, are those drawn by a Lixivium after Calcination, and called *Lixivious Salts*. Nature produces none of these *Salts* simple and unmixed, but we easily extract them by Art, from the Mixts wherein she has placed them. The Principal Natural *Salts* may be reduced to *Salt-petre*, *Sea-Salt*, and *Vitriol*. Each of which has its different Kinds; of the various Combination whereof, with different Oily Matters, all the Natural *Salts*, we know of, are compounded. These *Salts* are found, by Chymical Analyses, to consist of Aqueous, Earthy, Oily, or Sulphurous, and Acid Particles. The Acid Matter is the *Pure Salt*, or the *Salt-Principle*, and is the Base of all the rest. This M. *Homberg* observes, is pretty uniform, and nearly the same in all *Salts*, before the particular Determination to form this or that Salt, by the particular Admixture of the Sulphur, &c. *Salt petre*, *Sea-Salt*, &c. therefore are not Principles, but the *Acid Salts* distilled from them are, and the Water wherein these *Salts* swim, and the Earth, or *Fixed Salt*, remaining in the Retort after Distillation, are other Chymical Principles.

The Principal *Salt* is held a *Mean* between the *Active* and *Passive* Principles. The pure *Acid*, though accompanied with its sulphurous determinating Matter, never becomes sensible but when lodged in some earthy Matter, or artificially in some simple aqueous Matter. In the first Case, it appears under the Form of a crystallized *Salt*, as *Salt petre*, &c. In the second Case, it appears in the Form of an Acid Spirit, which, according to the Determination of the Sulphur that accompanies it, is either Spirit of Nitre, or Spirit of *Common Salt*, or Spirit of Vitriol; and what we have here observed of the three Simple, or *Fossile Salts*, may be applied to all other more Compound *Salts* of Plants, Animals, &c. with this difference, That when, in Form of a *Concrete Salt*, these last always take a greater Quantity of earthy Matter, and when in Form of an Acid Spirit, a great Quantity of aqueous Matter, than the Simple ones. Whence it follows, that the Acid Spirits of Compound *Salts* are always weaker, lighter, and less penetrating than those of *Fossile Salts*; and after Distillation leave a great Quantity of earthy Matter behind them.

We don't know precisely what Figures the three *Salt-Principles*, *Acid*, *Urinal*, and *Lixivial*, must have. But to judge by their Effects, one would conclude, the *Acids* to be pointed, only the Points sheathed in some sulphurous Matter. The *Urinous Salts* to be Spunges, containing some of the *Acid*, and some of the foetid Oil of the Animal or Plant : And the *Lixivious Salts* to be Spunges, only containing the remainder of the Acid, which the calcining Fire could not expel.

*Acid Spirits* may be conceived as pure, and without any Mixture; in which Case all Acids will be found of the same Nature : But if we consider them as Distillation gives them, we shall always find them accompanied with some sulphurous Matter, which we cannot separate from them, and which gives the Degree of Activity to the Acid Spirits. 'Tis this sulphurous Matter which characterizes them, and makes all the Difference we find between Acid Spirits. M. *Homberg* ranges all the Kinds of Acid Spirits under Three different Classes, according to the different sulphurous Matters which accompany them.

The First Class is of those which contained Animal or Vegetable Sulphur; under which come all Acids, distilled from Plants, Fruits, Woods, &c. as also Spirit of Nitre. 'Tis easy to conceive, that the Acids of Plants may have retained a Part of the Oil of the Plant, which is their Sulphur; since in reducing these Acids into *Salts*, we always find a little Oil therein; which can be nothing else but that of the Plants themselves. And for *Salt-petre*, as this is always drawn from Earths moistened with the Excrements of Animals, or from old Walls, Plaister, &c. full of the sulphurous Matters of the Animals that lived within them, the Soot, &c. 'tis thence, doubtless, *Salt-petre* borrows its Sulphur.

The Second Class is of those which contain a bituminous Sulphur: Under which come the Acids of Vitriol, Common Sulphur, and Alum. For those are all usually drawn from the same Mineral Stone, wherein the bituminous Matter, which makes one of the Principal Parts of Common Sulphur, predominates.

The Third Class is of those which contain a more fixed mineral, sulphurous Matter; approaching nearer the Properties of Metaline Sulphur : Under which Class come the Acids drawn from several Kinds of *Sea-Salts*, *Rock-Salts*, &c. For the *Rock-Salt*, or *Sal Gemmæ*, is always found in Places near Metallic Mines; and *Sea-Salt*, in all Appearance, is nothing but *Rock-Salt*, the Quarries whereof have been penetrated by Sea-Water, which has extracted all Saltness therefrom.

The sulphurous Matters of the First Class of Acids being very light, and taking up a deal of Place, must augment the Bulk of the Points of the Acids to which they are joined. And hence these Acids become disabled from penetrating very compact Bodies; but their Surface being increased from the same Cause, the Flame will have the greater Hold to drive them : And hence the Acids of this Class act more swiftly than any of the rest. The bituminous Sulphur is the least active of all the Sulphurs we know, as being loaden with a great Quantity of earthy Matter, which serves it as a Matrix. Hence it unites more difficultly with Saline Matters than any of the other Sulphurs; so that a less Quantity of it may be conceived to adhere to the Acids of this, than of either of the other Classes.

Accordingly we find, that the Acids of this Class, used alone, scarce dissolve any Metals; but mixed with the others, partake of their Sulphur, and thereby become enabled to dissolve all Metals. The Metalick-Sulphur is of all others the most fixed; that is, its Parts are the smallest , and most compact. Hence the Points of this Class of Acids will not be much swelled by it, and of consequence will be able to insinuate themselves into the most compact

Bodies, or those whose Pores are the smallest. And for the same Reason they will not give much hold to the Flame that agitates them, and will therefore act with less Violence than those of the First Class of *Salts*. Acids joined to *Fixed Salts*, compose *Mixed Salts*. Thus Spirit of *Nitre*, with *Salt* of *Tartar*, make *Salt-petre*; and Spirit of *Salt*, with *Salt* of *Tartar*, make a true *Common Salt*; and Spirit of *Vitriol*, with *Salt* of *Tartar*, a true *Vitriol*. However, the two ingredient Salts still remain, the one *Fixed*, the other *Volatile* : Acids joined with *Urinous Salts*, compose another Kind of *Salts*, called *Sales Ammoniaci*, which are always *Volatile*.

*Lixivious* and *Urinous Salts*, are called *Alcalies*, the first a *Fixed Alcali*, the second a *Volatile Alcali*. These *Alcalies* are usually esteemed Antagonists to the *Acid Salts*, because their Mixture always occasions a sudden Ebullition. But 'tis more probable this Ebullition is not the Effect of a Combat, but rather a Proper Junction and Union of two Matters which had been naturally united together, and only separated by the Fire, and now re-place themselves in the same Parts whence the Flame had tore them off. Hence, the one are compared to Sheaths, and the other to Points fit to be sheathed therein. Now, the Precipitation wherewith the Points of the *Acids* enter the Pores of the *Alkalies*, tears asunder their Contexture, and reduces them into minute Parts invisible to the Eye; and thus is the Business of *Dissolution* accounted for.

The Principal *Chymical Salts* of Use in Medicine are; Salt of *Urine*, of *Lavendar*, of *Viper*, of *Human Blood*, or *Wormwood*, of *Guayac*, of *Quinquina*, of *Tobacco*, of *Rhubarb*, of *Rosemary*, of *Calaureum*, of *Sage*, of *Juniper*, of *Vitriol*, of *Amber*, of *Saturn*, &c.

**SALT-PETRE**, called also *Nitre*, and by the Chymists *Dragon*, *Cerberus*, and *Salt of Hell*, a Kind of *Salt* either natural or factitious; of very great Use both in Chymical Preparations, in the Composition of Gun-powder, and in Dying, in the Glass-Manufacture, and in the making of *Aqua Fortis* for the Dissolution of Metals. Its minute Parts, or Crystals, are in Form of Needles; though some will have them Triangular, as those of Alum are Triangular, and those of *Common Salt* Cubical. When perfect they are said to be fistulous or hollow, like *Capulæ*.

Of Natural *Salt-petre* there are two Kinds : The first formed of a natural Crystallization of saline sulphurous Juices distilling in Caverns, or along old Walls. This is what they call *Salt-petre of the Rocks*; the same with the *Aphronitre* of the Ancients.

The second Kind of *Natural Salt-petre* is furnished by the Water of a dead Lake in the Territory of *Terrane* in *Egypt*, called the *Nitrian Waters*, exalted and concocted by the heat of the Sun, much after the manner of our *Bay-Salt*. This is the *Natrum*, or *Anatrum* of the Ancients, which our Druggists call *Natron*; now little used but in the bleaching of Linnens.

*Artificial*, or *Factitious Salt-petre*, is also principally of two Kinds. The first, called, by some, *Mineral Salt-petre*, is found in several Places in the Kingdom of *Pegu*, and about *Agra*, in Villages anciently populous, but now Desart. 'Tis also found in some Places along the Banks of the *Volga*, that famous River, which after watering a good Part of *Muscovy*, empties itself into the *Caspian* Sea. The *Natural Salt-petre* is drawn from three different Kinds of Mineral Earths, Black, Yellow, and White. The best is that drawn from the Black, as being purest from *Common-Salt,* and needing no purifying after it come to us, to fit it for making of Gun-powder; as the rest do.

The Method of working it is thus : Two flat Pits are dug; one of which they fill up with the Mineral Earth, turning Water upon it for some time, and then tread it with their Feet into the consistence of Pap, letting it stand two Days for the Water to imbibe, and extract all the *Salt* therein. They then pass the Water into another Pit, where standing some Time, it shoots and crystallizes into *Salt-petre.* This they boil once, or twice, as they would have it more or less white and pure, scumming it continually, and filling it out into Pots, holding 25 or 30 Pounds each, and exposing these to the Air, in clear Nights; by which Means if there by any Impurity, it sinks to the Bottom : They then break the Pots, and dry the Salt in the Sun.

All the *Salt-petre* we now have, M. *Homberg* observes, is drawn either from Earths moistened, and manured with the Excrements of Animals, or from old Walls, and the Plaister of ruin'd Buildings, which have been filled with Sulphurous Matters as well from the Animals which inhabited them, as the Soot penetrating them, and the Air incompassing them. However, we usually make a Division of *Salt-petre* into *Natural* and *Factitious.*

The second Kind of *Artificial* or *Factitious Salt-petre,* is that prepared from Nitrous Matters collected in old Buildings, Dove-houses, the Middle of ancient Ruins, &c. by means of *Lixiviums,* or Lyes made of Wood Ashes, and sometimes of those of Herbs. Of this there are great Quantities made in *France,* particularly in the Arsenal at *Paris,* where there is a Corporation of *Salt-petre* Makers appointed for the Purpose. The *Salt-petre* gained thus, they refine, by boiling it three or four times, and passing it successively through several Lyes.

Some Naturalists pretend, that the Earths, which have already serv'd for *Salt-petre,* may be re-animated, and made fit to serve again, by keeping covered for Twelve or Fourteen Years, and watering them with the Scum, &c. of the *Salt-petre,* and even with Brine.

Good common *Salt-petre* should be well clean'd, white, dry, and as free of *Salt* as possible. The best refined *Salt-petre,* is that whose Crystals are the longest, largest, and finest.

There are abundance of Chymical Preparations made with *Salt-petre,* as Spirit of *Nitre,* A*qua Regulis, Aqua-fortis, Crystal-Mineral, Sal-polychrest,* Butter of *Nitre,* &c.

The Philosophers generally allow the Air to be impregnated with a Volatile Nitre, or *Salt-petre,* which is thence communicated to Plaister, Mortar, &c. 'Tis probable it may derive from Soot and Smoak, which are actually found to abound with Volatile *Salt* of a Nitrous Nature. Dew and Rain are supposed to fertilize the Ground principally by their bringing down this Nitre.

*Salt-petre* has a Property of rarefying, or expanding itself to a prodigious Degree. 'Tis hence Gun-powder derives its Force, whereof *Salt-petre* is the Principal Ingredient. 'Tis computed, that when inflamed, it takes up above Ten Thousand Times the Space it possessed before.

**SAMIAN EARTH**, an Earth brought from the Isle of *Samos,* in the *Aegean* Sea. The best is called by *Dioscorides, Collyrium,* because used in the

Medicines of that Name. 'Tis white, very light, soft, friable, well-tasted, and a little glutinous on the Tongue. There is another Kind, harder and fouler, called *Ater-Samius*, in regard little shining Straws are frequently found in it, disposed like little Stars. Each Kind is esteemed very astringent, proper to dry, and draw Wounds.

There is also a *Samian Stone*, taken out of the Mines in the same Island. 'Tis white, and sticks to the Tongue when applied to it. 'Tis astringent and cooling, and is also used by the Goldsmiths to burnish their Gold, and give it a greater Lustre.

**SANDARAC**, or *Sandarach*, in Pharmacy, *Red Arsenic*, called also *Realgal* and *Red Orpiment*; 'tis sometimes also called *Sandaracha Græcorum*, in Opposition to the Gum.

**SANDARACH**, or *Gum-Sandarach*, called also *Sandaracha Arabum*, is a white Gum oozing out of the Trunk, and thick Branches of the great Juniper-Tree, by Incisions made in the Heats of the Summer. The little or common Juniper yields very little *Sandarach* : Its Fruit yields Oils, Waters, Salts, Spirits and Extracts of some Repute in Medicine.

The *Gum Sandarach* is an Ingredient in Varnish. 'Tis also reduced into an impalpable Powder, and used to prevent Paper from imbibing Ink. The best is in fine white Tears, free of Dust : The *English, Swedes*, &c. drive a considerable Trade therewith. Some will have it, that the *Sandarach* of the Juniper is not the right, but only that of *Oxycedron*, which see.

**SAND-HEAT**, or *Sand-Bath*, in Chymistry, one of the Chymists Fires, consisting of hot Sand, wherein Herbs, Flowers, &c. are infused in a Cucurbit. The *Sand-Heat* is esteemed gentle, digestive, and alterative.

**SANGUINE**, something abounding in Blood; hence *Sanguine* Temperament, or Constitution, is that where Blood and Heat predominate. *Sanguine* Constitutions require frequent Use of Phlebotomy. *Sanguine* People are usually observed to be brisk, bold, daring, and even presumptuous: Hence *Sanguine* Hopes, strong, assured, &c. Hopes.

**SANGUINE-STONE**, *Lapis Sanguinalis*, or *Blood-Stone*, a kind of Jasper brought from *New-Spain*, of a dark brown Colour, marked with Spots of a Blood-red; the *Indians* cut it in Form of a Heart, and use it in Hæmorrhages, immoderate Menses, and other Fluxes of Blood. The Patient applies it by grasping it in his Right Hand, having first dipt it in Water. 'Tis sometimes also hung on the Part whence the Blood flows.

**SANGUIS** *Caprinus*, or *Hircinus*, the Blood of the He-Goat, either wild or tame, which is prepared, with great Precaution, to be used in Medicine, and supposed to have very extraordinary Qualities. The principal Precautions are these : The Goat is not to exceed four or five Years of Age; 'tis to be fed a considerable Time with aromatic Herbs, and especially those of the Saxafrage Kind; to be drawn out of the Throat, or the Testicles, by cutting them; but neither what comes first, nor last to be used, the former being too full of Humidity, and the latter too thick; and that the Operations be only performed in *July*, and the Blood put into Earthen Vessels, and dried either in the Sun or the Shade, and, lastly, bottled up to be used occasionally.

Among other Specific Virtues attributed to Goats-blood, the two most considerable ones are, that it cures the Pleurisy without bleeding; and that it dissolves the Stone in the Bladder, by taking it in Vehicles proper for those Diseases. To be good, 'tis to be extremely hard and difficult to pulverize.

**SANIES**, in Medicine, a thin, serous Matter, issuing out of Wounds and Ulcers. *Galen* compares it to Whey. It differs from Pus, which is thicker and whiter : The *Greeks* call it ιχωρ, crude Blood.

**SANTALUM**, *Santal, Sandal* or *Saunders*, a hard, heavy, odoriferous, medicinal Wood, brought from the *East-Indies*. There are of three different Colours, Citron, White, and Red. The Trees whence they are taken are all of the same Kind; and 'tis supposed their different Colours only arise fro the Differences of the Climates where they grow. 'Tis about the Height of the *European* Walnut-tree. Its Leaves resemble those of the *Lentisk*, its Flowers Blue, bordering on Black; its Fruit of the size of our Cherry, green at first, but blackening as it ripens, and of a faint Taste.

The Citron *Santal* is esteemed the best. 'Tis brought from *China*, and *Siam*: Is yellow, heavy, and of a good Smell; 'tis used in Medicine, as also by the Perfumers. The *White-Santal* is less odoriferous' 'tis brought from the Isle of *Timor*. The *Red-Santal* has the least Smell of the Three : 'Tis brought from the Island *Tamassarin*, and the Coast of *Coromondel*.

The *Santals* are all held to be a little Astringent, to strengthen the Heart and Brain, and to stop Vomiting; and are frequently used in Diet-drinks, and medicated Ales, against Scorbutick Complaints.

**SAPPHIRE**, or *Saphir*, a precious Stone of a beautiful Azure, or Sky-blue Colour. The *Saphir* is transparent, yet exceedingly hard, so as scarce to bear being Engraven. Different Colours constitute different Kinds thereof; the deepest Blues being esteemed *Males*, and the whitest *Females*. The *Saphirs* of *Pegu* are the most esteem'd.

They are found in the same Mines with the Rubies. There are some also brought from the Kingdom of *Calecut, Cananor*, and *Ceylon*; from which last Place we should be furnished with abundance, if the King of the Island did not prohibit all Commerce thereof with Foreigners. The soft *Water Saphirs* of *Bohemia* and *Silesia* are of some Account, though far inferior to the Oriental ones. Many People value the *Saphir* beyond the Ruby and give it the second Place among precious Stones, *viz.* that next the Diamond : Others give that Place to the Ruby. Some Authors affirm, That a *Saphir* being heated to a certain Degree, between two Crucibles luted together, loses all its Colour, and becomes perfectly White; so as to deceive even the Jewellers themselves, and make it pass for a Diamond.

The Chymists make several Preparations of *Saphir*; as a Salt, a Tincture, an Essence, a Water, an Oil, &c. and there a few Diseases but they pretend themselves able to cure by Remedies composed thereof. The Superstitious attribute still more strange Virtues to it; as, that it grows foul, and loses its beauty, when wore by a Person that is letcherous, &c.

The Rabbins hold, That *Moses's* Rod, and the Tables he received on Mount *Sinai*, were of *Saphir*. The Word is derived hence, that in the *Hebrew* the finest Things are all called *Saphirs*; whence, in Scripture, the Throne of God is said to resemble a *Saphir*.

Our Druggists sell two Kinds of *Saphirs* used in the Confection of Hyacinth: The one red, the other blackish. The last, by reason of the deep tincture they give that Medicine, are very improperly used there : The former are little reddish Stones, of the Sine of Pins-heads, very hard, and difficult to pulverize.

There is a particular Kind of *Saphir*, called, by the *Latins*, *Oculus Felis*, *Cat's-Eye*, remarkable for a fine diversity of Colours, as well as for its Hardness, which bears a Polish equal with that of the true *Saphir*.

**SARCOCELE**, in Medicine, a fleshy Excrescence, very hard, yet indolent, rising up by little and little about the Testicles, or on the inner Membrane of the *Scrotum*. The Word is formed from the *Greek* σαρξ, *Caro*, Flesh, and κηλη, Tumor. Sometimes indeed it is painful, in which Case there is danger of its degenerating into a Cancer : It usually owes its Origine to some external Cause, as a Blow, a Bruise, or Contusion. Such Accidents occasion the nutritious Juices to stop, and to be collected in great Quantities in the relaxed, or compressed Pores of those Parts, by which Means is form'd that Kind of Flesh called *Sarcocele*. 'Tis a very troublesome and obstinate Disease, and is frequently incurable by any other Means than cutting off the Testicle.

**SARCOCOLLA**, a Gum oozing out of a thorny Tree, with or without Incisions. Neither Authors nor Merchants are agreed as to the Place where it grows : Some say 'tis in *Persia*, others, in *Arabia Deserta*. It comes either in Grains, or in Tears of different Colours; sometimes White, sometimes Yellow, and sometimes Red, but all equally good, provided they be very dry. Their Taste is bitter, accompanied with somewhat of a disagreeable Sweetness. 'Tis esteemed warm and drying; very good to consolidate and heal Wounds, whence its Name, which is from the *Greek* σαρξ, Flesh, and κολλα, Glue. 'Tis sometimes also used in Collyria to stop Defluxions, and take off Specks on the Eye.

**SARCOMA**, in Medicine, a fleshy Excrescence arising from the proper Nutriment of the Part where it grows, without any Defluxion, or Discharge of Humours from other Parts. If the Flesh be not repress'd and kept under, it frequently produces Pipes like Veins and Arteries, whereby it receives Nourishment, as we see in Wens. It yields a very fetid Sanies, and arises chiefly about the Fundament, the Neck of the Womb, Fractures of the Cranium, &c. The *Latins* call it *Fungus*.

**SARCOMPHALUM**, in Medicine, &c. a fleshy Excrescence of the Navel, from the *Greek* σαρξ, Flesh, and ομφαλος, Navel.

**SARCOTICKS**, in Medicine, Remedies proper to fill up Wounds and Ulcers with new Flesh; the same as Incarnatives. *Sarcoticks* should be detersive and moderately hot. Such are Sarcocolla, Dragon's-Blood, Incense, &c. The Word is form from the *Greek* σαρξ, Flesh.

**SARSAPARILLA**, or *Salsaparilla*, a Medicinal Plant, growing in *New Spain*, *Peru*, and the *East Indies*. Its chief Use is on Decoctions and Potions in the Venereal Disease, being esteemed a great Observant and Sweetner; and, on that score, sometimes used as a Tea.

Its Root, which is the Part in Use, divides its self into a great Number of Filaments, six or seven Foot long; of the Thickness of a Quill. 'Tis Grey without Side, and White within, only mark'd with Two Red Streaks. Its Branches creep on the Earth, or along the Trunks of other Trees, &c. as the Ivy does.

To be good, it must be very dry, its Filaments long, easy to cleave; and, in cleaving, must not yield any Dust : When boiled in Water, it must give it a Red Tincture. Some of the Modern Physicians doubt the Medicinal Virtue of this Root, as it does not discover much, either in Taste, Smell or Tincture.

There is another Kind, the Filaments of whose Root are thicker, growing in the Island *Maregnan*, on the Coast of *Brasil*. This is not esteemed so good as the former. There is a third Kind brought from *Muscovy*, the Roots whereof are still bigger, but good for nothing but to burn.

**SASSAFRAS**, or *Saxafras*, a Yellow odoriferous Wood, of a brisk aromatic Scent, somewhat resembling Fennel. 'Tis the Wood of a Tree growing in *Florida*, whereof there are whole Forests. The Natives call it *Pavama*, the *Spaniards* and *French* also, *Cinnamon-Wood*, because, at the Conquest of their Country, under *Ferdinand Soto*, in 1558, they imagined this to be the true *Cinnamon* Tree.

The Wood of *Sassafras*, chiefly its Bark, wherein its principle Virtue is supposed to reside, was formerly sold at an incredible Price, to be used with Sarsaparilla and Esquilina, in the Cure of the Venereal Disease.

'Tis very drying and hot, tho' not quite so much as the Guaiacum : It is somewhat come into Fashion in Families, as the common Tea, which the Shavings of it make agreeably enough; but the Scandal of being good in Venereal Cases, is a Detriment to it, and prevents a deal of Good being done by it.

Indeed, with some, it does not agree, especially at first, and in a Morning, as it affects the Head, like some Perfumes, and occasions Pains, Drowsiness and Vapours : But Use and drinking it, in the Beginning, and the Afternoon, will, with most Constitutions, wear out these Inconveniences.

'Tis esteemed in the Gout, Sciatica, and Green Sickness. Chuse that covered with a thick Bark, reddish, and rough, of a sharp Taste, and a strong aromatic Smell.

**SATURANTIA**, is sometimes used in the same Sense as Absorbent.

**SATURNINE**, a Term applied to Persons of dark, sullen, melancholic Complections; as being supposed under the Predominancy of *Saturn*, or at whose Birth *Saturn* was the Ascendant.

**SATYRION**, a Root called by this Name, because its fancied Promotion of Lust: *Dioscorides* distinguished this from the *Orchis*, but Mr. *Dale*[1] ranks it under that Tribe. It passeth for a great Cordial and Restorer; but its Shape, resembling an Human *Penis*, seems to be the only Foundation for the Whimsey of making it a Provoker to Venery, and to forward Conception.

**SAXIFRAGE**, a Medicinal Plant thus called from its supposed Virtue in dissolving the Stone in the Bladder, from the *Latin Saxum, & Frango*, I break. Its Leaves are almost round, indented, fat and shining, like those of Ivy. In the Middle of the Leaves rise Stalks, about a Foot high, which, at their Extremities, bear little white Flowers, consisting of five Leaves, disposed in Form of a Rose. Its Seed, which is very small, is inclosed in the *Capsulæ* of a roundish Pod. Its Root divides itself into several Fibres, at the Bottom, whereof are found little reddish Tubercles, like *Coriander* Seed.

'Tis these Grains are commonly called the Seed of the *Saxifrage*, and are used in Medicine. The best manner of using them is to take them infused in White-Wine, or in a Decoction in common Water. Some use the Decoction of the Root itself : 'Tis held a great Diuretick.

Dr. *Quincy* observes, That its Lithontriptic Vertue is but little seen in Practice. He adds, That the Simple Water thereof, sold in the Shops, is good for nothing; the Virtue of the Plant, if it have nay, consisting in something too gross to rise over the Helm.

Some take it to derive its Name from its growing in the Clefts of Rocks, which it seems to pierce through.

**SCABIOUS**, a Medicinal Plant, very common in the Fields, and flowers in *July*. It has a great Character amongst many Dispensatory Writers, but seems to grow much out of use to what it has been : It passes for a very great Pectoral, and to do great Things in Asthma's and Pleurisies, and *Etmuller* gives it Pre-eminence in inward Abscesses. It hath a Place also amongst the *Alexipharmicks*. But hardly any thing is in better Esteem for the Itch, and other cutaneous Foulnesses; whence it has its Name, *viz.* from *Scabies*, Itch, and upon which Account it is often met with in Decoctions, and sometimes in a Syrup, among such as are called Sweetners. Some call it the *Widow's Flower*.

**SCALPER**, *Scalprum*, or Scalping-Iron, a Surgeon's Instrument used to rasp, and scrape foul, carious Bones.

**SCAMMONY**, in Pharmacy, the inspissated Juice of the Root of a Plant of the same Name, growing in the *Levant*, particularly about *Aleppo*, and St. *John de Acre*. The Juice flows from an Incision made in the Root; and is afterwards thickened by the Sun, as 'twas pretended, but in reality by the Fire. The Tree is much like an Ivy, its Leaves in Form of Hearts, its Flowers white, and it creeps on the Ground, or mounts on other Trees, Walls, &c.

The good, genuine *Scammony* of *Aleppo*, is to be grey, tender, friable, and resinous; the Taste bitter, and the Smell faintish and disagreeable. The

[1] This might be Samuel Dale (1659 – 1739), an English physician and geologist.

*Scammony* of *Smyrna* and that of the *East Indies* are less valued. The first as being more heavy, hard, and black; the latter, though light, friable &c. is in reality only a Composition of common Rosin with some other violent Purgers. *Pomet* shews, that both Kinds are rather Poisons than Remedies.

The true *Scammony* is one of the surest Purgatives; but, at the same time, one of the most violent we have : Hence 'tis seldom used without Correcting it by some Preparation. *Scammony* now in Use, must be very different from that of the Ancients, at least in the Preparation; by reason the Ancients give it in much greater Doses : Hence *Fallopius* conjectures, the modern *Scammony* to be adulterated with Spurge.

Some give the Name of American *Scammony* to *Mechoacam.*

**SCAPUS**, in Botany, the strait Stalk, or Stem of a Plant, standing upright like a Pillar, or Column.

**SCARIFICATION**, in Chirurgery, an Operation whereby several Incisions are made in the Skin, with an Instrument proper for that Purpose. *Scarification* is chiefly practised in Cupping. It acts by stimulating and evacuating. *Salmasius* will have us write *Scarifatio* not *Scarificatio*, in regard the Word is derived from the *Greek* σκαφρος. See his Notes on *Solinus*, where he thus corrects the reading of *Plin. Lib.* XVIII. *F. Hardouin*[1] lets the old Reading *Scarificatio* stand; though he owns that the M.S.S. have it *Scarifatio*; but adds, That *Theod. Priscian* writes *Scarificatio.*

**SCARLET-GRAIN**, a Matter used to dye a *Scarlet* Colour, usually taken for the Grain of a Plant. This imaginary Grain, called by the *Arabs*, *Kermes*, is found on a kind of Holm, growing in great plenty in the uncultivated Parts of *Provence, Languedoc, Spain* and *Portugal.* That of *Languedoc*, passes for the best, being big, and of a very bright Red; that of *Spain* is the worst, being very thin, and of a blackish Red; 'tis to be gathered when ripe, and is only good while new, that is, within the Compass of the Year, after which time a kind of Insert is found in it, that eats out the Heart thereof.

*F. Plumier* has made some particular Discoveries on the Subject of *Scarlet-Grain.* The *Arabic* Term *Kermes* , which signifies little Worms, he observes, agrees perfectly to the Nature of this Drug; which is the Work of a Worm, and not the Grain or Seed of a Tree, as is generally supposed. The Shrub 'tis found on, is the *Hexaculeate Cocci Glandifera*; on the Leaves, and little Shoots whereof, are seen, in the Spring Time, a kind of little Vesicle, which is at first not bigger than a Grain of Millet, and is occasioned by the puncture of an Insect, which deposites its Eggs therein.

In Proportion as it grows, it becomes covered with a kind of Ash-coloured Down, which hides the red Colour underneath. And when 'tis arrived at Maturity, which those who gather them know very well, 'tis taken from the Tree, in Form of a little Gall. The Pod, or Skin, is very light and brittle, covered with a fine membranous Pellicle all around, except at the Place where it grows to the Leaf. A second Skin, under the first, is full of a kind of Dust, partly Red, and partly White. Assoon as the Gall is gathered, the Juice

[1] Jean Hardouin (1646 – 1729), a French Jesuit scholar.

or Pulp is expressed from it; 'tis washed in Vinegar to destroy the little Insect withinside, which, without such precaution, would grow, feed on the Dust, and, at last, be hatch'd, and leave no more than an empty Shell.

The *Scarlet-Grain* is also of considerable Use in Medicine, where 'tis better known under its *Arabic* Name *Kermes. Menage* derives the Word from the *German Scarlak*, or the *Flemish Scharlaken* : Whence the *English* have form'd the *Scarlet*, and the *French* their *Escarlate.* Others derive it from the *Celtic Squarlera. Dalechampius*[1] will have it called *Scarlatum*, by Corruption, for *Caculiatum*, a barbarous Word introduced into *Spain*; others fetch it from the *Arabic Yxquer late.*

**SCELOTYRBE**; from Σκελος, *Crus*, the Leg, and Τμρβη, *Tumultus*, Uproar, signifieth those Pains in the Legs, that generally attend Scorbutick Habits, whence it is also frequently used for the Scurvy itself, and applied to some Medicines contrived against such Disorders.

**SCHIRRUS**, in Medicine, called also *Schirrome* and *Schirrosis*, a hard, indolent Tumor, form'd gradually in the soft, glandulous Parts of the Body; sometimes internal, sometimes external. There are two Kinds of *Schirrus's*; the one only beginning, and frequently painful when press'd by the Fingers; the other, confirm'd and senseless.

The *Schirrus* arises from a thick, viscid, probably gritty Matter, detained and indurated in the Pores and other minute Passages of the Parts affected. There are some *Schirrus's* as hard as Stones; some are even painful in their confirm'd State, and partake of the Nature of a Cancer.

The Word is form'd from the *Greek* σκιρρος, hardness.

**SCILLA**, or Squill, a Medicinal Plant, of the Onion-kind, but very large; chiefly brought from *Spain* : Used only in Infusion, and that generally in Vinegar, which it renders Emetic. There are two Kinds, Male, and Female; the Male are whitish, and the Female reddish. Their Infusion, when boiled into the Consistence of a Syrup, with Honey, called *Oximel Sylliticum* in the Shops, retains the same Properties.

They wonderfully deterge and scour off the viscid adhesions in the Bowels, and gently irritate the Stomach to Ejection. They are also, as all of the Onion Kind are, very Diuretick, and therefore in great Esteem, with some, in Dropsies : For if their Infusion be mixed with Cinnamon Water, they will seldom vomit, but work downwards, and very forcibly, by Urine : In Asthmas, and all Obstructions, or Infractions of the Lungs, which are to be removed by Detersives and Expectoration, there is scarce any thing more effectual. They are also esteemed *Alexipharmicks*, and upon that Account have a Place in the *Theriaca Andromachi.*

**SCLEROPHTHALMIA**, a kind of Ophthalmia, wherein the Eye is dry, hard, red, and painful. And the Eyebrows likewise; so as not to be opened after Sleep, without great Pain, by reason of their excessive dryness.

[1] Jacobus Dalechampius, born Jacques D'Alechamps (1513 - 1588), a French physician and botanist.

**SCLEROTICKS**, in Medicine, proper to *harden* and consolidate the Flesh, &c. of Parts they are applied to. Such as Purslain, Jubarb or House-leek, Psyllium, Morel or Garden night-shade, &c.

**SCORBUTUS**, *Scurvy*, in Medicine, a Disease very frequent in the *Northern* Countries, particularly in fenny, wet, humid Places, open to the North, &c. 'Tis accompanied with a great variety of Symptoms attacking the several Parts of the Body all at once.

Hence *Willis* says, 'tis not any particular Disease, but a Legion of Diseases. The most usual are Bleeding, Coughing, Vomiting, Difficulty of Breathing, Looseness, a Relaxation of the Parts, Swetting, a fœtid smell of the Gums, a falling of the Teeth, stinking Breath, reddish or yellow livid Spots, Pains of the Arms and Legs, Weariness, Faintings, Head-ach, &c. Some distinguish it into *Hot* and *Cold*; but there is little Foundation for such a Distinction, as the Cause is the same in all, *viz.* according to *Barbette* and *Decker*[1], a too thick Pituitous Lymph; whence various Symptoms in various Temperaments.

*Charleton* observes, That it arises chiefly from sharp, saline Particles, taken in by Inspiration, from Salt and corrupted Meats eaten, from bad Waters drank, from Nastiness, deep Chagrins, &c. He adds, That 'tis contagious.

Dr. *Quincy* will have it to consist in such a Constitution, wherein the Blood is unequally Fluid. And hence he observes, 'tis best remedied by Stimuli, Exercise, and such means as promote Sanguification : 'Tis now become so frequent, that there is scarce any Disease appears, but 'tis judged to partake of the *Scorbutus*.

The Cure is very difficult; and when the Disease is rooted, next to impossible. It sometimes goes off in a Flux by Stool, sometimes by the Hæmorrhoids, and sometimes by Urine, but more often degenerates into a Dropsy, Atrophy, Apoplexy, Epilepsy, or Convulsions. A very exact Diet is held of more Effect than the best Medicines; without this, it becomes incurable. Bleeding does not avail; strong Purgatives are hurtful : So is Sugar, and all sugar'd Things, *Mercurius Dulcis* used internally, so as not to salivate, but only raise a Sweating, is excellent. *Dolæus* undertakes to cure any *Scorbutus* in twelve Days time, by the use of this alone; only the Patient to drink nothing all that Time, but a proper Decoction, and to abstain from Acids, and Hog's Flesh.

*Charleton* recommends a continued use of Milk, particularly Milk Emulsions of Sweet Almonds, Decoctions of China, Broths, and other Anti-acids, and Analepticks. *Etmuller* makes the Basis of the Cure of the *Scorbutus* and Hypochondriacal Diseases the same, *viz.* copious Vomiting. Strong Catharticks, he observes, are prejudicial but gentle ones good; for the Body is to be still kept open.

He adds, That Vinegar is hurtful, and yet the acid Juices of Fruits and Vegetables, wholesome. Accordingly the use of Lemon Juice is much recommended by *Lister*. Milk, and all milky Things, while the Stomach is yet able to digest, are excellent. So are Martials. *Etmuller*, instead of Mercurials, recommends Antimonials. Thus much in the general; for the particular

[1] Cornelius Decker (1648 – 1685), also known as Cornelius Bontekoe, a Dutch physician.

Symptoms, particular Medicines adapted thereto, are to be used; only mixing Antiscorbuticks with them all.

The chief simple Antiscorbuticks are, Horse-radish, sowre Sorrel, Butter-bur, Scorzonera, Sow-thistle, Zedoary, Polypody, Elecampane, Guaiacum, Sassafras, Mustard-Seed, Nasturtium Aquaticum, Trifolium Paludosum, Oranges, Lemons, Juniper-Berries, Cream of Tartar, *Tartarum Vitriolum*, &c.

**SCOTOMY**, in Medicine, a Dizziness, or Swimming in the Head, wherein the Animal Spirits are so whirl'd about, that external Objects seem to turn round. See Vertigo.

**SCROPHULÆ**, in Medicine, Schirrous Tumours, arising usually about the Neck, and sometimes on other glandulous Parts, called also *Strumæ*, and popularly the *King's Evil*, or simply, *Evil*. The Word is *Latin*, formed by Diminution, from *Scropha*, Sow.

**SCRUPULUS**, *Scruple*; the least of the Weights use by the Antients; and amongst the Romans was the twenty-fourth part of an Ounce. *Scruple* is still a Weight among us, containing the third part of a Dram, or 20 Grains. Among Goldsmiths, the *Scruple* is 24 Grains.

**SEAR-CLOTH**, or *Cere-Cloth*, in Chirurgery, an external Remedy somewhat harder than an Unguent, yet softer than an Emplaster; though 'tis frequently used, both for one and the other. The *Sear-cloth* is supposed to have Wax in its Composition, which distinguishes and even denominates it. In effect, when a Linament or Unguent has Wax in it, it does not differ from a *Sear-cloth*.

*Sear-cloths* are a kind of Substitutes to Friction, for the raising a Salivation. They are usually compounded of resolutive Drugs, as Saffron, Myrrh and Aloes, incorporated with Wax and Gums, as Galbanum, Gum Ammoniac, and Saga-penum. The whole temper'd with Wine.

The Word *Sear-cloth* is supposed to be a corruption of *Cere-cloth*, and to be derived originally from the *Greek* κηρος, *Wax*.

**SEBESTUM**, or *Sebestens*, in Pharmacy, &c. a Fruit resembling a little Plumb; which when ripe, is of a deep red Colour, bordering on Black; very sweet, and the Flesh, or Pulp, glutinous, or sticky. The *Syrians* make a kind of Glue or Birdlime, of the *Sebestum*, called *Glue of Alexandria*. The Fruit is esteem'd Pectoral; but is little used in Medicine. The Stone within it is Triangular. It brought its Name from *Arabia*, whence *Pliny* observes it came in his Time into *Italy*.

**SECONDARY** Fever, is that which arises after a Crisis, or the Discharge of some morbid Matter, as after the Declension of the Small Pox, or Measles; and such a Fever is frequently dangerous.

**SECUNDA AQUA**, among Chymists, &c. is *Aqua-Fortis*, which has been already used to dissolve some Metal, &c.

**SECUNDINE**, in Medicine, the several Coats or Membranes wherein the *Foetus* is wrapp'd up, in the Mother's Womb, as the Chorion, Amnios, the Placenta, &c. thus call'd, because they come out in the second Place, *i.e.* after the Child, in Delivery. The Matrons or Midwives call the *Secundine*, The *After-Birth*, as being esteem'd a second Burthen, whereof the Mother is freed. Others call it, The *Delivery*, because when this is out, the Women is reckon'd to be perfectly deliver'd.

The *Secundine* must never be left in the Matrix; 'tis a foreign Body, which would destroy the Mother : 'Tis dangerous even to have a Piece of it left behind. *Hippocrates* observes, That Twins have always the same *Secundine.*

Dr. *Grew*, in his Anatomy of Plants, applies the Term *Secundine* to the Fourth and last Coat or Cover of Seeds; by reason this performs nearly the same Office in Plants, that the Membranes investing the Fœtus do in Animals. Indeed *Pliny, Columella, Apuleus*, &c. have used *Secundine* in the same Sense.

**SEED**, a Matter prepared by Nature for the Re-production and Conservation of the Species, both in Men, Animals, and Plants : Some Naturalists add, That even Stones, Minerals an Metals them-selves have each their proper Seed in their Mines, and are produced and perpetuated thereby.

**SEED**, in Botany, a Product of a Plant, whereby the Species is propagated. The Seed is frequently the Fruit of the Plant, as in the Case of most Herbs. Sometimes it is only a Part inclosed in the Fruit, and that in Form, either of Grain, Pippin, Kernel, or Berry.

The *Seed* is the natural Off-spring of the Flower, and that for whose Production all the Parts of the Flower are intended; So that when this is once well form'd, these several Parts of the Flower dwindle and disappear.

'Tis produced from the Farina of the Apices, let fall on the Heads of the Pistil, and thence forwarded to an Uterus, at the Bottom thereof, divided into several Cells; where, coming to receive the nutritious Juice of the Plant, it is first soften'd, then swell'd, increased both in Matter and Bulk, and at length comes its State or Maturity.

That the whole Plant is contained in the *Seed*, is an Opinion as old as *Empedocles*, and is still the prevailing Doctrine among the Generality of the Naturalists. Experience, the Microscope, and the Modern Philosophy, give it great Countenance. In effect, by the Use of good Microscopes, we discover, in the *Seed*, several of the Parts of the future Tree, only in Miniature; particularly a Root called the *Radicle*, and the Stem called *Pumule*.

In *Malpighi's* Life, we have a Debate between him and Seignior *Triumphetti*[1], Provost of the Garden at *Rome*, Whether the whole Plant be actually contained in the *Seed* : The Affirmative is maintained by *Malpighi*, with cogent Arguments; among which is this one, That in a Kidney Bean e'er sown, the Eye, assisted with a Micro-scope, easily discovers Leaves, a Bud, and even Knots or Implantations of the Leaves on the Stem. The Stem itself is very conspicuous, and plainly consists of woody Fibres, and series of little

[1] This may be Giovanni Batista Trionfetti (1685 – 1708), an Italian botanist.

Utricles. And whereas Seignior *Triumphetti* had objected, That by Poverty, Transplantation, &c. several Plants degenerate into others, particularly Wheat into Tares, and Tares again into Wheat : In Answer to this, which is one of the strongest Objections against that Opinion, *Malpighi* replies, That he is not fully satisfied as to the Truth of the Objection, for that both himself, and his Friends, making the Experiment, no Metamorphosis of the Wheat succeeded : But granting the Metamorphosis, 'tis the Soil, or the Air, or the Culture, is in the Fault. Now, from a morbid, and monstrous condition of Nature, there is no inferring her genuine and permanent State.

To the same Effect, Mr. *Leowenhoeck*, after a nice Observation of an Orange Kernel he had made to germinate in his Pocket, &c. concludes, "Thus we see how small a Particle, no bigger than a coarse Sand, is increas'd." A plain Demonstration, that the Plant, and all that belongs to it, was actually in the *Seed, viz.* The Body, Root, &c. Mr. *Derham* adds, That of all the *Seeds* he has viewed, except the Maple, the Plant appears the plainest to the naked Eye in the Nux Vomica.

The Fecundity of Plants, in the Production of *Seeds*, is very surprizing. M. *Dodart*, in the Memoirs of the *French* Academy of Sciences, computes, That an Elm, living 100 Years, ordinarily produces of it self 33000000 Grains; and adds, That had its Crown, or Head, been cut off, it would have put forth as many Branches, within half an Inch o the place where it was cut, as it had before; and that at whatever Height it were cut off, the Effect would have been still the same.·Hence he concludes, That the whole Trunk, from the Ground to the Rise of the Branches, is full of the Principles, or little Embryo's of the Branches, which, it is true, cannot all appear at once, but which being conceiv'd, as separated by circular Rims, half an Inch high, compose so many Sets of Branches, each whereof is ready to appear, and will really appear if the Head be lopp'd off just over it. Now these invisible Branches exist as really as those which appear. For whence else should they come? The Trunk cannot produce them, as being it self more than a packet of Fibres, destitute of all Action : Nor can the Sap, which, like the Blood, is fit to nourish the Parts, but not to form any new ones. The Branches thereof existed before the Tree was lopped, and if they had appeared, would have bore an equal Number of Grains as those which did. These Grains, therefore, they must already contain in little. On this Footing, the Tree may be said actually to contain itself, 15840000000 *Seeds*, wherewith to multiply itself as many times : But what we shall say, if each *Seed*, or Grain of a Tree, contain in itself another Tree, containing the same Number of *Seeds*? And, if we can never come either at a *Seed* which does not contain Trees, nor at a Tree which does not contain *Seed*? By this Means we shall have an increasing Geometrical Progression, the first Term whereof is 1, the second 15840000000, the third, the Square of 15840000000; the fourth, its Cube, &c to Infinity.

Several Species of Plants have always been supposed to be destitute of *Seed*, in regard, no Observation, no Microscope, no Anatomy, discovered any Thing like them: Such are the *Capillaries*, the several Kinds of *Fuci*, Sea-Plants, Mosses, &c. But the happy Industry of the present Age has discover'd the *Seeds* of some of them; and has left us out of all Doubt, that the rest are not without the same. The *Seeds* of Fern, and the Capillary Plants, were first discovered by *Ceasius*; and since, more fully and critically by Mr. *W. Cole*. The *Seeds* of some Sea-Plants, were discovered by the Count de *Marsigli*, and those of others, by M. *Reaumur*[1], the first mentioned in the History of the *French* Academy, for the Year 1712, and the latter for the Year 1711. The *Seeds* of some Kinds of Fuci have been discovered by Mr. *Samuel Doody*[2]; those of Coralloid Shrubs by Dr. *Tanc. Robinson*[3], as also, those of several Fungi, particularly Truffles, and *Crepitus Lupi's*, or Puff-Balls; and those of some other by Dr. *Lister*.

**SEEDS**, in Pharmacy, &c. The *Seeds* used in Medicine, &c. especially those imported from the *Indies, Levant*, &c. are severally described under their respective Articles, which see. Among those cultivated at Home, the Principal are the four *hot*, and the four *cold Seeds*, as they are called. The first are of those of Annis, Fennel, Cummin, and Caraway; the latter, those of Gourd, Pumpkin, Melon, and Cucumber.

**SEMEIOSIS**, in Medicine. See Diagnosis.

**SEMEIOTICA**, that Part of Medicine, which considers the Signs or Indications of Health and Diseases; and enables the Physician to judge what is, was, or will be the State, Degree, Order, and Effect of Health or Sickness. The Word is form'd from the *Greek* Σεμειον, *Sign*.

**SEMETS**, in Botany; Dr. *Grew* uses the Word for the Apices of the Attire of Plants.

**SEMINALIS CAPSULA**, or Seed-Bag, is the Husk, that contains the Seed of any Plant.

**SEMINAL** *Leaves* : Much the greatest Part of all Seeds sown in the Earth, come up, or shoot forth at first with little, plain, soft, and undivided Leaves; which, because they usually very different from the Leaves of the succeeding Plant Magnitude, Figure, Surface, and Position, are called *Seminal Leaves* : As the little embrionated Plant, which lies in Miniature in every Seed, is called the *Plantula Seminalis*.

**SEMINATION**, in Natural History, &c. the Act of Sowing or Shedding *Seed*; particularly that of Vegetables.

Assoon as the Seed is ripe, Dr. *Grew* observes, Nature takes several Methods for its being duly *Sown* : Not only by the opening of the Uterus, but in the make of the Seed it self. Thus, the Seeds of many Plants, which affect a peculiar Soil or Seat, as Arum, Poppy, &c. are heavy and small enough, without farther Care, to fall directly down to the Ground. Others, that are large, and light enough to be exposed to the Wind, are often furnished with one or more Hooks to stay them from straying too far from their proper Place: Thus, the Seeds of Avens have a single Hook; those of Agrimony and

[1] Rene Antione Ferchault de Reaumur(1683 – 1757), a French scientist and naturalist.

[2] Samuel Doody (1656 – 1706), an English botanist and apothecary.

[3] Tancred Robinson (1658 – 1748), an English physician and naturalist.

Goose-Grass, many; both the former loving a warm Bank, and the last a Hedge for its Support.

On the contrary, many Seeds are furnished with Wings, or Feathers; partly with the help of the Wind to carry them, when ripe, off the Plant, as those of Ash, &c. and partly, to enable them to make their Flight more or less abroad, that they may not, by falling together, come up too thick; and, that if one should miss a good Soil or Bed, another may hit. So the Kernels of Pines have Wings, though short ones, whereby they don't fly in the Air, but only flutter on the Ground.

But those of Typha, Dandelion, and most of the pappous Kind, have numerous long Feathers, by which they are wasted every way. Others are sown by being laid in springy elastic Cases, which, when they crack and burst, dart their Seed at convenient Distances : Thus, Wood-Sorrel having a running Root, Nature sees fit to sow the Seed at some Distance, the doing of which is effected by a white, sturdy, tendinous Cover, which beginning to dry, bursts open on one Side in an Instant, and is violently turn'd inside outwards. The Seed of the Hart's-tongue, and codded Arsmart, is flung, or shot away, by means of a Spring, wound, or girt round the Seed-case. When the Spring is become stark and tense enough, it suddenly breaks the Case into two Halves, like little Cups, and so flings the Seed.

Other Notable means of *Semination* are observed by other Authors : A Quantity of Fern-Seed, Mr. *Ray* tells us, laid in a Lump, on a Paper, the *Seminal Vesiculæ* are heard to crackle, burst, and by a Microscope, the Seeds are seen to be projected to a considerable Distance from each other. Dr. *Sloane* observes, That the *Gentianella flore Coeruleo*, or Spirit Leaf, requiring we Weather to be sown in, assoon as the least Drop of Rain touches the end of the Seed Vessels, with a smart Noise, and sudden Leap, it opens it self, and, with a Spring, scatters its Seed. The Plants of the Cardamine Family, throw their Cods open, and dart out their Seed upon a slight Touch of a Hand. Nay, Mr. *Ray* adds, That the Pods of the *Cardamine Impatiens* not only bursts open upon the slightest touch, but even by an Approach of the Hand to touch them, without any real Contact.

Other Plants sow their Seeds by inviting Birds, by their agreeable Taste and Smell, to feed of them, swallow them, and carry them about; thereby also fertilizing them, by passing through their Bodies. In such Manner are Nutmegs, and Mistletoe, sown and propagated.

**SENA**, or *Senna*, in Medicine, a purgative Leaf, much used in Compositions of that Kind : The Shrub which bears it, is cultivated in several Parts of the *Levant*, and grows five or six Foot high. It puts forth woody Branches, furnished with Leaves on one Side : Its Flowers are yellow, and yield a Fruit in Manner of a greenish flat Pod, containing several Lodges or Cells of Seeds, resembling Grape-stones. These Pods some Physicians prefer to the Leaves themselves.

There is also a Kind of *Sena* cultivated about *Florence*, but 'tis inferior to that of the *Levant*, as is owned by the *Italians* themselves. Father *Plumier* mentions a third Kind growing in the *Antilles* Islands.

M. *Lemery* distinguishes three Kinds of *Sena* from the *Levant*. The first brought from *Seyda*, called *Sena of Appalto*, that is *Custom Sena*, by reason of the Custom paid the Grand Seignior, for the Privilege of exporting it. The second comes from *Tripoli* : The third is called *Sena of Mocha*. The best of these Kinds is the first, which *Pomet* directs us to chuse, in narrow Leaves, of a moderate Size, shaped like the end of a Pike, of a pale green Colour, a penetrating Smell, soft to the Touch, &c.

The *Sena of Tripoli* holds the second Rank in Goodness. Its Difference from that of *Seyda*, consists in its Colour, which is green; its Smell which is very weak; and in a certain Harshness, or Roughness, which its discovers upon the Touch. Besides these three Kinds of *Sena*, and their Pods; the Druggists sell the Dust found at the Bottom of the Bales; which is a very poor Commodity; and yet much better than what they call the *Small Sena*, which comes with in the Bales, by way of Package, and which many hold to be a Plant of no Virtue, put in by Chance, or, at best, to increase the Weight.

The best of *Sena*, ordinarily found in our Shops, Dr. *Quincy* observes, is that which is sharpest leaved, and which smells freshest. The brightness of its Colour, and Quickness of its Flavour, are the Indications of its Goodness; for when it has lost is Scent, and grows dusky, it is good for little : This Drug, at first taking, is apt to nauseate the Stomach; and therefore, if a little Cinnamon, or a Dram or two if its distilled Water, be added, it passeth thro' with less Sickness. This is exactly conformable to the Sentiments of *Ludovicus*, who says, That the purgative Quality of this Herb resides in its mucilaginous or gummy Juice; which, the more it is divided, gripes the less in its Operation. *Rulandus* imagined a Sudorifick Quality to be in it; and accordingly order'd it in some Compositions of that Intention.

**SENSITIVE PLANTS**, a Species of *Plants*, call'd by the Ancients *Æschynomenous*, and by us *Sensitive*, *Living* or *Mimic Plants*, as giving some Token of *Sense*. These are such whose Frame and Constitution is so nice and tender, that at the Touch, or least Pressure of one's Hand, they will contract their Leaves and Flowers, as if *sensible* of the Contact. Botanick Writers mention many Kinds hereof; some of which contract with the Hand or a Stick; others with Heat, others with Cold.

The Truth is, many, of not most, Vegetables expand their Flowers, Down, &c. in warm, Sun-shiny Weather, and again close them towards Evening or in Rain, &c. especially at the beginning of Flowering, whilst the Seed is yet young and tender : As is very evident in the Down of *Dandelion*, &c. and in the Flower of the *Pimpernel*, the opening and shutting, whereof are the Country-man's Weather-wiser; whereby, *Gerard* says, he foretells what Weather shall follow next Day; for if the Flowers be close shut up, it betokens Rain and foul Weather; if they be spread abroad, fair Weather. *Ger. Her. Lib.*

**SEPIÆ OS**, Skuttlefish Bone : This is white and Spongy, and seems almost to be calcined by the Sun. It is rough and abstersive, and chiefly used in Medicine as a Dentifrice.

**SEROSITY**, in Medicine, an aqueous Liquor, mixed with the Blood and other Humours, *Degori* defines it, a sharp, bilious Juice, approaching nearly the Nature of Blood; but which, being extravasated, does not coagulate like Blood. Disorders of the Spleen are attended with *Serosities*. The Kidneys help to purge off *Serosities*.

**SERPENTARY**, a Medicinal Plant, called by the Ancients *Pistolochia*, and *Dracunculus*, and now by the People, *Snake Root*, and *Dragons Wort*. The Ancients were only acquainted with two Kinds of this Plant; the *Great* and the *Small* : But since the Discovery of *America*, the Botanists have added several others; as, The *Serpentary*, or *Snake Root*, of *Virginia*, that of *Canada*, and that of *Brasil*. They are all supposed to be Alexipharmicks, or Counter-Poisons; and as such are Ingredients in Treacle.

The Great *Serpentary*, called by the Antients *Dracunculus Major*, has its Stem very straight, smooth, and mark'd with red Spots, like the Skin of a Serpent; whence, probably, as much as from its Virtues, it is, that it take its Name. Its Root is big, round and white, covered with a thin Skin.

The smaller *Serpentary* has its Stalk much like that of the larger, only its Leaves are like those of Ivy; whereas those of the larger are folded in one another, after the Manner of Bastard Rhubarb. Its Root is round and bulbous.

The *Serpentary* of *Virginia*, called also *Viperia*, *Dittany*, *Snake Root*, and *Contrayerva* of *Virginia*, has its Leaves green and large, almost in Figure of a Heart; its Fruits round, and its Root, which is of a very strong Aromatick Smell, has, at Bottom, an infinite Number of long small Filaments, representing a Kind of Beard.

'Twas first brought into *Europe* from *Virginia* by the *English*, where 'tis esteemed a sovereign Antidote against the Bite of the Rattle Snake. We are told by Travellers, That this *Serpentary* does not only cure the Bite of the Rattle Snake, but that that Animal flies the smell thereof : For which Reason, the Indian, and other Travellers, always carry it with them on the End of Staff, to present towards the Snake, when, by Chance, they meet it.

**SERPENTINE**, in Chymistry, a *Worm*, or Pipe of Copper, or Pewter, twisted into a Spiral, and ascending from the Bottom of the Alembick to the Capital, and serving as a Refrigeratory in the Distillation of Brandy and other Liquors.

**SERPIGO**, in Medicine, a kind of Herpes, popularly call'd a *Tetter* or *Ringworm*. It consists of a Number of very small Pustules, rising close to each other, sometimes in a circular Form, with great Pain and Itching. It never comes to Digestion, and is not cur'd without Difficulty. For after it appears to have been quite extinguish'd, it frequently breaks forth again at certain Seasons of the Year. The common People use to anoint it with Ink : But where the Disease is fix'd, some Universals should be first applied.

**SERUM**, a thin, transparent, watry Liquor, somewhat saltish, which makes a considerable Part in the Mass of Blood. The Blood consists of two Kinds or Parts; the *Cruor*, or red Part; and the *Serum*, or wheyish, limpid Part.

Mr. *Boyle*, and some others, have taken the *Serum* to be more ponderous than the *Cruor*; but Dr. *Jurin*, in the *Philosophical Transactions*, from repeated Experiments, assures us of the contrary.

The *Serum* is, in reality, the same with the Lympha : 'Tis carried by the Arteries throughout the several Parts of the Body; when it returns partly in the Veins, and partly in the Lymphatick Vessels.

The Use of the *Serum* is to nourish the Parts of the Body; and to render the Chyle and Blood more fluid. Urine and Sweat, are nothing but Serum drained of their nutritious Parts, by repeated Circulations, and Secreted from the Glands of the Kidneys an Skin. The Redundancy, and other Vices in the *Serum*, are the Cause of various Diseases.

**SETON**, *Setaceum*, in Chirurgery, &c. a kind of topical Remedy, used, like a Cautery, or an Issue, to divert Defluxions from the Eyes; by making a Wound, in the Skin of the Hind Part of the Neck, which is kept suppurating, by Means of a little Skein of Silk, or Cotton, passed through it.

'Tis also applied to such as are apt to fall into Epileptic fits : 'Tis of more Efficacy than a common Issue, but is prescribed with much the same Intention. The Operation is frequently practised on Horses, &c. and called, by the Farriers, *Rowelling*. *Setons* evacuate with a gentle Pain; shake the nervous Kind; evacuate *Serum*, and give vent to Repletions.

**SHANKER**, in Medicine, a malignant Ulcer, which gnaws and east the Flesh; usually occasioned by some Venereal Disorder.

**SHINGLES**, in Medicine, a kind of Herpes, call'd also the *Milliary Herpes*. It consists of innumerable little Pustules breaking out in various Parts of the Body, *viz*. the Neck, Breast, Loins, Thighs, &c. The Place affected is somewhat Inflamed, and the Patient a little feverish. White Pustules arise and suppurate, and are succeeded by little round Scabs resembling Millet Seeds.

It is to be attack'd with Discutients; and the higher Pustules cut off with Scissars, and a Cerate of Oil and Wax to be applied. *Wiseman* observes, the *Shingles* comes near the Nature of a Psora, and are therefore to be cured with Mercurial Catharticks.

**SIDERATION**, in Chymistry, a Mortification of some Part of the Body; called also *Sphacelus* and *Necrosis*.

**SIDERATION**, the blasting or blighting of Trees, Plants, &c. by Eastern Winds, excessive Heat, Draught, or the like. See Blight.

**SIDERATION** is also used for a being suddenly benumb'd, and deprived of the Use of one's Limbs, Senses, &c. which the People call being *Planet-Struck*.

**SIGHT**, the Exercise, or Action of the Sense of Seeing. Our *Sight*, the noblest and most useful of all our Senses, Father *Mallebranch* shews, deceives us in abundance of Instances; Nay, almost in all : Particularly with regard to the Magnitude, and Extent of Things; their Figures, Motions, &c. Our Eyes do not shew us any thing less than a Mite : Half a Mite is nothing, if we believe their report. A Mite is only a Mathematical Point, with regard thereto; and we cannot divide it without annihilating it.

In effect, our *Sight* does not represent Extension, such as it is in it self; but only the Relation and Proportion it has to our Body. Hence, as Half a Mite has no Relation to our Bodies, and that it cannot either Preserve or Destroy, our *Sight* hides it entirely. Were our Eyes made like Microscopes, or were we ourselves as small as Mites, we should judge very differently of the Magnitude of Bodies.

It may be added, That our own Eyes are really no other than a kind of natural Spectacles; that their Humours do the same Office as the Lens in Spectacles; and that, according to the Figure of the Crystallin, and its Distance from the Retina, Objects are seen very differently; inasmuch, as we are not sure, that there are any two Persons in the World, who see them equally big. 'Tis even very rare, that the same Person sees the same Object equally big with both Eyes; as both Eyes are seldom perfectly alike : on the contrary, we generally see Things bigger with the left than the right Eye; Of which we have some very good Observations in that Journal of the Learned at *Rome*, for the Year 1669.

**SIGILLATA TERRA**, a Kind of Earth or Clay, dug in the Isle of *Lemnos*, thence also called *Lemnian* Earth; of considerable Use in Painting, and Medicine.

'Tis of different Colours, but most commonly red; heavy, soft, and friable; held very astringent, and, as such, used in Hæmorrhages; as also against the Plague and Poisons. *Pliny* attributes several other Virtues, which Experience does not justify; nor is it in that Esteem it anciently was; yet is still an Ingredient in Treacle.

'Twas anciently found in a Mountain, in the Neighbourhood of the City *Hephæstia*; where *Diana's* Priests went at certain Times, with great Ceremony, to dig it up. After a little Preparation, they made it up into Troches, and seal'd them with *Diana's* Seal; whence the appellation of *Sigillata, Seal'd*. 'Tis now brought from *Constantinople* in little Cakes orbicular, on one Side flat, on the other sealed.

**SIGN**, in Medicine, some Appearance in the Body, distinguishable by the Senses : Whence, by just Reasoning, is inferred the Presence, Nature, State, Event, of Health, a Disease, or Death.

Those which denote the present Condition of a Body, whether sick or well, dying or the like, are called *Diagnostic Signs*. Those which foretell the future State thereof, are called *Prognostic Signs*. That *Sign* which is proper to the Disease, and inseparable from it, as arising from the Nature thereof, is called a *Pathogenomic Sign*.

As all these are Effects produced by the Cause of the Disease, the Disease it self, and its Symptoms; they usually note the present Condition of the Matter which first produced the Disease, and even of that produced by the Disease. On which Footing, the Signs are all reducible to these three Classes, *viz. Signs* of the Crudity and Digestion of the Disease; of its Event, whether in Health, a Disease, or Death; and of its Secretion and Excretion : Which last Signs are called *Critical* ones.

**SIGNATURE** is also used by some Naturalists for the resemblance of a Vegetable or Mineral bears to any Part of the human Body.

**SILIQUA**, in Botany, is the Seed-Vessel, Husk, Pod, or Shell of Plants, of the leguminous Kind. Whence *Siliquous Seeds.*

**SILVER**, in Chymistry, is called *Luna*, Moon; and several Preparations are made from it : Particularly a *Tincture of Silver*, by dissolving thin *Silver* Plates, or *Silver* Shot in Spirit of Nitre; and pouring the Dissolution in another Vessel full of Salt-water. By this means, the *Silver* is immediately precipitated in a very white Powder, which they wash several times in Sprint-water. This Powder they put in a Matras; and pour rectified Spirit of Wine, and volatile Salt of Urine upon it.

The whole is left to digest in a moderate Heat for fifteen Days; during which, the Spirit of Wine assumes a beautiful Sky-blue Colour, and becomes an Ingredient in several Medicines. This is also called *Potable Silver*, or *Argentum Potabile.*

*Silver* is likewise converted into Crystals, by means of the same Spirit of Nitre; and 'tis this is called *Vitriol of Silver*. The *Lapis Infernalis* is nothing but *Silver* dissolved in *Aqua Fortis*, and left to crystallize.

**SIMILAR** *Disease*, a Disease of some simple, solid Part of the Body; as of a Fibre, with regard to its Tension or Flaccidity; of a Membrane; a nervous Canal, &c.

**SIMPLE**, in Botany, is a general Name given to all Herbs, and Plants; as having each its particular Virtue, whereby it becomes a *Simple Remedy*. The Simples brought from the *Levant*, and the *East-Indies*, where not known among us until the Year 1200.

**SINAPISM**, in Pharmacy, &c. an external Medicine, in form of a Cataplasm; composed chiefly of Mustard-seed, pulveriz'd, and mix'd up with the Pulp or Flesh of Figs, or with Briony, Garlic, Onion, Nasturtium, Euphorbium, Ranunculi or the like. The *Sinapism* excites a Redness, Heat, itching Tumour, ands sometimes a Blister on the Place 'tis applied to. 'Twas anciently in great Request; and still continues in Use for inveterate Diseases of the Head; long, continued Defluxions, &c. The Word is form'd from the *Latin*, *Sinapis*, Mustard-Seed.

**SINGULTUS**, in Medicine, a convulsive Motion of the Midriff, commonly call'd *Hiccoup.*

**SINUS**, in Chirurgery, a little Bag or Sacculus, form'd by the Sides of a Wound, or Ulcer; wherein *Pus* is collected. *Sinus's* that slope downwards, *Scultet* observes, are difficult to heal : Yet that Surgeon undertakes to cure any *Sinus* in a Week, by the Medicaments he describes on Page 338, and an agglutinative Bandage. He adds, that he never comes to make an Incision, till he finds that the Pharmaceutic Applications are ineffectual; and that for the Dilatation of the *Sinus's*, he does not use the deceitful Scalpel; as being more apt to deceive the Operator than the Patient.

**SINUS**, in Anatomy, a kind of Cavity in certain Bones, and other Parts, the Entrance whereof is very narrow, and the bottom wider and more spacious.

Of these *Sinus's*, we find several in the several Parts of the Body; particularly in the Basis of the Skull, on the *Ossa petrosa*, where the Ancients imagined their Use was to render the Bones more light : In several of the Joints of the Body, they serve to receive the Apophyses of other Bones. In the Duplicatures of the *Dura Mater*, are several *Sinus's*, which Doctor *Drake* observes to be venous Channels, form'd for the Reconveyance of the Blood. Of these, four only are considerable, *viz.* the *Sinus Longitudinalis*, which running along the middle of the convex Part of the Brain, sends out a Branch on each Side, between the Brain and Cerebellum, call'd the *Lateral Sinus's* : And the *Torcular Herophili*, form'd out of a Concourse of the *Lateral Sinus's*, and Pineal Gland.

They are all formed of the several Venous Branches, which return the Blood from the Brain and Cerebellum, and deliver their Contents into the Jugular Veins; where they are, as it were, the Roots. The Coats of these *Sinus's*, are furnished with strong Fibres, by means whereof, they are dilated by the Influx of the Venal Blood, and again contracted with a reciprocal Motion, like the Pulse of an Artery.

**SMARAGD**, a precious Stone of a green Colour, very Beautiful and Brilliant. The Oriental *Smaragds* are in the most Esteem, as being the hardest, and their Splendour the most vigorous; so as even to tinge the ambient Air with their Greenness. Great Virtues are ascribed to the *Smaragd. Cardan* and others say, it resists Plagues, Poisons and Dysenteries; that it refreshes the Spirits, &c. The Word is formed from the Greek, σμαραλδος.

**SMELL**, *Odor*, with regard to the Organ, is an Impression made on the Nose, by little Particles continually exhaling from odorous Bodies. *Smell*, with regard to the Object, is the Figure and Disposition of the Odorous Effluvia, which sticking on the Organ, excite the Sense of *Smelling*. With regard to the Soul, *Smell* is the Perception of the Impression of the Object on the Organ, or the Affection in the Soul resulting therefrom.

The Chymists teach, that Sulphur is the Principle of all *Smells*, and that these are more or less strong, as the Sulphur in the odorous Body, is more or less dried and exalted. Sulphur, they say, is the Foundation of Odors, as Salt is of Savors, and Mercury of Colours,

*Smell*, like Taste, consists altogether in the Arrangement, Composition, and Figure of the Parts; as appears from the following experiments of Mr. *Boyle*;

1°. From a Mixture of two Bodies, each whereof, is, of itself, void of *Smell*; a very urinous *Smell* may be drawn : That is, by the Grinding of Quick-lime, with Sal-Ammoniac.

2°. By the admixture of common Water, which of itself is void of *Smell*, or inodorous; another inodorous Body may be made to emit a very rank *Smell*. Thus Camphor dissolved in Oil of Vitriol, is inodorous; yet mix'd with Water, immediately exhales a very string *Smell*.

3°. Compound Bodies may emit *Smells*, which have no Similitude to the *Smells* of the Simples they consist of. Thus Oil of Turpentine, mixt with a double Quantity of Oil of Vitriol, and Distilled; after Distillation there is no *Smell* but of Sulphur; and what is left behind in the Retort, being urged again by a more violent Fire, yields *Smell* like Oil of Wax.

4°. Several *Smells* are only to be drawn by Motion and Agitation. Thus Glass, Stones, &c. which even when heated, yield no *Smell*, yet when rubbed and agitated in a peculiar Manner, emit a strong *Smell*; particularly Beech-wood in turning, yields a kind of Rosy *Smell.*

5°. A Body that has a strong *Smell*, by being mix'd with an inodorous one, may cease to have any *Smell* at all : Thus if Aqua-fortis, not well dephlegmated, be poured on Salt of Tartar, till it cease to ferment; the Liquor, when evaporated, will yield inodorous Crystals, much resembling Salt of Nitre. Yet when burnt, will yield a most noisom *Smell.*

6°. Form a mixture of two Bodies, the one whereof Smells extremely ill, and the other not well; a very pleasant aromatic Odor may be gain'd, *viz.* by a Mixture of Aqua-fortis, or Spirit of Nitre, with an inflammable Spirit of Wine.

7°. Spirits of Wine, by mixing with an almost inodorous Body, may gain a very pleasant aromatic *Smell.* This inflammable Spirits of Wine, and Oil of *Danzic* Vitriol, mix'd in equal Portions, then digested, and at last distill'd, yield a Spirit of a very fragrant *Smell.*

8°. A most fragrant Body may degenerate into a fœtid one, without the admixture of any other Body. Thus if the Spirit mentioned in the former Experiment, be kept in a well closed Receiver, it will soon turn to the rankness of Garlic.

9°. From two Bodies, one whereof is inodorous, and the other foetid; a very pleasant *Smell* may arise, much resembling Musk, *viz.* by putting Pearls into Spirit of Vitriol : For when dissolved they yield a very agreeable *Smell.*

**SMELLING**, the Act whereby we perceive *Smells*; or the Act, whereby we become sensible of odorous Bodies, by means of certain Effluvia thereof, which sticking on the Olfactory Organ, and briskly enough to have their Impulse propagated to the Brain, excite a Sensation in the Soul.

The principal Organs of *Smelling*, are the Nostrils, and the Olfactory Nerves; the minute ramifications of which are distributed throughout the whole concave of the former.

*Smelling* is performed by the odorous Effluvia floating in the Aïr, being drawn into the Nostrils, in Inspiration, and struck with such Force against the Fibrillæ of the Olfactory Nerves which the Figure of the Nose, and the Situation of the little Bones, render opposite thereto, as to shake them, and give them a vibratory Motion; which Action being communicated thence to the common Sensory, occasion an Idea of a sweet, or fœtid, or sour, or an aromatic, or a putrified Object, &c.

The Matter in Animals, Vegetables, Fossils, &c. which chiefly affects the Sense of *Smelling*, *Boerhaave* observes, is that subtile Substance inherent in the oily Parts thereof, call'd *Spirit* : For that when this is taken away from the most fragrant Bodies; what remains has scarcely any smell at all; but this pour'd on the most smell-less Bodies, gives them a Fragrancy. *Instit. Cap. de Olfac.*

*Willis* observes, That Brutes have, generally, the Sense of *Smelling* in much greater Perfection than Man; as by this, alone, they distinguish the Virtues and Qualities of Bodies unknown before; hunt out their Food at a great Distance, as Hounds and Birds of Prey, or hid among other Matters, as

Ducks, &c. Man having other means of judging of his Food, &c. did not need so much Sagacity in his Nose : Yet we have Instances of a great deal, even in Man.

'Tis found that the Laminæ, wherewith the Upper Part of the Nostrils is fenc'd, and which serve to receive the Divarications of the olfactory Nerves, are always longer, and folded up together in greater Number, as the Animal has this Sense more Accurate. The various Windings and Turnings of these Laminæ, detain and fetter the more of the odoriferous Particles.

**SMOAK**, a humid Matter, exhaled in Form of Vapour, by the Action of Heat, either external or internal. *Smoak*, Sir *Isaac Newton* observes, ascends in the Chimney by the Impulse of the Air it floats in : For that Air being rarefied by the Fire underneath, has its specific Gravity diminished; thus, being determined to ascend, itself, it carries up the *Smoak* along with it. The Tail of a Comet, this great Author takes to ascend from the Sun after the same manner.

**SNUFF**, a Preparation of Tobacco, made by reducing it into a Powder, fit to be taken at the Nose; in order to purge or clear the Head of Pituita. Ordinarily, Tobacco is only the Basis of *Snuff*; other Matters being added to give it a more agreeable Scent, &c.

The kinds of *Snuff*, and their several Names, are infinite; and new ones are daily invented; so that it would be as impertinent as 'tis impossible, to give a Detail of them. We shall only say, that are three grand Sorts; the first granulated; the Second an impalpable Powder; and the third the Bran or the coarse Part remaining after sifting the second Sort.

**SOL**, Sun, in Chymistry, is Gold; thus called from an Opinion, that this Metal is, in a particular Moment, under the Influence of that Luminary.

What should have been the principal inducement of torturing this Metal, with so much Violence to obtain from it some medicinal Virtues, Dr. *Quincy* observes, is not easy to be guess'd; unless it was to keep up the Authority of an ill-deserved Regard, and a Jealousy, that they could not be well in the common Opinion for Physicians, who could not do extraordinary Things in their Profession with a Metal, which had such a prodigious Influence on other Accounts.

Many, indeed, there have been, who have honestly opposed this Artifice; but the Contrary Sides have a long Time prevailed, and to such a Degree, that this Metal itself has not only bee transformed into all the Shapes imaginable for medicinal Purposes; but even its Name has been transferr'd to do Honour to, and enhance the Price of many other worthless Preparations, that bore any Resemblance to its sensible Qualities.

Hence many Tinctures of a yellow Colour, are presently the *Golden Tincture* of something or other. Most, indeed, acknowledge, that Gold in Substance, or reduced into the smallest Particles by the Hammer, as in the Leaf-Gold, is not digestible in the Stomach, so as to be transmitted to the Blood, and be of any Efficacy there. But there are, nevertheless, many, who are confident of its doing extraordinary Matters, if reduced into a Powder, by Amalgamation with Mercury, and by evaporating the mercury afterwards.

*Zacutus Lusitanus*, is one of the smartest Pleaders on this side the Controversy, against *Musa*[1], *Picus Mirandola* and *Platerus*[2]; who, besides many Instances of its Efficacy, urges the Authority of *Avicen*, *Serapion*, *Geber*, and many of the *Arabian* Physicians, with those of other Countries, and of later Date. *Quercetan*, *Schroder*, *Zwelfer* and *Etmuller*, with many other more modern, practical Physicians, fell into the same Opinion. But which side soever is in the right, the present Practice rejects all Pretensions to Medicine from it.

**SOLUTIO** *Continui*, or *Solution of Continuity*, a Term used by Physicians, &c. to express a Disease common to the solid Parts of the Body, wherein their natural Cohesion is separated. If this happen to a simple, similar part of the Body; 'tis called, simply, *Solutio Continui*. If on a compound, or organical Part, it acquires a particular Denomination, from the Nature of the Part, the Difference of the Cause, or the Manner of the Application; as, a *Wound, Rupture, Fracture, Puncture, Fissure, Contusion, Ulcer, Corrosion, Dilaceration, Exfoliation, Caries*, &c.

**SOLUTION**, in Physicks, the Reduction of a Solid, or firm Body, into a fluid State, by means of some Menstruum.

**SOLUTION**, in Chymistry, is sometimes used for the Analysis, or Reduction of a natural Body into its chymical Principles. In this Sense, *Solution* is the same with what we otherwise call *Resolution*.

**SOMNAMBULI**, an Appellation given to People, who walk in their Sleep; more usually called *Noctambuli*. The Word is form'd from the *Latin*, *Somnus*, Sleep, and *Ambulo*, I walk.

**SOPHISTICATION**, in Chymistry, Alchymy, &c. a Term particularly applied to the Counterfeit Works of fraudulent Alchymists, who use indirect Means of whitening Copper, gilding Silver, and giving other superficial Tinctures; as also of making Augmentations, by divers Mixtures, and other illegal Operations, to delude those, at whose Expence they are employ'd.

Hence the Term is also applied to Merchandizes, and other Goods adulterated, mix'd or alter'd by the Deceit of the Seller. Musc, at present, is almost all *Sophisticated*, as well as Bezoard, Balm of *Gilead*, Lapis Lazuli, and other valuable Drugs, *Canary* Wines are *Sophisticated* on the Place, before ever they come near our Ports.

**SOPORIFIC**, *Soporiferous*, or *Soporative*, a Medicine that has the Faculty of procuring Sleep. Such are Opium, Laudenum, &c. The Word is form'd from the *Latin*, *Soper*, Sleep : The *Greeks*, in lieu hereof, use the Word *Hypnotic*.

**SOPOROUS** or *sleepy* Diseases, are the *Coma* or *Catephora*, *Lethargy* and *Caurus*, which rather appears to differ as to more or less, than as to Essence.

[1] Abu Musa Jābir ibn Hayyān (712 - 815), also known as Geber, a Persian physician and alchemist.

[2] Felix Plater (1536 – 1614), a Swiss physician.

In this they all agree, That they induce a morbific Sweat.

**SPAGYRIC**, an Epithet given to Chymistry; which is called the *Spagyric Art*, or *Medicina Spagyrica*; and to Chymical Physicians, who are also called *Spagyrists*. *Vossius* derives the Word from the *Greek*, σπαουν, to extract, and αγενρειν, *congregare*, to collect; which are the two principal Offices of Chymists. *Paracelsus* first introduced the Word.

**SPARADRAP**, in Pharmacy, &c. an antient Name for a Sear-cloth, or Cere-cloth; smear'd on each Side with a kind of Plaister. 'Tis prepared by melting a sufficient Quantity of some Plaister or Unguent, and dipping a linnen Cloth therein, till such time as it have imbibed its fill. 'Tis then taken out, cool'd and polish'd on a Marble. There are as many different Kinds of *Sparadrap*, as there are of Plaisters for the Cloth to be dipp'd in. 'Tis sometimes call'd *Tela Gualteriana*.

**SPASMA**, *Spasmus*, in Medicine, a *Greek* Term, σπασμα, of equal Import with the *Latin*, *Convulsio*, and the *English*, *Convulsion*. There are *Spasma's* peculiar to certain Members, and distinguished by their particular Names: That of the Mouth is called *Spasmus Cynicus*; that of the Penis, *Satyriasis*, &c.

*Cardan* distinguishes two Kinds of *Spasma's* : The first consisting in a constant Contraction of the Muscles, which renders the Members rigid, and inflexible. The Second, in sudden, unnatural Motions and Palpitations, frequently intermitting and beginning again.

Accidental *Spasmi*, are of little Continuance : There are some arising from Flatulences; from Bites of Venemous Beasts, from the Puncture of a Nerve, the Acrimony of the Humours vellicating the Stomach, Vapours of the Matrix, excessive Cold, &c.

A *Spasmus* happening after the taking of Hellebore, or any other violent Purgative, is mortal.

**SPASMODIC**, something belonging to a Spasma, or Convulsion; as a *Spasmodic Medicine*, *Spasmodic Disease*, &c. Hunger, according to M. *Hecquet*, is a *Spasmodic Affection* of the Fibres of the Stomach; unless it arises from the Fibres being to much moisten'd by the Liquor thereof, so as to incapacitate them for their Office.

**SPATULA**, an Instrument used by Surgeons and Apothecaries; made flat at one end, and round at the other. The Surgeons have their little Silver or Steel *Spatulas*, to spread their Plaisters and Unguents withal. The Apothecaries have large ones of Wood, to stir their Drugs in diluting, tempering or boiling them. The Word is form'd from the *Latin*, *Spathus*, of the *Greek*, σπαθιον.

**SPECIES**, an Idea, which relates to some other more general on; or is compriz'd under a more universal Division of Genus. *Species* is a mere Term of Relation : And the same Idea may be a *Species*, when compared to another more general one; and a *Genus* with regard to a more particular one. Thus Body is a *Genus* with regard to an animate and inanimate Body; and a

*Species*, with regard to Substance. The last *Species*, is that which can only be divided into Individuals. Animal is a *Species*, with regard to Body; and Man is a *Species* with regard to Animal. God destroy'd Mankind by the Deluge; but he preserv'd the *Species*.

**SPECIFIC**, in Medicine, a Remedy, whose Virtue and Effect is peculiarly adapted to some certain Disease; is adequate thereto; and exerts its whole Force immediately thereon. Thus Quinquina, or the Jesuits Bark, is held a *Specific* for intermitting Fevers or Agues; Mercury for the Venereal Disease.

Authors make mention of three Kinds of *Specific Medicines*.

1° Such as are eminently and particularly friendly to this or that Part, as the Heart, the Lungs, the Brain, to Stomach, &c.

2° Such as seem to attract, expell, or evacuate some determinate Humour, by a kind of Specific Power they are endowed withal; as Jalap is supposed to purge watery Humours, Rhubarb, Bile, &c. And,

3°, Such as remove the Cause of a Disease, by some sudden Property, without our knowing how or why; or the Manner of whose Operation we are entirely ignorant of, and have only learnt their Effects by Experience.

In the Use of these last, there is no Enquiry into the Nature of the Disease; no regard had to the Symptoms or Phænomena : Nor is the Medicine at all to be adapted to the particular Circumstances thereof. All that we regard, is the Name of the Disease, and that of the Remedy: As, immediately, upon finding an intermittent Fever, we prescribe the Bark; to assuage Pain, Opium; to expel Poison, some Antidote.

A *Specific* Medicine, therefore, stands in Opposition to a *Scientific* or *Methodic* Medicine.

**SPECULARIS** *Lapis*, in Natural History, is a kind of Stone, clear as Glass, used in several Countries where 'tis found, for Window-lights, &c. 'Tis a kind of Talc, splits easily into thin Laminæ or Plates; and is sometimes calcined to make a fine Plaister.

**SPERMA-CETI**, in Pharmacy, usually call'd *Parmasity*, is a Preparation made from the Brain, and Cerebel of a kind of Animal, call'd by some, the Male Whale, and by the *Latins*, *Orca*; only distinguish'd from the common Whale by its having Teeth, in lieu whereof, the Whale has a kind of Tufts in its Throat.

It had its Name *Sperma Ceti*, Seed or Sperm of a Whale, given it, no doubt, to raise the value, by a Notion of its Scarcity.

The Antients were great Strangers to the Nature of this Preparation; insomuch, that *Schroder* seems in doubt, whether to reckon it an animal or mineral Substance.

The Method or preparing it, is a Secret in the Hands of a very few: The Process is thus;

The Brain being taken out of the Animal, is melted over a gentle Fire, and pour into Moulds, like those wherein Sugar-Loaves are form'd. When cold and drain'd of its Oil, 'tis taken out and melted over again; and this they continue to do till it be well purified, and become white. 'Tis then cut with a

Knife for the Purpose, and reduced into Flakes, such as we have it from the Druggists.

It must be chosen white, clear and transparent, of a rankish Smell, which some fancy to partake of that of the Violet : some sophisticate it with Wax; but that Deceit is discovered, either by the Smell of the Wax, or by the Dullness of the Colour.

Some also sell a Preparation made from the Tail of the Whale, instead of that from the Brain; which last kinds turns Yellow, assoon as opened to the Air. In the General, there is no Merchandise that should be kept closer from the Air than *Sperma Ceti*.

'Tis of some Use in Medicine. Dr. *Quincy*, says, 'tis a noble Remedy in many Cases, as the Asthma, &c. though chiefly used in Bruises, inward Hurts, and after Delivery. But 'tis certain, its greatest Property, and that which makes it so much in vogue, is its softening the Skin, and resolving Tumours of the Breast. Whence it comes to be used by the Ladies in Pastes, Washes, &c.

**SPERMATOCELE**, in Medicine, a Rupture occasioned by a Contraction of the seminal Vessels, whereby they are let fall into the Scrotum.

**SPHACELUS**, in Medicine, a total Mortification of any Part, occasioned by an Interception of the Blood and Spirits. The Word is *Greek*, σφακελς, form'd perhaps of σφαττω, *I kill*.

The *Sphacelus* is distinguished from the Gangrene; which is only a Mortification begun, and, as it were, the Road to a *Sphacelus*, which is the State and Perfection thereof. The *Sphacelus* is distinguished by the Lividness or Blackness of the Part affected; its Softness, Insensibility and cadaverous Smell.

The other Causes of the *Sphacelus*, are close Ligatures, excessive Colds, great Inflammations, Bites of Mad Dogs. 'Tis sometimes, also, call'd *Necrosis*, and sometimes *Sideratio*.

A *Sphacelus* Foot, according to *Aquapendente*, ought to be cut off in the mortified Part, near the live Part. When the Foot is off, the dead Flesh left behind, is to be consumed by the Application of an actual Cautery, repeated several Times, till the Patient feel the Heat of the Fire. *Scultet*.

**SPICA-NARDI**, Spike-nard, a kind of Ear growing even with the Ground, and sometimes in the Ground; used in the Composition of Treacle. It likewise should be used in the Compound Syrop of Chicory, in lieu of Cinnamon, which the Apothecaries generally out for it, because cheaper.

The Ear or *Spica*, is about the Length and Thickness of a Finger; very light, covered with long reddish Hairs, of a string Smell, and a bitterish, sharp Taste. There rise several of these Ears from the same Root. The Stem is small, and the Root the Thickness of a Quill.

The *Spica-Nardi*, is usually reckon'd in the Number of Roots. 'Tis also call'd *Nardus Indicus*; because brought from the *East Indies*.

'Tis accounted a *Stomachic* and *Nephritic*, proper to strengthen the Stomach, and promote the Discharge of Urine.

There is also another Kind, call'd *Spica Celtica*, growing in the *Pyreneans*, and the Mountain of *Tirol.*

**SPINA** *Ventosa*, in Medicine, &c. an Ulceration, wherein the Bones are eaten by a malignant Tumour, without any Pain of *Periosteum*, or Membrane that covers the Bone. After which, an indolent swelling being risen, the Part affected is quite eat out with the Ulcer; whence frequently follows a necessity of Amputation.

**SPIRIT**, in Chymistry, is one of the Principles of natural Bodies, called also Mercury. The chymical Principle *Spirit*, is a fine, subtile, volatile, penetrating, pungent Liquor, which arises ordinarily before the Phlegm of Water, and sometimes after it.

The great Properties of this Liquor are, that it penetrates and opens solid Bodies, corrodes, breaks, dissolves, and even dissolves certain mix'd Bodies; coagulates others, and produces an Infinity of Effects; and those even contrary to one another.

In the general, the Chymists call *Spirits*, all the fine subtile, and not aqueous Particles, raised from Bodies by Heat, and reduced into Liquors by Distillation; such are *Spirit* of *Vitriol*, of *Salt-petre*, of *Salt*, &c.

They also call *Spirits*, those aqueous Liquors drawn by Liquidation, when they are impregnated with Salts, or other active Principles, raised, together with them, by the Violence of the Fire.

These, when they excite any Sensation of Heat on the Tongue, are particularly called *Acid*, or *Sharp Spirits*.

When they make any Erosion on the Tongue, they are call'd *Corrosive Spirits*. Such as Taste somewhat like common Salt, are call'd *Saline Spirits*. Such as partake of the Taste of common Sulphur, are *Sulphurous Spirits*. And when this Taste is very strong, *Urinous Spirits*. Such as take Fire readily, *Inflammable* or *Ardent Spirits*. Such where the Acid predominates, though qualified with a little Sulphur, are call'd *Mix'd Spirits*.

In this Sense, the Chymists are said to draw a *Spirit* from Sulphur, Salt, and other Bodies, when they extract the Essence, or the subtilest Part thereof, by Distillation or otherwise.

*Spirits* is also a general Name among Distillers, for all distill'd Liquors that are neither Oil nor Phlegm.

**SPIRIT** *of Wine*, is only Brandy rectified once or more times, by repeated Distillations. One may likewise make a perfect Rectification of Brandy into *Spirit of Wine*, at one single Distillation, by using a chymical Instrument, consisting of several Cucurbites, described by *Glaser*[1].

**SPIRIT** *of Sulphur*, is a *Spirit* drawn from *Sulphur* melted and inflamed; the most subtile Part whereof, is converted into a Liquor, by sticking to a Glass Bell suspended over it, whence it falls Drop by Drop, into a Trough, in the Middle whereof, is placed the Stone Pot wherein the Sulphur is burnt. This

[1] Christoph, or Christophle, Glaser (1615 – 1678), a Swiss chemist and apothecary.

*Spirit* is held specific for the same Diseases as *Spirit of Vitriol.*

**SPIRIT** *of Salt,* a yellow Liquor drawn, by Chymistry, from Sea Salt. The best is that prepared in *England.* 'Tis much used in Medicine; but has not, perhaps, the Virtues ascribed to it. The common *Spirit of Salt,* being very corrosive, may be dulcified, by letting it digest three Days on a gentle Sand heat, with an equal Quantity of *Spirit of Wine* mix'd therewith.

**SPIRIT** *of Vitriol,* is *Vitriol* dried in the Sun, or in Defect thereof, the Fire, and then distill'd by Chymical Operations several Times repeated; first by a reverberatory Fire, and then in *Balneo Mariæ.* 'Tis held excellent against the Epilepsy, as well as against burning and malignant Fevers. The last *Spirit* drawn from Vitriol, and which is improperly call'd *Oil of Vitriol,* is use din the Dissolution of Metals and Minerals.

**SPIRITS**, in Medicine, are the most subtile and volatile Parts, or Juices of the Body; by means whereof, all the Functions and Operations thereof are performed. The *Spirits* are usually distinguished into *Vital* and *Animal.*

The Ancients, indeed, made a four-fold Distinction of *Spirits*; into *Vital, Animal, Natural* and *Genital* : Whereof the First they placed in the Heart; the Second in the Brain; the Third in the Stomach and Liver; and the last in the Testicles : But as this Division is founded on a false Hypothesis; 'tis now deservedly set aside.

*Vital* Spirits are only the most finest and most agitated Part of the Blood; whereon its Heat, and Motion depend.

*Animal* Spirits, are an exceedingly thin, subtile, moveable Fluid, Juice, or Humour separated from the Blood in the Cortex of the Brain, hence received into the minute Fibres of the Medulla, and by them discharg'd into the Nerves, by which it is convey'd through every Part of the Body, to be the Instruments of Sensation, muscular Motion, &c.

The *Animal Spirits*, call'd also *Nervous Spirits* and *Nervous Juice*, only differ from the *Vital Spirits*, in that these last are still mix'd and blended with the grosser Parts of the Blood, and circulate along with it : Whereas, the *Animal Spirits* are secreted thence by the Glands whereof the cortical Substance is composed; and have a Motion, Circulation, peculiar to them selves.

Dr. *Willis* conceives, that the *Animal Spirits* are prepared by a proper Distillation of the subtilest Part of the arterial Blood, brought by the Carotides into the Cortex of the Brain; and shews, that the Blood contained in the Sinus's of the Dura Mater, acts in this Distillation in the same Manner as Fire does in the chymical Distillations perform'd by Defluxion, where being placed over the Matter to be distill'd, it makes the subtilest Parts thereof descend.

The existence of the *Animal Spirits* is controverted : But the infinite Use they are of in the Animal Œconomy, and the exceeding lame Account we should have of any of the Animal Functions without them, will still keep the greatest Part of the World on their Side. And, in effect, the learned *Boerhaave* had gone a good way towards a Demonstration of their Reality.

The Blood brought to the Brain by the Carotides, and Vertebral Arteries, he shews, is infinitely prepar'd, secreted, elaborated and changed from its natural State, e'er it arrives there, insomuch as, contrary to the Nature of the rest, instead of cohering by the Fire, it immediately resolves wholly into a thin Vapour, without any Fæces behind. And is thus exceedingly well fitted for the Formation of so extraordinary a Fluid.

He shews, further, That the *Animal Spirits* are not form'd from the Cruor, but the Serum of the Blood, which *Malpighi's* History of the Growth of the Fœtus in an incubated Egg, shews to be divisible into Parts or Corpuscles, inconceivably smaller than the Cruor.

He adds, That the Nature of the Juice is such, as that no Salts or Oils in the Body can contribute any thing to it; and that in all appearance, 'tis only a most subtile, pure Water; which Liquor is found to resemble these *Spirits* in its extraordinary Miscibility, Mobility, Solidity, Softness, Simplicity, and want of Elasticity.

The same Author shews, further, from the Magnitude of the Carotids and Vertebrals, their straight uninterrupted Course, the great Quantity of Blood they bring, the Bulk of the Cortex, &c. that there must be a very great Quantity of this Liquor; that there is fresh prepared every Moment of Life; and that it is driven, every Moment, by the Action of Heat, &c. from the Brain and Cerebrel, to all the Parts of the Body furnished with Nerves; which Motion, he shews from the exceeding Fineness, Crookedness, &c. of the Ramifications must be very gentle, equable and constant, one Part continually driving before it another. Upon the whole, 'tis no Wonder it escapes the Notice of our Senses; and that no Ligatures, Wounds, Punctures, Injections or the like, make either it or the Apertures of the Nerves which it flows, visible : Nor does it avail, what some, who allow the Existence of *Animal Spirits*, urge against there being any coherent Juice or Liquor, *viz.* That we should find it ooze out and wet the adjacent Parts, upon cutting a Nerve, as we do in cutting a Lymphatic, &c. that upon binding a Nerve, the upper Part would swell; that the Agitations which Objects make on the Filaments, would deaden, &c. that 'tis impossible a Liquor should have two opposite Motions at the same Time; and that the Velocity of Sensations, and that the Rapidity of Motions of Man, prove, that the *Animal Spirits* are rather Light than a Liquor. *Mem. de Trev.*

**SPIRITUALIZATION**, in Chymistry, the Action of extracting *Spirits* from natural Bodies. *Spiritualization*, is an Operation that belongs principally to fermented Salts; then to fermented Juices and Liquors; the Fermentation rendring the *Spirits* Volatile and Inflammable. Spirit of Wine, is sometimes *Spiritualiz'd* to that degree, that upon Throwing a Quantity into the Air, not a Drop shall fall down; but the whole evaporate and be lost.

**SPLEEN**, is also used for a Disease; by Physicians more usually called the *Hypochondriac Disease.*

**SPLENETIC**, a Person affected with Oppilations, and Obstructions of the Spleen. In *Splenetic* People, the *Spleen* is swell'd beyond the natural Bulk, or harden'd, so as to shew a Schirrous Tumour thereon. *Splenetic* People are distinguished by a Livid, Lead-coloured Complexion; their Character is to be very prone to Laughter; which is an Expedient Nature is supposed to make use of, to evacuate the too redundant Humour the *Spleen* is charged withal, whence it is that the Ancients made the *Spleen* the Organ of Laughter; and hence that popular Saying of a Person laughing heartily, *That he vents his Spleen.*

**SPODIUM**, in Pharmacy, a kind of Calx or Ashes, esteem'd an excellent Cardiac, and held to have the same Virtues as Coral. The *Spodium* of the Ancient *Greeks*, was a kind of Ashes found on the Hearths of Furnaces wherein Brass was made; call'd by them σποδιον, *q.d. Cinis*. That of the *Arabian* Physicians, as *Avicenna* and others, was made of the burnt Roots of Rushes and Reeds. The Moderns make their *Spodium* of Ivory burnt and calcined to a Whiteness. 'Tis sometimes counterfeited, by burning Bullocks or Dogs-bones; but these are of no Value. The *Anti-Spodium*, which the Ancients substituted for their *Spodium*, was made of Myrtle-Leaves, Galls and some other Ingredients, calcined.

**SPORADIC**, in Medicine, an Epithet given to such Diseases as have some special or peculiar Cause, and are dispersed here and there, regarding particular Constitutions, Ages, or other Circumstances. The Word is form'd from the *Greek* σποραϛ, dispersed, spread, &c. *Sporadic* stands in Opposition to *Epidemic* Diseases, which are those arising from a general Cause, and that are common to all Kinds of Persons, of what Complexion and Quality soever.

**SPUNGE**, or Sponge, a kind of Sea-Fungus or Mushroom found adhering to Rocks, Shells, &c. on the Sea-shore. The Ancients distinguish'd two Kinds, *Male* and *Female* : But the Moderns make only one Kind; which, however, they distinguish with regard to its Texture, into *Coarse* and *Fine*. The Naturalists have been embarrass'd in all Ages, whether to range *Spunges* in the Animal, Mineral or Vegetable Family. Some wou'd have it a Concretion form'd of the Sea-mud; and others an Animal, from its Motion of Contraction and Dilatation.

The greatest Part of our *Spunges* are brought from the *Mediterranean*; though there are considerable Quantities from *Vicaria*, an Island on the Coast of *Asia*. The Diving or Fishing for *Spunges* is there reckoned the top Qualification in the Youth, who all get the better Wives as they excel more herein. To this Proof, the Maids refer the Preference among several Suitors; placing themselves in the Brink of the Sea, to be Witnesses of the Address of each; and giving themselves as a Prize to the Conqueror.

The fine or small *Spunges* are the most esteem'd; and usually come to us from *Constantinople*. Their Goodness consists in their being very white, light, and the Holes small and close; the larger and coarser come from the Coasts of *Barbary*, particularly *Tunis* and *Algier*.

The *Spunge* is a very useful Matter in the Arts. In Physic, it serves to foment Parts inflamed. By Analysis, it yields a deal of volatile, sharp Salts, like other Sea-Plants. Taken inwardly it choaks; and is for that Reason cut small, and fried or dipt in Honey, and given to Quadrupeds to kill them, which it seldom fails to do, by swelling and preventing the Passage of Food into the Intestines.

In *Spunges* are found a kind of Stones call'd *Cysthoelithres*, held good for the Worms in young Children, and taken in Powder.

**SPURIOUS** *Diseases*, are such as in some Symptoms cannot be brought under any distinct Head, and therefore are call'd by the Name of some, with which they most agree; and hence, also, they are often denominated Bastards, *Nothi*; as a *spurious* or *bastard Pleurisy*, a *bastard Quinsy*, and the like.

**SPURIOUS** *Flesh*, among Anatomists, that which is of a Constitution quite different from all the rest; as the Flesh of the Lips, Gums, Glans, &c.

**SPUTUM**, in Medicine, &c. the Spittle, or Excrement voided at the Mouth. An Examen of the *Sputum*, is of great Consequence in Phthisical Cases; and *Bennet*[1], in his *Theatrum Tabidorum*, applies himself in a particular Manner thereto. The *Sputum Sanguinis*, is a very dangerous Symptom in that Disease.

**SQUAMMOUS**, in Anatomy, an Epithet given to the Spurious or false Sutures of the Skull; because composed of *Squammæ* or Scales like those of Fishes, or the like Tyles laid so as to reach over one another. The *Sutire Squammæ*, are also call'd *Temporales*, from their terminating the Temples, or *Ossa Temporis*.

**SQUINANCY** or *Esquinancy*, by the *Latins*, &c. call'd *Angina*, and by us, popularly *Quinzy*, a Disease which stops the Freedom of Respiration and Deglutination. The Word is form'd from the *Greek* συναγχειν, to *Suffocate*.

The *Squinancy* consists in an Inflammation of the Throat; and particularly of the Muscles of the Larynx or Pharynx, which exactly closing the Chinks thereof, prevent Air from passing and out of the Trachea, and the Food from being swallowed and convey'd into the Stomach.

The *Squinancy* is divided into *true* and *spurious*; the *true Squinancy* is always accompanied with a Fever; the *bastard* or *spurious Squinancy* is free from it. They are caused by a Defluxion of Blood, either pure of bilious, from the Branches of the Carotid Arteries; and there causing a Phlegmon, either a Simple or an Eresypetalous one.

The *Squinancy* is of all others the most dangerous, when the Tumour is neither perceivable on the inside nor the out. That appearing on the outside is the most curable. In violent *Squinancies*, recourse should be had to Laryngotomy or Bronchotomy, which though rarely practised, may yet be used with Safety.

**STAMINA**, in the Animal Body, are those simple, original Parts, which existed first in the Embryo, or even in the Seed; and by whose Distinction, Augmentation and Accretion, by additional Juices, the human Body, at its

[1] Christopher Bennet (1617 – 1655), an English physician.

utmost Bulk is supposed to be form'd. The Word is *Latin*, and signifies *Threads*. All that is essential to the Animal, are the *Stamina*, which exist, *in ovo*; the rest being foreign, additional and even accidental. The *Stamina* seem to coincide with the *Solids*, which are surprisingly small in Quantity.

**STAMINA**, in Botany, those fine Threads or Capillaments growing up within the Flowers of Tulips, Lillies, and most other Flowers, around the Style or Pistil.

On the Tops of the *Stamina*, grow those little Capsulæ or Knots, call'd *Apices*, which M. *Tournefort* makes essential to the Stamina; whence M. *Reaumur*, who assures is in the Memoirs of the *French* Academy, that he could never discover any Apices on the Threads of the *Fucus Marinus*, refuses to call them *Stamina*; though he adds, one may suppose that the Apices fall assoon as the Threads or *Stamina* being to be unfolded.

In some tubular Flowers, as the *Narcissus*, *Digitalis*, &c. M. *Geoffroy* observes the *Stamina* are exceedingly short; and in some Flowers there are no *Stamina* at all, as in the long *Aristolochia*, wherein the Apices are immediately fasten'd on the Capsula, which incloses the Fruit. In some other Flowers, as those of Thistles, Lettice, Chicory, &c. the Apices are inclosed in the *Stamina*; several of which uniting, form a little Tube in Manner of a Scabbard, in the Inside whereof are the Apices, furnished with their Farina : The rest of the Cavity being taken up by the Pistil, which is a little Thread placed on the Embryo of the Seed.

M. *Tournefort* takes the Use of the *Stamina* to be, as it were, so many excretory Canals, for discharging the growing Embryo of its redundant Juices; and of these Excrements of the Fruit, he takes that *Farina* or Dust, found in the Apices, to be form'd. But M. *Geoffroy*, Mr. *Bradley*, and other late Writers on Plants, as well as some former, assign the *Stamina* a nobler Use.

These Authors, explaining the Generation of Plants, in a Manner, analogous to that of Animals, maintain the Use of the *Stamina* to be to secrete, in their fine capillary Canals, a Juice, which being collected, harden'd and form'd into a Farina or Dust, in the Tips or Apices, is thence, when the Plant arrives at Maturity, discharged, by the bursting of the Apices, upon the Top of the Pistil; whence is a Passage for it to descend into the *Uterus* where being received, it impregnates and fecundifies the Plant.

On this Principle, it may be said, that the same Flower contains both Sexes, which contribute each their Part to the Generation : That the *Stamina* are the Male-part; and the Farina, which us always found of an oily, glutinous Nature, the seminal Liquor; and that the Pistil is the Female

**STAMINEOUS** *Flowers*, among Botanists, are such as are so far imperfect, as to want those colour'd Leaves, we call *Petalæ*; and which only consist of the *Stylus* and the *Stamina*.

Such Plants as bear their *Stamineous Flowers*, Mr. *Ray* makes to constitute a large Genus of Plants, which he calls *Herbæ flore imperfecto, sive apetalo, Stamineove*. And these he divides into such as,

1. Have their Fruit or Seed totally divided from the Flower; which are such

Plants as are said to be of different Sexes : The Reason of which, is, that from the same Seed, some Plants shall arise with Flowers, and no Fruit; and others, with Fruit, and no Flowers; As Hops, Hemp, Stinging-nettles, Spinach, Mercurialis and Phyllon.

2. Such as have their Fruit only a little disjoined from their Flowers; as the Ambrosia Bardana Minor, Ricinus, and the Heliotropium Tricoccon.

3. Such as have their Fruit immediately contiguous, or adhering to their Flower : And the Seed of these is either, 1. Triangular; and of this Sort, some are lucid and shining, as the Lapathum, Rhabarbarum, and Bistorta, to which also may be added the Persicaria : Others are rough and not shining, as the Helleborus Albus, Fegopyrum, Convolvulus Niger, and the Polygonum. 2. Such as have a roundish Seed, a little flatted or compressed, or of any other Figure but the former Triquetrous or Triangular one; and these have their Flower, or the Calyx of the Flower, adhering to the Bottom or Basis of the Seed or Fruit; as the Potamogiton, Blituma Sylvestre, Parietaria, Atriplex, Blitum Sativum, Amuranthes, Hoclocericus, and the Saxifraga Aurea. 3. Such whose Flowers adhere to the Top of the Seed; as the Beta, Asarum, Archimilla. And to these kind of Plants, Mr. *Ray* reduces also the Kaligeniculatum, Sedum Fruticosum, the Scoparia or Belvidere of the *Italians.*

**STATICKS**, *Statici*, in Medicine, a kind of Epilepticks, or Persons seiz'd with Epilepsies. The *Staticks* differ from the Catalepticks, in that, these last have no Sense of external Objects, nor remember any thing that passes at the Time of the Paroxysm: Whereas the *Statici* are all the while taken up with some very strong lively Idea, which they remember well enough, out of the Fit.

**STATOCELE**, in Medicine, a Rupture, or Tumour in the Scrotum, consisting of a fatty Substance resembling Suet.

**STEATOMA**; στεαρ, *Sevrum*, Suet; is a Swelling, consisting of a Matter much like Suet, soft, without Pain, and without discolouring the Skin; contained in a Cystis; and easily turn'd out upon Incision.

**STEGNOSIS**, from στεγω, *constipo*, I fix, or harden; is an Obstruction of the Pores; whence *Stegnoticks* are the same as *Astringents.*

**STEGNOTICKS**, in Medicine, Remedies proper to close and stop the Orifices of the vessels, when stretch'd, lacerated, &c. Such are Pomegranate Leaves, red Roses, Plantain Leaves, Tormentil Root, &c. *Stegnoticks* are proper in the Haemorrhoids, and other Fluxes of the Blood. The Word is form'd from the *Greek* στεγω, *impedro, constipio,* I hinder, close.

**STELLATE** Plants, such as have their Leaves growing on the Stalks, at certain Distances, in the Form of a Star with Beams; or such Flowers are Star-like or full of Eyes, resembling Stars, in the Thrum or Pendants. Mr. *Ray* makes this the Tenth Genus of *English Plants*; this Kind is Cross-Wort, Mollugo, wild Madder, Asperula, or Woodruff, Gallium or Ladies Bed-straw, Aparine or Cleavers, Rubia Tinctorum or Dyers Madder. To which he adds, as akin to this Genus, the Nasturtium Indicum, *Indian* Cresse, or yellow Lark-Spur.

**STERILITY**, the Quality of something *Barren*; in opposition to *Fecundity*. The Word is form'd from the *Latin Sterilitas*, of *Sterilis*, Barren. *Sterility* was held a grievous Affliction by the Wives of the antient Patriarchs. Nature has annex'd *Sterility* to all monstrous Productions, that the Creation might not degenerate. Hence the *Sterility* of Mules, &c.

The *Sterility* of Mercury, says the Alchymists, resembles that of Women who are too cold and moist; and who, by being purged and heated, wou'd be raised from their *Sterility*, as Mercury is when purged according to the Rules of Art.

**STERNUTATIVE**, or Sternutatory, a Medicine proper to occasion *Sternutation*, or Sneezing. *Sternutatories* are of two Kinds, gentle and violent: Of the first Kind, are Betony, Sage, Marjoram, Tobacco, &c. Of the latter, are Euphorbium, white Hellebore, Pellitory, &c. *Sternutatories*, have their Effects by their sharp, pungent Parts vellicating the inner Membrane of the Nose, which is exceedingly sensible, and occasioning a Serous Matter contained in the Glands of the Nose, and in several Sinus's situate in the Base of the Cranium, and the *Os Frontis*, to be expell'd.

**STIBIUM**, an ancient Name for Antimony, now seldom used.

**STILLATITIOUS** Oils; are such as are procured by Distillation, in opposition to those got by Infusion, Expression, &c.

**STOMACHIC**, a Medicine that strengthens the *Stomach*; and promotes the Office of Digestion. Of this Kind are Wormwood, Rhubarb, Mint, Mastic, Aloes, Pepper, Cinnamon, Aromatick Bitters, &c. good Wine is also a *Stomachic.*

**STONE**, in Medicine, a Disease call'd also *Calculus*, and *Lithiasis*; and, occasionally, the *Gravel.* It consists of a *stony* Concretion form'd either in the Bladder or Kidneys; which prevents the Discharge of Urine, and occasions violent Pains.

The *Stone* is generated, according to some Authors, of the earthy viscid Parts of the Blood, harden'd, in course of Time, by the Heat of the Kidneys; much after the manner as Brick is baked in a Furnace. Dr. *Quincy* supposes the *Stone* generated of the harder Parts of the Urine, pent up by the Straightness of the Ducts, and brought into Contact and Cohesion.

*Etmuller* ascribes the Stone, sometimes to the stony and metallick Particles of our Foods and Drinks, which the Reins, through Weakness and Relaxation thereof, cannot eject; but more usually to the unequal Strength of the Kidneys : Whence it is that we see one Kidney breed *Stones*, and the other sound.

The *Stone* in the Bladder, is first form'd in the Pelvis of the Kidneys, whence falling into the Bladder, it becomes augmented by new Lamellæ or Coats.

The Diagnostic Signs of the *Stone in the Kidneys*, are,

1° A fix'd obtuse Pain in the Region of the Loins, appearing like a Weight loading the Reins. As the *Stone* falls out of the Pelvis into the Ureter, the Pain is exceedingly acute and racking, which holds till either the *Stone* be got into the Bladder, or returned again to the Pelvis.

2° An Inflexibility of the Spina Dorsi, from the Extension and Compression of the Nerves.

3° A Stupor of the thigh and Leg of that Side, from the Consent of Parts.

4° A Retraction of the Testicle.

5° A very small Quantity of Urine, either thin and limpid, or bloody. But assoon as the *Stone* is got into the Bladder, the Urine becomes thick, turbid, blackish and in great Quantity.

The Diagnostics of the *Stone in the Bladder*, are a sense of Heaviness in the Perinæum and inguinal Region, a perpetual and troublesome Desire of making Water, which is followed with a sharp Pain, principally in the Glans of the Penis, whence a Prolapsus of the Anus. But the surest Way of finding it, is by the Touch, *viz.* by thrusting the Finger or a Catheter up the Anus.

The Cure of the *Stone*, is either by a Liquor that will dissolve or break the concrete Stone; so as it may be evacuated Piece-meal; which is call'd a *Lithontriptic*; or by enlarging the Capacity of the Vessels; or by the Operation of Cutting, call'd *Lithotomy.* We have yet no assured Lithontriptic known, how many soever pretend to it; the most noted, are *Daffey's* Elixir, *Tipping's* Liquor, and *Roger's* Powder. The most usual Cure is by Cutting; the various Manners whereof, see under Lithotomy.

In some desperate Cases, the *Stone* has been known to make itself a Way through the Spinal Muscles.

Dr. *Lister* observes, that *Stones* are found, not only in the Bladder and Kidneys, but also in the Pituitary Ducts, the Brain, Liver, Ventricle, Intestines and Joints of the Hands and Feet; to which may be added, that in the *Philosophical Transactions*, we have likewise Accounts of Stones in the Pineal Gland, the Heart, Gall, Bladder, &c.

The *Stone*, *Etmuller* says, is not Disease, but the Product of a Disease : The Disease, properly, is *Lithiasis*, or the Disposition of the Kidneys and Bladder to generate Stones.

*Stones* are distinguish'd into three Kinds, White, Red and yellow; which last are the most usual. *Deckers* recommends calcin'd Egg-shells as excellent in all Suppressions of Urine : *Hamilton*, Linseed Oil, and Mr. *Boyle*, the Herb Arsemart.

**STOOL**, in Medicine. A Thing is said to be *voided by Stool*, when it is discharged by the Anus or Fundament. In the *Philosophical Transactions*, we have Instances of sick Persons voiding factitious Stones, Balls, &c. by *Stool.*

**STORAX**, or STYRAX, a resinous odoriferous Gum, brought from Syria; whereof there are three Kinds, viz. the *red Storax*, *Storax Calamita*, and *liquid Storax.*

The *red Storax*, call'd also *Jew's Incense*, is a Gum or Resin oozing out at an Incision of a Tree, call'd *Storax*, not unlike our Quince Tree. Its Fruit is of the Size of a Filberd, and contains a white, oily Kernel, of a Smell perfectly like *Storax*. It must be chosen in a Mass, of a reddish Colour, soft and fat, and of an agreeable Smell, bearing no resemblance to *liquid Storax*.

That in Cakes, Balls, &c. is all sophisticated; and only a wretched Composition of *liquid Storax*, and the Impurities of the true *red Storax* and other Drugs. That in Powder is still worse.

*Red Storax* is of some use in Medicine; and is also used by the Perfumers, and often substituted for Incense.

The *Storax Calamita*, thus call'd from the Rushes or Quills, in *Latin*, *Calami*, it was anciently brought in, is, in reality, only a Composition of several Drugs, and among the rest, of *red Storax*, whence its Name; though Authors have hitherto taken it for a natural Gum, different from the *red Storax*. In must be chosen in fine white Tears, very dry, and not bitter; sometimes 'tis in reddish Masses, full of these whitish Tears, only mix'd with a ruddy Substance. These two Kinds are esteem'd excellent Pectorals, Stomachicks and Cephalicks.

*Liquid Storax*, is a find of factitious Rosin, of a greyish Colour, composed of true *Storax*, common Rosin of the Pine, Oil and Wine, beaten with Water, into the Consistence of an Unguent. The Druggists also call it *Stacte*, to distinguish it, and sell it for the better Price. The best is that of *Holland*. 'Tis easily kept in a Cellar, by pouring Water on it from time to time. 'Tis an Ingredient in an Unguent which Experience has shewn to be excellent against the Scorbutus and Gangrene.

**STRABISMUS**, an ill Disposition of the Eye, which makes it look a-squint. This Indisposition consists in the Retraction of the Ball of the Eye, towards one Side; occasion'd by Convulsion, or a Palsie of one of its Muscles.

Children are apt to acquire it through the Carelessness of their Nurses, in placing them always on the same Side the Light, or of any other remarkable Object that occasions them to turn their Eyes that Way.

To remedy it, Care is to be taken, that the Light, or other notable Body, be placed on the other Side of them; or else a Mask put on them, the Holes whereof are so disposed, as that to see through them, the Child be obliged to turn his Eye the opposite Way. The Word is form'd from the *Greek* στραβισμυς, which signifies the same.

**STRANGURY**, in Medicine, a Disease occasioning a very frequent and involuntary emission of Urine, in very small Quantities, and, as it were, Drop by Drop; with an intense Pain. The Word is form'd from the *Greek* στραγξ, Gutta, Drop, and ουρον, Urine.

It arises from the too great Acrimony of the Urine, which vellicating the Nervous Parts of the Bladder, occasions a continual Inclination to urine. The extreme sharpness of the Urine, sometimes produces an Ulcer in the Bladder.

New Beer and other Liquors not well fermented, are used to occasion the *Strangury*.

Some Authors confound the *Strangury*, which the *Latins* call *Urinæ*

*Stillicidium*, with the *Urinæ Incontinentia*.

The Difference between them, consists in this, that in the former, the Urine comes away with Pain, in the latter, without. The former proceeds from the Acrimony of the Urine; and the latter from a Relaxation of Palsy of the Sphincter of the Bladder, which cannot keep the Neck thereof close shut.

**STRATIFICATION**, in Chymistry, an Arrangement of different Matters, in several *Strata* or Layers, alternately; call'd by the *Latins*, *Stratum super Stratum*; and mark'd in Books of Chymistry with S S S. This Operation is used in calcining of Minerals or Metals with Salts or other Matters. To purify Gold by Cementation, they *Stratify* Laminæ, or Plates of Gold in a Crucible, with a dry Paste call'd *Cement*.

**STRENGTHENERS**, such Medicines as add to the Bulk and Firmness of the Solids. *Strengtheners* differ from Cordials, as a Bandage doth from a Flesh-brush : The latter are such that facilitate and drive on the vital Actions; but the former, such as confirm the Stamina, and maintain the Solids in such a Condition as to exert themselves into Action on all proper Occasions, with the greatest Force and Vigour.

The continual Waste, which constant Motion make in the Constitution, were it not for frequent and proper Supplies, would soon wear the Body quite out. The Attritions and Abrasions of the circulating Fluids, would quickly carry away the Canals in which they circulate, were not somewhat furnished in their Composition, which is suited to fall into, adhere with, and recruit that which is washed off. And those Particles must be much more disposed so to do, whose Adhesions are greatest, when once they come into Contact; such are those of Bodies we call Glutinous, and which easily form themselves into Jellies, and such-like Consistences; for the Parts of such Bodies are very light, by the over-proportion of their Surfaces to their Solitidies, whereby their Motions are both more languid, when in Circulation; and when the stop, their Cohesions will be much the stronger, with whatsoever they happen to call into Contact.

Medicines of this Tribe, are therefore of great Service in Hecticks; where the swift Motion of a thin, sharp Blood, wears away the Substance of the Body, instead of nourishing it; for they not only retard the inordinate Motion; but give such a Weight and Consistence to the Juices, as fits them also for Nourishment. There are likewise other Causes, which may weaken the Solids, by admitting, or occasioning them to relax too much. Whatsoever therefore acts as a Stimulus, and crisps and corrugates the Fibres into a more compact Tone, which most austere and pointed Bodies do, will remove such Weakness, and increase Strength: And as also, too much Moisture may contribute to such a Relaxation, what has no other Quality but absorbing, and drying up such superfluous Humidities, may deserve, though accidentally, to come under this Denomination.

**STROAKING**, a Method of Cure some People have given into, in certain Diseases; consisting in a mere application of the Hands to the Part affected, in the way of Friction or Rubbing. That Frication has considerable Uses in many Diseases, is allow'd. But, as to the particular efficacy of the *Stroak* of particular Persons; we see little Foundation for it in Nature. Experience, indeed, affords some; to which we don't know what to object.

Mr. *Thoresby*[1], in the *Philosophical Transactions*, gives several remarkable Instances of Cures perform'd by that famous *Stroaker*, Mr. *Greatrix*[2]. Mr. *Thoresby's* own Brother being seiz'd with a violent Pain in his Head and Neck; Mr. *Greatrix* coming accidentally thither, gave immediate Ease to his Head, by only *Stroaking* it with his Hand : He then fell to *stroak* his Back; whence the Pain immediately fled to his Right Thigh : Then he pursued it with his Hand to the Knee, from thence to the Leg, Ancle, Foot, and at last to the great Toe, where it grew more violent; but upon rubbing there, it vanish'd.

Another Relation of the same Author having a great Pain and Weakness in her Knees, which occasion'd a white Swelling, that had hung to her several Years, in spight of all Means; the same *Stroaker* rubbing both her Knees, gave her present Ease, the Pain flying downwards from his Hand, till he drove it out of the Toes, after which the Swelling soon went absolutely away.

Mr. *Thoresby* gives various other like Instances, all among his Acquaintance; and adds, That when Mr. *Greatrix stroaks* only for Pains, he uses nothing but his Hand; but that for Ulcers, or running Sores, he uses Spittle on his Hand or Fingers.

**STRUMÆ**, in Medicine, Tumours arising most usually on the Neck; call'd also *Scrophulæ*, and, popularly the *Evil*, or *King's Evil*. The Word is *Latin*, form'd, as some will have it, *a struendo*; because they insensibly, *Structium assurgunt*. The *Greeks* call them κοιραδες, Sores.

**STUM**, is the Flower of Wine, set a working. Hence to *Stum*, is to put certain Ingredients into sick and decay'd Wine, in order to revive it, and make it brisk.

**STUPIFIERS**, in Medicine, the same as Narcoticks and Opiates.

**STUPOR**, a Numbness, occasioned by any accidental Bandage that stops the Motion of the Blood and Nervous fluids, or by a Decay in the Nerves, as in a Palsy, &c.

**STYGIAN** *Liquors*, a Term some Chymists apply to acid Spirits, from their Efficacy in destroying or dissolving mixt Bodies.

**STYPTIC**, in Medicine, a Remedy that has the Virtue of stopping Blood, or of binding up the Aperture of a wounded Vessel. The Service, Nettle, *Solomon's* Seal, &c. are Stypticks. There are various *Styptic* Waters and Powders of surprising Efficacy, in most of which, Vitriol is the principal Ingredient. The usual *Styptic* Water is made of Colcothar calcined, or Vitriol dissolved with burnt Alum, Sugar-candy, the Urine of a young Man, &c.

Dr. *Colbatch's* Styptic Powder has been famed; though Mr. *Cowper*, in the

[1] Ralph Thoresby (1658 – 1725), an English antiquary.

[2] Valentine Greatrakes (1628 – 1683), an Irish empiric healer.

Philosophical Transactions, gives us a Number of Instances, wherein it was applied with very little or ill success in human Subjects; though he gives us others made in Dogs, where it answered well.

M. *Tournefort* observes, from the Analysis he has made of Styptic and Astringent Plants, that Acids and Earths prevail therein; though some of them yield an urinous Spirit. On this Principle, he asserts, That their Salt is analogous to Allum, and that there is somewhat of Sal Ammoniac in their Texture. *Chomel*[1] observes, that this does not hold universally.

**SUBLIMATE**, a chymical Preparation, the Basis whereof is Mercury, or Quick-silver. There are two Kinds of *Sublimate*, *Corrosive* and *Sweet*.

*Corrosive Sublimate*, is prepared of Mercury, either Crude or revived from Cinnabar, together with Spirit of Nitre, Vitriol lixiviated to a Whiteness, and Sea Salt decrepitated; the whole reduced into a white brilliant Mass by *Sublimation*.

*Sweet Sublimate*, is the same with Corrosive, only temper'd and sweeten'd by the Addition of *Mercurius Dulcis*, and thus reduced into a white Mass full of hard glittering Pieces, like little Needles, by being pass'd several times over the Fire, and through several Matrasses. To take away all its Malignity, it should be dulcified at least Thrice.

Corrosive *Sublimate* is White, and full of shining, crystalline Veins. It cannot act, unless it find some Humidity to act on; and is then a violent Poison, which corrodes and destroys the Parts of the Body with much Violence. Oil of Tartar *per Deliquium*, held the best Antidote against it.

Sweet *Sublimate*, is thus call'd, in Opposition to the Corrosive. 'Tis given internally, in the Cure of several Diseases, particularly Venereal ones.

**SUBLIMATION**, in Chymistry, an Operation which differs very little from Distillation, excepting, that in Distillation, only the Fluid Parts of Bodies are raised, but in this, the Solid and Dry; and that the Matter to be distilled may be either Solid or Fluid; but *Sublimation* is concerned only about solid Substances.

There is also another Difference, namely, that Rarefaction which is of very great Use in Distillation, has hardly any room in *Sublimation*; for the Sub-stances which are to be *Sublimed*, being Solid, are incapable of Rarefaction; and so it is only Impulse that can raise them.

However, it may not be improper, to inquire a little more nicely into the Reason of such a Diversity in the Elevation of Bodies; why some do ascend with a gentle Heat, and others are not to be raised by the most vehement Fire : And such an Enquiry will more properly come in here, because this Head contains all the Business of Volatility and Fixation.

The Cause of this Elevation, and Ascent in the Particles of Bodies, is to be ascribed to the Fire; not only on the account of Impulse, but of another Property the Fire has; namely, to insinuate itself into all the Interstices of these Bodies, and thereby break the Cohesion of their Parts, so that at last they may become divided into very small Parts, if not into the smallest that

1 Pierre Jean-Baptiste Chomel (1671 – 1740), a French physician and botanist.

Art can reduce them into.

Particles thus separated and divided, lose much of their Gravity. For the Gravity of the same Particle decreases in the same Proportion as the Cube of the Diameter is lessened. Suppose, therefore, a Body, whose Diameter is 12 : If, then, its Diameter be made less by 1, *viz.* 11, the Gravity of that Body will be only 9 1/4 or thereabouts : A Body, therefore, by being divided into very minute Corpuscles, is very easily *sublimed.*

Add, that the Surface of a Body decreases in a very different Manner from Gravity only as the Square of the Diameter is lessened. Where the Gravity decreases, in such a Series, as is express'd by the Numbers 1728, 1331, 1000, *viz.* 144, 121, 100; and when, upon reducing the Diameter to 6, the Gravity becomes less than 2, the Surface will still amount to 36.

How much this contributes to a quick Ascent, will appear from the *Sublimation* of Camphire, Benzoin and Arsenick; whose Particles, as they cohere but loosely, are, for that Reason, diffused into a larger Surface; upon which account they are the easiest to be *sublimed* of any; nay, these solid Particles, upon account of their Surface, will sooner ascend than some Fluids.

So Flower of Sulphur rises sooner than Oil, not only than that of Vitriol, but any other, though ever so light.

By this Contrivance of Nature, *viz.* that the Gravity of Bodies decreases in a triplicate, but their Surface in a duplicate Proportion of their Diameters; it comes to pass, that Bodies, which have a very different Gravity, may be raised with the same Force. Thus the Salts of Animals, as of Harts-horn, human Blood, of Vipers, &c. being composed of very minute Corpuscles, as is found by Experience, in distilling them, do easily ascend; because the Surface in them, is not lessened so much as the Gravity is; and the Salts of Vegetables, as of Tartar, Balsam, &c. which are of a more close Texture, by reason of their larger Surfaces, are without much difficulty raised.

The Corpuscles also of Minerals and Metals, though very compact and heavy, do, in some measure, give way to the Fire, and are capable of being *Sublimed.* In all these Instances, the Breadth of the Surface, which exposeth the Particles more to the Impetus of the Fire, is the Reason why they are raised with as much Ease, as if their Gravity had been lessened, by diminishing their Surface : So that Particles though ever so different in Weight, may be equally raised by the same Degree of Heat, id the Proposition of their Gravity be reciprocal to that of their Surfaces.

**SUBSTITUTE**, in Medicine, a Drug or Remedy that may be used in lieu of another; or that supplies the Place of another of like Virtue, which is not to be had; call'd also a *Succedaneum.* The Root of the great Centaureum, and sometime's Monk's Rhubarb, are used as *Substitutes* to Rhapontic.

**SUBTILE**, in Physicks, intimates a Thing exceedingly small, fine, and delicate; such as the Animal Spirits, &c. the Effluvia of odorous Bodies, &c. are supposed to be.

One kind of Matter is only more *subtile* than another, in that being divided into smaller Parts, and those, too, more agitated; on the one hand, it makes less Resistance to other Bodies; and on the other, insinuates itself more easily into their Pores.

The *Cartesians* suppose a *subtile Matter* for their first Element. This they lay down as so exceedingly Fine, that it penetrates the minute Pores of Glass and other solid Bodies; and from this they account for most of the Phænomena of Nature. Yet they don't pretend to prove the Existence of this Matter, otherwise than by Consequence.

**SUBTILIZATION**, the Act of *subtilizing*, or rendering any thing smaller and *subtiler*; particularly, the dissolving or changing a mixt Body into a pure Liquor, or a fine Powder.

**SUCCEDANEUM**, in Pharmacy, a Remedy substituted in the Place of another first prescribed, when the Ingredients are wanting, necessary for the Composition of that other. *Substitute* and *Succedaneum*, are of equal Import, unless, with some Authors, we chuse to use *Substitute*, where a Simple of like Virtue is put for another; and *Succedaneum*, where a Compound is used with the same Intention.

**SUCCINUM**, in Pharmacy, *Karabe* or *Amber*; a bituminous Juice or Resin, which from a Fluor grows hard and brittle. The Whitest, and most Transparent, is accounted best; it is of no great Use in Medicine, *per se*, as its Texture seems to compact to open and yield to the natural Elaborations; though some have a great Opinion of it, as a Balsamick, and gave it in Gonorrhea's particularly. But it is certain, that what Pharmacy extorts from it, is of wonderful Efficacy, especially in nervous Cases.

**SUCCISA**, a medicinal Herb, call'd also *Morbus Diaboli*, or the *Devil's Bit*. 'Tis a powerful Sudorific, inasmuch as *Theodore Mayerne* observes, in the *Philosophical Transactions*, laying a Person sick of the Plague, or other malignant Fever, on a Bed thereof, moderately hot; he shall sweat 'till they take him off; and much more, if he drink of the Decoction or Juice of the Herb. The *Succisa* is now little used.

**SUDAMINA**, little Pimples in the Skin, like Millet Grains, frequent in Youth, especially those of a hot Temperament, and that use much Exercise.

**SUDOR** *Anglicanus*, or the *English Sweat*, is an Epidemic Disease, first perceived in *England*, in 1485. 'Twas properly, a sort of Plague; thus call'd, because attended with an extraordinary kind of Sweat. It made its Return four Times in the space of 66 Years, *viz.* in 1506, 1517, 1528, and 1551.

It began with a Sweat, which never ended, but either with the Death of the Patient, or his Recovery. If he survived 24 Hours, he was safe. Few People escaped of it at first; too much Care, and too little, were found equally destructive.

The Patient was to wait, without stirring, either in his Bed, or in his Cloaths, according to the Condition Nature was surprised in; without burthening him either with Remedies or with Foods; without cloathing either too much or too little; and, if possible, without either eating or drinking. The Sweat to be kept up, without either promoting it, by any extraordinary Heat, or checking it by the least Cold.

This was what was found by Experience; and which was at length practised, with happy Success. The Disease was first felt on the 21st of *September*, and in the same Day, spread itself all over *England*; where, after a great Mortality, it stopp'd all at once, towards the End of *October*.

Its Ravages were so great, that in some Parts, it took off a Third Part of the People, in a very little Time. At its Return under *Henry* VIII. in 1516, it was as general, and as dangerous as before, and again disappeared all at once.

At the third Attack, in 1528, 'twas less fatal; insomuch that *Bellay*, Bishop of *Bayonne*, then Ambassador in England, who Sweat like the rest, tells us, tat of Forty thousand Souls, seiz'd with it in London, only Two thousand died. In 1534, it pass'd over into Ireland, where it kill'd great Numbers.

**SUDORIFIC**, in Medicine, a Remedy that causes, or promotes Sweat. *Sudorificks* only differs from Diaphoreticks, in the Degree of their Action; the one promoting sensible Perspiration, the other insensible.

To the Class of *Sudorifics*, belong, 1°, all Things that moving violently through the Body, attenuate the Humours, and accelerate their Motion. 2° Such Things, as at the same Time diminish the Resistance in the Sudatory Vessels about the Cutis.

To which some add a third Kind, *viz.* such as absorb the Acidities of the Blood, and thus set at liberty the Matter of the Sweat.

The first Intention is chiefly effected, by a copious drinking of very hot Waters; by Acids drawn from vegetables by Fermentation and Distillation; or those of Fossils, attenuated by repeated Distillations; especially if these be drunk mix'd with hot Water; by *Alcali's* both volatile and fix'd, diluted with hot Water; by all compound *Salts*, dissolved in Water; by Sapa's, metallic Crystals, or the attenuated Parts of Metals themselves, as *Stibium Diaphoreticum, fix'd Sulphur* of *Tachenius*; *Bezoardic Mineral, Diaphoretic Mercury, Diaphoretic Gold*, &c. by sharp, subtile, acrimonious Aromaticks, as *Absynthium, Abrotonum, Opium, Asparagus, Anis, Asclepias, Aristolochia, Gum Ammoniac, Carduus Benedictus, Caraways, Cinnamon, Camomile, Saffron, Capillus Veneris, China, Dittany, Eupatorium, Gentian, Hyssop, Laurel, Mint, Leek, Rosemary, Sage, Savin, Sassafras, Scordium, Thyme, Veronica, Nettle*, and other Medicines compounded hereof, as *Treacle, Mithridate, Diascordium, Orvietan*, &c.

The Second is chiefly effected, by cleansing the Skin, by *vaporous Lotions, Baths*, and *Frictions*; by relaxing the Cutaneous and Subcutaneous Vessels, which is best done by hot Water sprinkled over all over the Body, the Head excepted; by increasing the external Heat about the naked Body; as by the Warmth of a Bed, a Vapour-bath, &c.

The Third is effected by Absorbents, as *Corals, Crabs-Eyes, Diaphoretic Antimony, Bezoard*, &c.

**SUFFITUS**, or Suffimentum, in Medicine, a thickish Powder, &c. prepared of odoriferous Plants, Gums, &c. which being thrown on Coals, the Vapours or Steam thereof, are received by Smelling.

**SUFFOCATION**, in Medicine, &c. a Loss or Obstruction of Respiration. *Suffocations* sometimes arise fro a too great Abundance of Blood thrown on the Lungs, or the Muscles of the Larynx, and preventing the Ingress of the Air; as is the Case in Squinancies, *suffocating* Catarrhs, Peripneumonias, &c.

The fumes of Wines, or strong Beers, when boiling, cause *Suffocation*, by interrupting the Circulation of the Blood. And the same may be observed of the Fumes of Lime, wherewith Walls are whitened; and those of Charcoal, Antimony, Sulphur, Vitriol and Spirit of Nitre.

The *Suffocation* under Water, is owing partly to the passage of Air being stopp'd up; and partly to the Irruption of Water into the Breast. See Drowning.

The *Suffocation of the Womb or Matrix*, is a Disease pretty frequent in Women, call'd also, *Fits of the Mother*. In this, the Patient imagines a malignant Vapour rising from the Matrix, and so pressing against the Lungs and the Diaphragm, as to prevent the free Motion necessary to Respiration.

Its true Cause, is a Convulsion of the Muscles of the Larynx, which straighten the Wind-pipe, and prevent the Air's passing into the Lungs. Hence it is, that Hysteric Women feel Constrictions in the Throat, as if one were strangling them with a Cord.

In France, they dispatch their People that are raving Mad, by suffocating them between two Pillows.

**SUFFRUTEX**, in Botanists, a Name given to a low, woody, perennial Species of Plants, sending out no Leaves from its Roots, and beginning to be branched from the very bottom of the Stalk; such as Lavender, Rue, Sage, &c.

**SUFFUMIGATION**, in Medicine, a Term applied to all Remedies that are received into the Body in form of Fumes, *i.e.* of Smoak or Perfumes. These are composed of different Matters, according to the Nature of the Disease. *Suffumigations* are intended to soften sharp, serous Humours, to provoke or check the Course of the Menses, to raise a Salivation in venereal Evils, &c. The Word is form'd of the *Latin*, *sub*, under, and *fumus*, smoak.

**SUFFUSION**, in Medicine, an overflowing of some Humour, shewing itself in the Skin; particularly of the Blood or Bile. That Redness ordinarily arising from Shame, is only a *Suffusion* of Blood appearing in the Cheeks. The Jaundice is a *Suffusion* of Bile over the whole Body. *Suffusion* is also used for a little Film or Pellicle, form'd in the aqueous Humour of the Eye, before the Pupil; call'd, also, *Cataract*.

**SUGAR** *of Roses*, is white Sugar clarify'd, and boil'd into a Consistence, in Rose-Water; when boil'd, they form it into Lozenges, sometimes into little Hail, of the Size of Peas, by keeping it stirring till it be cold and dry. 'Tis reputed good to loosen and allay Acrimonies, &c. of the Breast.

**SULPHUR**, in Natural History, a fat unctuous Mineral Substance, fusible and inflammable in Fire, and not dissoluble or miscible in Water. It is particularly call'd *Fossil*, or *Mineral Sulphur*, to distinguish it from the *Sulphur of Metals*, or *of the Philosophers*. Sulphurs make a particular Class of Fossils, divided into Solid and Fluid. The Solid Sulphurs are, common Sulphur, or Sulphur properly so call'd, Arsenic and Ambar. The Liquid Sulphurs are, Asphaltum, or Pisasphaltum, Bitumen, Petroleum, Naptha, and Oleum Terræ, &c.

**SULPHUR**, properly so call'd, or *Brimstone*, is of three Kinds, *viz. Vivum, Mineral*, and *Common Sulphur*.

*Sulphur Vivum* is thus called, as being such as it is taken out of the Mine : It is a kind of greyish argillous Clay, which easily takes Fire, and, in burning, casts a string sulphurous Smell. Its Colour occasions its being sometimes call'd *Grey Sulphur*.

'Tis chiefly brought from *Sicily*; and is but little used, except in some Galenical Compositions, and to *sulphur* Wine, to make it keep in Carriage. The best is soft, smooth, friable, and shining, of a Mouse-Colour, and not too full of Smell.

*Mineral Sulphur*, call'd also *Yellow Sulphur*; is a Kind of hard, earthy Bitumen, of a shining yellow colour, a strong stinking Smell, easily taking Fire, and dissolving. 'Tis found in great Quantities in the Neighbourhood of Vulcanos or burning Mountains, as *Vesuvius*, *Aetna*, &c. yet is it likewise found in its particular Mines; and we have very good from several Parts of *Italy* and *Switzerland*, tho' the best us that of *Quitto* and *Nicaragua* in *America*.

'Tis from this *Sulphur*, that the *Common Sulphur* used in Gunpowder, and on divers other Occasions, is drawn, by Means of Fire and Whale Oil, which dissolving it, 'tis pour'd into Moulds; and thus form'd into those Cylinders we find it in.

This *Common Sulphur* is either better or worse, according to the Refinery it comes from. That of *Holland* has a long Time had the Vogue; the second Place has been given to that of *Venice*, and the third to that of *Marseilles*; but the Order seems to have been since chang'd, and that from *Marseilles* is no win the first Place. It is chosen on large thick Cylinders, of a gold yellow Colour, very brittle, and when broke, appearing all brilliant as if Crystallized.

Beside the Use of *Sulphur* in the Composition of Gunpowder, whereof it is one of the three Ingredients, and that which makes it tale Fire so readily, 'tis of some Use in Medicine, and more in Chymistry. 'Tis also used in whitening Silken and Woollen Stuffs; to which End, the Vapour thereof is contriv'd to be receiv'd by them.

Its Vapour also whitens red Roses, and even young Rooks, taken out of the Nest, and expos'd thereto, become perfectly white. It has the same Effect on Gold; which is to be restored to its Colour by boiling it in Water with Tartar.

The Chymical Analysis of *Sulphur* is very difficult; its Principles being so volatile, and withal so fast bound together, that they either rise all together, or are dissipated and lost in being separated.

M. *Homberg*, however, has at length found the Secret of separating the Principles, and of saving them at the same Time. He finds it consists of an Acid Salt, an Earth, and oily, bituminous, an inflammable Matter, and usually a little Metal.

The three first he finds, by a long Series of Operations, are in pretty equal

Quantities; but the last, which he finds to be Copper, inconsiderable. The Acid, he adds, is exactly the same wit that of Vitriol; the Oil thick and red as Blood, appears to be the inflammable Part, and that which constitutes the Chymical Principle of *Sulphur*, but that it retains some heterogeneous Matter in the Operation. The Earth is extremely fix'd, and unaltered by the strongest Fire.

M. *Geoffroy* tried the Recomposition of Sulphur on M. *Homberg's* Principles with Success. The pure Acid Salt of Sulphur, being mix'd with an equal Quantity of the oily Matter, and earthy Alcali, and a little Oil of Tartar, and the Operation conducted according to the Rules of Art, the Mixture was converted into a pure burning *Sulphur*.

This done, he attempted the Composition of Sulphur, not by recompounding it out of the same Matters it had been resolv'd into, but by using Matters judged of the same Nature. Thus, by substituting Oil of Vitriol for the Acid Salt, and Oil of Turpentine for the inflammable Part, he succeeded as before.

Again, he found that fixed Salts, as they are Acids absorb'd in Earth, serve for two Principles at once, and need nothing but an inflammable Oil to make Sulphur : And even in lieu of this Oil, M. *Geoffroy* imploy'd, with equal Success, Charcoal, Pit-coal, and other Solids.

Indeed, Mr. *Boyle* and *Glauber* had before made common *Sulphur*, and that by Mixtures, such as M. *Geoffroy* describes; but they were both mistaken as to the Reason thereof; the once concluding, that the Sulphur he thus got, had been contain'd in the fix'd Salts, and the other in the Coal; neither of them dreamed, that 'twas the Mixture of the three Principles that produced the Mixt.

*Flowers of* **SULPHUR**, are the purest and finest Part of *Sulphur*, gain'd by evaporating *Sulphur*, by Sublimation, or burning it in Pots made for that Purpose; and gather'd in the Capital of the Cucurbit, where the Vapour sticks.

This Preparation, as, indeed, *Sulphur* in most of its Forms, is found excellent for the Lungs. The best Flower of *Sulphur* is that of *Holland*, which is in Cakes, or Pieces, light, soft, friable, and rather white than yellow. If it be in Powder, it must be very fine, of a yellow Colour, that is both whitish and gilt at the same Time.

Instead of this, we have frequently put upon us a vile Mixture of *Sulphur*, exalted by Fire, and mix'd with Starch, or Wheat Flower; and sometimes only *Sulphur*-Dust well sifted.

By adding fix'd Nitre, or Sal Polychrest, to the Flowers of *Sulphur*, we have the white Flowers of *Sulphur*.

*Magistery*, or *Balm*, or *Milk*, of **SULPHUR**, is *Sulphur* dissolved in a sufficient Quantity of Water, with Salt of Tartar; and precipitated by Means of a Spirit of Vinegar, or some other Acid. 'Tis called *Milk of Sulphur* from its Whiteness; and *Balm of Sulphur*, or *of the lungs*, from its excellent Use in Diseases of the Lungs and Breast.

*Salt of* **SULPHUR**, is a Chymical Preparation, very improperly thus called, as being no other than the Sal Polychreston, impregnated with Spirit of Sulphur, and reduced to an Acid Salt, by evaporating the Humidity thereof. Some hold it a powerful Febrifuge.

**SULPHUR** *of Antimony*, is a sulphurous Matter drawn from Antimony by divers Operations. That drawn from the Fæces of the Crocus Metallorum, is by some called, *Golden Sulphur*.

**SULPHUR** *Metallorum*, or Sulphur of Metals, called also, Sulphur Figens, is used among the Chymists and Alchymists for a peculiar Matter, which enters the Composition of all Metals. Metals are suppos'd to consist of two essential Parts, or Principles; Mercury as the Basis, or Metallic Matter; and *Sulphur* as the Binder or Cement, which fixes the fluid Mercury into a coherent malleable Mass. Some of the latest and best Chymists, particularly Mons. *Homberg*, will have this Sulphur to be no other than Fire.

**SUPERFETATION**, in Medicine, an After-Conception; or a second Generation, happening to the Mother, already pregnant, conceives, of a later Coition; so that she bears at once Two Fætus's of unequal Age and Bulk, and is delivered of them at different Times. The Word is form'd from the *Latin*, *Super*, over, and *foetus*, Embryo.

We meet with Instances of *Superfetations* of Women, in *Hippocrates, Aristotle, Pliny, du Laurens*[1], &c. But they are much more frequent in hares and Sows. An Instance of an extraordinary Kind of *Superfetation*, we have in *Bartholin*; who tells us, That a *Danish* Girl was born being with Child.

*Menzelius*[2], a *German* Physician, adds, That in 1672, the Wife of a Physician, in *Thuringia*, was delivered of a Girl big with another; whereof she was delivered in Eight Days Time, and which was Baptized, and died a Day after her Mother.

In the History of the Royal Academy of Sciences, for the Year 1709, mention is made of a Letter from a very considerable Magistrate, to the Academy, containing a very remarkable Instance of a *Superfetation*; a Butcher's Wife of *Aix* being delivered in that Year of Nine Children, each about Two Days after other, all well form'd and alive.

The Naturalists hold, That Female Rats are frequently born with young rats in their Wombs. In the King of *Denmark's* Cabinet, is seen an Egg, in the middle whereof is another Egg perfectly form'd. We meet with something like a *Superfetation* in Plants too; there being a kind of Lemon found to grow inclosed in the Body of another.

**SUPER-PURGATION**, in Medicine, an excessive, over-violent Purging. A Man who had taken Powder of Diacarthamus inwardly, was sent by it to Stool an hundred times; and was cured of the *Super-purgation* by a Pound of Capon Broth, an Ounce of Saccharum Rosatum, five Grains of Laudanum, and the Yolk of an Egg. In lieu of Laudanum, they sometimes use a Drachm

[1] Andre du Laurens (1558 – 1609), a French physician and anatomist.

[2] Christianus Menzelius, born Christian Mentzel (1622 – 1701).

and a half of new Treacle.

**SUPPLANTALIA**, among Physicians, Plaisters apply'd to the Soles of the Feet, generally made of Leaves, Mustard, wild Radish, Salt, Soap, Gunpowder, &c.

**SUPPOSITORY**, in Pharmacy, a solid Medicine thrust up the Fundament, in lieu of a Liquid one, or Clyster, where that would not be so convenient. The *Suppository* was invented for the Convenience of such as have an Aversion to the taking of Clysters; or to be used where the Disease does not allow thereof. The *Latins* call it *Balanus*, because anciently made in Figure of an Acorn.

'Tis composed of common Honey, mix'd up with either Soap, or Oil, and form'd into Pieces of the Length and Thickness of the little Finger, only Pyramidal. To the Composition is sometimes added Powder of Scammony, Euphorbium, Colocynthis, &c.

On some occasions 'tis made simply of a Cut of Bacon, the Stem of a Leek, or the like Matter, thrust, like a Tent, up the Anus, to irritate the Sphincter Muscle, and oblige it to extrude the Excrements.

**SUPPRESSION**, in Medicine, is apply'd to the Humours that are retain'd in the Body by some Obstruction or Stoppage of the usual Outlets. As, a Suppression of Urine, of the Menses, &c.

**SUPPURATION**, in Medicine, the Action whereby extravasated Blood, or other Humours, are chang'd, in the Body, into *Pus*. The Word is form'd from the *Latin*, *sub*, under and *pus*, *puris*.

The Change is begin by a Dissipation of the most subtle and spirituous Parts of the Blood : What is left behind, thickens and purifies by little and little; that us, its Salts and Sulphurs disengage themselves from the grosser Parts wherein they were embarrass'd. These Parts thus disengaged, and acting on one another, bruise and break each other, and thus excite a Fermentation, which increases the Heat of the Part; whereby the Matter is further digested, and a Pain and Tension produc'd. At length the Blood loses its Colour, and becomes quite white, by the Mixture of its Acid, sulphurous and acrimonious Particles; as we see happens to sulphurous Alcalies, when mix'd with Acids.

**SUPPURATIVE**, a Medicine that promotes Suppuration. *Suppuratives* are all hot; by which Means, increasing the Heat of the Part, they resolve the Humour into a *Pus*. Such are Mallows, Lilly-Roots, Drachylon, &c.

**SWEAT**, a Moisture issuing out of the Pores of the Skins of Animals; thro' too much Heat, Exercise, or Weakness; or through the Action of certain Medicines call'd *Sudorificks*.

*Sweat* is either the Consequence of an Acceleration of the Blood's Motion, by Stimuli, or Exercise; or of a Relaxation of the Pores of the Cutis; by means of either whereof, the Matter which before perspir'd insensible, is now render'd sensible. The former is the Case in Natural and Medicinal *Sweats*, and the latter in morbid, fainting, and cold *Sweats*.

The principal Organ of *Sweat* are the milliary Glands; which are spread over the whole Ambit of the Body; and furnish'd, each with a Vein, Artery, and Nerve, besides an excretory Duct, thro' the Orifice whereof the *Sweat* is cast out under the Cuticle. This Duct is cover'd with a little round Valve, lying immediately under the Cuticle, whereby the *Sweat* is occasionally either retain'd or transmitted.

The *Sweat* thus secreted, is various, according to the Variety of the Weather, Soil, Sex, Age, Temperament, Emunctories, Diet, Time of Digestion, &c. as in the Urine.

In a sound Body, Sweat is scarce ever found, but from a Fault in some of the six Non-Naturals : Its immediate Effect is always hurtful; By Accident it sometimes does good.

The Physicians order *Sweats* in cold and inveterate Diseases, as the Palsy, Rheumatism, Sciatica, and many other Diseases. Diseases frequently have their Crises in *Sweats*.

*Sweating* is indicated by the Beginning of a critical *Sweat*, to carry off the Disease; by the Tenuity of the morbid Matter dispers'd thro' all the Vessels, as in the Plague, a venomous Bite, the *French* Disease, e'er yet fix'd; by the particular Temperature of the Patient, and by various Obstructions to be remov'd in the several Parts of the Body; particularly in subcutaneous Diseases, such as the Itch, Psora, Leprosy, &c.

*Matthiolus* tells us, That the *Sweat* of all Quadrupeds, as Horses, Asses, &c. is venomous; and that of other Beasts is unwholesome. *Tachenius* adds, that the *Sweat* of Horses, particularly, is so acid, that it pierces the strongest and firmest Boots, that are Proof against all Water. Some Naturalists affirm, that Dogs and Cats never *sweat*, how hot soever they be, because they are not found to have any Pores in the Cuticle.

**SWOONING**, a Kind of Syncope, or Fainting, wherein the Patient loses all his Strength, and his Understanding. *Swooning* may be occasion'd by any thing that alters, corrupts, or dissipates the Vital Spirits; as, long Watching, violent Pains, great and sudden Evacuations, putrid Vapours arising from Abscesses in the noble Parts.

**SYMPATHETIC**, something that has a Sympathy, or that acts by Sympathy. *Sympathetic* is particularly applied to all Diseases which have two Causes; the one remote, the other near. In which Sense, the Word is opposed to *Idiopathetic*.

Thus, an Epilepsy is said to be *Sympathetic*, when produced by a remote Cause; *i.e.* when the Disorder in the Brain, embarrass'd, and, as it were, mired with Blood, is preceded and produced by some other Disease.

There is a *Sympathetic* Palpitation of the Heart, and an *Idiopathetic* one. There is but one Idiopathetic Cause of the Palpitation; but there are several *Sympathetic* ones.

Among Chymists and Alchymists, the Term *Sympathetic* is principally applied to a kind of *Powder*, and a Sort of *Ink*.

**SYMPATHETIC POWDER**, a Powder once very much fam'd; supposed to have this wonderful Property, That if spread on a Cloth dipt in the Blood of a Wound, the Wound would be cured, though the Patient were any Number of Miles off.

This Powder, M. *Lemery* tells us, is nothing but *Roman Vitriol*, open'd by the Sun-beams penetrating it, and imperfectly calcining it, in the middle of Summer. But it is now generally allowed a mere Piece of Charletanery, whatever Sir. *Kenelm Digby* and others before him and after, plead in its Favour.

Sir *Kenelm*, in an express Treatise on the Subject, where he gives Instances of Cures perform'd by it, accounts for the Manner of its Operation thus : The Sun's Rays, says he, attract and draw the Spirits of the Blood, at a great Distance; by which means the Atoms thereof, are driven and dispersed far and near in the Air. Now, the Spirits of Vitriol, incorporated with the Blood, fly along with them, and the Two together form a kind of Train of Corpuscles. On the other Side, there is continually issuing and exhaling from the Wound, abundance of fiery Spirits, which attract the neighbouring Air, and this Air, by a continued Concatenation, attracting, still, the next Air, at length, meets the Atoms, with the Spirits of the Blood finding their Source again, re-enter into their primitive Seat, and being joined with the vitriolic Spirits, the Wound is comforted and healed, imperceptibly.

But to the Confusion of all this fine Reasoning; 'tis found by Experience, that the Powder is so far from this Effect at a great Distance, that 'tis scarce perceived, if done in the same Room with the Patient. Though 'tis possible, as the Parts of the Vitriol are in continual Motion, if the Cloth be applied just by the Patient, some of the Effluvia thereof, may enter the Wound, and help to stop the Bleeding.

**SYMPATHY**, in Medicine, an Indisposition befalling one Part of the Body, thro' the Disorder or Faultiness of another; whether it be thro' the Affluence of some Humour, or Vapour sent from elsewhere; or thro' the Want of the Influence of some Matter necessary to its Action.

**SYMPTOM**, in Medicine, is ordinarily confounded with *Sign*, and defin'd an Appearance, or Conjunction of Appearances, in a Disease, which shew or indicate its Nature and Quality, and whence one may judge of the Event thereof.

In this Sense, a Delirium is held a *Symptom* of a Fever; and Pain, Waking, Drowsiness, Convulsions, Suppression of Urine, Difficulties of Breathing and Swallowing, Coughs, Disgusts, Nauseas, Thirst, Swoonings, Faintings, Looseness, Costiveness, Dryness and Blackness of the Tongue, are held the principal *Symptoms* of Diseases.

But *Boerhaave* gives us a much more just and accurate Notion of a *Symptom*: Every præternatural Thing, says he, arising from a Disease, as its Cause, in such Manner, however, as that it may be distinguish'd from the Disease itself, and from its next Cause, is call'd a *Symptom* of the Disease.

If it arise after the same Manner, from the Cause of the Disease, it call'd a *Symptom of the Cause.* If it arise from some former Symptom as its Cause, it is call'd a *Symptom of a Symptom.* Whatever happens to a Disease, from any other Causes than those mention'd, is more properly call'd an *Epigenema*.

Hence it appears, that these former *Symptoms* are really Diseases themselves, very different as to Number, Effect, &c. tho', after the Ancients, they may be conveniently enough reduc'd to Faults in the *Functions*, *Excretions*, and *Retentions*.

Under the first come all Diminutions, Abolitions, Increases, and Depravations of Animal Actions, particularly with regard to *Hunger* and *Thirst*, *Sleeping* and *Waking*. Under the second come, *Nausea's*, *Vomitings*, *Lienteries*, *Coeliac Affections*, *Diarrheas*, *Disenteries*, *Iliac Passions*, &c. Under the third, come the *Jaundice*, *Stone*, *Dropsy*, *Fever*, *Ischuria*, *Strangury*, *Asthma*, *Catarrh*, &c.

**SYMPTOMATICAL**, in Medicine, is a Term often used to denote the Difference between the primary and secondary Causes in Diseases; as, a Fever from Pain is said to be *Symptomatical*, because it arises from Pain only; and therefore the ordinary Means in Fevers are not, in such Cases, to be had recourse to; but to what will remove the Pain; for when that ceases, the Fever will cease, without any direct Means taken for that.

**SYNAUCHE**, in Medicine, a kind of Squinancy, wherein the internal Muscles of the Fauces, or Pharynx, are attack'd. When the external Muscles of the same are seiz'd, it is call'd a *Parasynanche*. The Word is form'd from the *Greek*, συν, with, and αγχειν, to press, suffocate.

**SYNCOPE**, in Medicine, a deep and sudden Swooning; wherein the Patient continues without any sensible Heat, Motion, Sense, or Respiration; is seiz'd with a cold Sweat over the whole Body, and all the Parts turn pale and cold, as if dead. The Word is form'd from the *Greek*, συν, with, and κοπτειν, to cut.

There are several Causes of *Syncope's* :

1°. Too great an Exhaustion of Spirits; as after long Diets, excessive Evacuations, violent Exercises, long Bathings, &c.

2°. The irregular Motion of the Spirits preventing their due Influx into the Parts; as sometimes happens in Fear, Wrath, and other violent Passions.

3°. Immoderate Hæmorragies.

4°. An ill Constitution of the Blood; as in Cacochymies, or in Persons who have taken something that either dissolves or coagulates the Blood.

5°. Secret Diseases, as Abscesses, or Polypus's of the Heart, Worms, &c.

In very numerous crouded Assemblies, People sometimes fall into *Syncopes*, thro' the hot, thick, impure Air they breathe. Some Women are liable to them upon the Smell of Musk, Civet, &c.

For *Syncopes*, give volatile Spirits and Aromatics. *Heurnius*[1] recommends Treacle Water, and Cinnamon Water; and *Etmuller* the Volatile Salt of Vipers, Spirit of Sal Ammoniac, Oil of Ambar, and sometimes Bleeding.

**SYNDROME**, from συνδρομη, Concursus, a Combination of Diseases.

[1] Johann Heurnius (1543 – 1601), a Dutch physician.

**SYNOCHA**, and Synochos, in Medicine, are Terms borrowed from συνοχεω, *sustino*, I support, or hold up; or συνεχω, *continuo*, I continue. The Practice of Authors, with regard to these two Words, is whimsical enough : Literally they both signify the same Thing; yet is the former used to signify an intermitting, and the latter a continu'd Fever.

**SYNOVIA**, in Medicine, a Term used by some Authors for the nutritious Juice proper to each Part. Others use it for the Gout and other Diseases arising for a Vice in the nutritious Juice. Others restrain it to the oozing out of the nutritious Juice thro' the wounded Parts. *Van Helmont* defines it a kind of transparent Mucilage, like Seed, such as issues from the Legs of a Calf upon cutting off the Feet.

**SYNTECTOE**, in Medicine, a kind of Colliquation of the Solids of the Body; such as frequently happens in Inflammations of the Bowels, Colliquative Fevers, &c. wherein a fatty Uliginous is voided with the Excrements by Stool.

**SYPHILIS**, is a Term used for the *Lues Venerea*. Some will have it from συν, *cum*, with, and φιλια, *Amor*, or *Amicitia*, Love or Friendship; because it proceeds from the infectious Intercourses of Lovers in Coition. Others will have it from the Name of a Shepherd so called, who was remarkably afflicted with it. However, some Authors of Note use the Term; and *Fracastorius* a famous *Italian* Physician, gives it for the Title of a fine Poem, which he wrote upon that Distemper.

**SYRINGES** are of considerable Use in Medicine and Chirurgery. By them Clysters are administered : Injections of medicinal Waters, &c. made into Wounds, &c. They also serve to inject colour'd Liquors, melted Wax, &c. into the dried Vessels of the Parts of Animals, to shew the Disposition, Texture, Ramifications, &c. thereof. The Word is from the *Latin*, *Syrinx*, Pipe.

**SYSTOLE**, in Medicine, the Contraction of the Heart and Arteries of an Animal. The *Systole* of the Heart is well accounted for by Dr. *Lower*, who shews, that the Heart is a true Muscle, the Fibres whereof are acted on like those of other Muscles, by Means of certain Branches of the eight Pair of Nerves inserted into it, which bring the Animals Spirits from the Brain hither. By a Flux of these Spirits, the Muscular Fibres of the Heart are inflated, and thus shorten'd; the Length of the Heart diminish'd, its Breadth or Thickness increas'd, the Capacity of the Ventricles clos'd, the tendonous Mouths of the Arteries dilated, those of the Veins shut up by means of their Valves, and the contain'd Juices forcibly express'd into the Orifices of the Arteries.

And this we call the Συστολη, or Contraction of the Heart; the opposite State to which is call'd *Diastole*, or Dilatation of the Heart.

Dr. *Drake* adds to Dr. *Lower's*[1] Account, that the intercostal Muscles and Diaphragm, contribute to the *Systole*, by opening the Blood a Passage from

[1] Richard Lower (1631 – 1691), an English physician and anatomist.

the right Ventricle of the Heart, to the left thro' the Lungs, to which it could not otherwise pass : By which Means, the Opposition the Blood contain'd in that Ventricle must necessarily have made to its Construction, is taken off. *Lower* and *Drake* make the *Systole* the natural State of or Action of the Heart, and the *Diastole* the violent one : *Boerhaave*, on the contrary, makes the *Systole* the violent, and the *Diastole* the natural State.

**TABELLA**, or Tablette, in Pharmacy, a solid Electuary, or Composition of several Drugs, made up dry, and form'd into little Squares; more usually call'd *Lozenges*. Powders, Confections, Fruits, Salts, &c. are dissolved in Sugar, and made into *Tabulæ*; as those of the Juice Liquorice for Colds, &c. We have Cordial, Stomachic, Aperitive, Hepatic, &c. *Tablettes*. Jellies and Broths are sometimes reduc'd into *Tablettes*, to be carry'd in the Pocket. There are *Tablettes* of *Manus Christi*, or Sugar of Roses pearled. *Tabellae Magnanimitatus*, are those taken by feeble old Men, when match'd with young Wives, to assist and bear them out in the Affairs of Generation.

**TABES**, in Medicine, a general Name for Consumptions of all Kinds. *Tabes Dorsalis*, is a kind, or rather a Degree of Consumption : proceeding sometimes from an excessive Application to Venery. The Patient has neither a Fever, nor loss of Appetite; but a Sensation, as if there were a Number of Pismires running from the Head, down the Spinal Marrow; and when he evacuates, either by Urine, or Stool, there flows a liquid Matter like Semen. After any violent Exercise his Head is heavy, and his Ears tingle; and at length he dies of a Lipyria, *i.e.* a Fever, where the external Parts are cold, and the internal burn at the same time.

**TACAMACHA**, or Tacamahaca, a kind of resinous Gum, distilling from the Trunk of a very large Tree, growing in *New Spain*; but, in greatest Abundance, in the Island of *Madagascar*. 'Tis not unlike our Poplar Tree, only bigger and taller, its Leaves small and green, its Fruit red, of the Size of our Walnuts, exceedingly Resinous, and containing a Stone like our Peaches.

The Wood of the Tree makes good Timber for Ships, and the Gum it yields, serves for their Caulking; though its chief Use is in Medicine.

There are three Kinds of *Tacamacha*; the Sublime, call'd also the *Tacamacha* in the Pod; *Tacamacha* in the Mass; and *Tacamacha* in Tears.

The first is the Natural Resin, as it falls of itself, without any Incision being made in the Tree : The Good is dry, reddish, trans-parent, of a bitter Taste and string Smell, resembling that of Lavender. The Islanders gather it in little Gourds cut in two, and cover'd with a Palm Leaf.

The *Tacamachas* in *Tears*, and in the *Mass*, are those which flow from the Tree through Incisions : They must chosen dry and clear, and their Smell resembling that of the first Kind.

Gum *Tacamacha* is found good for digesting and resolving of Tumors, and assuaging Pains. Burnt upon Coals, 'tis reckon'd good for Hysteric Fits of Women, and likewise applied to the Belly in form of a Plaister. Some apply it to the Temples in the same Manner, and to the Nape of the Neck for Pains in the Head, Defluctions of Rheum upon the Throat, and Inflammations of the Eyes, as also in the Tooth-ach. It is of so subtle and penetrating a Nature, that it is greatly used in external Applications, to suppurate and disperse Tumours; and is accounted effectual, even in those which are Scrophulous.

It is likewise used externally in Arthritic Pains, with Success; in effect, the Indians use it for all Kinds of Pains. *Schroder* affirms, That he has seen intolerable Pains in the Leg removed by it.

**TALLOW-TREE**, in *China*, is a Tree growing in great Plenty in that Country, which produces a Substance like our *Tallow*, and serving for the same Purpose. 'Tis about the height of a Cherry-Tree; its Leaves in Form of a Heart, of a deep, shining, red Colour, and its Bark very smooth. Its Fruit is inclos'd in a kind of Pod, or Cover, like a Chestnut, and consists of three white round Grains, of the Size and Form of a small Nut, each having its peculiar Capsula, and within, a little Stone.

This Stone is encompass'd with a white Pulp, which has all the Properties of true *Tallow*, both as to Consistence, Colour, and even Smell : And accordingly, the Chinese make their Candles of it; which would, doubtless, be as those as good in Europe, if they knew how to purify their *Vegetable Tallow*, as well as we do our *Animal Tallow*.

All the Preparation they give it, is to mix a little Oil with it, to make it softer, and more pliant. 'Tis true their Candles made of it yield a thicker Smoak, and a dimmer Light, than ours; but those Defects are owing, in great measure, to the Wicks, which are not of Cotton, but only a little Rod, or Switch of dry light Wood, cover'd with the Pith of a Rush, wound round it; which being very porous, serves to filtrate the insensible Parts of the Tallow, attracted by the burning Stick, which by this Means is kept alive.

**TALPA**, in Medicine and Chirurgery, a Tumour thus call'd of the Oedematous Kind. The *Talpa*, and Nates, chiefly arise about the Head, as the Consequence of some Venereal Disorder. The *Talpa* elevate the Skin from the Pericranium; and generally denote a Foulness in the subjacent Bone of the Skull.

**TAMARINS**, or Tamarinds, a kind of Medicinal Fruit, of a tart, agreeable Taste; brought from the *East Indies*, and call'd by some *Indians Dates*, and by others the *Indian Acacia*.

The Tree which yields it, call'd by the *Indians Tamarinds*, and the *Portuguese Tamarindos*, is not unlike our Ash, or Walnut Tree; its Leaves resemble those of Female Fern; its Flowers are join'd eight or ten together, like those of the Orange Tree.

Its Fruit is in a Pod, the Length of a Finger, and the Thickness of the Thumb; cover'd at first with a green Rind, which afterwards becomes brown, and contains a blackish Pulp, among which are found Seeds resembling Lupines : 'Tis this Pulp alone that is brought to us, and us'd in Medicines.

The *Tamarinds* must be chosen big, of a Jet Colour, a brisk Taste, not too dry, and such as have not been laid in the Cellar, nor falsify'd with Molasses of Sugar and Vinegar. They are found laxative, cooling, and good to quench Thirst. In burning Fevers, they are prescrib'd to moisten and cool the Mouth.

**TARANTISMUS**, in Medicine, the Disease or Affection of those bit by the *Tarantula*. Dr. *Cornelio*[1], in the *Philosophical Transactions* represents this as an imaginary Disease; and tells us, that all those who think themselves seized with it (excepting such as for particular Ends feign themselves so) are most of them young wanton Girls, whom the *Italian* Writers call *Donne de*

[1] Tomasso Cornelio (1614 – 1684), an Italian physician.

*sale*, who falling, from some particular Indisposition, into a melancholy Madness, persuade themselves, according to the vulgar Prejudice, that they have been stung by a Tarantula. But the Evidence on the other side of the Question, is too strong to be thus overturned; as will appear from the following Article.

**TARANTULA**, or Tarentula, in Natural History, a venomous Insect, whose Bite gives Names to a new Disease. The *Tarantula* is a kind of Spider, denominated from the City *Tarentum*, in *Apulia*, where it is chiefly found : 'Tis about the size of an Acorn; and is furnish'd with eight Feet, and as many Eyes; its Colour various; but it is still hairy : From its Mouth arise two Sorts of Horns, or Trunks, made a little hooked, with the Tips exceedingly sharp; thro' which it conveys its Poison.

These Horns, M. *Geoffroy* observes, are in continual Motion, especially when the Animal is seeking for Food; whence he conjectures they may be a kind of moveable Nostrils.

The *Tarantula* is found in several other Parts of *Italy*, and even in the Isle of *Corsica*; but those of *Apulia* alone are dangerous : Even these, when remov'd thence, are said to become harmless : 'Tis added, that even in *Apulia*, none but those found on the Plains are much to be fear'd; the Air being hotter there, than on the Mountains.

M. *Geoffroy* adds it is an Opinion of some, that the *Tarantula* is never venomous but in the coupling Season; and *Baglivi*, that 'tis never so, but in the Heat of the Summer, particularly the Dog-Days, when, becoming enrag'd, it flies on all that pass by.

The Bite occasions a Pain, which at first appears much like that felt on the Stinging of a Bee, or an Ant : In a few Hours, the Patient feels a kind of Numbness; and the Part affected becomes mark'd with a little livid Circle, which soon after rises into a very painful Tumour : A little longer, and he falls into a profound Sadness, breathes with much Difficulty, his Pulse grows feeble, his Sight fails; at length he loses all Sense and Motion, and dies, unless reliev'd. But these Symptoms come somewhat differently, according to the Nature of the *Tarantula*, and the Disposition of the Patient. An Aversion for Black and Blue; and, on the contrary, an Affection for White, Red, and Green, are other unaccountable Symptoms of this Disease.

All the Assistance Medicine has been able to discover by Reasoning, consist in some Chirurgical on the Wound, in Cordials and Sudorificks; but these are of little Efficacy : A Thing that avails infinitely more, is, what Reason could never have thought of, Music.

As soon as the Patient has lost this Sense, and Motion, a Musician tries several Tunes on an Instrument; and when he has hit on that, the Tones and Modulation whereof agree to the Patient, he is immediately seen to make a faint Motion : His Fingers first begin to move in Cadence, then his Arms, then his Legs; by Degrees his whole Body : at length he rises on his Feet, and begins to dance; his Strength and Activity still increasing. Some will continue the Dance for six Hours without Intermission. After this he is put to Bed; and when he is judg'd sufficiently recruited of his first Dance, he is call'd out of Bed, by the same Tune, for a Second.

This Exercise is continu'd for several Days, six or seven at most; in which time the Patient finds himself exceedingly fatigu'd, and unable to dance any longer; which is the Characteristic of his being cured : For as long as the Poison acts on him, he would dance, if one pleas'd, without any Discontinuation, till he died of the mere Loss of Strength.

The Patient perceiving himself weary, begins to come to himself; and awakes, as out of a profound Sleep, without any Remembrance of what had pass'd in his Paroxysm, not even of his Dance.

Sometimes the Patient, this recovering from his first Access, is quite cured; if he ben't, he finds a melancholy Gloom hanging over him; he shuns the Sight of Men, and seeks Water; and if he ben't carefully look'd to, thrown himself into some River. If he don't die, the Fit returns at that Time Twelvemonth, and he is driven to dancing again. Some have had these returns regularly for 210 or 20 Years.

Every *Tarantatus*, or Patient in this Disease, has his particular and specific Tune; but, in the general, they are all very brisk, sprightly Tunes.

**TARTAR**, in Chymistry, &c. a Kind of Salt, which rises from famous Wines, and sticking to the Top and Sides of Casks, forms a greyish Crust, which hardens to the Consistence of Stone.

*Tartar*, says an ingenious Author, has the Juice of the Grape for its Father, Fermentation for its Mother, and the Cask for its Matrix. *Tartar* is either *white* or *red*, according to the Colour of the Wine it is rais'd in.

Its Goodness rather depends on the Number of repeated Fermentations, which a Succession of new Wines in the same Cask for several Years, makes, than on the Soil or Climate where the Wine is produc'd.

That brought from *Germany* is the best, as being taken out of those monstrous Tuns, some whereof hold a thousand Pipes of Wine; so that the Salt has Time to come up to its Consistence, one of the chief Qualities to be regarded in *Tartar*. That of *Montpellier* is the next in Order; then that of *Lyons*, *Paris*, &c.

*White Tartar* is preferr'd to red, and is really better : The Marks of good *Tartar* of either Kind, are, its being thick, brittle, brilliant, and very little Earthy.

*Tartar* is of considerable Use among the Dyers; as serving to dispose the Stuffs to take the Colours the better.

The Chymists make abundance of Preparations from *Tartar*; as *Cream*, or *Crystal of Tartar*, which is nothing but *Tartar* powder'd, and reduc'd by means of boiling Water, a straining Bag, and a Cellar, into little Crystals.

*Salt of* Tartar is made of *Tartar* wash'd, ground, purify'd, and calcin'd in Paper, by a reverberatory Fire; or 'tis made by pulverizing what remains in the Retort after the Distillation of *Tartar*. On the one or the other of these Preparations, they pour a great Quantity of hot Water, to make a Lye of it; this they filtrate, and evaporate the Liquor by a Sand Heat, till the fix'd Salt be found at the Bottom of the Vessel.

*Oil of* Tartar, is the Salt of *Tartar* expos'd to the Air for some Days, in an open Vessel, in a moist Place, till it dissolve into an Oil; tho 'tis improperly so call'd, being no more than a dissolv'd Oil.

Tartar *Vitriolated*, which some call *Magistery of Tartar*, is Oil of *Tartar* mix'd with rectify'd Spirit of Vitriol : Upon mixing the two, there arises a great Ebullition; by means whereof, of Liquids they become Solids.

Tartar *foliated*, is a Preparation of *Tartar* with distill'd Vinegar, which reduces it into white Leaves.

Oil of *Tartar per deliquium*, is held the best Remedy against corrosive Sublimate.

**TARTARIZING**, a Term used by some Writers, for the Act of Refining or Purifying, by means of Salt of Tartar.

**TASTE**, or Savour, a Sensation, excited in the Soul by means of the Organ of *Taste*; *viz.* the Papillae of the Tongue, &c.

Dr. *Grew*, in a Lecture on the Diversity of *Tastes*, before the Royal Society, distinguishes them into *Simple* and *Compound*.

By the former, he understands such as are Simple Modes of *Taste*, although mingled with others in the same; thus the *Taste* of a Pippin is Acidulcis; of Rhubarb, Amara-stringent, and therefore compounded, in both; but yet in the Pippin the Acid is one simple *Taste*, and the Sweet another; as distinct as the Bitter and Astringent are in the Rhubarb.

Two faults, he observes have here been committed : The first, a defective enumerating of simple *Tastes*, and reckoning them, indistinctly, among such as are compounded.

*Simple Tastes*, of which we usually only reckon six or seven Sorts, are at least sixteen; 1. *Bitter*, as in Wormwood; whose contrary is, 2. *Sweet*, as in Sugar. 3. *Sour*, as in Vinegar; whose contrary is, 4. *Salt*. 5. *Hot*, as in Cloves; to which is opposite, 6. *Cold*, as in Sal Prunella; for we may as properly say a cold *Taste*, as an hot one, since there are some Bodies which do manifestly impress the Sense of Cold upon the Tongue, tho' not to the Touch. 7. *Aromatick*; to which is contrary, 8. *Nauseous*, or malignant.

He thinks also that Tastes may be distinguish'd into such as are, 9. *Soft*, which are either Vappid, as in Water, Starch, Whites of Eggs, &c. or *Unctuous*, as in Oils, Fat, &c. 10. Or such as are *hard*; of which he reckons four Kinds, as, 11. *Penetrant*, which worketh itself into the Tongue without any Pungency; as is found in the Root and Leaves of wild Cucumber. 12. *Stupefacient*, as in the Root of black Hellebore; which being chew'd, and for some time retain'd upon the Tongue, affects that Organ with a Numbness, or Paralytic Stupor. 13. *Astringent*, as in Galls : And, 14. *Pungent*, as in Spirit of Sal Armoniac; which two last *Tastes* he makes contrary to the Unctuous, as Penetrant and Stupefacient are contrary to the Vappid one.

The *Compound Tastes* are very numerous; but we have Words to express but six of them, 1. *Austere*, which is astringent and bitter, as in the green and soft Stones of Grapes. 2. *Acerb*, properly so call'd, which is astringent and acid, is in the Juice of unripe Grapes. 3. *Acrid*, which is pungent and hot. 4. *Muriatick*, which is salt and pungent, as in common Salt. 5. *Lixivious*, which is Saltness join'd with some Pungency and Heat. 6. *Nitrous*, which is Saltness join'd with Pungency and Cold.

**TASTING**, the Sense whereby we distinguish Savours; or the Perception the Soul has of external Objects, by means of the Organ of *Taste*.

Authors have differ'd much as to the *Organ of Tasting*. *Bauhin, Bartholin, Vestingius*, &c. place it in the laxer fleshy Parts of the Tongue : Dr. *Wharton* in the Gland at the Root of the Tongue : *Laurentius*, in the thin Tunic covering the Tongue; others in the Palate, &c. But the great *Malpighi*, and, after him, all the latest Writers, place it in the Papillæ, chiefly lying about the Tip and Sides of the Tongue.

These Papillæ arise from the Corpus Nervosum that covers the muscular Flesh of the Tongue; whence, passing thro' the Corpus Reticulare, they stand up under the external Membrane of the Tongue, erect, cover'd with Vaginæ, or Sheaths of the said Membrane, to defend them from Objects too violent.

These Vaginæ are porous; and stick out so far, that when the Aliment is squeez'd, they enter within the same, to receive the Object, ort the Matter of *Taste*.

These Papillæ, *Boerhaave* conjectures, to arise from the ninth Pair of Nerves: And these he asserts, are the only Organ of *Taste* : Those others of the Tongue, Palate, Jaws, &c. he observes, contribute nothing thereto, tho' probably those of the Cheeks, next the Dentes Molares, may.

The *Object of Tasting*, is any Thing either in Animals, Vegetables, or Minerals, from which Salt or Oil may be extracted.

Tasting, then, is perform'd by the Objects being attenuated, and mix'd with Saliva, warm'd in the Mouth, and apply'd to the Tongue; where, insinuating into the Pores of the membranous Vaginæ of the nervous Papillæ, and penetrating to the Surface of the Papillæ themselves, it affects and moves them; by which Means a Motion is communicated along the Capillament of the Nerves to the common Sensory, and an Idea excited in the Mind, of Salt, Acid, Sweet, Bitter, Hot, Aromatic, Austere, or the like; according to the Figure of the Particles that strike the Papillæ, or the Disposition of the Papillæ to receive the Impulse.

**TEA**, or as the *Chinese* call it, *Tcha*, the Leaf of a Tree or Shrub, growing in several Provinces of *China*, *Japan*, and *Siam*.

The *Tea* Plant affects Valleys, and the Feet of Mountains, and a stony Soil. Its Seed is usually sown in Places expos'd to the South; and bears three Years after sown. The Root resembles that of the Peach Tree : The Leaves are green, longish at the Point, and pretty narrow, an Inch and half long, and jagged all around. The Flower is much like that of the wild Rose. The Fruit is of different Forms, sometimes round, sometimes long, sometimes triangular; of the ordinary Size of a Bean; containing two or three Peas, of a Mouse Colour, including each a Kernel. These Peas are the Seeds by which the Plant is propagated.

The Tree is of various Heights, from one Foot to an hundred : Some there are which two Men can't fathom, whiles others scarce exceed the feeblest Shrub in a Garden. The best Time to gather the Leaves of the *Tea*, is while they are yet small, young, and juicy: When gather'd, they are pass'd over the smoak of boiling Water to moisten them; then they are laid on Copper Plates, which are heated; and thus, the Leaves drying, they curl up in the Manner they are brought to us.

'Tis very rare to find Tea perfectly pure; the Chinese always mixing other Herbs with it, to increase the Quantity. Indeed, the Price 'tis sold for among them is moderate enough; usually 'tis about Three-Pence a Pound Sterling, never more than Nine-Pence.

The *Chinese* know nothing of *Imperial Tea*, *Flower of Tea*, and many other Names, which in *Europe* serve to distinguish the Goodness and the Price of this fashionable Commodity; and yet beside the common Tea, they distinguish two other Kinds, *viz. Voui* and *Soumlo*, which are reserv'd for People of the first Quality, and sick Folks.

We have three Kinds of Tea in *Europe*, *viz. Green Tea*; which is the common *Tea* of the *Chinese*, &c. F. *le Compte* calls it *Bing Tea*, and say 'tis gather'd from the Plant in *April*. 'Tis held very digestive, and a little corrosive: It gives a pale greenish Tincture to Water; and its Leaves are much twisted.

The second is *Bohea Tea*, which is the *Voui Tea*, or *Bou Tea*, of the *Chinese*. F. *le Comte* makes this only to differ from the *Green Tea*, by its being gather'd a Month before it, *viz.* in *March*, while in the Bud; and hence the Smallness of the Leaves, as well as the depth of the Tincture it gives Water. But 'tis much more probably the *Tea* of some particular Province; the Soil being found to make an Alteration in the Properties of the Tea, as much as the Season of gathering it. 'Tis all bought at *Nanquin*; and it is but lately that the *Dutch* have introduced it into *Europe*, where it begins to be much in vogue.

The third is *red Tea*, or *Tartar Tea*, or *Honan Tcha*, which tinges the Water with a pale red, and which is said to be extremely digestive : By means whereof, it is that the *Tartars* are said to be able to feed on raw Flesh. Its Taste is earthy; and much the least agreeable of them all; but little known in *England*.

*Tea* is to be chosen Green, of the brisket Smell, as whole as possible; and the greatest Care taken that it hasn't been exposed to the Air to pall, and evaporate.

The Drink, *Tea*, is made in *China*, and throughout the greatest Part of the East, after the same Manner as in *Europe*; *viz.* by infusing the Leaves in boiling Water, and drinking the Infusion hot. Indeed, among us, 'tis usual to temper its Bitterness with Sugar, which the Orientals use little or none of. However, the *Japanese* are said to prepare their Liquor a somewhat different Way, *viz.* by pulverizing it; stirring the Powder in hot Water, and drinking it as we do Coffee.

The *Chinese* are always taking Tea, especially at Meals : 'Tis the chief Treat wherewith they regale their Friends. The most moderate take it at least thrice a Day; others, ten times, or more : And yet 'tis computed, the Consumption of *Tea* among the *English* and *Dutch* is as great in Proportion as among the Orientals. In *France*, the use of *Tea* is much declin'd, and Coffee is now becoming the prevailing Liquor.

As to the Properties of *Tea*, they are strangely controverted : The Eastern Nations are at least as much possess'd with them as the *Europeans*; but 'tis, perhaps, because Imagination bears as great a Sway there as here. The

Reason why the Gout and Stone are unknown in *China*, is ascrib'd to the Use of this Plant; which is said further to cure Indigestions of the Stomach, to carry off a Debauch, and to give new Strength for Drinking, to dispel Wind, to cure the Vapours, &c.

*Sim. Paulli*, Physician of the King of *Denmark*, in an express Treatise on this Plant, endeavours to shew, that these virtues ascrib'd to it in the East, are local, and don't hold with the Inhabitants of *Europe*. He holds, that those past their 40th Year should never use it, as being too desiccative : That *Tea* has no other Virtues but those of Betony : And adds, with *Bauhin*, that 'tis only a species of Myrtle founding *Europe* as well as the *Indies*.

But this Opinion is refuted by *Pechlin*[1], in a Treatise of *Tea*, intitled, *Theophilus Bibaculus, sive de Potu* Theæ *Dialogus*; Where he maintains, That 'tis good to prevent Scorbutic Diseases; that its gentle astringent Virtues strengthens the tonic Motion of the Intestines, &c. But he blames the drinking it with Milk; and especially after a full Meal, or after much Wine.

**TEMPERAMENT**, in Medicine, is particularly understood of the Natural Habitat and Constitution of the Body of Man; or the Disposition of the Animal Humours.

The Notion of this *Temperament* arises hence, that the Blood flowing in the Veins and Arteries, is not conceived to be a simple Fluid; but a sort of imperfect Mixt, or an Assemblage of several other Fluids. For it does not only consist of the Four simple, or primary Qualities; but of Four other secondary Ingredients compounded thereof, into which it is supposed to be resolvable, *viz. Choler, Phlegm, Melancholy* and *Blood*, properly so called.

Hence, as this, or that Ingredient Humour prevails in a Person, he is said to be of a Choleric, Phlegmatic, Melancholic, Sanguine, &c. *Temperament*.

The ancient Physicians brought these Animal *Temperaments* to correspond with the universal *Temperaments* above described : Thus the *Sanguine Temperament* was supposed to coincide with *hot* and *moist*; the *Phlegmatic* with *cold* and *moist*, the *Melancholic* with *dry* and *cold*, &c.

*Galen* introduced the Doctrine of *Temperaments* into Physic, from the Peripatetic School; and made it, as it were, the Basis of all Medicine. The whole of curing Diseases, consisted in tempering the Degrees of the Qualities, Humours, &c.

On the Footing Medicine now stands, the *Temperaments* are much less consider'd. Dr. *Quincy* and other Mechanical Writers, pare away the greatest Part of the Galenic Notion, as useless and uncertain; and consider the *Temperaments* as no other but those Diversities in the Blood of different Persons, whereby it becomes more apt to fall into certain Combinations in one Body than another, whether into Choler, Phlegm, &c. whence, according to them, People are denominated *Choleric, Phlegmatic*, &c.

The Ancients distinguish'd two Kinds of *Temperaments* in the same Body; the one *ad Pondus*, in Weight; the other, *ad Justitiam*.

The *Temperament ad Pondus*, is, where the elementary Qualities are

[1] Johann Nicolaus Pechlin (1644 – 1706), a Dutch physician.

founding equal Quantities, and in equal Proportions; such is supposed to be in the Skin of the Fingers; without which they would want the Power of distinguishing Objects, with sufficient Accuracy. *Galen* observes, that the *Temperament ad Pondus*, is only imaginary; and that though it were real, it could not subsist above one Moment.

The *Temperament ad Justitiam*, is that which contains unequal Portions of those Qualities, but yet in such proportion as is necessary for the Discharge of the Functions proper to the Part: Such is the *Temperament* in a Bone, which contains more earthy than aqueous Parts, to make it more hard and solid, for its Office of sustaining.

Dr. *Pitcairn* looks on the *Temperaments* or Constitutions, as native Diseases; According to him, any one indued with whatever *Temperament*, hath the Seeds of a real Disease within him: A particular *Temperament*, supposing that some secretions are in greater Proportion that is proper for Life Indefinitely long.

As the Diversities of *Temperaments* are not other than Diversities of Proportions in the Liquids, which may be diversified infinite Ways; so there may be an infinite Number of *Temperaments*; though Authors have supposed Four. The *Sanguin*, which is reckon'd a *Temperament*, *Pitcairn* says, is no other than a Plethora.

**TENESMUS**, in Medicine, a continual Inclination to go to Stool; yet without voiding any Thing, unless, sometimes, a little purulent bloody Slime. The Word is form'd from the *Greek*, τεινειν, *tendere*, to bend, in regard those attack'd with this Disease, feel a continual Tension in the Fundament.

The Cause of the *Tenesmus*, is a sharp, pungent Humour, irritating the Intestinum Rectum, and exciting those troublesome Endeavours to evacuate. Those affected with the Stone, are also subject to the *Tenesmus*, from the Communication, or Consent between the Bladder and the Rectum.

The Cure of the *Tenesmus* depends on proper Evacuations and Astringents; the former always proceeding the latter; such are Bleeding, if Plethoric, gentle Cathartics, especially of Powder of Rhubarb, &c. An Emetic of the *Indian* Root, *Ipecacuanha*, has been found of great Service in a long standing *Tenesmus*; for the augmenting one Evacuation, is the lessening of another, and it becomes so much the more serviceable, as they happen to be Contraries.

**TERGIFÆTOUS** Plants, are such as bear their Seeds on the Backsides of their Leaves. Such are the Capillaries.

**TEREBINTHIA**, in Medicine, Natural History, &c. See Turpentine.

**TERTIAN**, a Fever or Ague intermitting but one Day; so that there are two Fits in three Days. The Method of curing *Tertians*, as well as other Agues, is by the Cortex, either given in Substance or Decoction. This last is best in weak Constitutions, and where the Fits are not so regular; but the Substance more to be depended on as to Certainty in other Cases.

**TESTACEOUS**, in natural History, an Epithet given to a Species of Fish, which are covered with a string, thick Shell; as Tortoises, Oysters, Pearl Fish, &c.

In Strictness, however, *Testaceous* is only applied to such Fish, whose strong and thick Shells are intire and of a Piece : Those which are soft, thin, and consist of several Pieces jointed, as Lobsters, &c. being called Crustaceous.

In Medicine, all Preparations of Shells, and Substances of the like Kind, are called *Testaceous Powders*. Such are Powders of Crabs Claws and Eyes, Harts-horn, Pearl, &c.

Dr. *Quincy*, and others, suppose the Virtue of all *Testaceous* Medicines to be alike; that they seldom or never enter the Lacteals; but that the chief of their Action is in the first Passages; in which Case, they are of great use in absorbing Acidities.

Hence they become of Use in Fevers, and especially in rectifying the many Distempers in Children, which generally owe their Origin to such Acidities.

**TESTUDO**, in Medicine, a soft broad Tumour, or gathering of impure Humours between the Skull and the Skin, call'd also *Talpa*, as resembling the Form of a Tortoise or a Mole.

**TETANOS**, in Medicine, a Term purely *Greek*, and signifying a kind of Tonic Spasmus, or Convulsion, wherein the fore and hind Muscles of the Head are render'd rigid and inflexible; so that it can neither bend one Way nor t'other. The Word is form'd from the *Greek*, τεινειν, to stretch. Some Authors also use *Tetanos*, or *Tetanus*, in a more general Sense. When a Convulsion is universal, they denominate it *Tetanus*; which they sub-divide into *Emprosthotonus* and *Opisthotonus*.

**TETRAPETALOUS**, in Botany, an Epithet given to Flowers that consist of four Petala, or Leaves, plac'd around the Pistil. These, M. *Jussieu* calls *Polypetalous* Flowers. Mr. *Ray* who calls them *Tetrapetalous*, makes them constitute a distinct Kind, which he divides into

1°. Such as have an uniform *Tetrapetalous* Flower, and their Seed-Vessels a little oblongish, which he therefore calls *Siliquose*; as the Keiri or Leucoium Luteum, and the other common Leucoium, the Dentaria, the Luecoium Siliquosum, Alysson, Viola Lunaris, Paronychia, Hesperis, Alliaria, Rapa, Napus, Sinapis, Rapistrum, Eruca Spuria, Erisimum, Cardamine, Turritis, Pilosella Siliquosa, and the Raphanous Rusitcanus and Aquaticus.

2°. Such as have their Seed Case or Vessel shorter, which therefore, for distinction Sake, he calls *Capsulæ*, and *Siliquosæ*; as the Myagrum, Draha, Leucoium, Siliqua subrotunda, Cochlearia, Nasturtium, Lepidum vulgare, Thlaspi, Brasica marina, Glastum, Eruca marina, &c.

3°. Such as have a seeming *Tetrapetalous* Flower, that is, a Monopetalous one, divided deeply into four Partitions; which he particularly calls *Anomalous*; as the Papaver, Agremony, Veronica, Tithymallus, Plantago, Coronopus, Psyllium, Lysimachia Siliquosa, Alsine spuria, &c.

**TETRAPHARMACUM**, from τετρα, *quater*, four, and φαρμακον, *Medicamentum*, is any Remedy consisting of four Ingredients.

**THERAPEUTICE**, Therapeuticks, that Part of Medicine which is employ'd in seeking out Remedies against Diseases, and in prescribing and applying them to effect a Cure. The Word is form'd from the *Greek*, θεαπευειν, to attend, to cure.

*Therapeutice* teaches the Use of Diet, Pharmacy, Chirurgery, and the *Methodus Medendi*. *Therapeutice* is also apply'd, figuratively, to the Mind, and to Discourses made to correct the Errors and Defects thereof.

Such is the *Therapeutice* of *Theodoret*; being a Treatise against the Errors or unwholesome Opinions of the *Greeks*, *i.e.* the Heathens.

**THERIACA**, Treacle, in Medicine, a Name the Ancients have given to various Compositions, esteem'd good against Poisons; but now generally restrained to what, by way of Distinction, we sometimes call *Theriaca Andromachi*.

This is a Compound of no less than 64 Drugs, prepared, pulveriz'd, and reduced, by means of Honey, into a liquid Electuary. The Basis, or Foundation, of the Composition is Vipers Flesh. M. *Charas* has wrote a particular History of the Animals, Plants and Minerals, which enter the Composition of this fam'd Remedy.

'Tis found sovereign against the Bites of venomous Beasts, and in the Wind-cholic; and is also used in intermitting Fevers, and in Cases requiring Perspiritives and Diaphoreticks; also in continual Fevers, especially such as are malignant, and where the Pulse is low and ticking; in the Small-Pox and Measles: And, as most of the Ingredients thereof, are very hot, for all Diseases, where the natural Heat s weak and languid.

*Andromachus*, *Nero's* Physician, passes for the Inventor of the *Theriaca*; at least, 'twas he gave the first Description thereof in Elegiac Verses; his Son did the same in Prose, and *Democrates* in Iambics.

Anciently, the Treacle made at *Venice* had all the Vogue; and many still retain the ancient Prejudice; but 'tis now prepared at *Montpellier*, *Paris*, and even at *London*, with as much Advantage as at Venice.

There is another vulgar kind of *Theriaca*, call'd *Diatessaron*, because only consisting of four Ingredients.

*Treacle Water* and *Treacle Vinegar* are found good Preservatives against putrid Air, whether by begin only smelt at, or by rubbing the Wrists, Temples, and Nose therewith.

**THISTLE**, *Carduus*, a name common to divers Plants, whose Flowers consist of several little narrow longish Leaves, in Manner of Tubes, rang'd close together like a Head, and whose Leaves are very prickly.

The most known of these Plants are

1° *Carduus Benedictus*. The Apothecaries distil a Water from it, said to be of great Service in pestilential Diseases, the worse Kind of Fevers, and particularly as a Sudorific. The Water is likewise accounted one of the four common Cordial Waters : Its fixt Salt is much of the same Nature as other fit Salts prepar'd from Wormwood, &c. *viz.* Anti-emetic, Diuretic, &c.

2° The *hundred-headed Thistle*, or *Eryngium vulgare*; the Root whereof boil'd in Wine, is us'd with good Success against Retention of Urine : This is not properly of the *Thistle* Kind.

3° Our *Ladies Thistle, Carduus Albis Maculis notatus vulgaris* C B, the Decoction whereof is recommended against the Dropsy, Jaundice, and Pains of the Kidneys.

**THYMUS**, in Medicine, is used for a kind of Wen, growing on the natural Parts, the Fundament, and several other Places of the Body, which cloven Asperities like those of the Herb *Thyme*, whence its Name. The ordinary Method of curing a Thymus, is by Ligature and desiccative Lotions, or by Caustics; and if large, by Incision; taking Care first to secure the greater Vessels by tying them.

**TIN**, a whitish Metal, softer than Silver, yet much harder than Lead. The Chymists, &c. hold *Tin* an imperfect Metal, generated of two different Seeds, *viz.* that of Silver and that of Lead; which renders it a kind of Compound of both; and accordingly it is frequently found in Lead and Silver Mines.

*Tin*, however, has also its proper Mines, of which our Counties of *Cornwall* and *Devonshire* are an abundant Evidence : The greatest Part of the *Tin* consumed in *Europe*, is procured from thence; and *Cambden* even supposes this Abundance of *Tin* in those two Provinces, to have given the original Denomination *Britain* to the whole Country. In the *Syrian* and *Chaldee*, *Tin* is call'd *Bragmanac*; the Primitive whereof is *Bratman* or *Britman*, whence *Britain*.

The principal Characters or Properties of *Tin*, enumerated by *Boerhaave*, are, That it is the lightest of all Metals; very little ductile or elastic; the most subtle and volatile of all Metals; scarce dissoluble by Acids, unless the weaker Sorts; and easily and intimately miscible with other Metals, the Ductility whereof becomes diminish'd by such Mixture.

The same Author concludes, that Sulphur is a prevailing Ingredient in *Tin*, and deduces several of its particular Properties therefrom. He adds, that could the Metal be perfectly purged of this heterogeneous Sulphur, 'tis probable it would be no other than Silver.

Several Authors had before noted a great Conformity, in divers Particulars, between the two Metals; as, that both grow bitter when dissolved by Acids; that when fused together, there is scarce any separating them again, not even by Lead. Add, that Mr. *Boyle* and others, give us several Instances of Silver being actually procured in considerable Quantity from *Tin* Ore.

Yet some Naturalists judge the Analogy greater between *Tin* and Lead; and contend that *Tin* is only Lead, under a less Degree of Coction; but if there be some Marks of Agreement between them, there are as many of Disagreement. The Calx of Lead for instance, easily fuses and vitrifies, but that of *Tin* not without the last Difficulty : If *Tin* and Lead be mix'd by a vehement Fire, a vehement Colluctation ensues, and they both run into a Calx : Add, that *Tin* is easily revivified; but Lead with great Labour.

The method of getting, preparing, &c. the *Tin* in the *Cornish* Mines, much the best and most considerable in the World; is given us in the *Philosophical Transactions.*

The working of the *Tin*-Mines is very hard and difficult; not only by the Reason of the great Depth which the Veins descend to, even as low as 50 Fathom; but also because the Rocks, through which Passages are frequently to be cut, are often so hard, that the Workmen can't dig a Foot in a Week. Nor is the soft, shaking Earth found in *Tin*-Mines, much less inconvenient to the Workmen; both by reason of foetid, malignant Vapours it exhales, and of the currents of Water often met withal therein : all these Disadvantages together render it impracticable for the Workmen to hold it above four Hours together.

The mineral Stones or Glebe being dug and drawn out of the Mine, is there broke into Pieces with large Iron Mallets; then brought to a Stamping Mill, where 'tis still pounded smaller with Stampers, much like those of Paper Mills; and the Water passing through it washes away the earthy Parts, leaving the Metallic ones behind : The Lotion is repeated twice, to make the better Separation.

This done, they dry it in a Furnace on Iron Plates; and grind it very fine in a Crasing Mill; then wash it again; then dry it : In this State, the metallic Matter is call'd *Block*, or *Black Tin.*

To convert it into *Tin*, *i.e.* into *white Tin*, they carry it to a Furnace or blowing House; where, by means of a Charcoal Fire, kept up by huge Bellows work'd with the Water, it is melted; after it has pass'd all these Preparations, and is become cold, they forge it; which is the last Thing done to it in the Works.

The Dross or Scoria scumm'd off the *Tin* in Fusion, being melted down with fresh Ore, runs into Metal; and even the Causalty; *i.e.* the Matter wash'd and separated from the Metal in the Mill, being thrown up in Heaps, after resting Six or Seven Years, they fetch it over again, and it yields as good *Tin* as any of that of *Germany.*

The Workmen distinguish several Kinds of *Tin*; as *Moor-Tin*, which is the best Sort, a Fool whereof, weighs 80 Pounds; and *Mine-Tin*, which is the next, a Fool thereof weighing about 52 or 50 Pounds. The Tin got from the soft, gravelly Earth, they call *Pryan Tin*, to distinguish it from that got from the Stones, which is better by almost half.

Two Pounds of *black Tin*, when melted, yield about one of *White.*

There is a Curiosity in these *Cornish* Mines, which the Lover of Natural History will be pleas'd to hear; and 'tis this : That in digging, at the Depth of 40 or 50 Fathoms, they frequently meet with large Trees, still entire.

*Childrey*[1], in his Natural History, goes back as far as the Deluge to place them there; but without having recourse to so great Antiquity, they who believe that the Mines, when exhausted of their Ore or Mineral Matter, renew and fill again in course of Time, will soon solve the Difficulty, by supposing, that in the first Working of these Mines, these Trees had been let down to

[1] Joshua Childrey (1623 – 1670), an English natural philosopher.

serve as Props and Pillars. But there are other People will think this Renewal of the Mines itself a Difficulty as great as the former. However, what the former Author adds, *viz.* that in some Places in the Mines, they likewise find Pick-Axes, &c. with wooden Shafts, as also brass Nails, and even a Medal of *Domitian*, seems to countenance the Opinion.

The Chymists call *Tin, Jupiter* : But from what Analogy between the Metal and the Planet, we leave them to explain. By the Analyses made of this Metal, they hold it compounded of Earth, Sulphur, a metallic Salt, and Mercury. The chief Preparations from *Tin*, are Salt of *Tin*, Flower of *Tin*, and Diaphoretic of *Tin*.

*Salt of Tin*, or of *Jupiter*, is *Tin* calcined; and distill'd Vinegar pour'd thereon; from which, by means of Fire, and then of a cool Place wherein 'tis put, a very white Salt is drawn.

*Flower of Tin*, is a kind of white Cosmetic, or Paint, for the Complexion; drawn with Sal Ammoniac, by means of Sublimation.

*Diaphoretic of Tin*, is fine *Tin*, and Regulus of Antimony melted, first together, and then both with Salt-petre. Whence, after various Lotions, is drawn a Powder, held to be sovereign against various Diseases.

*Ceruss of Tin*, is a white Powder, procured from *Tin*, whereof a Fucus is made, call'd *Spanish White*. This *Ceruss* is not made with Vinegar, as that of Lead is; but with the Urine of a young Person : The Powder is also used to colour *Delft* ware.

*Calx of Tin*, is what we properly call *Bismuth*.

**TINCTURE** or Essence, in Pharmacy and Chymistry, a Separation of the finer and more volatile Parts of a mixt Body, made by means of a proper Menstruum which takes away a Part of its purest Substance, and by that means becomes a sharer in its Colour, Virtues, &c.

Thus in Pharmacy, we have Cephalic *Tinctures*, Antiscorbutic *Tinctures*, Stomachic *Tinctures*, Anticholic *Tinctures*, Invigorating *Tinctures*, &c. *Tinctures* are also drawn from Roses, from Corals, &c.

To make a *Tincture*, the Matter is usually bruised, put in a Matrass, and the Menstruum, which commonly is Spirit of Wine, poured on it, to the Height of two or three Fingers above it. Then the Glass is closed, and set for Digestion, in a Sand Heat during four or five Hours, till the Spirit is well impregnated, and has received a high Colour.

Thus are *Tinctures* of odoriferous Vegetables, as Cinnamon, &c. drawn; and the same Menstruum serves for those of Metals and Minerals.

The *Tinctures* of Metals, so much talk'd of by the Chymists and Alchymists, are not proper *Tinctures*; they are only Dissolutions, where in the Metal is divided and attenuated to a greater Degree, than it is in its natural and ordinary Dissolvent.

If the *Tincture* were irreductible; that is, if the Metal were dissolv'd to such a Degree, as that it could not be brought back again into Metal; or, which comes to the same, if the Principles which compose it were disunited, it would be what the Chymists have so long and so earnestly wish'd for, and sought with such infinite Pains, especially with regard to Gold; the

*Irreductible Tincture* whereof, is what should be call'd *Aurum Potabile.*

But no such *Tincture* has ever yet been discover'd : The Potable Gold in use among us, being only Gold extremely divided; and the Case is the same with the *Tinctures* of other Metals.

The Intention of metalline *Tinctures*, is to rarify and extend the Sulphur of the Metal as much as possible; and so render the fix'd and earthy Parts, as subtle and volatile as may be : If they are designed to be of Use in Medicine, some harmless and agreeable Intermedium is to be used.

The Alchymists give the Name of *Grand Mineral Tincture* to the Philosophers Stone; from an Opinion, that all which is required to that Operation, is to give the Colour or *Tincture* of Gold to fix'd Mercury.

Marble, Alabaster and Bones, receive *Tinctures* from Lixiviums, and sharp Juices; and Mr. *Boyle* thinks there is reason to hope the same may be done of precious Stones; Rock Crystal, 'tis certain, is tinged by Subterranean Juices; to is Saphyr itself.

In the Memoirs of the *French* Academy, mention is made of certain Liquors, e.gr. Salts drawn from Wheat, which will extract *Tinctures*, even out of some precious Stones. 'Tis added, they are the more capable of producing this Effect, as they give a greater Degree of Redness to the Solution of Vitriol.

**TINEA**, in Medicine, a Diseases call'd by the *Arabic* Writers *Sahafati*, and in English usually a *scall'd Head*. The *Tinea* is a Disease of the Leprous Kind : Authors usually reckon three Species of it, *viz.* a *dry*, *moist*, and *lupinous*; which, in reality, are only so many Degrees of the same Disease.

*Turner*[1] defines it an Ulcer arising in the Heads of Children, from a viscous, corrosive, or saline Humour, which preying on the Cutaneous Glands, in Time destroys their Texture. In the first Stage it is cover'd with white, dry, scurfy, or squammous Matter : In the second the subjacent Flesh appears granulated : And in the third it is ulcerous.

The internal Remedies proper for the *Tinea*, are Mercurials, proper Cathartics, and Diuretics, or Edulcorants; and sometimes a Salivation, especially by Unction, has been efficacious, after all other Methods have prov'd vain. The Externals are Fomentations made of Roots of *Oxylapathum, Birthwort, Horse-radish, Wormwood*, &c. boil'd in Water and strain'd; to which are added, Spirits of Wine camphorated, &c. *Liniments* of Hogs Lard, white Precipitate Mercurial Ointments, with powder'd Brimstone; and sometimes Powder of *Roman* and white Vitriol, red Precipitate, &c.

It has its Name *Tinea*, Moth, from the Similitude of the Holes eat by that Insect on Paper, &c.

**TINNITUS**, *Auris*, *Tingling of the Ear*, a Disease pretty frequent in the Ear, consisting in the Perception of a Sound which is not, or, at least, which is not external. This Perception is occasion'd by the beating of an Artery in the Ear, by Inflammation, or Abscess of the Tympanum or Labyrinth, by the Admission of foreign Bodies, by Commotions of the Cranium, Blows on the Ear, &c. Extraordinary and irregular Motions of the Animal Spirits are also

[1] This is probably George Turner (1550 – 1640), an English physician.

found to occasion Tinnitus, as we find in Deliriums, Phrensies, Vertigos, &c. The Tingling of the Ear is one of the Diagnostic Signs of the Plague.

**TOBACCO** or Tabacco, a Medicinal Herb, not known in *Europe* till after the Discovery of *America* by the *Spaniards*; and first Imported about the Year 1560. The *Americans* of the *Continent* call'd it *Petum*; those of the Islands, *Yoli*. The *Spaniards*, who gave it the Name *Tabaco*, took it from *Tabaco*, a Province of *Jucatan*, where they first found it, and first learnt its Use.

The *French*, at its first Introduction among them, gave it various Names; as *Nicotiana*, or the *Embassador's Herb*, from *John Nicot*, then Embassador of *Francis* II. in *Portugal*, who brought some of it with him from *Lisbon*, and presented it to a Grand Prior of the House of *Lorrain*, and to Queen *Catherine de Medicis*; whence it was also call'd *Queen's Herb* and *Grand Prior's Herb*.

They also gave it other Names; which are now all reduced to the original Name, *Tobaco*, or *Tobacco*, for *Tabaco*, given it by *Hernandez de Toledo*; who first sent it into *Spain* and *Portugal*.

Besides the *Tobacco* of the *West Indies*, there are considerable Quantities cultivated in the *Levant*, the Coasts of *Greece* and the *Archipelago*, the Island of *Malta* and *Italy*. The Marks of good Twist *Tobacco*, are a fine shining Cut, an agreeable Smell; and that it have been well kept.

*Tobacco* is either taken by way of Snuff, as a Sternutatory; or as a Masticatory, by chewing it in the Mouth; or by smoaking it in a Pipe. 'Tis sometimes also taken in little longish Pellets put up the Nose, where 'tis found to produce very good Effects, to attract a deal of Water or Pituita, unload the Head, resolve Catarrhs, and make a free Respiration; for the subtile Parts of the *Tobacco* in Inspiration, are carried into the Trachea and Lungs, where they loosen the peccant Humours adhering thereto, and promote Expectorations.

Some have left this *Tobacco* in their Noses all Night; but this is found to occasion Vomiting the morrow Morning. Another thing charge on this Way of Application, is, that it weakens the Sight.

When taken in great Quantities in the way of Snuff, 'tis found to prejudice the Smelling, greatly diminishes the Appetite, and in time gives rise to a Phthisis.

That taken in the way of Smoak, dries and damages the Brain. *Borrheus* in a Latter to *Bartholine*, mentions a Person, who through excess of Smoaking had dried his Brain to that degree, that after his Death, there was nothing found in his Head but a little black Lump, consisting of mere Membranes.

Some People use the Infusion of *Tobacco* as an Emetic; but 'tis a very dangerous and unjustifiable Practice, and often produces violent Vomitings, Sickness and Stupidity.

*Bates* and *Fuller* give some Receipts, in which *Tobacco* is an Ingredient with mighty Encomiums in Asthmatic Cases.

A strong Decoction of *Tobacco*, with proper Carminatives and Catharticks, given Clyster-wise, sometimes proves of good Effect in what is usually called the *Stone Colic*; and also in the Iliac Passion.

A Drop or two of the Chymical Oil of *Tobacco* being put on the Tongue of a Cat produces violent Convulsions, and Death itself in the space of a Minute; yet the same Oil used in Lint, and applied to the Teeth, has been a Service in the Tooth-ach; though it must be to those that have been used to the taking of *Tobacco*, otherwise great Sickness, Reachings, Vomitings, &c. happens; and even in no Case is the internal Use of it warranted by ordinary Practice.

A strong Decoction of the Stalks, with sharp pointed Dock and Allom, is said to be of good Service, used externally, in Cutaneous Distempers, especially the Itch. Some boil them for that Purpose in Urine. The same is said to be infallible in curing the Mange in Dogs.

Sig. *Paulli*, Physician of the King of *Denmark*, in an express Treatise on *Tobacco*, observes that the Merchants frequently lay it in Bog-houses, to the End that becoming Impregnated with the volatile Salt of the Excrements, it may be rendered the brisker, more foetid and stringer.

*Amurath* IV. Emperor of the *Turks*; the Grand Duke of *Muscovy*, and the Emperor of *Persia* have prohibited the Use of *Tobacco* in their States. Our King *James* I. wrote a Treatise against *Tobacco*, entitled a *Counter-blast to Tobacco*. By a Bull of Pope *Urban* VIII. such are excommunicated, as take *Tobacco* in Churches.

**TOOTH-ACH**. The *Tooth-ach* usually proceeds from a Caries which rots the Bone, and east it hollow. Sometimes it proceeds from a Defluxion of a sharp Matter upon the Gums. For the *Tooth-ach*, a Paste made of soft Bread, and the Seed of Stramonia, laid on the Tooth affected, abates the Pain. If the Tooth be hollow, and the Pain great, a Composition of equal Quantities of Opium, Myrrh, and Camphor, made up into a Paste with Brandy or Spirits of Wine, and about a Grain or two put into the hollow Place, puts a stop to the Caries, and blunts the acute Pain of the Nerve; by which it often gives immediate Relief.

Chymical Oils, as those of Origanum, Cloves, Tobacco, &c. are also of Service, destroying, by their hot Caustic Nature, the Texture of the sensible Vessels of the Tooth affected; tho', from too liberal an Use of them, frequently proceeds a Defluxion of Humours, and Impostumation.

A Blister apply'd behind one or both Ears, seldom fails to cure the *Tooth-ach*, especially when attended with a hot Defluxion of Humours, and swelling of the Gums, Face, &c. Liniments of Rum, Brandy, or Spirit of Wine, camphorated, are good, us'd outwardly, to abate the Swelling.

Mr. *Cheselden* mentions one cur'd of *Tooth-ach* by applying a small cauterizing Iron to the Anthelix of the Ear, after he had undergone Bleeding, Purging, Salivation, Secretions, &c. to no Purpose : The Case was very remarkable; for when he was seiz'd with it, a Convulsion of that whole Side of his Face follow'd, whenever the Pain became acute, or he attempted to speak.

To prevent and cure the Scurvy in the Gums, 'tis recommended to wash the Mouth every Morning with Salt and Water; and to hinder the Teeth from spoiling or growing carious, some use only Powder of Hartshorn to rub the Teeth with, and then wash their Mouth with cold Water : 'Tis alledg'd, this is preferable to other Dentifrices, on this account, because their hard Particles are apt to abrade that fine smooth Polish, with which the Surface of the Teeth is cover'd, and which is their Preservative from the ill Effects of Air, Ailment, Liquor, &c. which occasion Ailments of the Teeth when wore off.

Dentifrices are usually compounded of Powders of Hartshorn, red Coral, Bone of the Cuttle Fish, burnt Alum, Myrrh, Dragon's Blood, &c. Some commend Powder of Bricks, as sufficient to answer all the Intentions of a good Dentifrice.

**TOPHUS**, in Medicine, a stony Concretion in any Part of an Animal Body; as in the Bladder, Kidneys, &c. or in the Joints.

Dr. *Rutty*[1], in a Treatise, just publish'd, of the Urinary Passages, takes the Stone to arise from the Attraction of volatile and saline Particles; of which Particles the Stone, when view'd with a Microscope, seems to be made up : He thinks the Fault of these Aggregates of saline Particles, ought generally to be suppos'd to begin in, or proceed from, the Papillæ of the Kidneys, and not from the Sediment of the Urine in the Bladder.

The Reason why Wine-drinkers are more subject to the Stone, and other Concretions, than Malt or Water-drinkers, he supposes to be the volatile and saline, or earthy Particles contain'd in the Wine, in greater Quantities than in the Ale, &c. A Calculus, observes, reduc'd to a Caput Mortuum, will, upon the Affusion of warm Water, dissolve, and entirely mix; but in a short Time will again settle, and the Particles thereof so closely unite or attract, as that, by repeated Affusions, they cannot be brought again to dissolve.

**TORCULAR**, or Torcularis, among Chirurgeons, a Contrivance for stopping of Bleedings in Amputations.

**TORMINA**, in Medicine, a Term used to express Pains in the general; but particularly a Species of Pain call'd *Tormina Ventris*, or *Alvi*; in *English*, the Gripes.

Young Children are very often troubled with Gripes; 'tis upon this account, that Nurses, in order to prevent or remedy them, usually mix with their Spoon-meats, a little Brandy or some Carminitive Seeds, as Carus Seeds, &c. Some Children breed their Teeth with violent Gripes, which is apt to turn to Convulsions of the Bowels.

In Adults, the dry Gripes, is usually cured by the Exhibition of warm Cath-articks, such are Tincture of Hiera Picra, Elixir Salutis, Tincture of Rhubarb, &c. with the Assistance of Opiats.

**TORREFACTION**, in Pharmacy, a kind of *Assation*, wherein a Drug is laid to dry on a Metal Place plac'd over Coals, till it become friable to the Fingers. The Word is form'd from the Latin, *torre-facere*, to roast.

*Torrefaction* is particularly us'd, when, after reducing some Drug, as Rhubarb, or Myrabolans into Powder, 'tis laid on an Iron or Silver Plate, and that plac'd over a moderate Fire till the Powder begin to grow darkish; which is Mark those Remedies have lost their purgative Virtue, and have acquir'd a more astringent one.

[1] William Rutty (1687 – 1730, an English physician.

Formerly, they us'd to *torrify* Opium, to get out some malignant Parts fancy'd to be in it, e'er they durst use it in Medicine; but the Effect was, that its volatile Spirits and Sulphur, wherein its greatest Virtue consists, were hereby evaporated.

**TRACHOMA**, in Medicine, a Roughness or Asperity of the inner Part of the Palpebræ; attended with an Itching, Redness, and frequently with Pustles, resembling Millet-Seeds. Its Degrees are the *Sycosis* and *Tylosis*.

**TRAFINE**, among Surgeons, an Instrument call'd also *Trepanum, Anabapiston, Modiolus*, &c.

**TRAGACANTH**, or Adraganth, a kind of Gum oozing out at Incisions made in the Trunk and larger Branches of a Plant, or little Shrub, of the same Name. The Word is form'd of the *Greek*, τραγος, Goat, and ακανθα, Thorn, by Reason the Plant is beset with Thorns.

The naked Hillocks of Mount *Ida* in *Candia*, M. *Tournefort* tells us, produce a deal of the Plant *Tragacanth*, which gives the Gum spontaneously towards the end of *June*, and in the following Months; when the nutritious Juice of the Plant, thicken'd by the Heat, bursts most of its Vessels it is contain'd in. The Plant grows also in several Places in the *Levant*, particularly about *Aleppo*.

This Juice coagulates in Threads, which make their Way into the Pores of the Bark, where being push'd forward by new Juice, they get thro' the Bark, and are at length harden'd in the Air, either into little Lumps, or into twisted Pieces in Form of little Worms, more or less long according to the Matter they are form'd of.

It should seem to that the Contraction of the Fibres contributes to the Expression of the Gum : Those fine Fibres, like those of Hemp, laid bare and trampled under Foot by Men and Horses, contract themselves, and facilitate the Expression of the extravasated Juice.

The Gum is of different Colours, and Qualities; some being white, other-some greyish, some red, and some almost black. The white is the best. It must be chosen clear, smooth, and twisted like little Worms.

It dissolves easily in any aqueous Menstruum, which it will give the Consistence of a Syrup to, in the small Proportion of a Dram to a Pint. It is smooth and softening, and therefore good to obtund the Acrimony of any Humours, which makes it of Service in such Coughs as proceed from Catarrhs and Defluxions of Rheum. It is also very strengthening in some Seminal Weaknesses, and prevalent against the Whites in Women.

**TRAGEA**, in Pharmacy, a Term frequently used to express Powders grossly beat; but now obsolete.

**TRANSLOCATION**, in Pharmacy, the same with Filtration or Percolation.

**TRANSMUTATION**, the Act of transforming, converting or changing one Nature into another. The Term is chiefly us'd in Chymistry and Medicine : 'Tis greatly question'd, whether the *Transmutation* of Silver into Gold, and of

Tin into Silver, so much sought by the Chymists, be possible or not.

Nature, Sir *Isaac Newton* observes, seems delighted with *Transmutations* : He goes on to enumerate several Kinds of *Natural Transmutations*; gross Bodies and light, he suspects, may be mutually *transmuted* into each other; and adds, That all Bodies receive their active Force form the Particles of Light which enter their Composition.

For all fix'd Bodies, when well heated emit Light as long as they continue so; and again, Light intermingles itself and inheres in Bodies as often as its Rays fall on the solid Particles of those Bodies.

Again, Water, which is a fluid, volatile, tasteless Salt, is by Heat *transmuted* into Vapour; which is a kind of Air; and by Cold, into Ice, which is a cold, transparent brittle Stone, easily dissolvable; and this Stone convertible again into Water by Heat, and Vapour is by Cold.

Earth, by Heat, becomes Fire; and by Cold, is turned into Earth again ; Dense Bodies, by Fermentation, are rarified into various kinds of Air; and that Air by Fermentation also, and sometimes without, reverts into gross Bodies.

Quicksilver sometimes puts on the Form of a fluid Metal; sometimes it appears in Shape of a pellucid, fragile Salt, called *Sublimate*; sometimes of a pellucid volatile, white, tasteless Earth, called *Mercurius Dulcis*; by Distillation it becomes Vapour, and by Agitation in vacuo, shines like Fire, &c.

All Bodies, Beasts, Fishes, Insects, Plants, &c. with all their various Parts grow and increase out of Water, and aqueous and saline Tinctures; and by Putrefaction, all of them revert into Water, or an aqueous Liquor again.

Further, Water expos'd a while to the open Air, puts on a Tincture, which is Process of Time has a Sediment and a Spirit; and before Putrefaction, yields Nourishment both for Animals and Vegetables.

**TRANSMUTATION**, in Alchymy, the Act of changing or exalting imperfect Metals into Gold or Silver. This is also call'd the *Grand Operation*, and is to be effected with the Philosophers Stone.

Some Alchymists hold, that the *Transmutation* should rather be call'd the *Perfection* of imperfect Metals; as holding all Metals intended by Nature to arrive equally at this Perfection, inasmuch as they are compos'd of the same Matter; and that 'tis only the Impurity of their Matrices, that is, of the Place wherein they are form'd by Nature, that has prevented their arriving thereat.

The Elixir being projected on any of those Metals, it is suppos'd to purge, and separate the impure Parts from the pure, and to join itself wholly to the Mercury (which is the pure Part,) as being of the same Nature.

Whether or no Metals are *transmutable* into one another, is a Point strongly disputed among the Philosophers; the Alchymists strenuously asserting the Affirmative.

Some Metals 'tis commonly allow'd many be chang'd into others, *e.gr*. Iron into Brass or Copper, and Lead into Tin; but *Cardan* and some others deny even this, and argue further, that tho' the Iron and Brass, as being nearly alike in Weight and Tenacity, &c. provided their Colour and Hardness could be chang'd, might be converted into one another, either really, or, at least, apparently, yet would the *transmuting* or ripening of other Metals into Gold or Silver be still impossible; both as those metals are all to be first calcin'd, after which they can never be brought again to their pristine Purity; and as there is a Generation requir'd, which is not the Work of Art, but Nature.

*Cardan de Metall. Lemery, Dickenson*[1], and others, give us Accounts of the various Impostures of *Adepti* in the Business of *Transmutation*; some, for Instance, fixing Mercury with Verdigrease, and then heightening the colour with Cadmia, Turmeric, &c. But this, if try'd with the Coppel, all goes off in Fumes; and, in effect, nothing produc'd this Way ought to be adjudg'd true Gold, unless it endure Coppelling, Cementation, Putrification, with Antimony and the Depart.

Add, that it must have the Malleability, extreme Ductility, and specific Gravity of Gold, which is to Water as 18 and half to 1.

The Trick of *transmuting* Cinnabar into silver is thus : The Cinnabar being bruis'd grossly, is stratify'd in a Crucible with granulated Silver, and the Crucible plac'd a in a great Fire; and after due Time for Calcination, taken off: then the Matter being pour'd out, is found to be Cinnabar turn'd into real Silver, tho' the Silver Grains appear in the Number and Form they were put into the Crucible; but the Mischief is, coming to handle the Grains of Silver, you find them nothing but light friable Bladders, which will crumble to Pieces in your Fingers.

Mr. *Boyle* in his *Scept. Chymist.* Tells us, that two Friends of his did, by urging Mercury in a skilfully manag'd Fire, turning almost Weight for Weight into Water; but does not say what was the specific Gravity of the produc'd Water, nor of the remaining *untransmuted* Mass of Mercury. He likewise assures us, that Rain Water being distill'd and re-distill'd by a Friend of his, near 200 times, did, after each Distillation, leave at the Bottom of the Glass Body, a considerable Quantity of a white Earth; and that more plentifully in the latter Distillation than the former.

This he believ'd to be a certain Quantity of Water actually transmuted into Earth; adding, that it was above twice as heavy specifically as common Water, and of so fix'd a Nature, that it lay a considerable Time in a red hot Crucible, without losing any of its Weight, or emitting any Smoak.

**TRANSPIRATION**, the insensible, or almost insensible Passage of an excrementitious Matter through the Pores of the Skin; called also Perspiring.

There are an Infinity of these *transpiratory* Pores in the Skin; the most considerable whereof, are the Orifices of the Ducts arising from the milliary Glands. The Cause of *Transpiration*, is the Circulation and Heat of the Blood.

Insensible *Transpiration* is found very much to exceed all the sensible Evacuations put together. *Sanctorius* even shews, in his *Medicina Statica*, that a Person loses more in one Day by *Transpiration*, than by all the other Outlets, in Fifteen. He adds, that if the Food taken in one Day weigh Eight Pounds, the *Transpiration* will be Five of them.

Cold prevents *Transpiration*, by its constringing the Pores of the Skin, and

[1] Edmund Dickinson (1624 – 1707), an English physician and alchemist.

thickening the Liquors circulating in the cutaneous Glands : Heat, on the contrary, augments *Transpiration*, both by its opening the excretory Ducts of the Glands, and by increasing the Fluidity and Velocity of the Humours.

M. *Dodart*, from a Number of Experiments made for 33 Years together, assures us that we *transpire* much more in Youth than in Age. In some Persons, the *Transpiration* is so copious, that they void but very little of the coarser Excrements, though they eat heartily.

*Transpiration* is absolutely necessary in the Animal Œconomy, to purify the Mass of Blood, and discharge it of a Number if useless heterogeneous Particles which might corrupt it. Hence it is, that upon a Stoppage of the usual *Transpiration*, there arise so many Indispositions, particularly Fevers, Agues, Itch, &c.

*Transpiration* is also of use to the Organ of Feeling, in that it prevents the Papillæ of the Skin from being dry'd, either by the Air, or by the continual Touches of external Bodies.

*Transpiration* is also used by some Authors, for the Entrance of the Air, Vapours, &c. through the Pores of the Skin into the Body.

*Cardan*, by this kind of *Transpiration*, accounts for the Prodigy of Women, whose daily Urines weigh'd 27 Pounds; though all the Foods she took, both dry and liquid, did not exceed Four Pounds. Dr. *Baynard* suspects some such *Transpiration* to be the Case in hydropical Persons.

**TRANSPLANTATION**, in Natural Magic, is used for a Method of curing Diseases, by transferring them from one Subject to another; much in vogue among certain Philosophers. This *Transplantation* is effected, either by the Use of a certain Medium; or without, by simple Contact.

The first Kind, which is that most properly call'd *Transplantation*, is when the Patient's Excrement being mix'd up with Earth, the Disease is transplanted into a Vegetable, arising from a Seed sown in the said Compost; or, when the Pairings of the Nails, of a Gouty Person, are inclosed in an Augur-hole made in a Plant, particularly an Oak.

The second Kind of *Transplantation*, properly call'd *Approximation*, is, when a Finger seiz'd with a Panaris or Whit-low, is cured by rubbing in a Cat's Ear, which is held to receive the Pain.

In this Case, the sound Subject receives the vital Spirits, unites with them, and corrects their morbific State : And, as certain Diseases are got by Approximation; the infected Spirits of a diseas'd Body, insinuating themselves into a sound one, and thus infecting the same; so they are cured by Approximation; when the Spirits of a diseased Person entering a sound Body, the latter corrects and retrieves the morbific State of the former.

*Transplantation*, by means of the Magnet, is of five kinds, *viz. Insemination, Implantation, Imposition, Irroration* and *Inescation*; each whereof, see under its proper Article.

**TRAUMATICKS**, τραυματικ, Vulneraries; are Herbs or Drugs good for the curing of Wounds.

**TREMOR**, Trembling, in Medicine, a Disease nearly akin to a Convulsion, wherein there is something of a convulsive Motion accompanying a voluntary or natural Motion. A *Tremor* is frequently found to arise upon the more violent Passions, particularly, Anger, Gluttony, Venery, &c. but hit is accidental and transitory. A *Tremor* is sometimes apt to degenerate into other worse Diseases, *viz.* Palsy, Apoplexy, Lethargy, Spasmus, &c. In old Men it is incurable.

The Medicine commonly made use of in *Tremors* and other nervous Distempers, by the name of *Palsey Drops*, is no other than *compound Spirit of Lavender*. The most successful Way of using it, is by taking 30 or 40 Drops twice or thrice a Day, dropt on Loaf Sugar or a little Bread. 'Tis supposed, that by this Way, the most spirituous and efficacious Parts make their Way directly by the Nerves of the Pallat, &c. without undergoing the Course of the Circulation, as it is said to do when taken in a liquid Vehicle.

**TREPIDATION**, in Medicine, a *Tremor*, or Trembling of the Members and Nerves of the Body. The first Symptom of Madness in Dogs, is a *Trepidation* of the Members, &c.

**TRIA** *prima*, among Chymists, the three Hypostatical Principles, *viz.* Salt, Sulphur, and Mercury; of which they hold all Bodies to be primarily made, and into which they are held resolvable by Fire.

**TRIFOLIUM**, or Trefoil, any three-leaf'd Grass : That which is most used in Medicine, is the *Trifolium Aquaticum*, or Buck-Bean, which is very detergent, and used with Success in Scorbutic, Rheumatic, and Scrophulous Habits. The way of using it is generally to make a pretty strong Infusion of the dry'd Herb, in form of Tea.

**TRIPLOIDES**, of the *Greek*, τριπλοος, a Surgeon's Instrument, with a three-fold Basis, us'd in the restoring great Depressions of the Skull.

**TRITURATION**, in Pharmacy, *Grinding*; the Act of reducing a solid Body into a subtile Powder; call'd also *Levigation*, *Pulverisation*, &c. The Word is form'd from *tri* and *tero*, I wear.

The same Term is also applied to the comminuting, bruising, and dividing of humid Matters, into little Parts : The *Trituration* of moist Bodies is perform'd in Marble, or Stone Mortars, with Pestles of Wood, Glass, Ivory, &c. The *Trituration* of Woods, Bark, Minerals, and other hard and dry Bodies, is perform'd in Metalline Mortars.

*Trituration*, *Boerhaave* observes, has a wonderful Force to dissolve some Bodies, and will render them as fluid, as if they were fused by the Fire. Thus if you grind the Powder of Myrrh, and Salt of Tartar together, they will dissolve each other. By rubbing new and bright Filings of Iron in a Mortar, with double their Weight of clean Sulphur, the iron will be dissolved, so as by diluting it with Water to afford the Vitriolum Martis.

Gold long ground in a Mortar, with Salt of Tartar, will yield a kind of Tincture; and rubbed with Mercury, in a Mortar of Glass, it entirely dissolves into a Purple Liquor, and becomes a most powerful Medicine.

Dr. *Langelotte*[1] has wrote a curious Treatise of the great Effects of *Trituration* in Chymistry; and describes a peculiar Way he employed to grind Gold, whereby he could render it as fluid as the Fire does, and make an Aurum Potabile, by the bare Motion of a Mill.

That Author, in the *Philosophical Transactions*, mentions his way of grinding Gold, and describes two Engines, or Philosophical Mills for the Purpose, with one of which, in the Space of Fourteen natural Days, he reduced a Leaf of Gold to a dusky Powder, and putting it into a shallow Retort placed in a sand Heat, he thence obtained, by gradually increasing the Fire and giving a string one at last, a few very red Drops, which, digested per se, or with tartarized Spirit of Wine, afforded a pure and genuine Aurum Potabile.

The Success of this operation, the Doctor attributes, in a great measure to the Salt of the Air, which in grinding, plentifully mixes and unites itself with the Gold.

**TROCHE**, *Trochiscus*, in Pharmacy, a Form of Medicine, made to be held in the Mouth to dissolve. *Latin* Authors call them *Pastilli, Rotulæ, Placentulæ, Orbes*, and *Orbiculi*; and the *English*, frequently, *Lozenges*.

The *Troche* is properly a dry Composition, the chief Ingredients whereof, after having been brought into a very subtile Powder, are incorporated with some proper Liquor as, distill'd Waters, Wine, Vinegar, or Mucilages; and reduced into a Mass, which is moulded into little Cakes or Balls of any Form, at Pleasure, and dried in the Air far from the Fire.

There are *Troches* of various Kinds, and for various Intentions; as Purgative, Alterative, Aperitive, Corroborative, &c. The chief *Troches* are of Agaric, Liquorice, Nutmeg, Amber, Rhubarb, Capers, Myrrh, Roses, Camphor, Squillæ, Vipers, &c.

Those of Coloquintida, are call'd *Troches of Alhandel*, from the *Arabs*, who call Coloquintida, *Handal*.

**TRYPHERA**, *Tryphere*, in Pharmacy, a Term us'd for several Kinds of Opiates. The *Great Tryphere* is composed Opium, Cinnamon, Cloves, and several other Ingredients : It is used to fortify the Stomach, to stop Fluxes, and for some Diseases of the Womb. There is also the *Saracenic Tryphere*, and the *Persian Tryphere*, thus call'd, because first introduced the one by the *Saracens*, and the other by the *Persians*; they both purge gently. The Word is form'd from the *Greek*, τρυφερος, delicate, soft, by reason it makes those who use it, rest.

**TUBER**, or Tubercle, in Botany, a kind of round turgent Root, in form of a Knob or Turnip. The Plants which produce such Roots, are hence denominated *Tuberose* or *Tuberous Plants*.

**TUBER** or Tuberosity, in Medicine, is used for a Knob or Tumour growing naturally on any Part; in Opposition to Tumors which arise accidentally, or from a Disease. The same Term is used for the Knot in a Tree.

[1] Joel Langelott (1617 – 1680), a German physician and alchemist.

**TUBERCULES**, Tubercles, are little Tumors which suppurate and discharge Pus; often found in the Lungs.

**TUMEFACTION**, the Act of swelling, or rising into a Tumor. Inflammations and *Tumefactions* of the Testes, frequently happen in the Gonorrhæa; either form the Weakness of the Vessels, violent Motion, unseasonable Use of Astringents, a Neglect of Purging, or the like.

**TUMOR**, or Tumour, in Medicine, &c. a preternatural Rising or Eminence on any Part of the Body. *Tumor* is defined by the Physicians, a Solution of Continuity, arising from some Humour collected in a certain Part of the Body, which disjoyns the continuous Parts, insinuates itself between them, and destroys their proper Form.

This has given occasion to the *Arabs* to define a *Tumor* to be an indisposition, composed of three kinds of Diseases, *viz.* an Intemperature, an ill Conformation, and a Solution of Continuity, all which they comprise under the Name *Aposthem*, from the *Greek*, αποθημ.

*Tumors* may proceed from various Causes. The Mass of Blood throwing off or discharging itself of any particular Humour, as sometimes happens in the Crisis of a Fever, Pleurisy, Empyema, Bubo, &c. will give rise hereto. And according to the Nature of Humour so discharged, whether Sanguinous, Watery, Bilious, &c. the *Tumor* is different.

Other *Tumors* there are, occasioned by Flatulency, as the Tympany, after the same Manner as hydropical *Tumors* are occasioned by a Collection of the Lympha, or Serum, in a particular Part. Ruptures of the Intestines, or their starting from their Places, will likewise cause a *Tumor*.

External Injuries are another general Cause of *Tumors*. Thus a Contusion, or a violent Stricture of any Part, a Wound, Fracture, Dislocation, &c. will make it swell, or rise above its natural Level. And the same thing may likewise happen from the Bites of venomous Creatures, &c.

*Tumors*, properly so call'd, *i.e. Humoral Tumors*, or those which contain a fluid Matter, arise either from a Stagnation, *i.e.* an Obstruction of the Passage of some Fluid, occasioning a slow Congestion; or a Tranflation or Fluxion of a Humor from some other Part; or a Generation of some new Humor.

*Tumors* of the first Kind are very numerous, and are usually divided, with regard to the particular Humors they are filled with, into Phlegmons, which come from the Blood.

*Erysipela's*, which are filled with the Bile. *Oedema's* filled with Pituita. And *Schirrus's* with Melancholy. To which may be added, *Flatulencies*, fill'd with Wind.

Of the second Kind, are *critical Tumors*. And of the third Kind, are *Cancer's*, *Ganglio's*, and all *Tumors* contain'd in a Cystis or Bag.

*Tumors* also frequently acquire peculiar Denominations from the Part affected, as *Ophthalmia*, if in the Eye; *Parotides* about the Ears; *Paronichia* in the Fingers, &c.

With respect to the Cure, all *Tumors* are divisible into *Simple* and *Compound*, *i.e.* into such as are of a kindly Nature, and go off, or are cured in a reasonable Time , by the use of common Means, without the Appearance of any violent or dangerous Symptoms; and such as are more malignant, or prove difficult of Cure, and are attended with bad Symptoms, and affect the adjacent Parts, or the whole Body. When a *Tumor* is form'd by Fluxion, a sudden Pain, Heat, Tension and Pulsation are felt in the Part, and manifest signs of a Fever appear.

In those form'd by Congestion, the Swelling rises slowly, and the Pain, and other Symptoms, come on gradually, and prove less violent; unless it happens in the Joints, and other of the more sensible Parts.

All *Tumors*, except those from Ruptures, terminate or are removed, either by Discussion, Suppuration, Putrefaction, Induration, or Translation.

When a *Tumor* is discussed, the Part that was affected, appears relaxed, or reduced to its natural Size and Figure, and is free from Pain and Hardness.

When a *Tumor* hastens to Suppuration, a considerable Degree of Heat, Pain, and Pulsation are felt in the Part, and if the *Tumor* be large, or lie deep, a Fever generally comes on : When the Matter is formed, these Symptoms commonly decrease, and sometimes totally vanish. And now, if the Situation of the Parts permits of it, the *Tumor* appears drawn to a Point, or becomes conical in the Middle, or most depending Part, where the Matter collected commonly proves White. At this Time, likewise, the *Tumor* appears to be more contracted, and the Skin of the Part more shrivelled or flaccid than before : And now, upon Pressure, if the *Tumor* be superficial, or by vibrating it between the Fingers, the matter may be felt to squash from Side to Side.

*Tumors* in the fleshy Parts of the Body, tend to their State, or suppurate faster than *Tumors* in the Joints, Glands, &c.

When a *Tumor* is resolved by Induration, the Swelling of the Part, and the Pain decrease, as the Hardness comes on. When in terminates in Putrefaction or Mortification, the Part grows senseless, and turns black and fœtid.

But when a *Tumor* goes off by Repulsion, or a Return of the Matter into the Blood, it disappears at once; upon which a Fever, or some other acute Disease presently ensues.

*Windy Tumors*, M. *Littre* describes as form'd of Air, inclosed under some Membrane, which it dilates more or less in proportion to the Quantity , and from which it cannot escape; at least not for some time.

The Difficulty is, to conceive how the Air should come to be collected here. M. *Littre* thinks that the most ordinary Cause of *windy Tumors*, is the gathering of Juice in some neighbouring Part, wherein there is an Obstruction. The Air which is intimately mix'd with all the Juices of the Body, continues to be so while they are in their natural Fluidity and Motion; but if they be collected in any Part, and, by Consequence, have their Fluidity and Motion diminished, the Air gets its Liberty, and disengages itself from them. Now the Membranes of the Part wherein the Liquor is collected, becoming dilated by this Collection, and their Pores enlarged; the disengaged Air escapes through them; but the Juice is left behind, as being too much thickened by its stay there : It therefore runs under some other neighbouring Membrane, which it raises, swells, and extends.

**TURBITH**, or Turpeth, *Turpethum*, a Medicinal Root, brought from the *East Indies*, particularly *Cambaya*, *Surat*, and *Goa*; tho' others will have it, that the true *Turbeth* comes chiefly from *Ceylon*. It is commonly suppos'd to take its Name *Turbith* from the Violence of its Operation, as disturbing the whole Œconomy.

The *Turbeth* of the Moderns bears so little resemblance to that of the Ancients, that 'tis difficult to suppose them the same. That sold by our Druggists is longish, about the Thickness of a Finger, resinous, heavy, and of a brownish hue without, and whitish within. 'Tis brought to us cloven in the Middle, length-wise, and the Heart or woody Matter taken out.

When in the Ground it shoots out Vines, some whereof creep along the Ground, and the rest wind about the neighbouring Trees and Shrubs.

It yields a deal of resinous Matter in a spirituous Menstruum, which Dr. *Quincy* observes, does not affect the larger Passages much; but is very active in the smaller Vessels, and glandulous Contorsions, which it wonderfully clears of all viscid Adhesions.

Some Apothecaries, either thro' Ignorance or Parsimony, substitute white Thapsia, which they call grey *Turbeth*, for the true *Turbeth*; tho' both as to Taste, Colour, and Quality, they are very different.

*Turbeth* is a violent Purgative, and is used in the Dropsy, Palsy, and Apoplexy.

*Mineral* **TURBITH**, or *Turpethum Minerale*, is a Name which the Chymists give to the yellow Precipitate of Mercury, which purges violently.

The Method of preparing it is thus : On the dry Powder gain'd by dissolving Mercury in Oil of Vitriol, pour a proper Quantity of warm Rain Water, and the Powder will immediately turn of a yellow Colour. Continue to wash this Powder by repeated Affusions of Water, till the Liquor comes away as insipid and colourless as it was pour'd on, leaving a beautiful yellow Calx at the Bottom of the Vessel, which being gently dry'd at the Fire, is call'd by the Name of *Turbith mineral*.

This Powder is call'd *Mineral Turbith* from the resemblance it bears to the vegetable *Turbith* of the *Arabians*, in strongly purging the most internal Recesses of the Body; for tho' it be insipid on the Tongue, yet it is possessed of very considerable Virtue. Being boil'd with Water, it loses more of its Salts, and thereby grows milder, and more safe; so it does by being deflagrated twice or thrice, or distill'd with Spirit of Wine.

A very few Grains of this *Turbith* will prove emetic and purgative. It is also accounted an excellent Medicine in the Cure of the Venereal Disease : But as it operates with considerable Violence, it ought not to be given, unless the Viscera are known to be sound.

This appears to have been the grand Secret of *Paracelsus*, which, in his scarce *German* Book of Hospital Medicines, he praises so extravagantly for the Venereal and all Chronical Diseases. *Sydenham* also commends it in Venereal Cases, given in the Quantity of six or eight Grains, in strong Habits of Body, so as to prove emetic; but when imprudently used, it is apt to give the Dysentery.

**TURGESCENCE**, a Swelling or growing turged or bloated. Form the *Latin*, *turgere.*

**TURMERIC**, a Root us'd by the Dyers to give a yellow Colour, call'd in *Latin, Curcuma Officinarum.* 'Tis brought chiefly from the *East Indies*; tho' the Island Madagascar does like-wise afford it. You are to chuse that which is big, new, resinous, hard to break, and heavy.

'Tis yellow both within and without Side, very hard, as if petrify'd and not unlike, either in Figure or Size, to Ginger. The Leaves it produces are like those of white Hellebore; its Flowers rise in Manner of a Spica or Ear; and its Fruit rough like our new Chestnuts.

Some People have mistakenly imagin'd there was a Native red *Tumeric*; their Error was owing to this, that the yellow Root, as it grows old, turns brown; and when pulveriz'd reddish.

'Tis much us'd by the Glovers, &c. to dye their Gloves; as also by the Founders, &c. to give a Gold Colour to their Metals. The *Indians* use it to dye their Rice, and other Foods, of a yellow Colour; when some call it *Indian Saffron.*

Our Dyers don't find that it gives so steady a Yellow as the Luteola or Greening Weed; but 'tis admirable to brighten and heighten the red Colours dyed with Cochineel or Vermillion; as Scarlets, &c.

*Tumeric* is us'd in Medicine by Way of Decoction, Infusion, Powder, &c. with other Ingredients, in the Jaundice, Hypochondriac, Leucophlegmatic, and Cachectical Constitutions.

**TURPENTINE**, *Terebenthina*, a transparent Gum or Resin flowing either Naturally or by Incision, from several fatty resinous Trees; such as the *Terebinthus*, Larch, Pine, Fire, &c. We can distinguish several Kinds of *Turpentines*; as that of *Chio*, that of *Venice*, that of *Bourdeaux*, that of *Cyprus*, *Strasbourg*, &c.

The *Turpentine* of *Chio*, which is the only genuine Kind, and that which gives the Denomination to all the rest, is a whitish Resin, bordering a little on the Green, very clear and a little odoriferous; drawn by Incision from a Tree called *Terebinthus*, very common in that Island, as also in *Cyprus*, and some Parts of *France* and *Spain.*

The Gum must be chosen of a solid Consistence, almost without either Taste or Smell, and not at all Tenacious, which distinguishes it from the false *Turpentine* of *Venice*, commonly substituted for it, which has a string Smell, a bitter Taste, and sticks much to the Finger. This *Turpentine* of *Chio* is indisputably the best; but its Scarcity occasions it to be little in use.

The *Turpentine* of *Venice*, is falsely so called, for though there was a *Turpentine* anciently brought form *Venice*, yet that now so called, comes al from *Dauphine.* 'Tis liquid, of the Consistence of a thick Syrop, and whitish; and flows either spontaneously, or by Incision from Larches, Firs and Pines, chiefly in the Wood *de Pilatze.*

That flowing naturally, call'd by the Peasants *Bijon*, is a kind of Balm not inferior in virtue to that of *Peru*, to which it is frequently substituted. That drawn by Incision, after the Tree has ceas'd to yield spontaneously, is of very considerable Use, in several Arts, and 'tis even of this Varnish is made.

It must be chosen White and Transparent, and Care be taken it hasn't been counterfeited with Oil of *Turpentine.*

The *Turpentine* of *Bourdeaux* is white and thick as Honey. It does not ooze from the Tree in the Manner it is sent to us; but is properly a Composition, wherein, among other Ingredients, is a white hard Sort of Rosin call'd Galipot.

The *Turpentine* of *Strasbourg*, *Dantzig*, &c. is that most commonly used among us; and is preferr'd, by our People, to that of *Venice*, which it is distinguish'd from, by its green Hue.

The Uses of Turpentine in Medicine are innumerable. 'Tis a great Vulnerary, and very Detergent, and as such is prescribed in all Abscesses and Ulcerations, &c. It promotes Expectoration, and as such is prescribed in Diseases of the Lungs and Breast : But it is most famous for clearing the Urinary Passages, and as such prescribe in Obstructions of the Reins, in Gonorrhæas, &c.

*Oil of* **TURPENTINE**. There are two Kinds of Oils drawn from *Turpentine* by Distillation; the first White, the second Red; both esteem'd as Balsoms proper for the Cure of Wounds, Chilblains, &c. But they are so little used among us, that 'tis not easy to procure either of them. What is commonly sold under the Name of *Oil of Turpentine*, or *Etherial Oil*, is only a Distillation of the Rosin called Galipot, fresh from the Tree. It is used with success in the Cure of green Wounds, as also by the Painters, Farriers, &c. To be good, it must be clear and white as Water, of a strong penetrating Smell, and very inflammable.

**TUSSIS**, in Medicine, a *Cough*; a Disease affecting the Lungs, occasioned by a sharp serous Humor, vellicating the Fibrous Coat thereof, and urging it to a Discharge by Spitting, &c. When the Humor is so subtile, that the Lungs cannot lay hold of it, to throw it off; or when the Humor is so thick that it will not give Way, it is said to be a *dry Cough.* Dry Coughs are the most dangerous. *Hippocrates* says, the Cough ceases, if the Testicles swell.

**TUTTY**, *Tutia*, or *Lapis Tutiæ*, a metallic Soot, thrown off from Brass, in the Furnace; and form'd into Concave Flakes of different Sizes and Thickness; very hard, greyish, and full of little protuberant Grains as big as Pins Heads. It is found adhering to Rolls of Earth suspended for that Purpose over the Furnaces of the Founders in Brass, to receive the Fumes of the melted Metal.

To prepare *Tutty* for Use, they heat it red Hot three times in a Crucible, among burning Coals; and quench it as often in Rose-water : Then they grind it on a Porphyry Stone, mixing with it as much Rose-water, or Plaintain-water as is necessary, till it be brought to a very fine Powder : Then they make it up into little Troches, and thus dry it.

*Tutty* is very desiccative. Its principal Use is in Diseases of the Eyes, particularly Inflammations; in order to which, it is diluted with Rose-water, or Plaintain-water, in form of a Coryllium. Some use it incorporated with fresh Butter, in form of an Unguent.

In the *London* Dispensatory, it gives Title to a Composition called *Ointment of Tutty*, good for Eye Diseases, and frequently used by Surgeons with other Desiccatives to cicatrize Ulcers. 'Tis also good in the Hemorrhoids.

*Tutty* is now brought chiefly from *Germany*. Anciently it came from *Alexandria*.

**TYMPANITES**, or Tympany, in Medicine, a flatuous Tumor, or Swelling of the Abdomen, or Belly; very hard, equable, and permanent; whereby the Skin is stretch'd so tight, that when struck, it give a sound like that of a Drum.

The *Tympanites* is a Species of Dropsy; but what the Cause or Seat of the Disease is, or what the morbific Matter is that occasions the Tumor, Physicians are not all agreed.

Wind certainly makes a principal Part of the morbid Matter; but this is scarce ever found without Water, excepting at the Beginning; so that some will not allow of any Difference between the *Tympany* and the *Ascites*.

Some suppose it to arise from a watery Humour extravasated and rarify'd into Vapour; and by a Property common to it with common Air, corrupting the Parts. But this *Boerhaave* makes a particular Kind of *Tympanies* or Wind Dropsy; and adds, that it is cured like Ascites or Water Dropsy, by Tapping, &c.

Others will have the *Tympanites* to arise from the Air's insinuating itself thro' Perforations in the putrefy'd Intestines. A *Tympanites* from this Cause, *Boerhaave*, who makes it a peculiar Class, observes, is almost always incurable.

*Willis* sets aside this latter Cause, and accounts for the Disease from an Irregularity in the Animal Spirits belonging to the Viscera, which rushing tumultuarily into the nervous Fibres, bloat them up : Thus is the Peritoneum inflated, the Intestines distended, and the Mesentery, and other Viscera, render'd turgid; and while this is doing, that the Vacuities left in the tumify'd Viscera may be fill'd up, a Quantity of the Humour contain'd in them is rarefy'd into Vapour, which presently spreads in Blasts through the vacant Places.

Others account for the *Tympanites* from a Convulsion of the Muscles of the Abdomen, &c.

M. *Littre* has propos'd a new System of the *Tympanites*, built on a great Number of Observations. According to him, it does not proceed from any Convulsion of the Abdominal Muscles, nor from any Air contain'd in the Cavity thereof, or in the Thorax, the Mesentery, or Epiploon; but from the Air inclos'd in the Stomach and Intestines, which swells them excessively.

This Air, always carry'd into the those Parts with the Food, maintains a kind of Equilibrium therein; opposing, on the one Hand, the too great Pressure on that long Canal when empty of Food; and finding, on the other Side, in the Spring of the Coats of the Stomach an Intestines, an Obstacle capable of preventing its too great Dilatation.

If this Equilibrium chance to be destroy'd by the Irritation of the Fibres, whose Spring in that Case prevails over that of the Air; this latter is expell'd either upwards or downwards, or both : (whence Belching, &c.) But if the Equilibrium come to be broke by the Force of the Air, render'd superior to that of the Fibres, by those latter being left destitute of Spirits, from the Blood's being impoverish'd after a long Sickness; in that Case, the Air, rarefying itself beyond Measure, swells the Cavities it is contain'd in.

If it be demanded, Why when the Stomach and Intestines are so full of Wind, none of the Wind escapes, either thro' the Anus, or by the Mouth, which uses to be expell'd by those Passages?

M. *Mery* solves the Paradox thus : According to this Theory, the Fibres, both of the Stomach and Intestines have lost their Spring, at least in Part, and are in an imperfect Palsy; but the Winds evacuated either by the Anus or Mouth, are Winds which those Viscera expel out of their Cavities, by putting them in a State of Contraction capable of surmounting the Forces which oppose the Egress of the Matters contain'd in those Cavities. These Forces are two Sphincters, one whereof shuts the upper Orifice of the Stomach, and the other the Anus : But paralytic Viscera, *i.e.* Viscera destitute of Spirits, in which alone consists the Strength of the Muscles, cannot overcome the Resistance of those two Muscles : Whence the Wind, therefore, cannot escape thro' its usual Out-lets.

The *Tympanites* rarely kills of itself; but frequently degenerates into an Ascites. Cathartics rather aggravate than alleviate it : Antihystericks, Anti-scorbuticks, Chalybeats, and Strengtheners are of use, before it be fallen into an Ascites. Equal Quantities of Leek and Elder Leaves mix'd analytically, is a fam'd Empirical Medicine, which has often prov'd effectual when every thing else has fail'd.

'Tis usual to apply Carminatives to the Belly, as the Emplaster of Cumin-Seeds, &c. and also to use Carminatives mix'd with Cathartics, Diuretics, &c. internally : But if the Disease proceed from a Paralytic Cause, destroying the Tone of the Fibres of the first Passages, what is of Use in rectifying of Paralytic Disorders, where the Tension of the Fibres are insufficient, will doubtless for the same Reason be of Use here.

**TYPHOIDES**, in Medicine, an ardent or burning Fever. See Fever.

**TYPHOMANIA**, in Medicine, a Disease of the Brain, wherein the Patient not being able to sleep, tho' greatly inclin'd thereto, lies with his Eyes shut, talks absurdly, and flings himself this Way and that. If he be pull'd, or the like, he just opens his Eyes, looks about, and sinks again into a kind of dozing, which is interrupted by a Train of disagreeable Imaginations. A *Typhomania* frequently takes place in Fevers, Phrenzies, and the like Diseases. 'Tis also call'd a *Coma Vigil.*

**TYROSIS**, in Medicine, a Coagulating or Curdling of Milk in the Stomach; after the Manner of Cheese. The Word is form'd of the *Greek*, τυρος, Caseus, Cheese.

**ULCER**, *Ulcus*, in Medicine, a Solution or Discontinuity of Texture, or a loss of Substance in the fleshy Parts of the Body, proceeding from an internal Cause. *Galen* defines it an inveterate erosion of the soft Parts of the Body, by which, instead of Blood, they are brought to yield a kind of *Pus*, or *Sanies*; which prevents the Consolidation. *Etmuller* defines an *Ulcer*, a Solution of Continuity from some corrosive Sharpness or Acidity, that takes away from the Parts, and turns the proper Nourishment of the Body into a sanious Matter. A like Solution of Continuity happening in a bony Part, is call'd a *Caries*.

*Galen* commonly uses the Words *Ulcer* and Wound, indifferently; but the *Arabs* and the Moderns after them, distinguish between the two.

Spontaneous *Ulcers*, are generally supposed to proceed from Acrimony, or a corrosive Disposition of the Humours of the Body, whether brought on by Poisons, the venereal Taint, or other Causes.

*Ulcers* are divided into *simple*, and *complicated* : They are again divided, with regard to their Circumstances, into *Putrid*, or *Sordid*, wherein the Flesh all around is corrupted and fetid; *Verminous*, where the Matter being thick, does not flow away, but generates Worms, &c. *Virulent*, which instead of Pus, or Sanies, yield a malignant *Virus*, &c. They are again distinguish'd, with regard to their Form, into *Sinuous, Fistulous, Varicous, Carious*, &c.

When an *Ulcer* happens in a good Constitution, and proves easy of Cure, 'tis said to be *Simple*. When attended with other concurring Symptoms, as a Cacochymic Habit, which greatly retards or obstructs the Cure, it is called a *Compound Ulcer*.

A *Simple Ulcer* is attended with no other Sign than that of Erosion; but *Compound Ulcers* happening in a Scorbutic, Dropsical, or Scrophulous Constitution, may be attended with Pain, a Fever, Convulsions, a large and emaciating Discharge of Matter, Inflammation and Swelling of the Part, Callosity of the Lips, a Caries of the Bones, &c.

A *Putrid* or *Sordid Ulcer*, is that whose Sides are lined with a tough, viscous Humour, and is also attended with Heat, Pain, Inflammation, and a large Flux of Humours to the Part : With time the *Sordes* increase and change Colour, the *Ulcer* corrupts, its Matter grow fetid, and sometimes the Part gangrenates. Putrid Fevers often give rise to this kind of *Ulcer*.

A *Phægenic Ulcer*, is an *Ulcer* of a corrosive Nature, eating away the adjacent Parts all a-round; the Lips thereof remaining tumified. When this kind of *Ulcer* eats deep, and spreads wide, without being attended with a Tumour, but putrifies and grows foul and fetid, 'tis call'd *Noma*; and both, on account of the Difficulty wherewith they heal, are also termed *Dysepulota*.

*Varicous Ulcers*, are such as being seated in the Veins, and becoming painful and inflammatory, swell up the Part they posses. These, when recent, being occasion'd by the Use of Corrosives, or proceeding from a ruptured Varix, are often attended with an Hæmorrhage. The Veins adjacent to the *Ulcers* are, in this case prætornaturally distended, and may sometimes be felt interwoven together, like net-work, about the Part.

*Sinuous Ulcers*, are such as run a-slant or side-ways from their Orifice, and may be known either by searching with the Probe, Wax-Candle, &c. or the

Quantity of Matter they discharge in proportion to their apparent magnitude. These sometimes lie deep, and have several Turnings : they are distinguished from *Fistulas* only by their want of Callosity, except in the very Orifice.

*Fistulous Ulcers*, are such as are sinuous, or winding, and attended with a great Callosity, and discharge a thin, serous, and fetid Matter.

Old *Ulcers* are rarely cured without the Use of Internals, which are to be such as absorb and destroy the Acidity; Sudorificks especially, Decoctions of the Woods, Antimonials, Viperines, and Volatiles; but above all things Vomitories often repeated: In the most obstinate *Ulcers*, mercurial Salivation is often required; Old *Ulcers* are frequently incurable without making an Issue in the opposite Part.

The Cure of simple, shallow *Ulcers*, is commonly affected by applying a Pledget armed with a *Liniment. arcaei*, or *Basilic. Flav.* To the Part, a Plaister of *Diachyl. simp.* or *de Minio*, being laid over it, and repeating the dressing once a-day, or seldomer.

If only the Cuticula be lost or eat away, nothing more than a little *Unguent. de Siccativ. Rub.* or *Diapomphol.* &c. spread thin upon Linen, need be applied.

If spongy Flesh should grow up, in either case it may be kept down with a little *Roman Vitriol*, &c. as in the case of healing up the *Simple Ulcers* made by the braking of the common Tumors.

Evacuations are indispensably necessary in the Cure of *Ulcers* of the compound kind, where the Constitution will admit thereof.

If the *Ulcer* be fistulous, sinuous, cancerous, &c. and the Matter fetid, thin, or sanious, it is found proper to join Calomel with Purgatives, or to give it in small Doses, between the repetitions thereof, so as not to salivate.

Besides the Use of evacuating Medicines, it will here also be proper to order a Course of Diet-drink, made with the Sudorifick Woods, especially where the *Ulcer* is suspected to be Venereal. In the mean time proper Dressings are to be used.

When the *Ulcer* obstinately resists this Treatment, a Salivation is generally proposed, and seldom fails to promote the Cure, tho all other Remedies should have been tried in vain. If the Patient be too weak to undergo the Fatigue of a thorough Salivation, it may be moderated, and kept up the longer, in Proportion to his Strength.

External Medicines for *Ulcers*, are Digestives, Cleansers, Sarcoticks, and Epuloticks. Monsieur *Belloste* gives us a Medicine of singular efficacy in the Cure of *Ulcers*; and it is no ore than a Decoction of Walnut Leaves in Water, with a little Sugar; in which a Linen Cloth being dipp'd, is to be laid on the *Ulcer*, and this to be repeated every second or third Day. This simple and vulgar Medicine he finds suppurates, deterges, incarnates, resists Putrefaction, &c. more than any other Medicine known.

An *Ulcer* in the Lungs makes what we call a *Phthisis*.

The *Venereal Disease* is a great Source of Ulcers; particularly in the Præpuce and Glans, in Men; the Vagina, &c. in Women; and in the Mouth and Palate in both. See Venereal *Disease*.

*Venereal Ulcers* are of various kinds; those that grow callus and cancrous, are call'd *Shankers.*

**ULCERATION**, a little Aperture, or Hole in the Skin, caused by an *Ulcer*. Caustic Medicines sometimes occasion *Ulcerations* in the Skin. Arsenic always *Ulcerates* the Parts it sticks to. A Flux at the Mouth *Ulcerates* the tongue and Palate.

**UMBELLÆ**, among Botanists, &c. is applied to the round Tufts or Heads of certain Plants, set thick together, and all of the same height. But *sparsed* or *thin Umbellæ*, is when they stand at a distance from one another, yet all of an equal height.

**UMBELLIFEROUS** Plants, are such as have their Tops branched, and spread out like an Umbrella; on each little Subdivision of which, there is growing a small Flower; such are Fennel, Dill, &c. This Flower is always *Pentapetalous*; and is succeeded by two naked Seeds adjoining to each other, which are the true Characteristicks that distinguish these Plants from others.

The *Umbelliferous* are a very large Genus of Plants, and are distinguish'd by Mr. *Ray* as follows :

1°, Such as have a compounded Leaf, of a triangular and pinnate Form. The Seeds of these are either broad, flat and plain, almost like Leaves; as the *Sphondylium, Pastinaca Latifolia, Panax Heracleum Tordylium, Orcoselinum, Thysselinum, Apium Cicutæ foliis, Daucus Alsaticus carvifolia, Anethum, Pucedanum, Thapsia, Ferula*, &c. Or with a Seed more tumid, and less compressed and flat than the former; as the *Cachrys, Laserpitium, Cicutaria vulgaris, Scandix, Cerefolium, Myrrhis Sativa Angelica, Levisticum, Siler Montanum, Bulbocastanum, Sisarum, Œnanthe, Sium, Pimpinella, Apium, Cicuta Visnaga, Saxifraga, Crithmum, Fœniculum, Daucus vulgaris, Anisum, Caucalci, Coriandrum, Pastinaca Marina*, &c.

2°, Such as have a simple, or undivided Leaf, or at least one only a little jagged; as the *Perfoliata, Buplerum, Anstrantia niger, Sanicula*, and the *Seseli Aethiopicum.*

**UNGUENT**, *Unguentum*, in Chirurgery, a topical Remedy, or Composition, used in the dressing of Wounds and Ulcers.

*Unguents*, Liniments, and Curats are external Forms applied on divers Parts of Body, both to cure, and to ease and relieve 'em. They only differ from each other in Consistence, with regard to which *Unguents* hold the Medium; being stiffer than *Liniments*, but softer than *Cerats*.

Oils are ordinarily the Bases of all three; to which are added Wax, *Axungia*, and several Parts of Plants, Animals, and Minerals, both in respect of the Virtues they furnish, and to give a Consistence to the Oils, and to keep 'em longer on the Parts, that they may have more time to act.

The principal *Unguents* are *Unguentum Rosatum, Unguentum Album*, or white Unguent of Ceruss; the *Populeum* made of the Buds of the Poplar-Tree; the *Unguentum Apostolorum*, so call'd from the twelve Drugs it consists of, a Cleanser; the *Unguentum Basilicum*, a Suppurative; the *Unguentum Egypticum*, Caustic; the *Unguentum Aureum*, Incarnative and Cicatrizing;

the *Unguent. de Apio*, Mundicative; the *Unguent. Agrippæ*, said to be discover'd by King *Agrippa*. *Pomatums* are also ranked in the Number of *Unguents*.

**UNGUIS**, in Medicine, a Disease of the Eye, occasion'd by a nervous Excrescence on the *Conjunctiva*, beginning at the great *Canthus* and spreading insensibly till it reach the *Pupil*, and at last quite cover it. The *Greeks* call it πτερυγον The ordinary Cause of the Unguis is an excessive Acrimony in the Tears, which corrode the Conjunctiva, as is often the Case in an Opthalmia, or after the small Pox.

**UNGUIS**, or *Unguiculis*, among Botanists and Florists, is a little Speck, or a different Colour from the rest of the *Petala*, or Leaves of Flowers. It has the Figure of a Nail of the Hand : Its place is at the Origin, or Root of those Leaves; as we see in the Rose, Poppy-flowers, and dives others. In preparing of Medicines, the *Ungues*, or *Unguiculi*, are pull'd off the Flowers that enter the same.

**UNGULA**, among Surgeons, a sort of hooked Instrument where withal to extract a dead Fœtus out of the Womb.

**UREDO**, is sometimes used by Physicians for an Itching or Burning in the Skin.

**URENTIA**, is sometimes used for Medicines of a hot or burning Quality.

**URINE**, a liquid Excrement, or Humour, separated from the Blood in the Kidneys, convey'd thence into the Bladder, and discharg'd by the *Urethra*. The Word *Urine* is form'd from the Greek υορον, which signifies the same thing.

The *Urine* is secreted from the Arterial Blood in the Glands of the *Kidneys*; from which arise numerous little pellucid Pipes and Veins, which receiving the secreted *Urine*, at length join into twelve *Papillæ*, out of which the Urine oozes into a Cavity call'd the *Pelvis*, from whence it runs into the *Ureters* of either side, and thro' them into the *Bladder*; and from that, at length, thro' the *Urethra*, out of the Body.

The secretion of *Urine*, then, is not perform'd by any Attraction, as some will have it; or by any Emulsion, as others; or any Fermentation, as others; or any Precipitation, as others : but by the Force of the Heart, and Arteries, whereby the Blood is driven thro' innumerable Turnings and Windings of the Vessels; attenuated by Resistances, opposite Motions, violent Concussions, and various Mixtures, till the more liquid and serous Part thereof, is forc'd thro' Canals smaller than the Blood-Vessels, and so collected and discharg'd.

'Tis more than probable, that the Blood of the Emulgent Artery, convey'd thro' all the little Branches that spread thro' the exterior Membranes of the *Vesiculæ* whereof the Kidneys are compos'd, being by this means exceedingly divided, and as it were attenuated, enters the *Vesiculæ* themselves, and gives them their red Colour; that it is there filtrated, and the serous or urinous Parts secreted; and that this Filtration is promoted by the alternate

Contractions and Dilatations of the fleshy Fibres that inclose the little Vesicles; and that after the Filtrations, the Parts that remain Blood are resum'd by the Capillary Branches of the Veins; the rest entering the excretory Ducts of the *Vesiculæ*, which are the first Receptacle of the *Urine*. *Hist. Acad. de Sciences*, An. 1705.

Monsieur *Morin*, in the *Memoirs of the* French *Academy*, marks out a new Rout or Course for the *Urine*. The *ordinary* one, which is the Passage of any Liquor we drink thro' the Stomach, into the Intestines, thence into the Lacteals, thence into the Receptacle of the Chyle, thence into the Subclavian Vein, thence into the *Cava*, thence into the right Ventricle of the Heart, thence into the Lungs, and thence into the left Ventricle of the Heart; thence into the *Aorta*, thence into the Emulgent Artery, thence into the Kidneys, thence into the Ureters, and at last into the Bladder; seems too long and circuitous; considering how readily Mineral Waters pass, and what a speedy effect Asparagus is found to have. Besides, that in this Principle, the Liquors we drink mixing with so many other Liquors in their Way, should be greatly alter'd thereby; whereas we frequently find a Tincture of Cassia, render'd by *Urine* almost as black as when first taken : and the like is observed of divers other Liquors.

M. *Morin*, therefore, maintains, that a good part of the Liquor we drink, oozes thro' the Membranes of the Stomach, and falls into the Pelvis; where it enters the Bladder thro' the Pores thereof, without getting into the Intestines, which are lined with too thick and viscid a Humour to allow it Ingress.

This System is confirm'd hence, That both the Stomach and Bladder, even of a dead Animal, are found easily permeable to Water.

Accordingly, Dr. *Morgan* assures us, that if the Contents of the Abdomen be taken out of an animal Body, after it is just open'd; and the Stomach be fill'd with warm Water, while the Parts are yet reaking; the Liquor will pass into the Bladder, which will visibly receive it, and be fill'd in proportion as the Stomach empties.

The same Author adds, that if a Ligature be made upon the Ureters, while the Animal is yet living, and the Blood continues to circulate; tho this must cut off all Communication from the Kidneys to the Bladder; yet any Liquor with which the Stomach is fill'd will pass into the Bladder.

From the whole, tho some of our best Anatomists hold that a Circulation of the whole mass of Blood is effected in five Minutes, and others in two; which might account for the quick Passage of the *Urine*; 'tis hard to conceive, but that part of it must go immediately from the Stomach to the Bladder.

The general Design of Nature in this new *Urinary* Drain, is supposed to be to prevent any sudden Plethora, or immoderate Distension of the Vessels upon Drinking.

As a necessary Consequence of this System, the Author establishes two kinds of *Urines*; the one filtrated immediately out of the Stomach into the Bladder; the other making the long Course of the Circulation.

*Urines* are of various Kinds and Properties. After drinking plentifully of any aqueous Fluid, the *Urine* is crude, insipid, void of Smell, and easily retain'd. That yielded by Chyle well concocted, is sharper, more saline, less copious, somewhat fetid, and more stimulating. That from Chyle already converted into Serum, is more redder, sharper, salter, and more fetid and stimulating. And that secern'd after long Abstinence, from Humours well concocted and wore off the solid Parts, is the least copious, sharpest, saltest, reddest, most fetid, almost putrify'd, and of all others the hardest to retain.

The *Urine*, therefore, contains the watery Part of the Blood, its sharpest, subtilest, and most volatile Salt, and that nearest to the alkaline Kind; its sharpest, smallest, and most volatile Oil, and that nearest to Putrefaction; and its smallest most volatile Earth.

The Sal Armoniac of the Antients was prepar'd from Camels *Urine*. And the Phosphorus, in use amongst us, from human *Urine*. Salt-petre is likewise prepar'd from the *Urine*, and other excrements of Animals.

The *Indians* scarce use any other Medicine but Cows *Urine*. The *Spaniards* make great use of Urine to clean their Teeth withal : So did the *Celtiberians* of old.

*Urine* is also used in Dying, to ferment and warm the Woad. Old *Urine*, tinges Silver with a fine gold Colour.

**URINE**, in Medicine. The *Urine* affords one of the principal Criterions, or Signs whereby Physicians judge of the State of the Patient, and the Course of the Disease. In casting, or examining *Urine*, the Things to be consider'd, are, its *Quantity, Colour, Smell, Taste, Fluidity,* and the Matters swimming therein.

An abundance of *Urine*, indicates a Looseness of the Renal Pipes, a Diminution of Perspiration; Sweat; Saliva; an imperfect mixture of the Blood, whereby the watery Parts separate easily from the rest; a nervous Indis-position;a copious drinking of some aqueous Liquid, or some Diuretic taken. Such *Urine* presages a Thickness of what is left behind, and its Acrimony; Thirst, Anxiety, Obstructions, and their Effects, a dry, thirsty, hot Consumption.

A contrary State of the *Urine* indicates the Contraries; and presages future Repletions, Heaviness, Drousiness, Convulsive Tremors, &c.

A thin, limpid, insipid, colourless, tasteless *Urine*, denotes a great Constriction of the Renal Vessels, and at the same time, a brisk Agitation of the Humours; a strong Cohesion of the Oil, Salt, and Earth in the Blood it self, and an imperfect Mixture of the aqueous Parts therewith; some grievous Indis-position of the Mind, a hysteric or hypochondriac Fit; a Debility of the Viscera; Crudity, Pituita, Obstructions of the Vessels; and, in acute Diseases, a want of a Coction and Crisis. Such *Urine* portends much the same as a too copious *Urine*; and in acute inflammatory Diseases, a bad Condition of the Viscera, Deliria, Phrensies, Convulsions, Death.

*Ruddy Urine*, without any Sediment, in acute Diseases, indicates a violent Motion and Attrition among the Parts that constitute the Humours, and between the Vessels and the Humours; a close intimate Mixture of the Oil, Salt, Earth and Water in the Humours : and hence a great Crudity of the Disease, and its long Duration, and great Danger. Such *Urine* presages gangrenous Destructions of the finest Vessels; chiefly those of the Brain and *Cerebel*, and thence Death : a difficult Coction; a slow, doubtful Crisis : And, all these the worse, as the *Urine* is redder, and freer of Sediment. If there be a heavy copious Sediment, it shews a string antecedent Attrition; loose Vessels; sharp, saline, colliquated Blood, unfit for Nutrition,; intermitting Fevers; and Scurvy.

The Presages are, the Durableness of the Disease, wearing of the Vessels, Weakness, colliquative Sweats, Saliva, &c. Atrophy, and Dropsy. If the Sediment in such *Urine* be branny, scaly, filmy, &c. it presages the like, only worse.

A *yellow Urine*, with a Sediment as before, denotes a Jaundice, and the Symptoms thereof in the Cutis, Stools, Hypochondriums, &c.

A *green Urine*, with a thick Sediment, denotes an atrabilary Temperature, and that the Matter thereof is resolved, and now excreted : consequently Anxieties about the *Præcordia*, Perturbations of Stool, Iliac and Colic Pains. *Black Urine*, denotes the same with green, only in a greater and worse degree.

Blood, Pus, Caruncles, Filaments, Hairs, Anguillæ, Grumæ, Sand, Parts of Stone, and a mucus at the bottom of the *Urine*, denote some disorder in the Kidneys, Ureters, Bladder, Testicles, Seminal Vesicles, *Prostratæ*, and Urethra.

*Fatty Urine*, generally breeds small Sands, adhering to some viscid Matter, and thus produces a sort of oily Membrane, or Pellicle, which denotes an abundance of Earth, and a heavy Salt in the Blood, and presages the Scurvy, Stone, &c.

*A Fœtid Urine*, denotes the Salts and Oils to be attenuated, dissolv'd, and almost purify'd; whence very great danger, both in chronic and acute Diseases.

*Urine* which when shook, retains its Froth long, denotes a Tenacity of the Mixture, and thence a difficulty of Crisis; and pulmonick Diseases, or Catarrhs in the Head.

But the *Urine* is chiefly consulted in acute Fevers, where 'tis a very sure Sign : For, 1°, *Urine* with a white, light, equable, turbinated, inodorous Sediment, thro' the whole Course of the Disease to the Crisis, is a very good Presage. 2°, Copious, white, strangurius *Urine*, with much white Sediment, emitted at the time of the Crisis, cures and takes away Abscesses. 3°, A thin, ruddy *Urine*, that does not subside; a white, thin, watery *Urine*; a thin, equable, yellow Urine; a turbid *Urine* that does not subside, denotes, in acute Diseases, a great Crudity, a difficult Crisis, and a durable dangerous Disease.

**URINOUS** *Salts*, are the same with what we otherwise call *Alcali Salts*, or *Alkalies*. There are two Kinds of *Urinous Salts*, the one *fix'd*; the other *volatile*. The fix'd prevail in Plants, and the volatile in Animals. They are called *Urinous*, in respect of their Taste and Smell, which bear some resemblance to those of Urine.

**UROCRITERIUM**, a *Casting of Water*, a giving Judgement of Diseases by the Sight of the Urine. The Word is compounded of ουρον, *Urine*, and κριτηριον, *Criterion, Mark, Sign*. Hence also the Words Uromancy, Uroscopy, &c.

**USNEA**, in Natural History, a sort of Plant of the Moss Kind, growing on the Oak, Cedar, and dives other Trees.

**USNEA** *Humana*, is a small greenish Moss, growing on human Skulls, than have lain a long time exposed to the Air. 'Tis very astringent, and held proper to stop Hæmorrhages. It is also an Ingredient in the *Weapon-Salve* of *Paracelsus* and *Crollius*.

**USTION**, in Pharmacy, the preparing of certain Substance by burning them. The Word is form'd from the Latin *urere*, to burn. The Antients made use of the *Ustion* of Horns, Nails, Feathers, and other Parts of Animals, for divers Remedies : And the Moderns still use *Aes Ustum*, which is burnt Copper, or Copper that has undergone the *Ustion*, with Sulphur. The *Ustion* of Minerals is a more imperfect kind of Calcination.

**UTERINE**, *Uterinus*, something belonging to the Uterus, or Womb of Women. Thus Uterine Brothers or Sisters, are those born of the same Mother, but different Fathers.

*Furor* **UTERINUS**, in Medicine, is a kind of Madness, attended with Lascivious Speeches and Gestures, and an invincible Inclination to Venery. The *Furor Uterninus*, is a complication of Hysterical Symptoms, arising from a Turgescency or Inflation of the Uterine Vessels.

It is usually supposed to consist in some irregular Motion of the Spirits, occasion'd by a hot, lustful Temperament, the Conversation of debauch'd Persons, or the reading of wanton Books, hot Foods, the Abundance and Acrimony of the serous Matter which moistens the Pudendum, Suppression of the Menses, large Doses of Cantherides, &c.

It has been frequently found, that Maids that were held to be possess'd, were only seiz'd with the *Uterine Fury*.

Before the Paroxysm, the Patient often appears silent, with Flushing in the Face, and a Respiration and Pulse frequently intermitting, and suddenly varying. During the Paroxysm they burst sometimes into Laughter, and then into a Fit of Tears, &c.

Bleeding, fœtid Suffiments, and other hysterical Medicines, are proper during the Fit.

Men are subject to the Disease as well as Women; so that it might with more Propriety be call'd the *Furor Venerus*, or *Venereal Fury*.

It had its Name *Furor Uterinus*, from an Opinion, that it proceeded from Vapours rising from the Womb to the Brain.

**UTERUS**, in Anatomy, the *Matrix* or *Womb* of a Women; or that Organ of Generation wherein the Business of Conception is perform'd, and wherein the Embryo or Fœtus is lodg'd, fed, and grows, during the time of Gestation, or till its Delivery.

**VALERIAN**, the *great Set-wall*, a Plant, whose root is of considerable use in Medicine. There are various Kinds of *Valerian*; but the only one in use is that cultivated in Gardens, call'd the *large Valerian*, or *Valeriana Hortensis*; and by *Dioscorides*, *Phic folio olisatri*. It has its Name, according to some, from one *Valerius*, who first brought it into use; according to others, from *Valere*, to have great Virtues.

It is warm and aromatick, but somewhat of a fetid Scent : Its efficacy, as a Sudorific, is supported by the Testimony of both antient and modern Practice. It has been reckon'd by some Detersive, so much as to make it Diuretick, and good in all Obstructions of the *Viscera*. It is extoll'd also for strengthening the Optic Nerves, and restoring decay'd Sight; but the present Practice acknowledges it not in any such Intentions. It sometimes does Wonders in hysterical Affections; especially where those of the fetid kind are good, and the Spirits too impetuous in their Motions, so as to occasion Convulsions. It is also assisted with Camphire, and some other things of the like Nature which are very powerful in breaking thro' the minutest Obstructions, to cure obstinate Agues.

It is efficacious in all nervous Cases; and particularly the Epilepsy: which Virtue in it seems to have been first discover'd by *Fabius Columna*, who prescrib'd it for that Purpose in Pouder.

M. *Marchant*[1], in the Memoirs of the Academy of Sciences, has confirm'd this Virtue by many Instances within his Knowledge : And what is very remarkable, is, that in the two Observations he enlarges most upon, the Patients voided great Quantities of Worms. His Custom was, always to purge before he administer'd it.

**VALETUDINARY**, *Valetudinarius*, a Term sometimes used by the writers of Medicine, for a Person of a weak, crazy, sickly Constitution, frequently out of order, &c. Dr. *Cheyne*, by all means, directs the weakly, the studious, the sedentary, and the *valetudinary*, to a low, spare Regimen.

**VANILLA**, or Banilla, a little black Seed, growing in longish Pods; used in the *West Indies*, *France*, *Spain*, &c. as a principal Ingredient in the Composition of Chocolate; to give it Strength, and an agreeable Flavour. It is also used to perfume Tobacco withal. It is supposed to strengthen the Brain, and Stomach; to attenuate viscid Humours, provoke Urine, and the Menses.

**VAPORATION**, in Chymistry, a Term applied to the Action of *Vapour*. The Chymists have a Bath call'd a Vaporatory, or *Balneum Vaporationis*, or *Vaporis*; whereby the Warmth or Humidity of a *Vapour* is made to act on some other Body, that is to be warm'd, or moisten'd.

**VAPOROSUM** *Balneum*, or Vapour-*Bath*, in Chymistry, a Term applied to a Chymist's Bath, or Heat, wherein the Body is placed so as to receive the Fumes of boiling Water. The *Balneum Vaporosum* consists of two Vessels, disposed over one another in such manner, as that the *Vapour* rais'd from

[1] Jean Marchant (1650 – 1738), a French botanist.

the Water contain'd in the lower, heats the Matter enclosed in the upper. The *Vapour-Bath* is very commodious for the distilling of odoriferous Waters, and the drawing of Spirit of Wine. We also use the Term *Vapour-Bath*, when a sick Person is made to receive the *Vapours* arising from some liquid Matter placed over a Fire.

**VAPOURS**, in Medicine, a Disease, call'd popularly the *Hypo*, or *Hypochondriacal* Disease; and in Men, particularly, the *Spleen*. 'Tis supposed to be owing to a subtle Vapour, rising from the lower Parts of the Abdomen, particularly the *Hypochondrium* to the Brain; which it disturbs, and possesses with wild, delirious, but generally disagreeable Imaginations. Vapours, supposed to be emitted from the Womb, in Women, are what we otherwise call *Hysterical Affections*, or *Suffocations*, or *Fits of the Mother*.

**VARI**, in Medicine, little, hard, ruddy Tumors, whitish about the Tips, and of the size of a Hemp-seed; frequently found on the Face and Neck of young People; chiefly such as are much addicted to the Venery. If the red be very lively, the Cure is somewhat difficult; and tho the Pustles be taken away, the Redness remains. To which, if an Inflammation and Hoarseness be added, 'tis a Symptom of an approaching Leprosy.

**VARIOLÆ**, in Medicine, a contagious Disease, popularly called the *Small* Pox. It is call'd *Variolæ*, as shewing it self in Pustles, or little Tumors like *Varices*; or as *variegating* the Skin.

**VARIX**, in Medicine, a little Dilatation of a Part of a Vein, so as to make it bulge out, or thrust the Skin above its natural level. Sometimes, it is confined to one single Branch of a Vein; and sometimes it extends to several; and sometimes runs crooked, and bent, in various Knots and Circumvolutions.

It happens oftenest to the Crural and Hæmorrhoidal Veins; sometimes, also, to those in the Testes, and frequently in the Abdomen and Breasts of pregnant Women, and such as give suck.

It is supposed owing to the too great abundance or thickness of the Blood : or to the Relaxation of the Membranes of the Veins; immoderate Labour, Sprains, Cramps, too great Pressure or Stricture by Bandages; and Stagnations of the Blood from a Plethora, Cacochymia, &c. may give occasion thereto.

Melancholic Persons, and those who feed on coarse Meats, are most subject to them : The generality of Women with Child have *Varices* on their thighs and Legs, occasion'd by the *Fœtus* compressing the Iliac Veins; and by that means preventing the Reflux of the Blood to the Heart.

*Varices* happening spontaneously, and proving of a moderate size, are rarely dangerous; but even are allow'd serviceable in the case of the Hemorrhoids. When immoderate, they sometimes occasion a Cachexy, Dropsy, or Consumption.

The Cure is to be attempted by Evacuations, as Phlebotomy and Catharticks; external Applications, as discutient Fomentations, Cataplasms, Embrocations, Bandages, &c. Or, lastly, where the Case grows dangerous, by Incision.

The Word is pure *Latin*, form'd from the Verb *Variare*; by reason of the Turns and Meanders of the Veins, which the Tumor sometimes follows.

*Hernia* **VARICOSA**, in the Testes, is known by the Situation of the Tumor, the Course of the Vein, Relaxation of the Part, or its appearing inflated with Air, distended, and painful. It is remedy'd by a proper Truss, or Bandage, with the Medicines abovemention'd.

**VASCULIFEROUS** Plants, are, according to the Botanists, such as besides the common Calyx, have a peculiar Vessel or Case to contain the Seed; which is sometimes divided into Cells. These have always a Monopetalous Flower; either *uniform*, or *difform*.

The former have their Seeds all divided, 1°, into two Partitions, as the *Hyoscyamus, Nicotiana, Priapæia*, and the *Gentiana*. 2°, Into three Partitions, as the *Convolvulus, Speculum Veneris, Trachelium, Rapunculus Campanula, Rapunculus Corniculatus*, &c. 3°, Into four Partitions; as the *Stramonium*.

Those of the latter Kind, which have a difform Monopetalous Flower, as the *Linaria Pinguicula, Antirrhinum, Aristocholia, Scrophularia, Digitalis, Pedicularis, Melampyrum, Euphrasia*, &c.

**VASE** is sometimes used among Florists, for what they otherwise call the Calyx. The *Vase*, or rather Calyx of a Tulip, is the top, or Head of a Tulip; the Leaves whereof form a kind of *Vase*, or Cup.

**VEGETABLE**, in Physiology, a Term applied to all Plants, consider'd as capable of growth, *i.e.* to all natural Bodies which have Parts organically form'd for Generation, and Accretion, but not Sensation. In *Vegetables*, there is supposed to be a Principle of Life, commonly call'd the *Vegetative Soul*.

*Boerhaave* very scientifically defines a *Vegetable* to be a Body generated of the Earth; to which it adheres, or is connected, by Parts called Roots, thro' which it receives the Nourishment, and Increase; and consists of Juices, and Vessels, sensibly distinct from each other : Or a *Vegetable* is an organical Body, compos'd of Vessels, and Juices, every where distinguishable from each other; to which grow Roots, or Parts whereby it adheres to some other Body, from which it derives the Matter of its Life, and growth.

This Definition furnishes a just and adequate Idea of a *Vegetable* : for by its consisting of Vessels and Juices, it is distinguish'd from a Fossil; and by its adhering to another Body, and deriving its Nourishment therefrom, it is distinguish'd from an Animal.

A *Vegetable* is defined *an Organical Body*, because consisting of different Parts, which jointly concur to the Exercise of the same Function.

*Adhering by some of its Parts to another Body*; for we know of no Plant that is so absolutely vague and fluctuating, but has still a Body it adheres to; tho that Body may be various, *e.g.* Earth, as in our common Plants; Stone, as in Rock Plants; Water, as in Sea Plants; and Air, as some Mucilages.

As to those few Plants which appear to float with the Water, their manner of growth is somewhat anomalous : M. *Tournefort* has shewn, that all Plants do not arise strictly from Seeds; but that some, instead of Semen, deposite, or let fall a little drop of Juice, which sinking in the Water, by its Gravity reaches the bottom, or some Rock, &c. in its way; to which it sticks, strikes Root, and shoots into Branches : Such is the Origin of Coral.

Add, that the Root of a Plant may have any Situation at pleasure, with respect to the Body thereof; nor needs it either lowest, or highest, &c. Accordingly, in Aloes, Coral, Mosses, Fungus's, &c. the Root is frequently uppermost, and its growth downward.

The vascular Structure of *Vegetables*, is render'd very apparent, by an Experiment of Mr. *Willoughby*[1] : Cutting off some pretty big Branches of Birch, and making a sort of Bason, or Reservoir on the End thereof with some soft Wax; upon filling this with Water, and holding the Branch upright, the Water, in a few Minutes, sunk into the Vessels of the Wood, and running quit thro' the Length, dropp'd out considerably fast; continuing to do so, so long as the Water was pour'd on. The same succeeds in a Sycamore, Walnut, &c. tho the Flux is not so copious. *Phil. Transact.* No. 70.

There are Secrets whereby the Growth of *Vegetables* is surprisingly promoted. Mr. *Boyle* mentions a Virtuoso, who entertain'd his Friends at the End of their Meal, with a Salad of Lettices, which he sow'd in their presence, immediately before they sat down to table.

The Chymists have furnish'd us with some very extraordinary *Vegetables*; as the *Arbor Dianæ, Arbor Martis*, &c.

In effect, Gold, Silver, Iron, and Copper, being prepared in Aqua fortis, there rises out of 'em a kind of Tree, which *vegetates*, or grows, to the naked Eye, and spreads into Branches, Leaves, &c. the whole Height of the Water; till all the Matter is spent therein.

The Water the Chymists call *Flint-Water*; the Secret whereof has been communicated by *Rhodes Canasses*, a *Greek* Chymist.

**VEGETATIVE**, a Term applied to that Principle, or Part in Plants, by virtue whereof they receive Nourishment, and *grow*, or *vegetate*. The Philosophers speak of three Kinds of Souls, the *Vegetative*, *Sensitive*, and *Rational*. The *Vegetative Soul*, is that Principle whereby Trees and Plants live, grow, produce their Kind, &c.

This *Vegetative* Principal is differently seated in different Plants : An ingenious Author observes, that, generally speaking, its Place is exactly between the Trunk, and Root; at least this appears to be the Place in most of the Seminiferous Tribe; which, if cut down near that Place, rarely shoot again.

In other Plants, as the Elm, and many edible Plants, it seems to reside wholly in the Roots; which, if cut into ever so many Parts, yet, those being planted in the Ground, soon grow.

In others, as the Willow Kinds, it seems to be diffus'd all over, both Root, Trunk, and Branches; insomuch that if cut into a thousand Pieces, there is no destroying 'em without splitting them in the middle; and scarcely then.

[1] Francis Willoughby (1635 – 1672), an English naturalist.

Lastly, in others, as the Cereus's, Ficus's, &c. it is seated in the Body, Branches, and Leaves; any of which being put into the Ground, strike Root immediately, and grow.

The Office of this *Vegetative* Principle, is to concoct the indigested Salts which ascend thro' the Roots; and to assimilate 'em to the Nature of the Plant.

**VELLICATION**, among Physicians, the Act of Twitching. *Vellications* are particularly used for sort of sudden Convulsions that happen to the Fibres of the Muscles.

**VENEREAL DISEASE**, call'd also *the Lues Venerea, French Disease, Foul Disease, French Pox, Great Pox*, &c. is a contagious Disease, contracted by some impure Humour, generally receiv'd in Coition; and discovering itself in Ulcers and Pains, about the Genital and other Parts.

It is generally said to have made its first Appearance in *Europe*, in the Year 1493; tho others will have it much older, and contend for its being known to the Antients, only under other Names.

Mr. *Becket*, particularly, has attempted to shew, that it is the same with what among our Forefathers was call'd the *Leprosy*; and which in many of our antient *English* Writings, Charters, &c. is called *Brenning*, or *Burning*.

In order to prove his Point, he has search'd the Records relating to the Stews antiently kept on *Bankside, Southwark*, under the Jurisdiction of the of the Bishop of *Winchester*.

Among other Constitutions of these Stews, dated 1162, it was appointed, *That no Stew-holder should keep any Woman that hath the perilous Infirmity of* Burning. And in another Vellum Manuscript, dated 1430, it is again order'd, *That no Stew-holder keep no Woman within his House that hath any Sickness of* Brenning, *but that she be putte out, upon the Peyne of making a Fine unto the Lord of a hundred Shillings*.

To confirm this Account, Mr. *Becket* quotes a Description of the Disease from a Manuscript of *John Arden* Esq. Surgeon to K. *Richard* II and K. *Henry* IV. *Arden* defines the Disease called *Brenning, Incendium*, to be, *a certain inward Heat and Excoriation of the Urethra* : which Definition, Mr. *Becket* observes, gives us a perfect Idea of what we now call a *Clap*; agreeable to the latest and most exact anatomical Discoveries, and free of all the Errors of *Platerus, Rondeletius*[1], *Bartholin, Wharton*, and other later Writers on this Disease.

As to the Leprosy being the same with this *Venereal Disease*, it must be own'd, there are a good many Symptoms in the one Disease, which quadrate well enough with those in the other; but then the Symptoms in each are so precarious, that a great deal of Stress can't be laid hereon.

The common Tradition is, that the *Venereal Disease* first broke out in the *French* Army, when it lay encamp'd before *Naples*; and that it was owing to some un-wholesome Food : On which Account, the *French* call it the *Neapolitan Disease*; and the *Italians*, the *Mal Francese*.

[1] Gulielmus Rondeletius, born Guillaume Rondelet (1507 – 1566), a French naturalist.

But others go much higher, and suppose it to be the Ulcer *Job* complain'd of so grievously : and accordingly, in a Missal printed at *Venice* in 1542, there is a Mass in honour of S. *Job*, to be said by those recover'd of this Disease; as being supposed to owe their Deliverance to his Intercession.

But the Opinion which prevails most among the more knowing of our Physicians, is, that the Disease is of *Indian* Extraction; and that it was brought hither by the Spaniards from the *American* Islands, where it was very common, before ever the *Spaniards* set footing there : Whence the Spaniards call it *Sarva des Indias*, or *Las Buvas* : notwithstanding what *Herrera* says, that the *Spaniards* carry'd it to *Mexico*, instead of bringing it thence.

*Lister*, and others, take it to have had its first Rise from some of the Serpentine Kind; either from a Bite thereof, or from some of their Flesh taken as Food : This is pretty certain, than Men bitten or stung by Scorpions, are greatly eas'd by Coition; but the Woman, *Pliny* assures us, receives a deal of damage thereby : which is no slender argument, of the Disease arising from some Person so poison'd.

He adds, there is no room to doubt, but that the *Lues* arose from some such Cause; for upon any venomous bite, the Penis becomes vehemently extended; and the Patient being seiz'd with a *Satyriasis*, breaths nothing but Rage and Lust : Nature, in effect, seeming to direct him to Coition for a Remedy.

But what proves a Remedy to the wounded Person, proves a Disease to the Woman: And from Women thus infected, other Men, who have to do with 'em, become infected in their turns; and thus has the Disease been propagated.

The first Symptoms generally arising after an Affair with an infected Person, are a Heat, Swelling, and Inflammation about the Penis or Vulva, with a hotness of Urine.

The second or third Day usually brings on a Gonorrhæa, or Dripping, which denominates it a *Clap*; and which in a few Days more is follow'd by a Cordee.

Tho sometimes there is no Gonorrhæa or Cordee; but the Poison rather make sits way thro' the Cutis to the Groin; and there arise Bubos, with various malignant Pustles in all Parts of the Body.

Sometimes, also, there happen callous Ulcers, call'd *Shankers*, in the *Scrotum* and *Perinæum*; and sometimes a cancerous and callous Ulcer between the Prepuce and Glans; and in some the Testicles swell.

Add to these, violent nocturnal Pains, Nodes, Heats in the Palms of the Hands, and Soals of the Feet; and hence Fissures, Excoriations, Condylomata, &c. about the *Anus*; falling of the Hair; ruddy, yellow, or livid Spots, Hoarseness, Relaxation and Erosion of the Uvula; Ulcer of the Palate, Ozæna, tingling of the Ears, Deafness, Blindness, Itch, Consumption, &c. But 'tis rare all these Symptoms happen to the same Person.

The *Venereal Disease*, *Sydenham* observes, is communicated by Copulation, Lactation, Handling, Saliva, Sweat, the genital Mucus, and the Breath : And in whatever Part it is first receiv'd, it there discovers it self first. When the Infection is receiv'd along with the Milk from the Nurse, it commonly shews it self in Soreness and Ulcers of the Mouth.

The Method of Cure is various, according to the various Symptoms and Stages: For the first Stage, *viz.* a *Gonorrhæa, Virulenta*, or Clap.

Dr. *Pitcairn's* Method is this : After two or three Vomits, he directs *Mercurius Dulcis*, for some Days, twice a Day; when the Mouth grows sore, let alone the Mercury for three or four Days, and purge every other Day. As the Mouth grows well again, repeat the use of Mercury, and thus alternately, till the Symptoms cease.

For a confirm'd *Lues*, Mercurial Salivation is a generally held the only effectual Cure : Tho Mercurial Frictions, applied in such Quantity, and at such Intervals as not to raise a Salivation, is held by some to be not only easier and safer, but even more successful, in this Disease, than Salivation it self.

Dr. *Sydenham* tells us, he uses to salivate immediately, without any preliminary Evacuation, or preparation of the Body at all. His Method is this; He prescribes an Unguent of two ounces of Axang. Porcin. Swines-seam, and one ounce of Mercury. With a third Part of this, he orders the Patient to anoint his Arms and Legs, for three Nights successively, with his own Hands; so as not to touch either the Arm-pits, the Groin, or the Abdomen. After the third Unction, the Gums usually swell, and a Ptyalism comes on. If it does not come in the time, he exhibits Turbith Mineral gr. viii. in Conserve of Red Roses; which occasioning a Vomiting, raises the Ptyalism. And, if afterwards, the Salivation abate, ere the Symptoms are quite disappear'd, he orders it to be promoted with a fresh Dose of *Mercurius Dulcis*. The Diet and other Regimen, to be the same as in a Catharsis.

**VENTER**, *Belly*, in Anatomy, a Cavity in the Body of an Animal, containing Viscera, or other Organs, necessary for the Performance of divers Functions. Physicians divide the human Body into three *Venters*, Regions, or Cavities; the first is the *Head*, containing the Brain, &c. The second the *Breast*, or *Thorax*, as far as the Diaphragm; containing the Organs of Respiration. The third is what we commonly call the *Venter*, or *Belly*, is that wherein the Intestines and the Organs of Generation, and Digestion, are contain'd; called by Anatomists the *Abdomen*.

This last, call'd also the *lower Venter*, is subdivided into three Regions; the first and highest whereof, call'd the *Epigastric* Region, reaches from the *Cartilago Xiphoides* near to the Navel; the second, call'd the Umbilical, comprehends the Space of three or four Fingers breadth, about the Navel, containing the Reins and Loins; and the third, the Hypogastric, which reaches to the Pudenda, and is what we properly call the lower Venter : *Hippocrates* calls it ητρον.

Its two sides are call'd *Ilia*, the *Flanks*; and its lowest extreme the *Groin*; in Latin *Inguen*, and in *Greek* βουβον.

**VENTER**, or *Belly*, is also popularly us'd for the exterior Part of the lower *Venter* : In which sense, we say, the Navel is in the middle of the *Venter*, &c. It is also used for the *Ventricle*, or Stomach; because that Part is enclosed in the Cavity thereof. It this Sense it is, that Jonah is said in Scripture to have been three Day's in the Whale's Belly. Lastly, *Venter* is also used for the Womb, or *Uterus* of Women And hence the Writ *De Ventre Inspiciendo*.

Hence, also, in the Civil Law, we say, *Partus Sequitur Ventrem*, the Child follows the Belly; meaning, that its condition is either free or servile, according to that of its Mother. They also say, to *appoint a Curator for the Belly*, with regard to posthumous Children yet in the Mother's Womb.

**VENUS**, in Chymistry, is used for the Metal Copper. Its Character is ♀; which, say the *Adepti*, expresses it to be Gold, only join'd with some corrosive and arsenical Menstruum; which removed, Copper would be Gold.

*Venus* is universally allow'd, by the Chemists, &c. to be one of the most powerful Medicines in Nature : Of this, is said to have been compos'd the famous *Butler's Stone*, which cured most Diseases by only licking it. Of this is compos'd that noble Remedy of *Van Helmont, viz.* the Sulphur of Vitriol, or *Ens Vitrioli*, fix'd by Calcination, and Cohobation. Of the *Ens Vitrioli* of *Venus*, is likewise composed Mr. *Boyle's* Arcanum, the *Colcathar Vitrioli.*

'Tis certain, Copper is a most excellent Emetic, and a noble Antidote against Poisons; for it is no sooner taken than it exerts its force : whereas other Vomitories lie a while in the Stomach : But one single Grain of Rust of Venus immediately Vomits. Hence, syrups that have stood over-night in Copper Vessels, create a vomiting.

It is also an excellent Medicine in Chronical Cases : Hence a famous Physician is recorded to have cur'd *Charles* V. of a Dropsy by the Use of *Copper.*

*Venus* is dissoluble by all the Salts known, both Acid, Alkaline, and Nitrous; nay, even by Water and Air, consider'd as they contain Salt.

'Tis from this common Reception of all Menstruums, that Copper is call'd *Venus, q.d. meretrix publica*, a common Prostitute; The others take the Denomination to have been occasion'd by its turning of a Sea-green Colour, when dissolved by Acids.

**VERDEGREASE**, *Ver-de-Gris*, a kind of Rust of Copper, of great use among Painters, for a green Colour. *Verdegrease* is prepar'd from Copper Plates, and Husks of Grapes well saturated with Wine, put up in earthen Pots; and ranged *stratum super stratum*, that is, first Husks, then Copper; and so alternately.

When the Pots are fill'd, they are set in the Cellar; whence, after some time, they are taken out, to gather the *Verdegrease*, which is a green Rust, covering the Plates all over.

Some talk of *Verdegrease* made with Vinegar, and other corrosive Salts; but 'tis a Mistake : the best Wine being nothing to good for the purpose.

Accordingly, the greatest Part of the *Verdegrease*, consum'd in *Europe*, is made in *Languedoc*, of the Wines of that Country; and is exported in Cakes, about 25 Pounds weight each. There is but very little quite pure; To be good, it must be very dry, of a deep green, and pretty clear of white Spots.

The Word is form'd from the *Latin Viride æris* : 'Tis also call'd *Ærugo*. Others call it the *Flower*, and others the *Vitriolic Salt of Copper*; tho, in reality, it be the proper Substance thereof.

The Apothecaries use to dissolve *Verdegrease* in distill'd Vinegar, and the filtrate, and evaporate it in the Cellar; upon which it shoots into Crystals.

These Crystals are used among Chirurgeons, &c. to eat off the fungus Flesh.

**VERMES**, in Medicine, a Disease popularly call'd *Worms*; arising from some of those Reptiles being generated, and growing in the Body : whence, frequently, dire Symptoms proceed.

The ordinary Place of Worms is in the Intestines : Tho there is scarce any Part of the Body but is sometimes infected with 'em : For besides the *Vermes Intestinales*, there are *Dentales, Gingivales, Pulmonarii, Cardiaci, Sanguinarii, Urinarii, Cutaneous, Umbilicales*, Worms *in the Liver*, the *Saliva*, &c.

They are all ingender'd from the Eggs of some Insect, deposited in something that is taken into the Body by way of Food, or some other way.

There are three Species of Worms, most frequent in the human Body : The *Teretes*, or round and long, mostly found in the *Duodenum*; the *Latus*, or flat, call'd *Toenia*; and the round and short, found in the *Rectum*, call'd *Ascarides*. Sometimes, indeed, there are anomalous Worms expell'd; as horned, hairy, four-footed, two-headed, &c.

The Symptoms of the Disease are, Vomiting, Head-ach, Heart-burn, Sighing, Swooning, feeble Pulse, heavy Sleep, Deliria, Squinancy, Pleurisy, canine Hunger, and innumerable others; occasion'd by the animals sucking, moving, vellicating, gnawing, consuming the Chyle; irritating the Nerves, wounding the Solids, &c.

As to the *Latus*, beside the other common Symptoms, those affected with this have one peculiar to 'em; which is, that with their Stools they discharge several little Bodies, like Gourd-Seeds.

Dr. *Tyson*[1], in the *Philosophical Transactions*, No 146. gives a curious account of the flat Worm, or *Lumbricus latus*; call'd by *Hippocrates* Ταινια, and in *English*, ordinarily, the *Tape-Worm*, or *Jointed Worm*. This Worm is always single : It lies variously convoluted; being sometimes as long as all the Guts, and sometimes vastly exceeds that length.

*Olaus Borrichius* assures us, a Patient of his, in a Year's time, voided 800 Foot of this sort of Worm, tho he had not yet met with the Head : in voiding, the Patient always perceiv'd to break it off. Dr. *Tyson* parallels this Case with that of a Patient of his, who voided vast Quantities of this Worm, for several Years together : but in various Pieces; some two, three, four, six, or more Yards long : But all put together, he says, would much exceed the length of that of *Borrichius*.

The Joints in this Worm are very numerous : In one of 24 Foot long, Dr. *Tyson* number'd 507 Joints. Above the middle of the Edges of each Joint, he observ'd a protuberant Orifice. Those Orifices he takes for so many Mouths; the best Microscopes discovering no Mouth in the Head.

The Worm is frequent enough in most Kinds of Animals; as Dogs, Oxen, Crabs, Herrings, Pikes, &c.

Some Authors assert, that it is not one, but many Worms link'd together, and included in a *Spolium* of the Intestines; and that this *Spolium* is not

[1] Edward Tyson (1649 – 1708), an English physician and anatomist.

animated, but receives its Sense and Motion from *Vermiculi*, or *Cucurbitini* inclosed in it. This, *Gabucinus*[1], *de Lumb. Com.* says, he has plainly discover'd : But Dr. *Tyson* abundantly evinces the contrary.

**VERMICULAR**, an Epithet given to any thing that bears a relation, or resemblance to Worms, *Vermiculi*. Anatomists particularly apply it to the Motion of the Intestines, and certain Muscles of the Body. The *Vermicular*, or Peristaltic Motion of the Intestines, is perform'd by the Contraction of the Fibres thereof, from above, downwards; as the Antiperistaltic Motion is by their Contracting from below, upwards. The Contraction happening in the *Peristaltic*, which others call the *Vermicular* Motion, as resembling the Motion of Worms, does not affect all Parts of the Intestines at once; but one part after another.

**VERMIFORMIS**, in Anatomy, a Term applied to various Parts in the human Body; bearing some resemblance to Worms. Such are the *Processus*, or *Apophyses Vermiformes*; which are the two Extremities of the *Cerebellum*, situate near the fourth Ventricle.

**VERMINATION**, is sometimes also used among Physicians, for a sort of *Tormina Ventris*, or wringing of the Guts; wherein the Patient is affected, as if Worms were gnawing his Intestines.

**VERRUCA**, in Medicine. Hence, *Verrucous* is applied to any Excrescencies which have resemblance to Warts.

**VERTICILLATE** Plants, are such as have their Flowers inter-mix'd with small Leaves, growing in a kind of Whorls about the Joints of a Stalk; as Penny-royal, Hore-hound, &c.

The peculiar Characteristick of this Genus of Plants, according to Mr. *Ray* is, that their Leaves grow by Pairs, one just against another, on the Stalk : the Flower monopetalous, but usually hanging down with a kind of Lip, or turned something like the form of an Helmet : Four Seeds after each Flower; to which the Periantheum of the Flower serves instead of a *Capsula Seminalis*.

The same Author makes two Species of these *Verticillate* Plants.

1°. The *Fruticosæ*, or such whose Superficies is Perennial : These, again, have either a plain Flower, as the *Chamædrys Vulgaris*, *Thucrium*, and the *Marum Syriacum*; or a Flower with a Lip, which they call a *Labiated Flower*; or one some-thing in the form of an Helmet, which they call *Galeated*; as the *Sacria Staechas, Hyssopus, Rosmarinus, Satureia, Marum vulgare, Thymum vulgare*, and the *Polium Montanum*.

2°. The Herbacæ, or such whose Stalks are not Perennial; these are the *Menthae, Verbena, Dictamnus Creticus, Origanum, Marjoram, Ocimum, Horminum, Galeopsis, Nepeta, Betonica, Prunella, Stachys, Clinopodium vulgare, Lamium, Moluca Hedera Terrestris, Galericulata, Calamintha, Melissa, Marrubium Commune, nigrum* and *aquaticum; Chamæpetys, Scaradonia, Scordium, Bugula, Syderitis, Cardiaca*.

[1] Girolamo Gabuccini was a sixteenth century Italian physician.

**VERTIGO**, in Medicine, an Indisposition of the Brain, wherein the Patient sees the Objects about him as if they turn'd round, and fancies he turns round himself; tho all the while at rest. The Word is form'd *à vertendo*, from turning.

Physicians distinguish two Kinds, or rather, two Degrees of *Vertigoes* : The first, call'd a *Simple Vertigo*, is when the Body and external Objects appear to turn round, without any great dimness of Sight. The other, call'd *Scotomia*, or *Vertigo Tenebrosa*, is when the Eyes are darken'd, and as it were cover'd with a Mist. Some make a third Stage, *viz.* a *Vertigo Caduca*, wherein the Patient actually falls down : But this seems scarce to differ from an Epilepsy.

Sometimes the *Vertigo* is seated in fore-part of the Head, and sometimes in the hind-part : whereof, the latter is much the more dangerous.

*Bellini* accounts for the *Vertigo* very well, from a preternatural Motion in the *Retina* : for 'tis evident, an Object will seem to move circularly, if the Images thereof, painted on the *Retina*, fall successively on different Parts of the *Retina*.

This they may do, either by the Objects moving while the Eye is at rest, or from the Eye moving while the Objects rest; or, lastly, the Object and Eye being both at rest, the Rays falling on the same Place by the Optic Nerve's being alone in Motion. For since a right and an oblique Incidence do not excite the same Tremors in the Nerves, and the same species of Motion; if the Optic Nerve only be moved, and the Object be at rest, it will appear to shift its Situation, by the Change of Place in which it was represented.

External Causes of *Vertigines*, are a continued turning round of the Body, Drunkenness, too long Fasting, immoderate Exercise, Surprize, Voracity, much use of Pulse, Onions, Leeks, Raddishes, Cabbages, Mustard, &c. and in the general, whatever may press, distend, or contract the Arteries.

**VESICA**, in Anatomy, a Bladder; a membranous or skinny Part, in which any Humor is contain'd.

**VESICA**, among Chymists, is a large Copper Vessel, tinn'd on the inside; used in distilling ardent Spirits : so called, as resembling the Figure of a blown Bladder.

**VESICATORY**, an external Medicine, serving to raise a Blister; whence also it is it self, tho improperly, call'd a *Blister*. *Vesicatories* are a stronger sort of *Sinapisms*. *Vesicatories* are Unguents, Cataplasms, or Plaisters made of sharp, irritating Medicaments, which have a Faculty of drawing the Humours from within, outwards; inflaming and ulcerating the Skin, and raising *Vesicæ*, or Bladders; whence the Name of *Vesicatory*.

We have *Vesicatories* made of Cantharides, Euphorbium, Figs, Sublimate of Mercury, *Lapis Infernalis*, Mustard, Anacardium, Scillæ, Briony, Vinegar, Pepper, Leaven, &c. which are incorporated and made up with Honey, Gums, Resins, &c. to bring them to the Consistence requir'd.

**VESICULA**, *Vesicle*, a Diminutive of *Vesica*; signifying a little Bladder. The Lung consists of *Vesiculæ*, or *Lobules* of *Vesiculæ*, admitting Air from the *Bronchiæ*; and not only Air, but also of Dust, &c.

**VETERNUS**, is used by some Physicians for a Lethargy, or other drousy Disease.

**VIA PRIMÆ**, among Physicians, are the Stomach and Guts; including the whole Length of the Alimentary Duct or Canal, from the Mouth to the *Sphincter Ani*. In this sense, we say, An Obstruction in the *Primæ Viæ*. Purging and Emetic Medicines operate chiefly in the *Primæ Viæ*. Sudorificks, Alteratives, Cardiacks, &c. suspend their action till after they have passed the *Primæ Viæ*.

**VIAL**, or Phiol, a small thin glass Bottle.

**VIBEX**, is sometimes used by Physicians for a black and blue Spot, occasion'd by a Flux of Blood.

**VICTUS** *Ratio*, among Physicians, a particular manner of living, for the Preservation of Health, and Prevention of Diseases.

**VIGILIA**, the State of an Animal which is opposite to Sleep, and popularly call'd *Waking*, or *Watching*.

**VINEGAR** *of Antimony*, is an acid Spirit, drawn by Distillation from the *Marcasite* of Antimony. Its use is commended in continued and malignant Fevers. The Apothecaries likewise make a kind of Theriacal *Vinegar* of Dittany, Angelico, Valerian, Cardimums, Oranges, &c.

**VINOUS**, *Vinosus*, something that relates to Wine; particularly the Taste, and Smell thereof. All Vegetables, by a due Temperament, afford a *Vinous* Liquor; as Corn, Pulse, Nuts, Apples, Grapes, &c. And a second Fermentation, duly manag'd, turn any *Vinous* Liquor into an acetous one.

The proper Character and Effect of Fermentation, is to produce either a *Vinous* or an acetous Quality in the Body fermented.

Some of our Countrymen, bound on a Voyage to the *East Indies*, having fill'd several Casks with *Thames*-Water, to carry along with 'em; observed an intestine Motion in it, when they came to the Equator; and found it afterwards turn'd into a kind of *Vinous* Liquor, capable of affording an inflammable Spirit by Distillation.

This, without dispute, proceeded from the Flowers, Leaves, Roots, Fruits, and other vegetable Matters, continually falling or wash'd down into that River. Such Waters are always found in a State of Putrefaction, ere they put on a *Vinous* Nature.

**VINUM**, in Medicine, or *Vinum Medicatum*, is particularly applied to several *medicated Wines*, *i.e.* Medicinal Preparations, whereof that Liquor is the Basis; such as the *Vinum Marinum*, Sea-Wine; made by casting Sea-Water on the Grapes in the Vat. *Vinum Cydonites*, Quince-Wine; made of slices of that Fruit, steep'd in Must, or new Wine.

*Vinum Rosatum*, Rose-Wine; made by steeping Roses for three Months in

Wine. *Vinum Strobilites*, or Pine-Apple Wine. *Vinum Hysopites*, Hysop-Wine. *Vinum Aromaticum*, made by infusing Aromaticks, or Spices, in new Wine or Must. *Vinum Picatum*, pitch'd Wine; made of Pitch infus'd in Must. *Vinum*, call'd also *Acetum, Scilliticum.*

*Vinum Absynthites*, or Wormwood-Wine; is made of the great or little Absynthium, by taking the Apices or Tops of the Flowers, putting them in a Sacculus, or Bag, and suspending it in the middle of a Vessel of Wine; which fermenting, extracts the Taste, Smell, and Virtues of the Wormwood.

*Vinum Emeticum*, Emetic Wine; is Wine wherein Glass, Regulus of Antimony, and Crocus Metallorum have been steep'd. It only takes a certain degree of Efficacy from the Matters; nor is it found any stronger at three Months end, than at the end of eight Days. It purges both upwards and downwards.

*Vinum Hippocraticum*, or Hippocras; so called of *Manica Hippocratis*, or *Hippocrate's* Sleeve, thro' which it is strain'd; is a sort of spiced Wine, in which Sugar and Spices have been steeped for some time.

**VIPER**, in Natural History, a kind of Serpent, famed not only for the exceeding Venomousness of its Bite, which is one of the most dangerous Poisons in the Animal Kingdom, but also for the great usefulness of its Flesh in Medicine.

*Vipers* make a considerable Article in Medicine. Most Authors agree, that there is no Part, Humour, or Excrement, not even the Gall it self, of a *Viper*, but may be swallow'd without much harm. Accordingly, the Antients, and, as several Authors assure us, the *Indians* at this day, both of the East and West, eat 'em as we do Eels.

*Caro Viperina*, Viper's Flesh, either roasted or boil'd, the Physicians unanimously prescribe as an excellent Restorative; particularly in the Elephantiasis, incurable Consumptions, Leprosy, &c. Dr. *Mead* thinks they might be less sparing in the Quantity than they are; instead of a little *Viper's* Flesh, he recommends the Broth or Gelly of *Vipers*; or, as the Antients did, to boil and eat them as Fish, or at least to drink *Vinum Viperinum*; *i.e.* Wine wherein they had been long infused.

*Viper's Flesh* is an Ingredient in several of our best Antidotes; as the *Theriaca Andromach.*, &c. The Apothecaries also sell the *Pulvis Viperinus*, which is only dried *Vipers* pulveriz'd, Heart, Liver, and all, and pass'd thro' a Sieve. This, to heighten the Price we suppose, they call *Animal Bezoard.*

The *Salts of Vipers*, whether volatile or fix'd, also their fat or *Axungia*, and their *Oil*, chymically drawn, are Drugs in good repute.

**VIRGINEUS** *Morbus*, the *Virgin's* Disease; the Green Sickness, or Chlorosis.

**VIRIDE** *Æris*, the same as *Ærugo*, or *Verdegrease.*

**VIRULENT**, a Term apply'd to any thing that yields a Virus; that is, a corrosive or contagious Pus. The *Gonorrhæa Virulenta*, is what we popularly call a Clap.

**VISCERA**, in Anatomy, a Term of equal import with Entrails, or Bowels; including the Heart, Liver, Lungs, Spleen, Intestines, and other inward Parts of the Body. The Word is also frequently used singularly, *Viscus*, to express some particular part of the Entrails; by reason the Word *Entrails* has no Singular. The Term *Viscus* is pure *Latin*, being form'd of *Vesci*, to feed; by reason, the Foods, call'd in *Latin*, *Vesca*, undergo divers Preparations in the *Viscera*.

**VITA**, *Life*, is a very ambiguous Term : For both God and Man, and a Soul, and an Animal, and a Plant, are said *to live* : yet there is not any thing common to *all* these, beside a kind of active Existence, which, however, is very different. *Life*, then, in the general, expresses a kind of active, operative Existence; and is therefore conceiv'd to consist in Motion. But, particularly,

*Vita Corporis, the Life of a Body*, consists in an uninterrupted Motion therein. A Body, therefore, said to be living, must consist of various Parts or Members, both internal and external, so framed and put together, as to constitute one Whole. And these Members must be moved and warm'd by some fluid Substance, permeating the whole Frame; by which Heat and Motion, the vital Functions are to be perform'd. Such are Nutrition, Generation, Local Motion, &c.

*Vita Mentis, the Life of a Mind*, is held by the *Cartesians* to consist in a perpetual Cogitation, or uninterrupted Course of Thinking; which seems likewise to have been *Aristotle's* meaning, when he call'd the Soul εντελεχεια; which his Interpreters call *Actus* : Thinking being the only proper Act of the Mind. But Dr. *Locke* endeavours to refute this Principle.

*Vita Hominis, Life of a Man*, consists in a continued communication of Body and Mind; or in Operations to which both the Motions of the Body, and Ideas of the Mind, contribute.

Thus, *e.g.* the Mind now thinking of something, on Occasion of that Thought, there arises a certain Motion in the Body : And, now, again, the Body moves first, which Motion is follow'd by some Thought of Mind.

In such alternate or reciprocal Operation, does the Life of Man consist; consider'd as he is a Compound of Body and Mind.

**VITAL**, in Anatomy, something that ministers principally to the constituting or maintaining of Life in the Bodies of Animals. Thus, the Heart, Lungs, and Brain, are called *Vital* Parts. Vital *Spirits* are the finest and most volatile Parts of the Blood.

Vital *Functions*, or *Actions*, are those Actions of the *Vital Parts*, whereby Life is affected; so as that it can't exist without 'em. Such are the musculous Action of the Heart; the secretory Action of the *Cerebellum*; the respiratory Action of the Lungs; the Circulation of the Blood and Spirits, thro' the Arteries, Veins, and Nerves.

**VITRIFICATION**, or Vitrification, the Act of converting a Body into Glass, by Fire. Of all Bodies, Fern-Ashes, Sand, Bricks, and Pebbles, *vitrify* the most easily. Accordingly, it is of the first of these that Glass is principally made.

Gold, held by M. *Homberg* near the Focus of the Duke of *Orleans's* large, burning, concave Mirror, at first smoak'd, then changed, all of it that did not go off in Fumes, into Glass, of a deep violet Colour. The Glass of Gold weighs less than Gold. *Memoirs of the* French *Academy*, 1702.

All Metals, and even almost all Natural Bodies, sufficiently heated, *vitrify* : And this *Vitrification* is the last Effect of the Fire; after which the most intense heat of the largest Burning-Glass, will make no further Alteration.

*Vitrification*, some Authors will have to be chiefly effected by the Salts uniting and incorporating with the metalline Particles.

But, according to M. *Homberg*, all *Vitrification* results from the Earth, which being exposed to a violent Fire, and intimately penetrated by some other Dissolvent, commences Glass. Thus, supposing the Principle of Gold to be Mercury, a metallick Sulphur, and an Earth; the *Vitrification* of Gold is easily conceived; the Mercury, being volatile, exhales in Smoke, and leaves behind it the Earth, and Sulphur, which are fix'd; the Sulphur dissolves the Earth and vitrifies it.

**VITRIOL**, in Natural History, a kind of Fossil, or mineral Salt, chiefly found in Copper Mines. *Vitriol* is more properly rank'd among the Class of Semi-metals, as having a metallic Matter mixt or combined with its Salt. *Vitriol* is defined by *Boerhaave*, a saline, metallic, transparent Glebe; dissoluble in Water, and fusible and calcinable by Fire.

It acquires different Names, according to the different Places where it is dug : and the *Vitriols* of those also, differ from each other in Denomination and Colour, some being *White*, others *Blue*, and others *Green*.

*Roman Vitriol*, for instance, is White; that of *Cyprus*, Blue; and that of *Pisa* and *Germany*, Greenish. *White Vitriol* partakes but little of any Metal, *Blue* partakes of Copper, and *Green* of Iron. See Iron, &c.

Monsieur *Geoffroy*, the elder, observes, that they all consist of an acid Salt, like that found in Alum and Sulphur; excepting that in Alum, the Acid is mixt with an absorbent Earth, or Calx : in Sulphur it is united with certain fat, bituminous Parts; and in *Vitriols*, with metallic Parts. According to *Boerhaave*, *Vitriols* consist of a metallic Part with a Sulphur adhering, a menstruous Acid, and Water.

In *Blue Vitriol*, the Metal, wherewith the Acid, &c. is join'd, is Copper. In *White Vitriol*, commonly call'd *White Copperas*, it is mixt with *Lapis Calaminaris*, or some ferruginous Earth, intermix'd with Lead or Tin. In *Green Vitriol*, the Acid is join'd with Iron.

The Antients give the Name *Chalcitis*, or *Chalcite*, to *native Vitriol*; or that which acquires its full Perfection in the Entrails of the Earth, and which is a kind of mineral Stone, of a reddish Colour. Of this they observ'd three different States, or Transformations : *Chalcitis*, in its first State, they call'd *Misi*; this afterwards turn'd into *Melanteria*, and that into *Sori*.

The Moderns take this *Chalcitis* to be the same with the *Colcothar* brought from *Sweden* and *Germany*, the best whereof is of a brownish-Red Colour, and a *vitriolic* Taste, and dissolves easily in Water; and, when broke, is of the Colour of shining Copper.

All the other *Vitriols* above-named, are really factitious, being only a kind of Crystals, drawn by means of Water, from a sort of Marcasite ordinarily found in Mines, and call'd, by Naturalists, *Pyrites* or *Quis*.

*Roman Vitriol* is made by exposing these *Pyrites* to the Air, till such time as they calcine, and change into a greenish, acid, *vitriolic* Calx, or Dust; in such State they are thrown into the Water, and afterwards, by boiling and evaporation, reduced into that kind of Crystals sent to us from *Italy*.

All the other *Vitriols* are made after the same manner, that is, much after the same manner as Alum is made in *England*, or Salt-petre in *France*.

For *Green Vitriol*, they add a great number of pieces of Iron to the Liquor in the boiling; these raise a great Ebullition. As soon as the Iron is dissolved, the evaporate the Dissolution to a certain Degree; and so let it crystallize. The Crystals being form'd, there remains a thick, reddish unctuous Styptic, and astringent Liquor, which Monsieur *Geoffroy* calls *Eau-mere de Vitriol*, as containing all the Principles of the Mineral, tho dis-united.

The Powder of this *Vitriol* is exceedingly styptic, and excellent for the cure of Wounds, and the stopping of Blood. Its Effects this way, have been rais'd by the knavery of some, and the credulity of others, to a kind of Miracle; it being that this makes the basis for the famous *Sympathetic Powder*.

The medicinal Virtues of *Vitriol* are very great; but all owing to the Iron, or other metallic Parts mixt with it, and therefore follow the kind of Metal. Thus, those of *Green Vitriol* depend on the stypticity or astringency of Iron, or *Mars*.

The *Eau-mere* drawn from the *Green Vitriol*, Monsieur *Geoffroy* observes, does not differ any way, essentially from a great Number of Preparations which the Chymists have given us of *Vitriol*, *Iron*, and the *Lapis Hæmatites* : As the fix'd and *anodyne Sulphurs of Vitriol* or *Mars*; Arcana, and Magisteries of *Vitriol*; Tinctures, &c. of *Vitriol, Mars*, &c. The common Basis of all which is Iron exceedingly subtilized and attenuated.

A Solution of *Vitriol* mix'd with a Tincture of Galls, becomes instantly exceedingly Black : and 'tis this is the common Writing-Ink.

Monsieur *Lemery*, the younger, has a pretty Hypothesis to account for this Blackness : he imagines, that as the *Vitriol* whereof Ink is made, is Iron dissolved by an Acid, and intimately mix'd therewith; and as Gall is an Alkali, or Absorbent, this Alkali meeting the Acids which hold the Iron dissolved, unites with them, and makes them let the Iron loose, which thereupon revivifies, and resumes its natural Blackness. So that in strictness, 'tis Iron we write withal.

This system is confirm'd hence : that of the five sorts of *Vitriol*, that of *Cyprus* or *Hungary* is the only one whose base is Copper; that of the rest is Iron : and accordingly they all serve to make Ink withal; excepting that.

*Vitriol* also enters the Composition of *Aquafortis*. What we call *Calcanthum* is only *Vitriol* rubified, and is not the same with *Colcothar*, as some have imagined.

Some take the Word *Vitrolium* to be used, *quasi vitri oleum*, because of its shining Colour; but *Menage* rather derives its Name, *a vitreo colore* : The *Latins* call it, *Atramentum*; and the *Greeks*, *Calcanthus*.

Some Naturalists hold *Vitriol* to be the Root, or Matrix of Copper; because in the Copper Mines they never dig deeper than the Glebe out of which the

*Vitriol* is drawn.

*Vitriol* affords several Chymical Preparations, as *Spirit of Vitriol*, procured by first Calcining, then Distilling it. *Oil of Vitriol*, which comes out after the Spirit, by heightening the Fire wherewith that had been rais'd. What remains after both, is the *Colcothar of Vitriol. Tartar of Vitriol* is had by mixing *Oil of Vitriol* with *Oil of Tartar per deliquium*; a Salt precipitating to the bottom, which being set to exhale and crystallize, is the *Tartar of Vitriol.*

*Metallic* **VITRIOLS** : All Metals, it is to be observed, may be converted into *Vitriols*, by dissolving 'em with acid Spirits, and letting 'em stand; tho 'tis very difficult to obtain *Vitriol* of Gold and Silver, by reason these Metals are not easily dissolved by the Spirit; but *Vitriols* of Iron and Copper are easily had.

**VITRIOL** *of Mars*, is a Preparation made by dissolving Iron, or Steel, in a proper acid Menstruum, then evaporating or drawing off the Moisture, and bringing the Matter to crystallize, *viz.* by setting it in a cool place. It is also called Salt of Steel.

**VITRIOL** *of Luna*, or *the Moon*, is the Body of Silver chymically opened, and reduced into the Form of a Salt by the sharp Points of *Spirit of Nitre.*

**VITRIOL** *of Venus*, is a Preparation made by a solution of Copper in the *Spirit of Nitre*, evaporated and crystallized, to gain the Salt; call'd also *Vitriol of Copper*. These factitious *Vitriols* being only Metals dissolved and crystallized in saline Menstruums, are frequently call'd, by way of distinction, *Metallic Vitriols*, and *Metallic Salts*.

**VITRIOLIC**, something that as the Quality of *Vitriol*; or partakes of the Nature of *Vitriol*. In this Sense we say, a *Vitriolic Spring, Vitriolic Stone, Vitriolic Spirits*, &c. If Iron be thrown into a *Vitriolic Water*, and the red Rust arising in on the Surface be melted down, it will be found real Copper; which is an Instance of the Transmutation of one Body into another.

**VITRIOUS HUMOUR**, in Anatomy, is the third Humour of the Eye, called *Vitrious, i.e. glassy*, from its resemblance to melted Glass. It lies under the Crystalline; by the impression of which, its fore-part is rendred Concave. Some Authors call the Coats or Membranes that contain this Humour, the *Vitrious Tunics.*

**VIVIFICATION**, in Medicine, the Art of *Vivifying*, that is, of contributing to the Action that gives Life, or maintains Life. The Chymists also use the Word in speaking of the new Force, Vigour, and Lustre by which this Art they give to natural Bodies, particularly to Mercury; which after having been fix'd or amalgamated, they restore to its first State.

**VOLATILE**, in Physicks, is commonly used to denote a mix'd Body whose integral Parts are easily dissipated y Fire, or other Heat; but is more properly used for Bodies whose Elements, or first component Parts, are easily separated from each other, and dispers's in Air.

For, as any mix't Body is said to be fix'd in a double Sense; so may it be said to be *Volatile* two ways : whence the same Body, *e.g.* Mercury, is both *volatile*, and fix'd at the same time.

Since, as its Integral Parts, or those which still retain the Nature of Mercury, are easily separable by Fire, and readily fly away; it is said to be *Volatile* : And yet as 'tis very difficult to destroy its Contexture, and resolve it by Fire, or any other Menstruum, into its first Elements, it is said to be *fix'd*. The same may be said of Sulphur, Antimony, &c.

Minerals, for the generality, are less *volatile* than Vegetables, and Vegetables less than Animals.

The Chymists distinguish between *Volatile* Salts, and Fix'd Salts.

The Capitals of Alembicks stop and collect the *Volatile* Parts of Substances in Sublimation; and make what we call Flowers.

"The Particles of Fluids which do not adhere very strongly together, and are of such Smallness, as renders them most susceptible of those Agitations which keep Liquors in a Fluor, are easily rarify'd into Vapour; and, in the Language of the Chymists, are Volatile. Those which are grosser, and so less susceptible of Alterations; or cohere by a stronger Attraction, do not evaporate without a stronger Heat, or perhaps not without Fermentation : These are what the Chymists call Fix'd Bodies." *Newton. Optic.* P. 371.

**VOLATILE**, in Chymistry. When the Fire decompounds any mix'd Body, the Parts most disposed to receive a great Motion, are soonest loosen'd, and rise up in the Order which their difference in their Disposition give them; the rest remaining immoveable at the bottom of the Vessel. Those that rise first, are called *Volatile Parts*; such are *Phlegm, Oil, Spirits*, and *Salts*, both urinous and alkalious. The Parts remaining, *viz. Earth*, and *Lixivial Salts*, are call'd *Fix'd*.

**VOLATILISATION**, the Act of rendering Fix'd Bodies *Volatile*; or of resolving 'em by Fire into a fine, subtile Vapour, or Spirit, which easily dissipates, and flies away. All Bodies, even the most fix'd, as Gold may be *volatiliz'd*; either of themselves, or with the Admixture of some volatile Substance, or Spirit; by Distillation, or Sublimation.

In the *Memoirs of the* French *Academy*, we have a Discourse on the *Volatilisation of the fix'd Salts of Plants*, by M. *Homberg*. That admirable Chymist, it seems, by an odd Accident, found fix'd Salts spontaneously *volatiliz'd* in Soap : Now Soap, we know, is a Composition of Oil, and the alkalous lixivial Salts of the Plant *Kali*. Upon this, M. *Homberg* conjectur'd, that the Oil from which the volatile Salts seem to derive their *Volatility*, being intimately mix'd with the fix'd Salts of the Kali in the Soap, had render'd them *volatile* : So that they cease to be Alkalious, by reason their Pores are now fill'd with the Oil which they have absorb'd. Oil, in effect, has always somewhat of an Acid in it; which Acid, being join'd to the Alkali, the whole is render'd a kind of intermediate Salt; which yet, as the Acid and Alkali were only join'd by means of this oil, is still Oily or sulphureous.

In consequence of this View, he made divers chymical Operations, whereby he found, that to dispose the fix'd Salts of Plants to *volatilise*, the Process is to be begun by making them into a Sapa, and letting that Sapa shoot out little saline Points, or Crystals on its Surface; which Crystals are no other than fix'd Salts already *volatiliz'd*. Then, the Remainder of the Matter is to be set over the Fire, after being well imbib'd and penetrated by some new Liquor, proper to assist in a new Sublimation of more fix'd Salts to be *volatiliz'd* : and this is to be repeated till no more Salts will rise.

The Choice of the Liquor wherewith the Sapa is to be saturated, is not indifferent. Water is, of all other, the least fit for the Effect : Oil does well; yet distill'd Oil better than that drawn from Expression : and Spirit of Wine best of all.

By such means, M. *Homberg volatiliz'd* almost half a Quantity of Salt of Tartar, which is a fix'd Vegetable Salt.

**VOLVULUS**, in Medicine, a *Latin* Name, which some Authors have given to a Disease other wise call'd the *Iliac Passion*; and by others the *Miserere mei*. 'Tis a kind of Cholic, wherein the Patient voids his Excrements by Mouth, instead of the *Anus*; by Reason the Membranes of the Intestine *Ileon* are drawn within one another, and form Knots, which prevent the ordinary Course of the *Fæces*.

**VOMICA**, in Medicine, a Collection of Pus in any Part of the Body. When this Mass or Collection is in the Lungs, 'tis called *Vomica Pulmonum*. When in the Kidneys, *Vomica Renum*, &c. The *Vomica* of the Lungs differs from an *Empyema*, which is a Collection of Pus in the Cavity of the Thorax.

*Nux* **VOMICA**, *Vomiting Nut*, is a little, round, woolly Fruit, half the bigness of a Farthing; hard as Horn, of a Mouse-colour without, but of various Colours within : sometimes yellow, sometimes white, and sometimes brown. 'Tis not know what Plant is that bears it. 'Tis a Poison for Dogs, and divers Quadrupeds, which it kills presently, thro' excessive *Vomiting*.

**VOMITING**, *Vomitus*, the Act of casting up, or evacuating by Mouth what is contain'd in the Stomach. This Action has been generally allow'd to be owing principally, to the Contraction of the Fibres of the Stomach, when irritated by the acrimonious Quality, or oppress'd with the Quantity, of Contents.

But M. *Chirac*[1], and after him M. *du Verney*[2], and others, set aside the Fibres of the Stomach; and advance, That *Vomiting* is produced wholly by the extraordinary Motions of the Diaphragm, and the Muscles of the lower Venter. So that the Stomach is here supposed destitute of all Action, and casts back its Contents only by its being compress'd and flatted, from some foreign and accidental Causes.

However, *Boerhaave*, and most of our latest Writers, allow both the Stomach, the Diaphragm, and the Muscles of the Abdomen, to have their share in the Action of *Vomiting* : Accordingly, that excellent Author makes *Vomiting* to consist in a convulsive and retrograde Motion of the muscular Fibres of the Gullet, Stomach, and Intestines; as well as those of the

[1] Pierre Chirac (1650 – 1732), a French physician.

[2] Joseph Guichard du Verney(1648 – 1730), a French physician and anatomist.

Abdomen, and the *Septum Transversum*; which, when in a less degree, produce a *Nausea*, and in a greater a *Vomiting*.

By the Contraction of so many Parts, the Stomach comes to be squeez'd, as in a Press; whence it is obliged to give up what is contain'd in its Cavity, and the neighbouring Parts; just as Water is in a Bladder or Sponge , when squeez'd between the Hands.

The Evacuation, too, must be upwards, rather than downwards; by reason the Passage is more open and easy that way, and that the Intestines are press'd by the Diaphragm, and the Muscles of the lower Venter.

The primary Cause of *Vomiting*, uses to be the too great Quantity, or too much Acrimony of the Contents, arising from Poisons, Contusions, Compressions, Inflammations, and Wounds in the Brain, Inflammations of the Diaphragm, Stomach, Intestines, Spleen, Liver, Kidneys, Panchreas, and Mesentery; unusual Agitations in Coaches, at Sea, &c. and *vomitive* and *emetic* Medicines.

**VOMITIVE**, or *Vomiting Medicines*. See Emetic.

**VULNERARY**, in Medicine, an Epithet given to Remedies proper for the Cure of Wounds, and Ulcers. The Word if form'd from the Latin *Vulnus*, Wound. There are divers *Vulnerary* Herbs; as *Aristolochia*, or Birthwort; *Sanicle*, or Self Heal; *Plantain, Mouse-Ear, Veronica*, or *Fluellin, Agrimony, Vervein*, or Holy Herb, &c. There are also *Vulnerary* Potions, composed of various Simples. *Vulnerary* Balms, Unguents, Plaisters, &c.

**WATER**, *Aqua*, in Physicks, a simple, fluid, and liquid Body; reputed the third of the four vulgar Elements. Sir. *I. Newton* defines Water to be a fluid Salt; volatile and void of Taste : But this Definition *Boerhaave* sets aside, inasmuch as Water is a Menstruum or Dissolvent of Salts and saline Bodies, which does not agree with the Notion of its being a Salt it self; inasmuch as, we don't know of any Salt that dissolves another.

*Whether* Water *be originally fluid*? Tho *Water* be defin'd a *Fluid*, 'tis a Point controverted among Philosophers, whether Fluidity be its Natural State, or the Effect of Violence : We sometimes find it appear in a fluid, and sometimes in a solid form; and as the former in our warmer Climates is the more usual, we conclude it the proper one, and ascribe the other to the extraneous Action of Cold. *Boerhaave*, however, asserts the contrary, and maintains Water to be of the Crystalline Kind; since, wherever a certain degree of Fire is wanting to keep it in fusion, it readily grows into a hard Glebe, under the Denomination of Ice.

Mr. *Boyle* is much of the same Sentiment. Ice, he observes, is commonly reputed to be *Water* brought into a preternatural State by Cold : But, with regard to the Nature of Things, and setting aside our arbitrary Ideas, it might as justly be said, That *Water* is Ice, preternaturally thawed by Heat. If it be urg'd that Ice, left to it self will, upon the Removal of the freezing Agents, return to *Water* : It may be answer'd, that, not to mention the Snow and Ice which lie all Summer long on the *Alps* and other high Mountains, even in the Torrid Zone, we have been assur'd, that in some Parts of *Siberia*, the Surface of the Ground continues more Months of the Year frozen by the natural Temperature of the Climate, than thaw'd by the Heat of the Sun; and a little below the Surface of the Ground, the *Water* which chances to be lodg'd in the Cavities there, continues in a state of Ice all the Year round : So that when in the heat of Summer the Fields are cover'd with Corn, if you dig a Foot or two deep, you shall find Ice, and a frozen Soil.

*No pure* Water *in all Nature. Water*, if it could be had alone, and pure, *Boerhaave* argues, would have all the requisites of an Element, and be as simple as Fire; but there is no expedient hitherto discover'd for making it such. Rain-*Water*, which seems the purest of all those we know of, is replete with infinite Exhalations of all kinds, which it imbibes from the Air : So that filter'd and distill'd a thousand times, there still remains Fæces. Further, the Rain-*Water* gather'd from the Roofs of Houses, is a Lixivium of Tyles, Slate, or the like, impregnated with the Dungs and Faeces of the Animals, Birds, &c. deposited thereon; and the Exhalations of numerous other Things. Add, that all the Rain-*Water* gather'd in Cities, must at must be saturated with the Smoke of a thousand Chimnies, and the various Effluvia of Numbers of Persons, &c. Beside that there is Fire contained in all *Water*; as appears from its Fluidity, which is owing to Fire alone.

As what is in the Air necessarily mixes it self with *Water*, it hence appears impossible to have such a thing as pure *Water*. If you percolate it thro' Sand, or squeeze it thro' Pumice, or pass it thro' any other Body of the like kind, you will always have Salt remaining. Nor can Distillation render it pure; since it leaves the Air therein, which abounds in Corpuscles of all sorts.

The purest of all *Waters* we can any way arrive at, is that distill'd from Snow, gather'd in a clear, still, pinching Night, in some very high Place; taking none but just the outer or superficial Part thereof. By a Number of repeated Distillations hereof, the greatest part of the Earth and other Fæces, may be separate herefrom : And this is what we must be contented to call *pure Water*.

Mr. *Boyle*, indeed, relates, that a Friend of his, by distilling a quantity of *Water* an hundred times, found at length that he had got six tenths of the first Quantity in Earth: Whence he concludes, that the whole *Water*, by further prosecuting the Operation, might be converted into Earth.

But is should be consider'd, that the *Water* cannot be removed, or poured into a Vessel, without the Mixture of some Dust therewith; so, neither can the Luting of the Vessel be distill'd without losing something every time. *Boerhaave*, therefore, rather concludes, that the *Water* thus often distill'd, might acquire still new Earth from the Dust floating in the Air, and the Instruments employ'd in the Operation.

That Author assures us, that after distilling some very pure *Water*, by a gentle Fire, the space of four Months, it appear'd perfectly pure; and yet leaving it to rest in Vessels exactly closed, it would conceive a slender kind of weedy Matter, somewhat like the *Stamina* of Plants, or the little Tufts of a Mucilage : and yet, *Schottus* saw *Water*, in *Kircher's Musæum*, that had been kept in a Vessel hermetically seal'd, upwards of fifty Years, yet still remained clear and pure, and stood to the same height in the Vessel as at first, without the least Sign of Sediment.

*Boerhaave* adds, that he is convinced no body ever saw a Drop of pure *Water*; that the utmost of its purity known, only amounts to its being free of this or that sort of Matter : and that it can never, for instance, be quite deprived of Salt; since Air will always accompany it, and Air has always Salt.

Water *in all Places and Bodies*. *Water* seems to be diffused every where, and to be present in all Space where there is Matter. Not a Body in all Nature but will yield *Water* : 'Tis even asserted that Fire it self is not without *Water*. A single Grain of the most fiery Salt, which in a Moment's Time will penetrate thro' a Man's Hand, readily imbibes half its weight of *Water*, and melts, even in the driest Air imaginable. Thus, Salt of Tartar, placed near the hottest Fire, will attract or imbibe *Water*; and by that means, increase considerably its weight in a small time : So in the driest Summer's Day, a pewter Vessel with Ice in it, brought up from some cold subterraneous Place into the hottest Room, will immediately be cover'd over with little Drops of *Water*, gather'd from the contiguous Air, and condens'd by the Coldness of the Ice.

'Tis surprizing to consider the plenteous Stock of *Water* which even dry Bodies afford. Oil of Vitriol, being exposed a long time to a violent Fire, to separate all the *Water*, as much as possible, from the same; will afterwards, by only standing a few Minutes in the Air, contract fresh *Water* so fast, as soon to afford it as plenteously as at first. Hartshorn, kept forty Years, and turn'd as hard and dry as any Metal; so, that if struck against a Flint, it will yield Sparks of Fire; yet, being put into a glass Vessel, and distill'd, will afford one eighth of its Quantity of *Water*. Bones dead and dried twenty five Years, and thus become almost as hard as Iron; yet, by Distillation, have afforded half their weight of *Water*. And the hardest Stones, ground and distill'd, do always discover a Portion thereof.

Eels, by Distillation, yielded Mr. *Boyle* some Oil, Spirit, and Volatile Salt, besides the *Caput Mortuum*; yet all these were so disproportionate to the *Water*, that they seemed to have been nothing but that coagulated : The same strangely abounds in Vipers, tho esteemed very hot in operation; and will, in a convenient Air, survive for some Days the loss of their Heads and Hearts. Human Blood it self, as spirituous and elaborate a Liquor as it is reputed, so abounds in *Water*, that out of seven Ounces and an half, the same Author, by Distillation, drew near six of Phlegm; before every any of the other Principles began to rise.

*Whether Water be the common Matter of all Bodies?* Form Considerations of this kind, *Thales*, and some other Philosophers, have been led to hold, That all Things were made of *Water* : Which Opinion, probably, had its rise from the Writings of *Moses*, where he speaks of the Spirit of God moving upon the Face of the *Waters*. But Mr. *Boyle* does not conceive the Water here mention'd by Moses as the Universal Matter, to be our Elementary *Water* : we need only suppose it an agitated Congeries of a great Variety of seminal Principles, and of other Corpuscles fit to be subdu'd and fashion'd by them; and it may yet be a Body fluid like *Water*, in case the Corpuscles it was made up of, were, by their Creator, made small enough, and put into such an actual Motion, as might make them roll, and glide easily over one another. However, *Basil Valentine, Paracelsus, Van Helmont, Centivoglio*, and others, have maintained the same Principle, *viz.* That Water is the Elementary Matter or *Stamen* of all things, and suffices alone for the Production of all the visible Creation. Thus, Sir *I. Newton*, "All Birds, Beasts, and Fishes, Insects, Trees, and Vegetables, with their several Parts, do grow out of *Water*, and *watery* Tinctures, and Salts; and by Putrefaction return again into watery Substances."

*Helmont* endeavours to prove this Doctrine from an Experiment; wherein, burning a quantity of Earth, till all the Oil was consum'd, and then mixing it up with *Water*, to draw out all the Salt; and putting this Earth, thus prepared, into an earthen Pot, which nothing but Rain-*Water* could enter; yet a Willow, planted therein, grew up to a considerable height and bulk, without any sensible Diminution of the Earth : Whence he concluded, that the *Water* was the only Nutriment of the Vegetable Kind, as Vegetables are of the Animal. The same thing is infer'd by Mr. *Boyle* from a parallel Experiment : And the whole is countenanc'd by Sir. *I. Newton*, who observes, that *Water*, standing a few Days in the open Air, yields a Tincture, which, like that of Malt, by standing longer, yields a Sediment, and a Spirit; but before Putrefaction, is fit Nourishment for Animals and Vegetables.

But Dr. *Woodward* endeavours to shew the whole a Mistake : *Water* containing extraneous Corpuscles, some of these, he shews, are the proper Matter of Nutrition; the *Water* being still found to afford so much the less Nourishment, the more it is purify'd by Distillation. Thus, a Plant in distill'd *Water* will not grow so fast as in *Water* not distill'd; and if the Water be distill'd three or four times over, the Plant will scarce grow at all, or receive any Nourishment from it. So that *Water*, as such, does not seem the proper Nourishment of Vegetables; but only the Vehicle thereof, which contains the nutritious Particles, and carries them along with it, thro' all the Parts of the

Plant.

Hence, a Water-Plant, *e.g.* a *Nasturtium*, brought up in a Vessel of *Water*, will be found to contain the more Salt and Oil, the muddier the *Water* is : In effect *Water* nourishes the less, the more it is purged of its saponaceous Salts; in its pure State, it may suffice to extend or swell the Parts, but affords no new Vegetable Matter.

*Helmont*, however, carries his System still further, and imagines, that all Bodies may be re-converted into *Water*. His Alkahest, he affirms, adequately resolves Plants, Animals, and Minerals, into one Liquor, or more, according to their several internal Differences of parts : And the Alkahest, being abstracted from these Liquors, in the same Weight and with the same Virtues as when it dissolv'd them; the Liquors may, by frequent Cohobations from Chalk, or some other proper Matter, be totally depriv'd of their seminal Endowments, and return at last to their first Matter, insipid *Water*.

Thus much is confess'd, that mix'd Bodies do all resolve by Fire, into Phlegm or *Water*, Oil, Spirit, Salt, and Earth; each of which is found to contain *Water*.

Spirits, for instance, cannot be better represented by Spirit of Wine, which of all others seems freest from *Water* : yet, *Helmont* affirms, it may be so united with *Water*, as to become *Water* it self. He adds, that 'tis materially *Water*; only under a sulphurous Disguise. According to him, in making *Paracelsus's Balsamus-samech*, which is nothing but *Sal Tartari* dulcify'd by distilling Spirit of Wine from it till the Salt be sufficiently saturated with its Sulphur, and till it suffers the Liquor to be drawn off as string as it was poured on; when the Salt of Tartar, from which it is distill'd, hath retained, or deprived it of the sulphurous Parts of the Spirit of Wine, the rest, which is incomparably the greatest Part of the Liquor, will turn to Phlegm. In effect, corrosive Spirits, according to Mr. *Boyle's* Observation, abound in *Water*; which may be observed, by entangling, and so fixing their saline Parts, as to make them corrode some proper Body; or else by mortifying them with some contrary Salt: which will turn them into Phlegm.

And as to Salts; Salt of Tartar well calcin'd, being laid to liquefy in the Air, will deposite an Earth; and if it be then committed to Distillation, will yield a considerable Quantity of insipid *Water*; insomuch, that if it be urg'd with a vehement Fire, the Salt will almost all vanish, and nothing saline remain, either in the *Water*, or the Earth. Whence *Helmont* concludes, that all Salts might be converted into *Water*. Add, that Sea Salt, recover'd from its own acid Spirit and Oil of Tartar, melts into *Water*, as much as into Oil of Tartar.

Lastly, Oils run, in great measure into Water; and 'tis probable, might be converted wholly into the same.

*No Standard for the Weight and Purity of* Water. *Water* scarce ever continues two Moments exactly of the same weight, being always varying, by reason of the Air and Fir therein. Thus, a piece of pure limpid Ice, laid in a nice balance, never continues *in Aequilibrio*. In effect, the Expansion of *Water* in boiling, shews what effect the different degree of Fire has on the Specific Gravity of *Water*. This makes it difficult to fix the specifick Gravity of *Water*, in order to settle its degree of Purity; but this we may say in general, That the purest *Water* we can procure, is that which is 880 times as heavy as

Air. However, neither have we any tolerable Standard in Air; for *Water* being so much heavier than Air, the more *Water* is contain'd in the Air, the heavier of course must it be : As, in effect, the principal Part of the Weight of the Atmosphere, seems to arise from the *Water*.

*Properties and Effects of* Water.

1°, *Water* is found the most *penetrative* of all Bodies, after Fire, and the most difficult to confine; so that a Vessel thro' which *Water* cannot pass, may retain any thing. Nor is it any Objection, that Syrups and Oils will sometimes pass thro' Bodies which will hold *Water*; this is not because owing to the greater Subtility and Penetration of their Particles, but to the Resin wherewith the Wood of such Vessels abounds, to which Oils and Syrups are as Menstruums; so that dissolving the Resin, they make their way thro' the Spaces left thereby; whereas *Water*, not acting on Resins, is retained.

And yet, *Water* gradually make its way, even thro' all Woods, and is only retainable in Glass and Metals; nay, it was found by Experiment at *Florence*, that when shut up in a spherical Vessel of Gold, and then press'd with a huge force, it made it's way thro' the Pores even of the Gold; so that the most solid Body in Nature is permeable to *Water*.

*Water* is even found more fluid than Air; a Body being reputed more fluid than another, when its Parts will find way thro' smaller Pores : now Air, 'tis known, will not pass thro' Leather, as is evident in the Case of an exhausted Receiver cover'd therewith; whereas *Water* passes with ease. Again, Air may be retain'd in a Bladder, but *Water* oozes thro'. In effect, 'tis found, that *Water* will pass thro' Pores ten times smaller than Air will.

It must not be omitted, however, that M. *Homberg* accounts for this passage of Water thro' the narrow Pores of animal Substances which will not admit the Air, on another Principle, *viz.* its moistening and dissolving the glutinous Matter of the fine Fibres of the Membranes, and rendering them more pliable and distractile; which are things that the Air, for want of a wetting Property, cannot do. As a Proof of this Doctrine, he filled Bladder, and compress'd it with a Stone, and found not Air to come out; but placing the Bladder thus compress'd in Water, the Air easily escap'd. *Hist. de l'Acad.* Ann. 1700. p. 45.

2°, *Water*, then, may even hence, *viz.* from its penetrative Power, be argu'd to enter *the Composition of all Bodies*, both Vegetable, Animal, and Fossil; with this peculiar Circumstance, That it is easily, and with a gentle heat, separable again from Bodies it had united with; which cannot be said of any other Body. Fire, indeed, will penetrate more than *Water*; but 'tis difficult to procure it again from the Bodies it is once fixed in, as is evident in Read Lead, &c.

This Property of *Water*, join'd with its Smoothness and Lubricity, fits it to serve as a Vehicle, for the commodious and easy Conveyance of the Nutritious Matter of all Bodies : being so fluid, and passing and repassing so readily, it never stops up the Pores, but leaves room for the following *Water*, to bring on a new Supply of nutritious Matter.

3°, And yet the same *Water*, as little cohesive as it is, and as easily separated from most Bodies, will *cohere firmly with some others*, and bind them together into the most solid Masses : Tho it appears wonderful, that *Water*, which will be shewn an almost universal Dissolvent, should withal be a great Coagulator.

*Water*, we see, mixed up with Earth or Ashes, gives them the utmost Firmness and Fixity. The Ashes, *e.g.* of An Animal, incorporated with pure *Water* into a Paste, and bak'd by a vehement Fire, grow into a Coppel; which is a Body remarkable for this, that it will bear the utmost Effort of a Refiner's Furnace. 'Tis, in effect, upon the glutinous Nature of *Water* alone that our Houses stand; for take but this out of Wood, and it becomes Ashes; or out of Tyles, and they become Dust.

Thus, a little Clay dry'd in the Sun, becomes a Pouder, which mix'd with *Water* sticks together again, and may be fashion'd at pleasure; and this dried again by a gentle Fire, or in the Sun, and then baked in a Potter's Oven, by an intense Fire, becomes little other than a Stone. So the *Chinese* or *Japan* Earth, whereof our Porcelain Vessels are made, which hold all Liquors, and even melted Lead it self, is diluted and wrought up with Water.

To say no more, all the Stability and Firmness seen in the Universe is owing to *Water* alone. Thus, Stone would be an incoherent Sand, did not *Water* bind it together; and thus, again, of a fat gravelly Earth, wrought up with *Water* and baked or burnt, we make Bricks, Tyles, and earthen Vessels, of such exceeding Hardness and Closeness, that *Water* it self cannot pass thro' them. And these Bodies, tho to appearance perfectly dry, and destitute of *Water*, yet, being pulveriz'd and put in a Retort, and distill'd, yield an incredible quantity of *Water*.

The same holds of Metal; for the Parings of Filings of Lead, Tin, Antimony, &c. by Distillation, yield *Water* plentifully; and the hardest Stones, Sea Salt, Nitre, Vitriol, Sulphur, &c. are found to consist chiefly of *Water*, into which they resolve by force of Fire.

The *Lapis Calcarius*, or Lime-stone, being expos'd to the Fire, affords a prodigious Quantity of pure *Water*; and the more of this *Water* is express'd, the more friable does it become, till at length it commences a dry Calx or Lime; wherein, in lieu of *Water* so expell'd, the Fire, in the Course of Calcination, enters; which is expell'd again, in its turn, by pouring on cold *Water*. Yet, the same *Water* and Calx, temper'd together, produce a Mass, scarce inferior, in point of Solidity, to the primitive Lime-stone.

4°, That *Water* is *not elastick*, is evident hence, that it is incompressible, or incapable by any Force, of being reduced into less compass : This easily follows from that famous Experiment abovemention'd, made by order of the great Duke of *Tuscany*. The *Water*, being incapable of Condensation, rather than yield, transuded thro' the Pores of the Metal, so that the Ball was found wet all over the outside; till at length, making a Cleft in the Gold, it spun out with great vehemence. From this last Circumstance, indeed, some have weakly concluded it was elastick. For the *Impetus* wherewith the *Water* darted forth, was more probably owing to the Elasticity of Gold, which communicated that Impression to the *Water*.

And hence we see the Reason why Blocks of Marble sometimes burst in cold weather; and why a Vessel fill'd with *Water*, and afterwards, by any means, reduced to a less compass, bursts the Vessel, tho ever so strong. This is observable in a piece of brass Canon, which being filled with *Water*, and the Mouth exactly stopp'd, so as to prevent all egress of *Water*; if a cold Night happens, sufficient to contract and constipate Bodies; the metallick Matter undergoing the common Fate, and the *Water* refusing to give way, the Cannon is burst asunder with incredible violence.

Some bring an Argument for the Elasticity of *Water* hence, that hot *Water* takes up m ore room than cold; but no legitimate Conclusion can be form'd from hence : for in the hot *Water* there is a good quantity of Fire contain'd, which interposing between the Particles of *Water*, makes it extend to a greater Space, without any Expansion of Parts from its own Elasticity. This is evident hence, that if *Water* be once heated, there is no reducing it to its former Dimensions, but by letting it cool again : which plainly shews, that the Expansion depends not on the Elasticity of Parts, but on the Presence of Fire. *Water*, then, tho incapable of Compression or Condensation, may yet be rarefied by Heat, and contracted by Cold.

It may be added, that a further degree of Cold, that is, such a one as congeals *Water*, or turn it into Ice, does expand it. There are other ways to manifest this Expansion of *Water* by Freezing. Mr. *Boyle* having poured a proper quantity of *Water* into a strong cylindrical earthen Vessel, exposed it, uncover'd, both to the open Air in frosty Nights, and the Operation of Snow and Salt; and found, that the Ice produced in both Cases, reach'd higher than the *Water* before 'twas froze. Add, that it has been found, that the Rain soaking into Marble, an violent Frosts coming on, have burst the Stones : And even Implements made of Bell-Metal, carelessly expos'd to the wet, have been broken and spoiled by the *Water*; which entering at little Cavities of the Metal, was there afterwards froze, and expanded into Ice.

From the whole, we may be enabled to settle something as to the Nature of the component Particles of *Water*; and, 1°, That they are, as to our Senses, infinitely small; whence their penetrative Power : 2°, Exceeding smooth and slippery, void of any sensible Asperities; witness their Fluidity, and their being so easily separable from other Bodies which they adhere to : 3°, Extremely solid: 4°, Perfectly transparent, and as such invisible; which we gather hence, that pure *Water*, inclos'd in a Vessel hermetically seal'd, projects no Shadow; so that the Eye shall not be able to discover whether the Vessel have *Water* in it or not; and in that the Crystals of Salts, when the *Water* is separate from them, lose their Transparency. 5°, Hard, rigid, and inflexible; as appears from their not being compressible.

If it be ask'd, How a Body so light, fluid, and volatile, and which so easy a Fire suffices to rarefy, should be so stubborn and incompressible? We see no other Cause to assign, but the Homogeneity of its Parts. If *Water* be consider'd as consisting of spherical or cubical Particles, hollow withinside, and of a firm Texture; here will be enough to account for the whole : Its Firmness and Similarity will make it resist sufficiently; and its Vacuity render it light enough, &c. The little Contact between Spherules, will account for the Weakness of its Cohesion, &c.

Salt melted in *Water*, does not fill the Vessel in proportion to its own bulk : Whence it follows, that there are little Spaces between its Particles, to admit those of the Salt. And hence, again, we gather, that the *watry* Particles are extremely solid, and inflexible; since, tho they have intermediate Spaces, no force or weight can compress, or crows them nearer.

5°, *Water* is the most *insipid* of all Bodies; the Taste we sometimes observe therein, arising not from the mere *Water*; but from Salt, Vitriol, or other Bodies mixed therewith : And accordingly, all the sapid *Water* recommended for Medicinal Uses, are found to deposite a Quantity of some of those Fossils.

6°, *Water* is perfectly inodorous, or void of the least Smell. *Water*, then, neither affects Sight, Taste, nor Smell, provided it be pure; and consequently might remain for ever imperceptible to us, but for the Sense of Feeling.

**WATER**, in Natural History, &c. is distinguish'd into *Pure*, call'd also *Elemental*; *Mineral*; and *Artificial* or Factitious.

As to the Pure, we have already observ'd, that there is, perhaps, none absolutely so; all Water being found to contain more or less Particles, such as are in terrestrial Bodies; not earthy Particles, we mean, but Oils, Salts, &c.

*Mineral* Waters, are those which contain such and so many Particles of different Nature from *Water*, as thence to derive some notable Property beyond what common Water has : Or, *Mineral Waters* are those which have contracted some Virtue extraordinary, by passing thro' Beds of Minerals, as Alumn, Vitriol, Sulphur, &c. or by receiving the Fumes thereof.

The Kinds of *Mineral Waters* are various, as they are the Kinds of Compositions of the Minerals they are impregnated withal.

Some are *Simple*, as only containing mineral Particles of one sort; others *Mix'd*, of two, three, four, or more sorts.

Hence, we have, 1°, Metallick Waters, viz. in different Parts, *Golden, Silver, Copper, Tin, Leaden*, and *Iron Waters*. 2°, Saline Waters, viz. *Nitrous, Aluminous, Vitriolate,* and those of common Salt. 3°, *Bituminous, Sulphurous, Antimonial, Cabronaceous*, and *Amber Waters*. 4°, *Earthy* and *Stony Waters*, viz. *Lime, Chalk, Oker, Cinnabar, Marble*, and *Alabaster Waters*. 5°, Mercurial Waters. See Mercury, Quicksilver, &c.

This Division of *Mineral Waters* is taken from their Essences; that is, from the Mineral Particles they contain : but the most usual and celebrated Division, is borrow'd from the manner wherein they affect our Senses; with regard to which there are ten Kinds; viz. *acid, bitter, hot, very cold, oily and fat, poisonous, colour'd, boiling, petrifying, incrusting*, and *saline*.

*Acid Waters*, called also *Acidulæ*, arise from the Admixture of Vitriol, Nitre, Alumn, and Salt. These are cold, and very frequent, there being not reckon'd less than 1000 in *Germany* alone : Some of which are sower as Vinegar, and used instead thereof; others vinous, and serving for Wine; others astringent, &c.

*Hot Waters*, called *Thermæ*, arise from the admixture of sulphurous Particles and Fumes. Of these, the hottest is that in Japan, which no Fire can bring *Water* to equal; and which keeps hot thrice as long as our boil'd *Water*.

*Oily* and *Fat Waters*, arise from a bituminous and sulphureous Matter; as Amber, Petroleum, Pitch, Naphtha, &c.

*Bitter Waters* are produced from an impure Sulphur, Bitumen, Nitre, and Copper. Such is the *Lacus Asphaltites*.

*Very cold Waters*, have their rise from a Mixture of Nitre and Alumn; or of Mercury, Iron, &c. The Depth of the Source or Spring too, has some effect.

*Poisonous Waters* are occasion'd by their creeping thro' Arsenical, Antimonial, and Mercurial Earths, or being impregnated by the Fumes. Such is the *Lacus Asphaltites*, and divers others about the *Alps*, &c. which immediately kill those who drink : But these are most of 'em fill'd up with Stones; which is one Reason so few are known.

*Saline Waters* are generated two ways; either they are deriv'd from the Sea, by some subterraneous Passage; or are generated from the Mineral Salts, which they meet withal in their passage ere they arrive at their Springs.

*Boiling* or *Bubbling Waters*, are produced either by a sulphureous, or a nitrous Spirit, mix'd with the *Water* in the Earth : If it be sulphurous, the *Water* is hot; if nitrous, cold. For all the *Waters* that boil as if hot are not so, but some few are cold : We read both of *Thermæ* and *Acidulæ* that boil.

There are divers other *Waters* that have very singular Properties, not reducible to any of these Classes : Such, 1°, is that Spring in *Portugal*, which absorbs all Bodies cast into it, tho the lightest : And not far from it there was antiently another, in which no Bodies, not the heaviest, could sink. 2°, In *Andulusia*, we are assur'd by *Euseb. Nierembergensis*, there is a Lake which foretells approaching Storms, by making a terrible bellowing, that may be heard 18 or 20 Miles distance. 3°, In *Granada*, is a Well whose *Water* dissolves Stones. 4°, We read of a Spring in *Arcadia*, which render'd those who drank of it abstemious. 5°, In the Island of *Chio* is a Spring, which converts those who drink of it into Fools. 6°, There are Springs in divers Parts of *England*, *Wales*, *Spain*, &c. which ebb and flow daily with the Flux and Reflux of the Sea; and some are even said to ebb and flow against the Tide. Add, 7°, *Stalactical Waters*.

**WATER**, in Chymistry, by the Chymists called more usually *Phlegm*; is the fourth of the five chymical Principles, and one of the passive ones. It is never pure and unmix'd; which, Dr. *Quincy* observes, make sit usually a little more detersive than common *Water*.

This Principle, probably, contributes much to the Growth of Bodies, in that it both renders and keeps the active Principles fluid; so that they are capable of being convey'd by Circulation into the Pores of the mixed : and also because it tempers their exorbitant Motion, and keeps them together; so that they are not so easily and soon dissipated.

In all such Bodies whose active Substances are join'd and united pretty closely together, as in common Salt, Tartar, all Plants that are not odoriferous, and in many animal Bodies; this Principle is the first that comes in Distillation : But when Water is mixed with volatile Salts, or with Spirit of Wine, or is in any odoriferous Mixture; then the volatile Particles will rise and come away first.

**WATERS**, in Medicine, Pharmacy, Chymistry, &c. call'd also *Artificial*, *Medicinal*, &c. *Waters*; are a Kind of Liquors, procured or prepared by Art from divers Bodies, principally of the Vegetable Tribe; having various Properties, and serving various Purposes. These Waters are either *Simple*, or *Compound*. *Simple* Waters are those procur'd from some one Vegetable

Body.

A *Simple Water*, is not supposed to be the mere *Water* or Phlegm of the Body it is drawn from, as is evident from the Taste and Smell thereof. The Intention of making such *Water*, is to draw out the Virtues of the Herb, Seed, Flower, Root, or the like, so as it may be more conveniently given in that form than any other. But the Phlegm, or watery Parts of any Medicinal Simple, is no better than common *Water* undistill'd : So that all those Ingredients which in Distillation raise nothing but Phlegm, as may be discover'd from the Scent and Taste of what comes over, are not fit for the Still. On this Principle, a great part of the *Waters* retained in the Dispensatories will appear good for nothing, at least not worth distilling.

The Means whereby this Separation is effected, are either *Evaporation, Infusion, Decoction,* or *Distillation.*

The first is perform'd by exposing the Vegetable in a cold Still to a gentle Heat, like that of a Summer's Sun; and catching the Effluvia which exhale from it. The Effect of this Operation, is a *Water*, or fluid Matter, which is the most volatile, fragrant, and aromatick Part of the Plant; and that wherein its specifick Virtue resided. And thus is it that the aromatick or odoriferous *Waters* of Vegetables are procured.

The second Means, *viz. Infusion*, is perform'd by putting the Vegetable in hot Rain-*Water*, below the degree of boiling; keeping it to this degree by an equable heat, for the space of half an Hour; and then straining our pouring it off. The only *Waters* procured this way in much use in the modern Practice, are those of Frog-spawn, and Oak-buds.

The third Means, *viz. Decoction*, only differs from the second in this, that the Water is kept to the degree of boiling.

The fourth Means, *viz. Distillation*, is perform'd by infusing the Subject in an Alembick, by a gentle warmth, for some time, and then increasing the Heat so as to make it boil; and lastly, catching and condensing the Steam or Vapour arising therefrom. This Process furnishes what we call the *Distill'd Waters*, of so much use in Medicine, &c.

The Vegetable Subjects best fitted for it, are the sapid and odorous, or those of the aromatick Tribe; as Angelica, Aniseed, Baum, Carraway, Coriander, Cumin, Dittany, Fennel, Hyssop, Marjoram, Mint, Roses, Rosemary, Saffron, Sage, Scurvygrass, Thyme, Cinnamon, Citron, Juniper, Lime, Myrtle, Orange, Peach, &c.

The Medicinal Virtues of *Waters* prepared after this manner, are the same as those of the respective Plants, &c. they are drawn from. Thus, the distill'd *Water* of Mint is Stomachic; that of Wormwood, Vermifugous, &c.

The *Materia Medica*, it may be observ'd, affords no Remedies in this way, but for the Intentions either of Cordials, Diureticks, or Diaphoreticks. Were it practicable to raise a Balsamick, Cathartick, or Opiate in this way, yet would those Properties be much more conveniently brought forth by other Processes; so that nothing is to be look'd for in a distill'd *Water*, but such subtile and light Parts of a Medicinal Simple, as may fall in with the forementtion'd Intentions : Indeed, very little comes over under that Division, weighty enough to affect even the urinary Secretions.

The Simple Waters of chief Virtue are the following ones, *viz.* Dill-*Water*,

*Aqua Anethi*; Baum-*Water, Aqua Melissæ*; Angelica-*Water, Aqua Angelicæ*; Mint-*Water, Aqua Menthæ*; Rosemary-*Water, Aqua Anthos*; Orange-Flower-*Water, Aqua Naphæ*; Black-Cherry-*Water, Aqua Cerasor. nig.*; Parsly-*Water, Aqua Petroselini*; Camomile, *Chamom.* Pennyroyal, *Pulegii*; Fennel-*Water, Aqua Fæniculi*; Damask-Rose-*Water, Aqua Rosarium dam.*; Hyssop-*Water, Aqua Hyssopi*; Rue-*Water, Aqua Rutæ*; Juniper-*Water, Aqua Juniperi bac.*; Eldar-*Water, Aqua Sambucifior.*; Lovage-*Water, Aqua Levistici*; Carminative-*Water, Aqua Carmnitiva*, &c.

It may be proper here to note, That whatever Properties any Simple has from the Grossness or Solidity of its Parts, which make it act as an Emetick, Cathartick, or Astringent; the Residue left after Distillation will remain in full possession thereof. Thus, the purging Syrup of Roses, is as well made after the Damask-Rose-*Water* is drawn off, as if the Flowers were juiced, or put into Infusion; because nothing of a Cathartickal Quality rises with the *Water*.

Sometimes, the Subject is fermented by an Addition of Yeast, Honey, or the like Ferment, to the hot *Water*, before the Distillation begin : In which Case, if the Ferment added were in sufficient quantity to effect a thorough Fermentation, the Liquid afterwards exhal'd and drawn off would be thin and inflammable; which makes what we call a *Spirit*; otherwise, thick, white, sapid, &c. and call'd a *Water*.

The *Waters* procured in this manner, contain the Oil of the Plant in great Perfection; which makes 'em of considerable use in Medicine, further than those rais'd without Fermentation; beside tat they keep better and longer; the Spirit in 'em preventing their corrupting or growing mothery.

*The Compound* **WATERS**, or those wherein several Ingredients are used, are very numerous, and make a large Article in Commerce; some prepared by the Apothecaries, according to the Dispensatory Prescripts, for medicinal Uses; others by the Distillers, to be drank by way of Dram, &c. and others by the Perfumers, &c.

They are distinguish'd by different Epithets, taken from the *Latin, Greek, Arabick, English*, &c. in respect of the specifick Virtues of the Waters; or the Parts of the Body for the Cure whereof they are intended; or the Diseases they are good against; or the Ingredients they are compounded of; or their different Uses, &c.

The most considerable among the Class of *Compound Waters*, we shall here enumerate. The manner of making 'em, 'tis true, is not always the same; especially those intended for drinking; for which, every one gives his own Method as the best. Those we here deliver, are taken from such as have the greatest Reputation, in preparing these things; or from those who have wrote best of 'em.

We have only three general Remarks to add, with respect to those intended for drinking :

1°, That such wherein any thong is infused, as broken Fruits, pounded Herbs, or ground Spices, are always pass'd thro' a Strainer, to make 'em finer and purer.

2°, That those made with Brandy or Spirit of Wine, are usually distill'd after the mixing of their Ingredients; which renders those liquors exceeding strong and dangerous, and confirms the Proverb; *Plures occidit Gula quam Gladius.* In effect, some of 'em as so penetrating, that they burn the Tongue when taken.

3°, That the *Waters* that take their Name from any particular thing, as Cinnamon, &c. have always some other Ingredients joined with 'em, according to the Taste or Smell requir'd.

*Alexipharmic*, or *Alexiterial Waters*, are *Waters* that resist Poisons and the Plague. Such are those of Angelica, Scorzonera, Citron, Orange, Scordium, Rue, &c. Such also are Treacle-Water, Plague-Water, Milk-Water, Poppy-Water, &c.

*Alumn* Water, is a vulnerary *Water*, thus call'd by reason the Basis or principal Ingredient thereof is Alumn.

*Angelica* Water, is usually prepar'd of Brandy, Angelica Roots and Seeds, Carduus, Baum, Fennel-Seed, &c. the whole beat together in a Mortar; infused for a Night, and then distill'd. It is reputed a good carminative, and Cordial, as also a Cephalic, &c.

*Aniseed* Water. To eight Parts of Essence of Anis-seed distill'd, put three Parts of Brandy, with one of *Water* boil'd; mix the whole together : and if you require it sugar'd, add half a Pint of clarify'd Sugar; but many prefer it without : and strain the whole.

*Apricot* Water. To a Quart of Water put six or eight Apricots, sliced; boil the whole, to extract the Taste; and when cold, add four or five Ounces of Sugar. When that is dissolved strain it.

*Arthritick* Waters, are *Waters* good the Gout, Palsy, Tremors, Pains in the Joints, &c. Such are those of Piony, Chamæpetis, Betony, Rosemary, &c.

*Bryony* Water, is one of the *Compound Waters* prescrib'd in the College Dispensatory; prepared from Bryony-Roots, Rue, Mugwort, Savin, Feverfew, Dittany, &c. It is a good Hysteric, opens Menstrual Obstructions, &c.

*Carduus* Water, is made from *Carduus Benedictus* pounded in a Mortar, and put in an Alembick. Then, a sufficient quantity of the Juice of the same sort of Plant, drawn by Expression, is pour'd into the Alembick, that the Herbs swimming in the Juice may be in no danger of sticking to the bottom of the Cucurbit in Distillation. Lastly, fitting on a Capital, and luting the Joints, distil half as much Juice as you put in. This *Water* is sudorifick; and good against the plague, Malignant Fevers, &c.

Water of *Separation*, or *Depart*, is only *Aqua fortis*; thus call'd, because serving to separate Gold from Silver. It is also called

*Caustic*, *Burning*, or *Strong Water*, and is prepared of a Mixture of Spirits of Nitre and Vitriol, drawn by force of Fire; to which are sometimes added Alumn and Arsenic. It dissolves all Metals, Gold only excepted. The Invention of Aqua fortis, is usually referr'd to the XIIIth Century : Tho some hold it to have been known in the Times of Moses.

*Cephalic* Waters, are Waters proper to strengthen and comfort the Brain. Such are those of Rosemary, Marjoram, Sage, Pyony, Bettony, Baum, &c.

*Chalybeat* Water, is a *Water* wherein red-hot Steel has been quenched. It is astringent, and good, like Ferruginous or Iron-*Waters*, for Diarrhæas, &c.

*Cherry* Water. In a Quart of *Water* crush half a pound of Cherries, with four or five Ounces of Sugar. Strain the whole thro'; a Cloth, till it be very clear.

*Cinnamon* Water. In a Quart of *Water* boil half an Ounce of broken Cinnamon; and taking it off the Fire, add a quarter Pound of Sugar : Let it cool, and strain it. *Or thus*: Take a Pound of Cinnamon, three Pounds of Rose-Water, and as much White wine : bruise the Cinnamon, infuse it fourteen Days, then distil it. The first *Water* that rises is the best; then the second; then the third.

*Clary* Water, is composed of Brandy, Sugar, and Cinnamon, with a little Ambergrease dissolved in it. It helps Digestion, and is Cardiack. This *Water* is render'd either purgative or emetic, by adding Resins of Jallap and Scammony, or *Crocus Metallorum*. Some make *Clary Water* of Brandy, Juice of Cherries, Straw-berries and Gooseberries, Sugar, Cloves, White Pepper, and Coriander-Seeds; infused, sugar'd, and strain'd.

*Clove* Water, is prepared of Brandy, and Cloves bruis'd therein, and distill'd.

*Cordial* or *Cardiac* Waters, are *Waters* proper to strengthening, and comfort the Heart. Such are those of Endive, Chicory, Bugloss, Burridge, Marigolds, &c.

*Fennel* Water. Infuse a Handful of Fennel in a Pint of cold *Water*, for an Hour or an Hour and a half : add three or four Ounces of Sugar. Strain it, and drink it.

*Gentian* Water. Take four Pounds of Gentian Roots, either green or dry'd; mince them small, infuse them in White-wine, or only sprinkle them therewith; then distil them, with the Addition of little Centaury the lesser. It is frequently used as a Stomachic, and is also commended for a Deterger; serving in Dropsies, Jaundice, Obstructions of the Viscera, &c.

*Gum* Water, is that made by letting Gum-Arabick, inclos'd in a linen Rag, infuse in common Water. The Ladies also make *Water* to gum their Hair, of Quince-Kernels steep'd in *Water*.

*Hepatic* Waters, are those used to cleanse, strengthen, and refresh the Liver., Such are those of Chicory, Capillaries, Purslain, Agremony, Fumitory, &c.

*Honey* Water, is a *Water* prepar'd in Places where much Honey is made, by washing out the Honey-Combs, and the Vessels they have been in, in common *Water*. This gives it a Honey-Taste, and it afterwards becomes very clear, and the People use it as their common Drink.

*Horse-raddish* Water, *Aqua Raphani*, is prepar'd of the Juices of Scurvygrass, Boork-Line, Water-Cresses, White-wine, Lemon-Juice, Bryony-Root, Horse-raddish, Winter's Bark and Nutmeg, digested and distill'd. It is a good Diuretic; cleansing, and removing Obstructions of the Viscera, promoting Perspiration, &c.

*Hungary* Water, is a Liquor distill'd *in Balneo Mariæ*, from Rosemary-Flowers, and Sprit of Wine well rectify'd. It has its Name from the wonderful Effects it is said to have had on a Queen of *Hungary*, at the Age of 72 Years. 'Tis good against Faintings, Palsies, Lethargies, Apoplexies, and hysterical

Diseases. There are divers ways of preparing it.

*Hysteric* Waters, are those proper to strengthen the Matrix, or Womb, and remedy the Disorders that befall it. Such are those of Bryony, Matricary or Motherwort, Hyssop, Fennel, Baum, Mugwort, Smallage, &c.

*Iced*, or *Frozen* Waters, are certain agreeable and wholesome *Waters*, as Orange-*Water*, or the like, artificially froze in Summer-time, particularly in hot Countries, to be used in Collations, &c. as Coolers. The way of making 'em is thus : The Vessels containing the Liquors design'd to be froze, as first set in a Pail, in such a manner as not to touch each other; then cover'd up, and the void Space in the Pail fill'd with common Ice, beaten, and mix'd with Salt. Every half Hour they clear out what Water the thawing Ice sends to the bottom of the Pail, by means of a Hole at bottom; and at the same time stir up the Liquors with a Spoon, that they may freeze into Snow; For were they to shoot in form of Ice, or Icicles, they would have no Taste. Then, covering the Vessels again, they fill up the Pail with more beaten Ice, and Salt, in lieu of that dissolved and evacuated. The more expeditious the Freezing is requir'd to be, the more Salt to be mix'd with the Ice.

*Imperial* Water, *Aqua Imperialis*, is a *Water* distill'd from Cinnamon, Nutmeg, Citron-Bark, Cloves, *Calamus Aromaticus*, Santal, and divers other Simples , infus'd in White-wine and Baum-Water. It is a pleasant Cordial-Dram, good against Diseases of the Brain, Stomach, and Womb.

*Juniper* Water, is a Compound *Water*, made of Brandy, and Juniper-Berries beaten therein, and distill'd.

*Lime* Water, is common *Water*, wherein Quick-lime has been flak'd, and afterwards filter'd.

*Milk* Water, *Aqua Lactis*, is prepared of Mint, Wormwood, Carduus Benedictus, Goats-Rue, and Meadow-sweet, bruis'd, infus'd in Milk, and drawn off by Infusion. It is held Alexipharmic and Cephalic.

*Aqua Mirabilis*, or *the Wonderful* Water, is prepared of Cloves, Galangals, and Spirit of Wine, digested 24 Hours, then distill'd. It is a good and agreeable Cordial; Carminative, &c.

*Nephritic* Waters, are such as strengthen the Reins, and help 'em to discharge by Urine any Impurities therein. Such are those of the Honeysuckle, Pellitory, Raddish, Beans, Mallows, &c.

The *Nephritic Water* of Dr. *Radcliff*[1], popularly called Dr. *Radcliffe's Water*, is taken into the last Edition of College Dispensatory. It is prepar'd from the Kernels of Black Cherries, Peaches, and Bitter Almonds, beaten in a Mortar into a Paste, with Rhenish Wine; and Seeds of Smallage, Treacle, Mustard, Gromwel and Parsley, beaten likewise, and added thereto : To the Mixture are put Juniper-Berries, Garlick, Onions, Leeks, Pimpernel, Horse-raddish, Calamus Aromaticus, Cinnamon, Wall-Rue, Mace, and Nutmegs : the whole macerated in Rhenish, Spirit of Black Cherries, &c. and thus distill'd. It is one of the most powerful Detergers and Cleansers known; good in the Dropsy, Jaundice, Asthma, Pleurisy, &c.

*Ophthalmic*, or *Eye* Waters, are such as are good in Disorders of the Eyes.

[1] John Radcliffe (1652 – 1714), an English physician.

Such are those of Eyebright, Fennel, Vervain, Plantain, Celandine, Cyanus, &c.

*Orange-Flower* Water, is made of common *Water*, Sugar, and Orange-Flowers, infuses for about two Hours. After the like manner, one may make Waters of divers other Flowers; as Violets, Jonquils, Jessamins, Tuberoses, &c.

*Peach* Water, is made after the same manner as *Apricot Water*; only with Peaches.

*Phagænic* Water, is Lime-*Water*, to every Pound whereof is added twenty or thirty Grains of Corrosive Sublimate, in Pouder. It serves to cleanse old Ulcers, to eat off fungous Flesh, &c.

*Plague* Water, *Aqua Epidemica*, is prepar'd from the Roots of Masterwort, Angelica, Pyony, and Butter-bur; Viper-Grass, *Virginia* Snakeroot, Rue, Rosemary, Baum, Carduus, Water Germander, Marigolds, Dragons, Goats-Rue, and Mint; the whole infus'd in Spirit of Wine and distill'd. It is of frequent Use as an Alexipharmic: It revives the Spirits, and promotes a Diaphoresis. It is the Basis of most Juleps now prescrib'd, especially in feverish Cases.

*Poppy* Water, is prepared from the Flowers of wild Poppies, infus'd in White-wine, or Brandy, and drawn off in a cold Still. It is a Cordial, good against the Colic, and by some call'd *Red Plague-Water*.

*Pyony* Water, is made of Pyony and Lime-Flowers, Lilly of the Valley steep'd in Canary, and distill'd : to the Water thus procured, are added the Root of Male Pyony, White Dittany, Birthwort, Mistletoe, Rue, Castor, Cubebs, Cinnamon, Betony, &c. IT is a good Cordial, and much used in nervous Cases.

*Rose* Water. Take of Roses three Parts, and of Fennel and Rue each, one Part; chop 'em small, and mix 'em well together; then distil 'em. This *Water* is excellent for the Eyes, &c.

*Scordium* Water, is prepared from the Juices of Goats-Rue, Sorrel, Scordium, Citrons and Treacle, digested and distill'd. It is an Alexipharmic.

*Specific* Waters, are such have some peculiar Virtue, appropriate to certain Diseases. Thus Purslain *Water*, wherein Mercury has been infused, is a Specific against Worms in young Children.

*Splenetic* Waters, are those proper against the Diseases of the Spleen. Such are those of Tamarisk, Cuscuta, Hartstongue, Hops, &c.

*Stephen's* Water, *Aqua Stephani*, is made from Cinnamon, Ginger, Galangals, Cloves, Nutmegs, Paradise Grains, Anis-seeds, Sweet Fennel, Carraway, Thyme, Mint, Sage, Pennyroyal, Pellitory, Rosemary, Red Roses, Camomile, Origany and Lavender, steep'd in *Gascoign* Wine, or Spirit of Wine, distill'd. It is a good Cephalic and a Cardiac, and is also reputed Hysterical.

*Stomachic* Waters, are such as have the Virtue to cleanse, strengthen, and confirm the Stomach. As Red Rose-*Water*, Mint-*Water*, Aniseed-*Water*, &c.

*Stygian* Water. See *Aqua Regalis*.

*Styptic* Water, is a Dissolution of Red Vitriol, or the Colcothar remaining in the Retort after the Spirit has been extracted; with burnt Alum and Sugar-candy. With thirty Grains of each of these three Drugs, they mix half an Ounce of Urine of a young Man, as much Rose-*Water*, and two Ounces of Plantain-*Water*. It is used to stop Bleeding. See Styptic.

*Treacle* Water, *Aqua Theriacalis*, is directed by the College Dispensatory, to be made of green Walnuts, Rue, Carduus, Marigold, Baum, Butter-bur-Roots, Burdock, Angelica, Masterwort, Water-Germander, Venice Treacle, Mithridate, Canary, Vinegar, and Lemon-Juice, steep'd and distill'd. It is the most used of any in the Shops; tho Dr. *Quincy* decries it as one of the worst concerted of all. Its Intention is to be an Alexipharmic and Sudorific.

Other Dispensatories give a more simple *Treacle-Water*, made from Treacle, with an equal quantity of Brandy and Vinegar. It is good for Ulcers, and Erosions of the Mouth; especially if a little *Armenian* Bole be dissolv'd therein.

*Vulnerary* Water, is a *Water* proper for healing of Wounds, prepared from the Juice of Vulnerary Plants.

**WATER**, in Anatomy, &c. is applied to divers Liquors or Humours in the human Body. Such is the *Aqua Phlegmatica*, Phlegmatic *Water*; which is a soft serous Humour, contained in the Pericardium, and wherein the Heart swims.

Anatomists are divided about it; some will not have it natural, but suppose it separated forcibly during the Pangs of Death : Their Reason is, the difficulty they meet withal in tracing its Passage, or how it is carried off. The latest Anatomists, however, seem to agree to its being a natural and necessary Humour : and one Reason is, that it is found even in the Pericardium of *Fœtus's*.

It has likewise been disputed whence it should be separated. The freshest Opinion is, that it is secreted by some Glands about the Basis of the Heart; and that it distils thence drop by drop, into the Cavity of the Pericardium, in such Quantity, as just to supply what is expended daily by the Motion and Warmth of the Heart; and so needs no Evacuation. Its Use is, to moisten, lubricate, and cool the Heart, and prevent any Inflammation that might arise from the dry Friction of Heart and Pericardium. So that it does the same Office to the Heart, that the Water does wherein the *Fœtus* swims; which without it would not have liberty to move at all.

**WEAPON-SALVE**, a kind of Unguent, supposed to cure Wounds sympathetically, by being applied, not to the Wound, but to the Weapon that made it.

**WEN**, a Tumor, or Excrescence growing on divers Parts of the Body; consisting of a Cystis, or Bag, fill'd with some peculiar Matter. Of this, Physicians usually reckon three Kinds, according to the matter it is form'd of, *i.e.* the Humour contain'd therein. If soft, resembling a Pulp, the *Wen* is call'd *Atheroma*; if Honey, *Meliceris*; and if Suet, *Steatoma*.

M. *Littre*, in *Mem. de l'Acad. des Sciences*, adds a fourth Kind, which he calls *Lipoma*; by reason, the *Wen* is form'd of soft Fat.

They are all, usually, of the like Colour with the rest of the Body; begin from very little, and grow gradually. They are not dangerous, but frequently last a long while. Sometimes they degenerate into Abscesses. The Cure is, to cut off the Cystis at the Root, which is always narrow.

*Spanish* **WHITE**, is a kind of Fucus used by the Ladies to whiten the Complexion, and hide the defects thereof. 'Tis made of Tin of Glass dissolved in Spirit of Nitre, and precipitated into a very fine Powder, by means of Salt water.

**WHITLOW**, in Medicine, a Tumor, by Physicians commonly call'd Paronychia.

**WINE**, is also a Name used in Medicine and Pharmacy, for divers Mixtures or Compositions, wherein the Juice of the Grape is a principal Ingredient.

These *Medicated Wines* make a considerable Article in our Dispensatories, in quality of Diet-Drinks; some being denominated from the Ingredients used in 'em; some from the Intentions wherewith they are prescribed; and some from their Qualities, &c.

*Bitter* Wine, *Vinum Amarum,* is an Infusion of certain bitter Stomachic Herbs, as Gentian-Root, Juniper-Berries, Tops of Centaury, Orange and Lemon Peel, in white Port, or other white *Wine*; taken by way of Whet in a Morning, to restore the pall'd Stomach after a Debauch, and bring the Fibres to their due Tension.

*Chalybeat,* or *Steel* Wine, is prepared of Filings of Steel, and Saffron infused, and filter'd. It is good for removing Obstructions in the Viscera, as in the Chlorosis, &c.

*Vinum Benedictum, the blessed* Wine, is made of *Crocus Metallorum* and Mace infused in Wine. It was formerly a celebrated Emetic, but now almost out of use for its roughness.

*Elecampane* Wine, *Vinum Enulatum,* is an Infusion of the Root of that Plant with Sugar and Currants, in white Port. It cleanses the Viscera, prevents Disorders and Obstructions of the Lungs; and is good in Asthmatic Cases, Cachexies, &c.

*Hog-lice* Wine, *Vinum Millepedum,* is prepared of Hog-lice put alive in white Port; and after some infusion, press'd and strain'd out : To the Liquor is added Saffron, Salt of Steel, &c. It is recommended against the Jaundice, Dropsy, Cachectic Habits, &c.

*Pectoral* Wine, *Vinum Pectorale,* is prepared of Liquorice, Saffron, Coriander-Seeds, Carraway, Anise, Salt of Tartar, Penny-royal, and Hyssop-Waters, digested with Canary *Wine,* and strain'd. It is a good Expectorant; helping to deterge and clean the lungs.

*Viper* Wine, *Vinum Viperinum,* is a Preparation of female Vipers, infused six Months in *Canary Wine.* It is a great Restorative, and provokes to Venery; good against Cutaneous Eruptions, &c.

*Vinum Scilliticum,* Wine *of Squills,* is an Infusion of those Onions in white *Wine* for forty days, and then the Squills strain'd out, and the Liquor preserv'd for use. It is a gentle Emetic, good against Inundations of Rheum,

&c.

**WORM**, in Chymistry, a long, winding Pewter-Pipe, with Distillers and Apothecaries place in a Tub of Water to cool and condense the Vapours in the Distillation of Spirits. See Alembic, Distillation, &c. Formerly, this *Worm*, or something like it, was placed above the Head of the Still, with a Refrigeratory at the upper end of it, which is useful enough in the Distilling of Wine. This is what the Chymists call a *Serpentine*.

**WORM-SEED**, a kind of Worm-Powder, call'd also *Barbotine, Semen contra, Semen sanctum, Semen santonicum,* and *Abrotonum*, is a kind of Seed proper to destroy *Worms* generated in a human Body, particularly in Children. This Seed is small, of a brownish Colour, an oblong Figure, a bitter Taste, and a string Smell.

The Place where it is produced, is *Persia*, about the Frontiers of *Muscovy*. It is brought to us from *Aleppo*, &c. Naturalists are not agreed about the Plant that produces it. *J. Bauhin* has a large Dissertation on the Subject. Some will have it the Species of *Absynthium*, or *Wormwood* call'd *Santonicum*, or *Marinum Absynthium*; others will have it the *Tanacetum*, other the *Aorotonum*.

Mons. *Tournefort* gives us the following Account of this notable Drug, in the second Volume of his Travels. The *Sementine* or *Worm-Powder*, is not gather'd like other Seeds. The Plant grows in the Meadows, and must be let ripen; and the mischief is, that as it grows near to Maturity, the Wind scatters a good part of it among the Grass, where it is lost; and this it is makes it so dear.

As the dare not touch it with the Hand for fear of making it spoil the sooner; when they would gather what is left of the Ear, they have recourse to this Expedient. They take two Hand-Baskets, and walking along the Meadows, sweep the Baskets the one from right to left, the other from left to right, as if they were mowing; by this means the Seed is shook out into the Baskets.

It must be chosen new, greenish, of a sharp, bitter, aromatic Taste, yet disagreeable.

**WORMWOOD**, a Medicinal Herb, among Physicians, &c. call'd *Absynthium*.

**WOUND**, *Vulnus*, in Medicine and Chirurgery, a recent Separation made in the soft or fleshy Parts of the Body, from an external Cause, and particularly the Action of some hard and sharp Instrument.

Or, it is a Solution of the Continuity of a fleshy Part, made by some penetrating Body; while yet it remains fresh, bloody, and without putrefaction : By which circumstances it is distinguish'd from an *Ulcer*. A like separation happening in a bony Part, is call'd a *Fracture*.

All *Wounds* proceed either from Puncture, Incision, or Contusion, according to the Nature and Make of the Instrument they were caus'd by.

*Wounds* are usually divided, with respect to their Cause, Circumstances,

Cure, &c. into *Simple* and *Compound. Simple Wounds* are those made by Puncture, Incision or Contusion separately; those of the outer Skin, without any considerable loss of Substance, or hurting any remarkable Vessel; and those not complicated with any dangerous Symptoms.

*Compound* Ulcers are those made by Puncture and Incision at the same time, to which is sometimes also added Contusion; those attended with great loss of Flesh, or the hurt of some considerable Vessel; and those made by envenom'd Instruments, or attended with violent Symptoms.

The History of a *Wound* is thus deliver'd by *Boerhaave*. Immediately upon the Solution, the *wounded* Parts recede further and further from each other. The Blood gushes out, at first, with some violence; but stops of itself : then a bloody scab is form'd in the Cavity of the *Wound*, and a thin ruddy Humour oozes out; the Lips of the *Wound* begin to redden, heat, ake, swell, and turn back; and (in great *Wounds*) a Fever and Thirstiness succeed. On the third or fourth day, there is found a white, viscid Pus; upon which, the heat, redness, tumor, &c. abate, and the Cavity gradually fills up from the bottom upwards, and from the Circumference to the Centre, with growing Flesh. Lastly, the *Wound* dries, and cicatrises.

But note, these Symptoms vary according to the Nature and Cause of the *Wound*. Thus, if it be by Incision, and a large Blood-Vessel be cut, the Hæmorrhage is more violent; especially if it be an Artery; in which case, florid Blood flies out impetuously and by starts : If only a Vein be cut, the Flux is more moderate and equable, and the Blood of a darker Colour. If the *Wound* be attended with Contusion, the Hæmorrhage is small.

In *Wounds*, where any large Artery is quite cut in two, the Flux usually proves mortal. A lesser Artery cut transversely, flies back against the solid Parts, and will have its Mouths stopp'd : If an Artery be not quite cut off, there arises a perpetual Flux; or if that be stopp'd, an Aneurisma. A Nerve being cut off, flies back, produces a Pain, and Obstruction about the *Wound*; and below it a Numbness, and wasting Immobility : The case is much the same in *wounded* Tendons and Membranes. *Wounds* of the temporal Muscles are rarely cured; but generally bring on horrible Convulsions.

The following *Wounds* are commonly reputed mortal; *viz.* those of the *Cerebellum*, and of the *Cerebrum*, if they be deep enough to hurt the *Medulla oblongata*; deep *Wounds* in the spinal Marrow, especially the upper part thereof; those of the Heart, Lungs, Liver, Spleen, Kidneys, Pancreas, Mesentery, Stomach, Intestines, &c. Those of the *Cava, Aorta, Carotides*, pulmonary, and other large Veins and Arteries. Those of the *Bronchia, Thorax, Diaphragm*; large *Wounds* of the *Oesophagus, Trachea*, and the Bladder, and all invenom'd *Wounds*.

In young Children and aged Persons, *Wounds* frequently prove mortal which seem'd but slight. Those *Wounds* generally prove troublesome which happen in an ill state of Body, and especially a low or hardy Diet. All *Wounds* are reputed more dangerous and difficult of Cure in Winter than Summer; in *August* than in Spring.

The Cure of *Wounds* consist sin the Uniting of the divided Parts; which is the work of Nature alone, and which the Chirurgeon can only contribute to by removing external Impediments, and applying Medicines familiar to the Part, call'd *Vulneraries* and *Basalmicks.*

The first Step, then, to be taken in a simple Wound, is to cleanse it, and extract any heterogeneous Body that may chance to be lodged therein. Next, the Cavity to be gently wiped with Dofils dipt in warm red Wine. The Lips now to be brought together by the Bandages or Sutures; and the Wound to be covered with a Pledget dipt in Balm of Peru, or Oil of sweet Almonds. The Pain thus eased, and the Symptoms removed, the Wound is to be suppurated, deterged, incarned, and cicatrized after the manner of Tumors and Ulcers.

If the *Wound* be dangerous, the Symptoms violent, and the Body Cacochymic, more powerful Means are had recourse to; as, first, Phlebotomy, then gentle Cathartics or Clysters, then vulnerary Drinks, Apozems, and Ptisans, with Cardiacs and Paragorics interposed.

In internal *Wounds*, Vulneraries and Alcalies do well, particularly *Album Græcum*, River Lobsters, Mercurials, &c.

Fresh *Wounds* are cured ordinarily in three or four days, without any other means than applying a few Drops of Balsam of *Peru*. Sometimes, however, Digestives are required.

Gun shot *Wounds* are usually the worst of all, by reason of the violent Contusion and Secretion of the Parts; which prevent their coming to Digestion for the Space of three or four days.

In the Cure of large *Wounds*, Bandages and Sutures are required, to fit and dispose 'em for healing.

**WRECK**, or *Sea*-Wreck, in Natural History, a kind of Herb, growing in the Sea, upon Rocks, and which the Waves tearing off, cast upon the Shore. In some Places it is used to manure the Ground. In *Normandy* and other Parts they burn it, and of the Ashes make a kind of Suude or Salt-wort, which they use in making of common green Glass, to promote the Fusion or Vitrification of the Matter.

**XEROMYRON**, formed of ξηρο, *dry*, and φαγω, *I eat*, a Word used by the Ancients to express what they do at other Times call in express Words a dry Ointment. It was a Composition of warm and aromatic Drugs, or of other Things fit for external Use, but without the fatty Ingredients, by which they were usually reduced into the form of Ointments.

**XEROPHTHALMIA**, a kind of Ophthalmia, wherein the Eyes itch, and are red, but without swelling or watering. The Word is compounded of ξηρος, dry, and οφθαλμος, Eye.

**XEROTRIBIA**, formed of ξηρο, *dry*, and τριβω, *I rub*, a Term used by Authors to express a dry Friction, a rubbing of some affected Part with the Hand or otherwise, to recall the Warmth and Circulation.

**XIR**, a Word used by the Chemists to express Mercury.

**XISINUM**, a Word used by some of the chemical Writers to express Vinegar.

**XYLO-ALOES**, in Medicine, &c. the Lignum Aloes : call'd also *Agillochum*. The Word is compounded of ξυλον, *Lignum* ,Wood, and αλοη, Aloes.

**XYLO-BALSAMUM**, a Name which Naturalists, &c. give to the Wood of the Tree which yields that precious Gum known to the *Latins* by the Name of *Opo-Balsamum*, and among us by the Name of *Balm of Gilead*.

We have Branches of this Tree brought us from *Cairo*. They are very streight, brittle, unequal, and full of Knots; their Bark reddish without, and greenish within. The Wood is whitish, and full of Pith, and when broke, yields an agreeable smell resembling that of the Balm.

The *Xylo-Balsamum* is reputed good to strengthen the Brain, and Stomach, and to expel Poison.

**XYLOCARACTA**, or Xylocaracte, in the Materia Media, a Name by which some Authors have called the Carob, or *siliqua dulcis*, the sweet-pipe tree. This was called by some of the Greek writers *xyloceraton*, the Tree bearing Pods, and from a corruption of this Name the other has been formed.

**YARROW**, *Achilla*, or Millefolium, in Botany. The Leaves and Flowers of the common *Yarrow*, or *achillæ millefolium* of Linnæus, which is in flower on our Ditch-banks, and in dry Pastures, the greatest part of the Summer, are greatly recommended by some of the *German* Physicians, as mild Corroborants, Vulneraries, and Antispasmodics, in Diarrheas, Hæmorrhages, Hypochondriacal, and other Disorders. They promise, says Dr. *Lewis*[1], by their sensible Qualities to be of no inconsiderable Activity.

They have an agreeable, though weak, aromatic Smell, and a bitterish, roughish, somewhat pungent Taste. The Leaves having the greatest Bitterness and Austerity, are chiefly directed for medicinal Use; the Flowers have the strongest and most subtile Smell, are remarkably acrid, and promise to be of great Efficacy, if the plant has any such Efficacy, as an Anodyne or Anti-spasmodic.

The Virtue of both Leaves and Flowers is extracted by watery or spirituous Mentrua; the Astringency the most perfectly by the Former; their aromatic Warmth and Pungency by the Latter; and both of them equally by a Mixture of the two.

The Flowers distilled with Water, yield a penetrating essential Oil, possessing the Flavour of the *millefoil* in perfection; in Consistence somewhat thick and tenacious; in Colour very variable, from a greenish yellow to a deep green, and bluish green and fine blue, which Differences depend in great Measure on the Soil in which the Plant is produced; the Flowers gathered from the moist, fresh Grounds, yielding generally a blue Oil, and those collected from dry Commons a green one, with a greater or less admixture of yellow. The Extract, obtained by inspissating the yellowish Tincture made in rectified Spirit, is more agreeable in Smell than the Flowers; of a moderately warm, penetrating Taste, somewhat like that of Camphor, but much milder, accompanied with a slight bitterishness and subastringency.

The *achillea pharmica* of *Linnaeus*, called *sneezewort*, or *bastard pellitory*, is perennial, grows wild on Heaths, and in moist shady Grounds, and is found in Flower from June to the end of Summer. The Roots of this Plant have a hot, biting Taste, approaching to that of Pellitory of Spain, with which they nearly agree in their pharmaceutic Properties, and for which they have been sometimes substituted in the Shops. They are by some recommended internally as a warm Stimulant and Attenuant; but their principal Use is as a Masticatory and Sternutatory.

**YAWNING**, *Oscitatio*, an involuntary opening of he Mouth, occasion'd by a Vapour or Ventosity, endeavouring to escape; and generally witnessing an irksome Weariness, or an Inclination to Sleep. The Remedy *Hippocrates* prescribes against continual *Yawnings*, is to make long Breathings, or Respirations. The same he recommends against the Hiccough.

The nervous Membrane of the *Oesophagus* is the Seat of Yawning, which is certain to be produced whenever any irritation determines the Spirits to flow

[1] William Lewis (1708 – 1781), an English physician.

thither in too great abundance. The Cause of the Irritation is supposed to be some troublesome Humour wetting the inner Membrane of the *Oesophagus*; which Humour proceeds either from the Glands spread throughout that Membrane, or from acid Vapours rising from the Stomach, as from a Boiling-Pot, and which condense on the Sides of the *Oesophagus* as on a Pot-Lid.

On such occasions, the nervous Fibres of the Membrane of the Gullet being irritated, dilate the Gullet; and the Mouth is constrain'd to follow the same Motion, as being lined with the same Membrane.

**YQUETAYA**, in Natural History, a Plant in *Brasil*, long used as a Medicine in that Country; and lately discovered to the *Europeans* by a *French* Surgeon. It has been since founding *France*, where being cultivated and examined by M. *Marchant*, it appears to be a kind of Scrophulary or Blood-Nettle.

It has this remarkable Property, that it takes away from Senna all its ill taste and smell, which Property of correcting the Infusion of Senna was unknown in the Scrophulary.

To use this Plant, it must be dried ten or twelve days in the Shade, and afterwards exposed to the Sun till quite dry.

**YSAMBRA**, a Word used by some as a Name for Hellebore, and by others to express a Species of Poison prepared in Spain, of which Hellebore is an Ingredient.

**YXIR**, a Word used by some of the old Chemists, to express anything good in Medicine.

**ZEDOARIA**, Zedoary, a Medicinal Root belonging to a Plant growing in the *East Indies*, whose Leaves are like those of Ginger, only longer and broader. *Zedoary* is of an Ash Colour, has an Aromatic, bitterish Taste; and comes into the Class of Cephalics : But it is also reckon'd by many amongst the Alexipharmics, whereupon it comes to have a Place in the Capitals; and is even said to prevent Infections by holding it only in the Mouth. On account of its agreeable Bitter, it also is prescribed among Stomachics; and for its spicy Warmth is commended in Cholics, and Hysterical Affections, for promoting he Menses, &c.

**ZINK**, or *Zaim*, a kind of Mineral, or Semi-Metal, which some confound with *Bismuth*, and others with Spelter. Others call it *Female Antimony. Zink* is a kind of Mineral Lead, very hard, white, and brillant; and which, tho' not ductile enough to denominate it a Metal, yet stretches a little under the Hammer.

'Tis found in great Quantity in the Mines of *Gosselaar* in *Saxony*. That commonly sold is in large, thick, square Cakes; which would make one suspect it had been melted when taken out of the Mine, and cast in Moulds of that Form.

*Zink* is used to purge and purify Tin; much as Lead is used to purify Gold, Silver, and Copper. Founders, Toy-men, &c. also use it with Turmeric to tinge Copper, &c. It gives a fine Gold Colour, tho' not a very lasting one.

M. *Homberg* conjectures, with a good deal of Probability, that *Zink* is no other than a natural Mixture of two real Metals, viz. Tin and Iron. What led him to the opinion was, that *Zink* yields precisely the same Fumes by the Burning-Glass, as such a Mixture does. Accordingly, he assures us, he often substituted the one for the other; and this always with the very same Effect.

The *Flowers of Zinc* were first used as an internal Medicine by the celebrated Chemist *Glauber*, but were little known in practice, till Dr. *Gaubius*[1], of *Leyden*, gave an Account of their Virtues., in his *Adversaria*. They have since been much employed in convulsive and spasmodic Diseases, and sometimes with good Effects. Even obstinate Epilepsies have been rendered much less violent by the Use of them.

**ZIZYPHUM**, a Name sometimes given to a kind of Fruit usually call'd *Jujubes*.

**ZOPISSA**, a kind of Mixture of Pitch and Tar; scraped off Ships that have been long time at Sea. The Word is form'd from ξεειν, *bullire*, to boil, and πισσα Pitch, *q. d. boil'd Pitch*. This Matter by being gradually penetrated by the Salt of the Sea, becomes partake of its Qualities; and being apply'd to the Body, externally, is found Resolutive and Desiccative.

**ZYTHUM**, a sort of Malt-Liquor, in use among the antient *Germans*. *Matthiolus* represents the antient *Zythum* and *Curmi* as the same with our Beer and Ale.

[1] Hieronymus David Glabius (1705 – 1780), a German physicin and chemist.

# HISTORICAL INDEX

Made in the USA
Coppell, TX
05 November 2026

11365030R00389